SHOCK AND RESUSCITATION

NOTICE

Medicine is an ever-changing science. As new research and clinical experience broaden our knowledge, changes in treatment and drug therapy are required. The editors and the publisher of this work have checked with sources believed to be reliable in their efforts to provide information that is complete and generally in accord with the standards accepted at the time of publication. However, in view of the possibility of human error or changes in medical sciences, neither the editors nor the publisher nor any other party who has been involved in the preparation or publication of this work warrants that the information contained herein is in every respect accurate or complete, and they are not responsible for any errors or omissions or for the results obtained from use of such information. Readers are encouraged to confirm the information contained herein with other sources. For example and in particular, readers are advised to check the product information sheet included in the package of each drug they plan to administer to be certain that the information contained in this book is accurate and that changes have not been made in the recommended dose or in the contraindications for administration. This recommendation is of particular importance in connection with new or infrequently used drugs.

SHOCK AND RESUSCITATION

EDITED BY

EVAN R. GELLER

Associate Professor of Surgery
Chief, Division of Trauma
The State University of New York
Stony Brook, New York

McGRAW-HILL, INC.

HEALTH PROFESSIONS DIVISION

New York St. Louis San Francisco Auckland Bogotá
Caracas Lisbon London Madrid Mexico Milan
Montreal New Delhi Paris San Juan Singapore
Sydney Tokyo Toronto

SHOCK AND RESUSCITATION

1234567890 KGP KGP 9876543

ISBN 0-07-023500-7

This book was set in Meridien by Compset, Inc.

The editors were Michael J. Houston and Susan Finn.

The production supervisor was Clare Stanley.

The cover was designed by Pat Nieshoff.

The project was supervised by Editorial Services of New England, Inc.

R. R. Donnelly & Sons was the printer and binder.

Library of Congress Cataloging-in-Publication Data

Shock and resuscitation / edited by Evan R. Geller.
    p.   cm.
   Includes bibliographical references and index.
   ISBN 0-07-023500-7 : $70.00
   1. Shock—Treatment. I. Geller, Evan R.
   [DNLM: 1. Shock—therapy. 2. Resuscitation. QZ 140 S5597 1993]
RB150.S5S483 1993
617.2'1—dc20
DNLM/DLC
for Library of Congress   93-7888
                             CIP

This book is dedicated to my wife, Sheri,
and children, Kaitlin, Sarah, and Ethan,
for giving me purpose;

and to the memories of my father, Milton Geller,
and friend, David Kreis, Jr., M.D.,
for giving me perspective.

CONTENTS

CONTRIBUTORS

ARTHUR E. BAUE, MD, FACS
Professor of Surgery
St. Louis University Medical Center
St. Louis, Missouri

THOMAS M. BIANCANIELLO, MD
Associate Professor
Department of Pediatrics
The State University of New York
Stony Brook, New York

IRSHAD H. CHAUNDRY, PhD
Professor, Department of Surgery
Michigan State University
East Lansing, Michigan

DONALD E. FRY, MD, FACS
Professor and Chairman
Department of Surgery
University of New Mexico
Albuquerque, New Mexico

EVAN R. GELLER, MD, FACS
Associate Professor of Clinical Surgery
Chief, Division of Trauma
The State University of New York
Stony Brook, New York

LEWIS R. GOLDFRANK, MD, FACEP
Director, Emergency Medicine
Associate Professor of Clinical Medicine
Medical Director, NYC Poison Center
Bellevue Hospital Center
New York, New York

JAMES M. HARKEMA, MD, FACS
Professor of Surgery
Department of Surgery
Michigan State University
East Lansing, Michigan

ALAN R. HARTMAN, MD
Clinical Associate Professor
Department of Surgery
The State University of New York
Stony Brook, New York

GLENDON C. HENRY, MD
Senior Administrative Attending Physician
Department of Emergency Services
New York City Poison Control Center
New York, New York

ROBERT S. HOFFMAN, MD
Clinical Assistant Professor of Surgery/Emergency Medicine
New York University School of Medicine
New York, New York

ZELMA H. T. KISS, MD
Division of Neurosurgery
University of Toronto
Toronto, Ontario, Canada

ANNA M. LEDGERWOOD, MD, FACS
Professor of Surgery
Department of Surgery
Wayne State University
Detroit, Michigan

WAYNE LIPSON, MD
Department of Surgery
The State University of New York
Stony Brook, New York

CHARLES E. LUCAS, MD, FACS
Professor of Surgery
Department of Surgery
Wayne State University
Detroit, Michigan

CAROL L. MILLER-GRAZIANO, PhD
Director, Division of Research
Department of Surgery
University of Massachusetts Medical Center
Worcester, Massachusetts

ROY PATTERSON, MD
Ernest S. Bazley Professor of Medicine
Chief, Section of Allergy/Immunology
Department of Medicine
Northwestern University Medical School
Chicago, Illinois

BASIL A. PRUITT, JR, MD, FACS
Commander and Director
United States Army Institute for Surgical Research
Professor of Surgery
Uniformed Services University for the Health Sciences
Fort Sam Houston
San Antonio, Texas

LORING W. RUE, III, MD, FACS
Assistant Professor of Surgery
University of Alabama at Birmingham
Birmingham, Alabama

JONATHAN M. SAXE, MD
Assistant Professor of Surgery
Wayne State University
Detroit, Michigan

STEVEN R. SHACKFORD, MD, FACS
Professor and Chairman
Department of Surgery
College of Medicine
University of Vermont
Surgeon-in-Chief
Medical Center Hospital of Vermont
Burlington, Vermont

KATHY R. SONENTHAL, MD
Section of Allergy-Immunology
Department of Medicine
Northwestern University Medical School
Chicago, Illinois

CHARLES H. TATOR, MD, PhD, FRCS (C)
Professor and Chairman
Division of Neurosurgery
The Toronto Hospital
Toronto Western Division
University of Toronto
Toronto, Ontario, Canada

DONALD D. TRUNKEY, MD, FRCS
Professor and Chairman
Department of Surgery
Oregon Health Sciences University
Portland, Oregon

STEPHEN A. VITKUN, MD, PhD
Associate Professor of Clinical Anesthesiology
    and Medicine (Pulmonary/Critical Care)
The State University of New York
Stony Brook, New York

ROBERT L. WAGUESPACK, MD
U.S. Army Institute of Surgical Research
Fort Sam Houston
San Antonio, Texas

STEVEN L. WALD, MD, FACS
Associate Professor of Surgery
Division of Neurosurgery
Department of Surgery
University of Vermont
Burlington, Vermont

ROBERT F. WILSON, MD, FACS
Professor of Surgery
Department of Surgery
Wayne State University
Detroit, Michigan

PREFACE

Any text on the subject of shock must choose a viewpoint and carefully consider its limitations. This text is directed at the practitioner caring for the patient in the early phases of shock from various causes. Given the basis of the most recent understanding of the biochemistry and physiology of the shock state, this text seeks to provide that rational treatment regimen which the practitioner must apply to effect resuscitation during the critical early hours of shock. It is clear that shock, in all its various forms, is treated most effectively by prevention. Failing this, an understanding of the earliest stages of shock and the required emergent interventions will allow the greatest chance of successful resuscitation. It is with this purpose that this text is written.

The treatment of the patient has long been of keen interest to many practitioners. The pervasive nature of the shock condition has made the understanding of its physiology and expertise in its treatment critical to a broad spectrum of treating physicians. In recent years, however, burgeoning research in the field of shock physiology and treatment has led to an explosion of new knowledge concerning shock and resuscitation. Much of this information has been gleaned through the efforts of the increasing legion of scientists who have turned their attention to the investigation of shock at the most fundamental biochemical and physiologic levels. The implication of this newly found knowledge is not always obvious to the practitioner struggling to provide his or her patient with the most effective means of resuscitation. This book seeks to address that dilemma. A conscious effort has been made to integrate the thoughts and efforts of prominent treating clinicians and scientists active in the field of shock and resuscitation. This combination of efforts begins with the latest verified research conclusions and is carried forward into the clinical arena. Specific effort has been made to include a thorough and current reference list within each chapter. Additionally, contributors of diverse backgrounds and opinions have been selected to provide several viewpoints regarding controversial areas of shock research and resuscitation. Points of vigorous investigation and debate—e.g., crystalloid versus colloid resuscitation and third space fluid dynamics—are addressed from multiple perspectives and related to recent investigative and clinical efforts. In this manner, it is hoped that the reader may gain an understanding of the most critical recent concepts relating to shock and utilize this knowledge to effect improved treatment.

The transition from laboratory investigation to clinical practice is nowhere more dynamic than in the field of shock and resuscitation. Recent bench-top discoveries have rapidly been applied in the emergency department and critical care units, often with conflicting results. It is necessary, therefore, for the clinical practitioner to possess a clear understanding of the basic scientific roots underlying modern resuscitative practice. Only through such a thorough understanding is the clinician equipped to properly evaluate and apply new techniques and therapeutic discoveries. This text emphasizes the most current basic understanding of shock physiology. Concepts are dissected to the most fundamental levels of current understanding and thoroughly referenced to the studies upon which such understanding is based. Historical sections emphasize the origins of the primary concepts in each field. In this manner, the clinician may appreciate the thread of scientific investigation underlying new treatment modalities. Such new modalities may then be evaluated and applied in a more rational manner. Conversely, the text provides for the researcher a broad overview of our current understanding of shock investigation. It is of benefit for the investigator to gain both a panorama of shock research and an appreciation for the clinical implications of his or her work.

It is hoped that this text will fulfill the needs of both clinician and researcher alike. In such a dynamic field, the danger lies in allowing the text to become dated in route to publication. Every effort has been made to maintain the timeliness of the work. In addition, emphasis has been placed throughout on recent advances and future directions. Armed with the knowledge gained by those who worked so diligently to lay the foundations of our understanding, it is sincerely hoped that both the researcher and clinician may continue to expand our knowledge and abilities relating to shock and resuscitation.

SHOCK AND RESUSCITATION

1

INTRODUCTION

Evan R. Geller

Shock is that critical condition of the patient which, if uncorrected, leads to death. Shock has many causes, comes at times expected, or appears by surprise. It assumes faces inscrutable and subtle or the ghastly obvious. Shock is calamitous, it is epidemic, it is inevitable. Every patient will be afflicted, if only as a harbinger of their imminent death. When treating shock successfully, the physician has rescued the patient from certain demise. For this reason, in the successful resuscitation of the shocked patient, the physician achieves his or her greatest victory.

Every physician must be knowledgeable regarding the condition of shock and skilled in its treatment. Those caring for the critically ill or injured will face this condition on a daily basis. However, even the most banal of practitioners will have occasion to confront a patient in shock, will need to recognize its signs, and must be able to call on techniques and medicines for its successful treatment. The rural family practitioner is called to the bedside of a victim of a toxic ingestion. An allergist responds to a nurse's cry for help to find a recently inoculated patient wild-eyed and stridorous. The radiologist responsible for a contrast injection, the surgeon, the anesthesiologist, the intensivist—all must have at their disposal the skills to rescue their patients from life-threatening shock. Should they fail, through ignorance or inability, the patient is lost.

The importance of shock goes beyond the bounds of the doctor-patient relationship. The resuscitation from shock of the acutely ill patient is always challenging, often expensive, and at times, futile. Frequently, the need for resuscitation occurs during the final stages of life. The resources required for resuscitative care are rarely trivial. The patient subjected to resuscitation is often compromised and seldom able to act on his or her own behalf. For all these reasons, the care and resuscitation of the patient in shock must involve difficult issues of ethics and economics. The paternalistic physician, acting at all times to do everything possible to preserve life, now becomes entangled in a dense and complex thornbush of advanced directives, health care proxies, and "springing powers of attorney." At the patient's bedside, the physician is told that care is conditional, with treatments titrated to an alchemy of prognosis mixed with palliation. At the other side, the doctor is asked to justify the patient's need for such extraordinary care by the director of the intensive care unit, a utilitarian by nature and necessity. "If the care of the unit is intensive," he or she might ask, "why is the resuscitation of my patient so extraordinary?" But the modern resuscitation of the patient in shock, requiring specialized hospital units and fantastic machinery, sees the physician and patient at the eye of a turbulent storm. This storm will increasingly affect all who treat this extraordinary condition.

HISTORY

SHOCK

The condition of shock has been recognized since antiquity. Astute clinicians over the past 200 years have recognized a severe condition, often brought on by injury or stress and frequently leading to death. Battlefield observation led to the appreciation that a wounded individual may often survive his initial injury to achieve control of his hemorrhage, only to subsequently exhibit a progressive malaise and deterioration resulting in the patient's death. The term *shock* appears to have been first employed in 1743 in a translation of the French treatise of LeDran regarding battlefield wounds.[1] These observations led to a multitude of explanations, most theorizing a circulating toxic agent thought secondary to the initial insult. For this reason, Napoleon's distinguished surgeon general, Ambroise Paré, advocated phlebotomy as a method of treatment.[2] Such humoral theories persisted until the late nineteenth century, when Crile's investigations documented lowering of the central venous pressure in the shock state in animal experiments. He concluded that this lowering was due to a failure of the autonomic nervous system.[3]

Shock research was intensified by the advent of World War I. Cannon, the American physiologist, studied both the clinical data available from wartime experience and animal experimentation in a careful examination of the shock state. These studies led Cannon to theorize that toxins and acidosis contributed to the previously described lowering of vascular tone.[4]

Following World War I, attention was turned by Blalock and others to theories regarding hypovolemia and occult plasma loss rather than toxins.[5] These efforts continued at a heightened pace during World War II and led to the institution of blood banking and transfusion. Aggressive resuscitation of battlefield casualties, accompanied by shortened periods between injury and definitive treatment, resulted in dramatic improvements in survival following injury (Table 1–1).

RESUSCITATION

Reports of the assisted revitalization of the dead date back at least to the seventeenth century.[6] Resuscitative infusions were first utilized clinically in the

TABLE 1–1. Relation of Treatment Interval to Mortality

Conflict	Interval to Treatment (hours)	Mortality (%)
World War I	12–18	8.5
World War II	6–12	5.8
Korea	2–4	2.4
Vietnam	1–2	1.8

treatment of the more obvious hypovolemia of cholera.[7] As noted, shock accompanying injury was previously thought secondary to toxins and more often was treated by phlebotomy than by volume restoration. With the work of Cuthbertson in the period between the world wars and a developing appreciation of the occult hypovolemia associated with tissue injury during the mid-twentieth century, aggressive fluid resuscitation became standard.[8] Wiggers first noted, however, that in his standardized dog model of hemorrhagic shock a point was reached where shock became irreversible despite volume restoration.[9] This finding foreshadowed the experiences of later conflicts in the twentieth century in Korea and Vietnam. Despite aggressive and apparently successful resuscitation of severely injured patients, death ensued as a consequence of organ failure syndromes. The Korean conflict saw the description of shock-induced acute renal failure. With still more aggressive fluid resuscitation during the Vietnam war, survivors of once-fatal injuries went on to succumb to "shock lung." Initially, this entity was feared to be the result of overly aggressive fluid resuscitation. Subsequent study utilizing the newly developed pulmonary artery catheter of Swan and Ganz demonstrated, however, that pulmonary edema developed not as a consequence of supranormal fluid volumes but rather as a result of alterations in pulmonary tissue permeability.[10] This finding has led a return to the search for circulating toxins associated with shock. The last two decades have witnessed an explosion of information regarding alterations of homeostasis and cellular physiochemistry during shock. The scientific investigations of Shires, Carrico, Baue, and countless others have shed light on the basic mechanisms underlying the resuscitation from shock.[11] Modern resuscitation, however, has seen the progression in civilian practice from the shock lung of Da Nang to the multiple organ failure syndrome seen now in every intensive care unit. Attention has focused on biochemical perturbations and altered mediators as sites for resuscitative interventions.[12–14] These subtle pharmacologic therapies, it is hoped, will prove effective in the successful resuscitation of those patients now surviving severe shock as a result of the practices learned from those who preceded us.

DEFINITIONS AND CLASSIFICATION OF SHOCK

The pathophysiology of the shock state has proven difficult to characterize with any consistency. These historical aspects are dealt with from several perspectives in the following chapters. Many reasons for shock have been put forward through the years, including theories relating to humors, imbalances, or central nervous system (CNS) mediation. It is testimony to the challenge that shock presents to the modern practitioner that there continue to exist a plethora of theories regarding the etiology and pathophysiology of shock. Indeed, the modern medical and investigational literature is replete with theories of humoral mediators, physiologic imbalances, and, most recently, a resurgence of the theory of CNS mediation. The historical "bad humor" thought circulating in the shock victim now finds its modern equivalents in the elusive "myocardial depressant factor of shock," nitrous oxide, and superoxide radicals. As new biologic substances and interactions have recently been discovered, again inappropriate and inharmonious balances between cytokines or prostanoids have been implicated in the shock state. Most recently, the discovery of endogenous opioids within the CNS and the relation of these substances to metabolism have reopened the question of the role of the CNS in the shock state.[15]

At the clinical level, most practitioners continue to define shock as that state when perfusion of tissues is inadequate to meet physiologic requirements.[16] This definition is by far the most frequently cited and serves as a common basis for the understanding of a variety of shock states. However, this definition offers little insight into the pathophysiology underlying this perfusion inadequacy. Indeed, in its strict sense, this perfusion definition may be simply untrue, since many tissues continue to be adequately perfused in shock. In some shock states, tissues may be overperfused, but cellular ischemia and shock persist. Although less than accurate, the perfusion definition remains the best unifying definition of shock for the clinician.

An alternative to the broadly unifying definition described above has been to break shock down into various states based on etiology. This approach, popularized by Blalock, acknowledges the fundamental differences in the various clinical conditions that we have traditionally referred to as shock. Septic shock, induced by infection or overwhelming inflammation, is recognized to be a distinct entity from hypovolemic shock, which, in turn, is quite a different condition from that shock which accompanies severe tissue injury. This division has allowed investigators to study the pathophysiology underlying each of these states, and each is found to be unique. Utilizing an etiologic classification, particular physiologic perturbations characterize each of the various shock states (Table 1–2). Diagnosis and treatment may be guided by this classification. While certain factors are common to each of these etiologies, to date, little in the way of a "unifying theory" accounting for all shock states can be claimed.

John Collins Warren referred to shock as "a momentary pause in the act of death."[17] More recently, we have seen described a syndrome of multiple organ failure (MOF), and in this entity we have begun to see unity between many types of shock. Severe shock, regardless of the etiology, leads to a "total body inflammatory syndrome," and the multiple organ failure syndrome results as a common final pathway. In the investigation of this syndrome, it is felt, one may discover some fundamental truths relating to shock. However, if shock is but a momentary pause, the MOF syndrome appears to be the process of death itself, now seen in slow motion as a result of the ministrations of the intensivist— death by individual organ system and by degree, but no less fatal. It would seem that the successful resuscitation of the patient suffering from shock will be di-

TABLE 1–2. Classification of Shock

Etiology	Syndrome	Characteristic Physiologic Parameters
Hypovolemia	Hemorrhagic shock	↓ CVP, ↓ CO, ↑ SVR
	Traumatic shock	↓ CVP, ↕ CO
Inflammation	Septic shock	↑ CO, ↓ SVR
Inadequate cardiac output	Cardiogenic shock	↓ CO
	Cardiac compressive shock	
Loss of vasomotor tone	Neurogenic shock	↓ SVR

Note: CO = cardiac output; CVP = central venous pressure; SVR = systemic vascular resistance; ↓ = decreased; ↑ = increased; ↕ = increase and/or decrease.

rected at the condition prior to the final common pathway of the MOF syndrome.

CONSIDERATIONS

INITIATION OF TREATMENT

Shock represents the process of dying. The ability to successfully intervene in that process clearly depends on the complex interaction of many factors. Effective resuscitation depends on the early and accurate diagnosis of the etiology of the shock state and the aggressive application of appropriate treatment. These diagnostic and therapeutic efforts are demanding. Resuscitative efforts are invasive, often painful, and always expensive. The resources needed to resuscitate the patient in shock will always be in short supply, demand always far outstripping available intensive care beds. Clearly, circumstances at times conspire to make resuscitation futile, death inevitable. That moment when treatment becomes inappropriate has proven even more difficult to define than shock itself. Indeed, that moment seems to shift with increasing frequency. The octogenarian, who, in a previous day, might be allowed to quietly succumb to pneumonia, is now subjected to the call of "code blue," crash endotracheal intubation, mechanical ventilation, and a prolonged stay in the invasive care unit. The outcome may not be altered, only painfully and expensively delayed a brief while. There is general agreement that resuscitation must be rationed, but no rationale exists for doing so. Every effort to save every life! The emergency medicine physician greets the young, bloodied victim of a high-speed motor vehicle accident. The patient is pulseless and unresponsive. He is dead, but can he be resuscitated? And does the possibility of resuscitation demand an attempt at resuscitation? In the ICU, death has been slowed to a weeks-long process, but in the emergency room, the concept of death has met its own demise. No one is dead until he or she has been unsuccessfully resuscitated.

It is clear that this approach is unacceptable medical practice. The thoughtless application of resuscitative therapy carries a great many consequences, not just for society on an economic basis. The consequences are felt by the family of the young accident victim "successfully" resuscitated to a persistent vegetative state. The consequences are felt by the practitioner accidentally inoculated during the conduct of another unsuccessful resuscitative thoracotomy. Therapy without consideration is bad medicine.

How then are we to decide who to resuscitate and who is dead? Really and finally dead, not just recently and briefly dead. While it is clear that successful resuscitation from traumatic shock is inversely proportional to the length of time before definitive treatment,[18] it is difficult to quantify exactly when treatment becomes futile and, therefore, inappropriate. Criteria are available, however, and careful study of their application on the part of the practitioner is needed. An example of such a criterion may be found in the Seattle experience, where it was found that resuscitation was not successful when the pulseless trauma victim presented without electrocardiographic activity.[19] Such a standard may be rationally applied by the practitioner in this setting. Similar appropriate criteria may be applied to other causes of shock, utilizing probabilities of success based on established medical experience. Existing literature supports a rational approach to the patient suffering a myocardial infarction and known to be pulseless for a prolonged period of time without CPR.[20] Similar parameters surround the septic patient in the ICU exhibiting failure of multiple organ systems[21] or requiring suprapharmacologic doses of vasopressive agents to maintain blood pressure.[22] In these and other circumstances, criteria exist for the knowledgeable practitioner to make a rational decision regarding resuscitation of the patient in shock. Although the considerations of patient, family, and other health care agents are involved, the decision and responsibility regarding resuscitation of the patient in shock rest with the attending physician.[23]

TERMINATION OF RESUSCITATION

Just as the attending physician shoulders the responsibility for the initiation of resuscitative efforts, he or she is also responsible for the difficult decisions regarding the termination of those efforts. Often resuscitation is instituted by prehospital care providers, bystanders, or health care workers at the bedside of the victim. Again, rational guidelines exist regarding the probability of successful resuscitation in various circumstances (Table 1–3).

Primary consideration should be paid to the patient's stated wishes. At times, resuscitative efforts will have been initiated, inappropriately or unknowingly, in the face of a "do not resuscitate" order or advance directive to the contrary. It is the responsibility of the physician to then discontinue resuscitative efforts. The temptation must be avoided, however, to abrogate the physician's responsibility toward appropriate medical care to the uninformed desires of the patient or family. One hears with increasing frequency in the ICU that the physician's "hands were tied" by the insistence of family, either for "too much" resuscitation or "too little." Such a situation almost always exists as a result of the failure of the physician to adequately inform the family and/or the patient regarding the clinical situation and alternatives of therapy. It is the responsibility of the attending physician to obtain, when at all possible, informed consent regarding resuscitative efforts.

TABLE 1–3. Predictors of Mortality Following Cardiac Arrest and Attempted Cardiopulmonary Resuscitation

Prearrest

Homebound lifestyle
Cancer
Cerebrovascular accident with residual neurologic deficit
Renal failure
Sepsis
Left ventricular dysfunction
Hypotension (systolic blood pressure less than 100 mmHg)
Metabolic acidosis
Recurrent cardiac arrest during the same hospital stay

Arrest

Unwitnessed collapse
CPR delayed more than 4 min
Bradyasystolic arrest rhythms (aystole/electromechanical dissociation/pulseless idioventricular rhythm)
Fine ventricular fibrillation (ventricular fibrillation amplitude <0.2 mV)
CPR for more than 15 min
Dilated pupils despite adequate ventilation and external chest compression
Endotracheal intubation

Source: Adapted from Bickell W, Rice M, Dellinger R: Termination of resuscitation, in Civetta J, Taylor R, Kirby R (eds): *Critical Care Medicine*. Philadelphia, Lippincott, 1988, chap 13, p 122, with permission.

Age is often cited as a criterion for the degree of aggressiveness regarding resuscitative efforts. Younger patients are generally regarded as worthy of greater resuscitative effort, with older patients felt to be less likely to survive. However, this does not appear to be a reasonable criterion for resuscitation. Studies have failed to substantiate the belief that older patients have a higher mortality or worse quality of life following resuscitation.[24,25] On the contrary, evidence exists that the opposite may be true (see Chap. 13). It would appear that age as an independent factor is not appropriate as a criterion for resuscitation.

EPIDEMIOLOGIC CONSIDERATIONS

While it is impossible to state accurately the prevalence or mortality of shock as a clinical entity, it is clear that shock, in all its forms, represents a leading cause of death in this country across all age groups. Indeed, it may be viewed as a nearly universal premortal condition, but this viewpoint contributes little to our understanding. Rather, one may examine the contribution of individual causes and forms of shock to overall mortality and then pursue therapies directed toward improving patient outcome. Traumatic shock, for example, is the third leading cause of death overall, behind myocardial infarction and cancer.[26] It accounts for more years of lost life than cancer and heart disease combined. The pathophysiology underlying this statistic is well known. As a consequence, the treatment of traumatic shock has progressed significantly in the past 30 years.

However, repeated studies have documented that 15 to 40 percent of patients succumbing to death from injury do so needlessly.[27] The mechanisms for alleviating these preventable deaths are known and proven. Efforts to implement public health systems that will optimize resuscitative efforts following injury are being actively pursued. Such efforts carry intrinsic commitments of valuable resources.[28]

FUTURE CONSIDERATIONS

Substantial progress is being achieved with increasing rapidity toward the understanding and treatment of shock. As new information is developed, previously accepted approaches are being modified and innovative therapies appear. Recently, critical studies of prehospital resuscitative regimens have begun to challenge existing dogma regarding the use of pneumatic compression devices.[29] Basic research into the cellular and biochemical alterations attending shock and the transition to irreversibility show promise of extending the period of successful resuscitation.[30]

Shock due to sepsis has now become the leading cause of death in the intensive care unit setting. The hypotensive septic shock state carries an 80 percent mortality.[22] This is despite the most prolific introduction of antimicrobial agents in history. While revolutionary advancements in the understanding of the molecular biology of sepsis occur now on an almost daily basis and new and novel agents of intervention in the treatment of septic shock appear on the clinical horizon, it may be that the death by degree evidenced in the MOF syndrome common to this type of shock is not amenable to reversal. It may be necessary, rather, to develop an understanding of the causes of the septic shock condition and its early pathophysiology so that novel diagnostic and therapeutic approaches may be directed at preventing the MOF syndrome. Indeed, the paradigm for future successful resuscitation may well focus on our ability to diagnose and treat shock at its earliest and most fundamental biochemical level.

REFERENCES

1. Simeone FA: Shock, trauma, and the surgeon. *Ann Surg* 158:759, 1963.
2. Paré A: *Oeuvres Completes d'ambroise Paré.* Paris, JB Bailiniers, 1840.
3. Crile GW: *An Experimental Research into Surgical Shock.* Philadelphia, Lippincott, 1899.
4. Cannon WB: *Traumatic Shock.* New York: Appleton and Company, 1923.
5. Blalock A: Experimental shock: The cause of low blood pressure produced by muscle injury. *Arch Surg* 20:959, 1930.
6. Hughes JT: The miraculous deliverance of Anne Green: An Oxford case of resuscitation in the seventeenth century. *Br Med J* 285:1792, 1982.
7. Howard-Jones N: Cholera therapy in the nineteenth century. *J Hist Med* 27:373, 1972.
8. Cuthbertson DP: The disturbance of metabolism produced by bony and non-bony injury, with notes on certain abnormal conditions of bone. *Biochem J* 24:1244, 1930.
9. Wiggers CJ: The present status of the shock problem. *Physiol Rev* 22:74, 1942.

10. Blaisdell FW, Lewis FR: *Respiratory Distress Syndrome of Shock and Trauma.* Philadelphia, Saunders, 1977.

11. Shires GT, Carrico CJ, Canizaro PC: *Shock.* Philadelphia, Saunders, 1973.

12. Lefer AM: Leukotrienes as mediators of ischemia and shock. *Biochem Pharmacol* 35:123, 1986.

13. Filkins JP: Monokines and the metabolic pathophysiology of septic shock. *Fed Proc* 44:300, 1985.

14. Lefer AM: Eicosanoids as mediators of ischemia and shock. *Fed Proc* 44:275, 1985.

15. Radosevich PM, Lacy DB, Williams PE, Abumrad NN: Glucoregulatory changes during hyperglycemia induced by intracerebroventricular beta-endorphin in the conscious dog. *Surg Forum* 36:22, 1985.

16. Kreis DJ Jr, Baue AE: *Clinical Management of Shock.* Baltimore, University Park Press, 1984.

17. Warren JC: *Surgical Pathology and Therapeutics.* Philadelphia, WB Saunders, 1895.

18. Trunkey DD: Trauma. *Sci Am* 249:28, 1983.

19. Harnar TJ, Oreskovich MR, Copass MK, et al: Role of emergency thoracotomy in the resuscitation of moribund trauma victims. *Am J Surg* 142:96, 1981.

20. Stueven H, Troiano P, Thompson B, et al: Bystander/first responder CPR: Ten years experience in a paramedic system. *Ann Emerg Med* 15:707, 1986.

21. Moyer E, Cerra F, Chenier R, et al: Multiple systems organ failure: VI. Death predictors in the trauma-septic state—The most critical determinants. *J Trauma* 21:862, 1981.

22. Ruiz CE, Weil MH, Carlson RW: Treatment of circulatory shock with dopamine: Studies on survival. *JAMA* 242(2):165, 1979.

23. Bioethics Committee, American College of Emergency Physicians: Medical, moral, legal, and ethical aspects of resuscitation for the patient who will have minimal ability to function or ultimately survive. *Ann Emerg Med* 14:919, 1985.

24. Bedell SE, Delbanco TL, Cook EF, et al: Survival after cardiopulmonary resuscitation in the hospital. *N Engl J Med* 309:569, 1983.

25. Peatfield RC, Sillett RW, Taylor D, et al: Survival after cardiac arrest in hospital. *Lancet* 1:1223, 1977.

26. *Accident Facts.* Chicago, National Safety Council, 1984.

27. Cales RH, Heilig RW: *Trauma Care Systems.* Rockville, Md, Aspen Publishers, 1986.

28. Kreis DJ Jr, Fine EG, Gomez GA, et al: A prospective evaluation of field categorization of trauma patients. *J Trauma* 28(7):995, 1988.

29. Mattox KL, Bickell WH, Pepe PE, Mangelsdorff AD: Prospective randomized evaluation of antishock MAST in post-traumatic hypotension. *J Trauma* 26(9):779, 1986.

30. Maitra SR, Krikely M, Dulchavsky SA, et al: Beneficial effects of diltiazem in hemorrhagic shock. *Circ Shock* 33:121, 1991.

2

HOMEOSTASIS

James M. Harkema
Irshad H. Chaudry

The basic living unit of the human body is the cell. Indeed, the cell determines organ function and ultimately the survival of the organism. Thus, for an organism to function most efficiently, optimal conditions must exist for cell life. For aerobic organisms this requires the delivery of oxygen from the atmosphere and substrates from external food sources to peripheral tissues for the production of energy by mitochondria. Body fluid constitutes the transport system, as well as the medium for metabolic processes within the cell. The movement of blood around the circulatory system is the initial step in the delivery of oxygen and nutrients. However, it is the microcirculation where transport of these substances to the cells occurs. Body fluid is essential in this stage as well. The cells are bathed in fluid that functions as the vehicle for the delivery of substrates, ions, and oxygen necessary for the maintenance of cell life. A continuous exchange of fluid between the plasma portion of blood and the interstitial fluid that surrounds cells facilitates this transport. Equally important for efficient cell function is the constancy of this fluid's composition. Thus it is not surprising that the body has complex and sensitive controls and regulatory devices that maintain the volume and composition of extracellular fluid within very fine limits.

The concept of an internal environment with a closely regulated composition was first introduced by French physiologist Claude Bernard.[1] He observed the stability of various physiologic parameters and concluded that "all the vital mechanisms, however varied they may be, have but one end, that of preserving constancy in the internal environment."[1] Thus he introduced the concept of a friendly *milieu intérieur* which allows the organism to function independent of the external environment. Walter B. Cannon, the American physiologist, also recognized the complexity and interaction of various physiologic processes in maintenance of the internal environment.[2] He introduced the word *homeostasis* as a description of this constant state and also as indicative of the regulatory mechanisms necessary to maintain it. Cannon placed emphasis on the dynamic equilibria and variability of this environment. As he stated, "The word does not imply something set and immobile, a stagnation. It means a condition—a condition which may vary, but which is relatively constant."[2] Guyton[3] further defines *homeostasis* as the "maintenance of static, or constant, conditions in the internal environment. Essentially all the organs and tissues of the body perform functions that help to maintain these constant conditions."

The concept of homeostasis, therefore, implies several regulatory processes. The variable that is to be regulated must be monitored, and changes in the variable must be detected. In addition, this sensory information must be interpreted and integrated so that appropriate corrective responses can occur. Finally, mechanisms must be present to correct the abnormality in the variable that is regulated. Thus negative feedback has acquired a prominent role in the control mechanisms within the body. That is, if there is a deviation in one direction, there is a reaction in the opposite direction that restores the variable to normal. For example, excessive water loss from the gastrointestinal tract via vomiting or diarrhea temporarily disrupts body water balance. However, the gastrointestinal tract is not a primary factor in water regulation. The kidney is the organ that controls water loss and thus restores water balance by promoting the reabsorption of water from the renal tubules. This response is negative with respect to the initiating stimuli, fluid loss. Although most regulatory mechanisms appear to depend on negative feedback, several investigators have emphasized that homeostasis does not involve negative feedback exclusively.[4,5] McFarland states, "The term feedforward is used for situations in which feedback consequences of behavior are anticipated and appropriate action is taken to forestall deviations in physiologic state."[4] Indeed, some physiologic mechanisms appear to actively promote change. One such phenomenon appears to be the changing of set points. For example, when pressure in the renal artery falls, renal blood flow decreases and renin is released. This results in the production of angiotensin II. Angiotensin II causes vasoconstriction and an increase in arterial pressure. However, independent of this increase in pressure, angiotensin II resets the baroreceptor-mediated decreases in heart rate toward higher pressures.[6] These actions tend to restore blood flow through the kidneys while imposing the elevated blood pressure in the general circulation on the rest of the body. In this regard, Mrosovsky[5] has introduced the term *rheostasis*, which he defines as "a condition or state in which, at any one instant, homeostatic defenses are still present but over a span of time there is a change in the regulated level. Therefore rheostasis includes a change in set point, both when the term is used descriptively without specifying a mechanism and when it is used to indicate a mechanism comprising negative feedback with a reference signal."[5] With regard to the mechanisms that are operative in maintaining the extracellular fluid volume and composition, negative feedback appears to play the predominant role. The mechanisms involved in positive feedback at present are, however, poorly defined. Nonetheless, rheostasis may have survival value when the organism is faced with extreme stress and different regulatory systems are in conflict. This chapter will deal primarily with the known mechanisms that maintain the internal environment. However, as our knowledge increases concerning the regulation of the internal environment, particularly when these mechanisms are stressed by volume loss or sepsis, it will be increasingly necessary to understand not only mechanisms that seek constancy in the internal environment but also those which promote change.

This chapter reviews body fluid compartments and their composition. In addition, it discusses homeostatic mechanisms for the maintenance of body fluids under normal conditions. Since most mechanisms involved in normal fluid homeostasis are also involved to some degree in the response to hemorrhage, some background information will be provided concerning hemorrhage. The last section of this chapter describes the mechanisms that promote restoration of the circulation and body fluids after hemorrhage.

BODY FLUID COMPARTMENTS

The internal environment is essentially fluid. This fluid environment is necessary for cell life and organ function. Indeed, the primary concern of control mechanisms involved in body fluid is to support a constant environment for cell function despite alterations in water and ion intake. Before discussing the mechanisms intrinsic to this process, a thorough understanding of fluid compartments and their composition is mandatory.

TOTAL BODY WATER

Water accounts for the largest proportion of body mass, constituting between 45 and 75 percent of body weight.[7,8] The variability in body water in relation to body weight is a function of the amount of fat. Water composes 70 to 80 percent of most tissues but only 10 percent of fat.[9] Thus water accounts for a lower percentage of body weight in the obese and in women, who have greater fat stores than men.[10] In the newborn infant, 75 percent of body weight may be water. Despite variations in fluid intake and loss, the total water content remains constant in the normal adult. Indeed, lean body mass and water content parallel each other and are remarkably constant.[11] Thus, in a man with an average weight (70 kg), the total body water is approximately 40 liters.

The volume of the fluid compartments of the body can be measured by the dilution technique. By placing a substance in the fluid compartment, allowing it to disperse throughout the fluid, and then measuring the extent that it has been diluted, the volume of the compartment can be calculated. This is expressed by the following formula:[12]

$$\text{Volume (ml)} = \frac{\text{quantity of test substance instilled}}{\text{concentration per milliliter of dispersed substance}}$$

Since there is continual movement of water throughout its total body distribution, tritium (H^3) or deuterium (H^2) can be used for measuring total body water using the dilution technique.[13] The drug antipyrine is also distributed evenly throughout the total body water and can be used for this determination as well. Marker substances are also useful in the determination of the volumes of the different compartments of body water.

EXTRACELLULAR AND INTRACELLULAR COMPARTMENTS

Total body water exists in two major compartments: intracellular and extracellular (Table 2–1). By definition, *extracellular fluid* includes all fluid outside the cells, including fluid in the plasma portion of blood, fluid between cells or in the interstitial space, and fluid in body cavities, such as the gastrointestinal tract and cerebrospinal fluid. This latter body fluid fraction also includes intraocular, synovial, pleural, and peritoneal fluids and has been designated as *transcellular water*.[14] This fluid is separated from the plasma not only by the capillary endothelium but also by an epithelial cell layer. Therefore, it is not as continuously in exchange with plasma as the interstitial fluid compartment, which is separated only by the capillary endothelium.

Since the extracellular fluid compartment is not homogeneous and does not have precise borders, accurate measurements of its volume are difficult. This compartment has been estimated by the use of markers that only slowly or incompletely enter the cell.[15,16] Not only must the marker not enter cells, but it also must reach every portion of the extensive interstitial space as well as plasma. It also should be excreted slowly and, ideally, would not be secreted into digestive fluids. Since no such marker has been identified, this compartment is less precisely measurable than total body water. Nevertheless, several markers have been investigated.[16,17] Hays[17] compiled a list of extracellular fluid compartment measurements and found that 15 to 28 percent of body weight is extracellular fluid. When corrections were made for intracellular chloride, Yasumura et al.[16] found that, using chloride as a marker, the extracellular water accounted for 40 to 50 percent of total body water. Thus, in a 70-kg adult, the extracellular fluid compartment would be approximately 15 liters.

The two major compartments of the extracellular fluid are the plasma and interstitial fluid. Plasma volume can be determined by a radioactively labeled protein that remains in the circulation or by a vital dye that attaches to plasma protein. It also can be calculated using labeled erythrocytes as the dilutional marker. Estimation of the plasma volume also may be determined using the equation

$$\text{Plasma volume} = \text{total blood volume} \times (1.00 - \text{hematocrit})$$

TABLE 2–1. Body Water Compartments

	Percent Body Weight	Volume (liters)
Total body water	60	40
Extracellular water	20	15
Plasma	7	5
Interstitial fluid	15	10
Intracellular water	35	25

Note: Water constitutes the major portion of the body mass and exists in two compartments: extracellular and intracellular. The extracellular compartment may be further divided into intravascular and extravascular. The extravascular water is that found between cells as well as in the body cavities.

This calculation probably underestimates the true plasma volume because the hematocrit in small capillaries may be considerably smaller than in large vessels, where blood is obtained for the hematocrit determination. It also should be noted that plasma is approximately 93 percent water. Plasma volume measurements obtained by a number of investigators averaged 4.5 percent of body weight, or 7 percent of total body water.[17] Thus, for a 70-kg adult, there is slightly less than 5 liters of plasma.

Measurement of the interstitial fluid compartment would require the use of a marker that would leave the plasma but not enter the cell. It also would require a technique to obtain interstitial fluid samples for dilution measurements. Since a marker has not been identified that meets these criteria, estimates of interstitial fluid volumes are derived from other fluid compartment determinations. Interstitial fluid volume is equal to the difference between extracellular water and plasma water. Edelman and Liebman[14] determined that interstitial and lymph water was 20 percent of total body water or about 12 percent of body weight. They further stated that water in connective tissue and bone each accounted for an additional 4.5 percent of body weight.[14] These transcellular fluids are not measured by extracellular dilutional measurements. Since in a 70-kg man total extracellular fluid is approximately 15 liters and plasma volume is 5 liters, then the calculated interstitial fluid is 10 liters.

The volume of *intracellular fluid* cannot be measured directly; therefore, intracellular water volume has been calculated as the difference between total body water and extracellular body water. Using these calculations, 30 to 40 percent of body weight is intracellular water, or approximately two-thirds of total body water is intracellular fluid. This amounts to 25 liters in a normal 70-kg male.

Although each marker used in the measurement of the various compartments has its limitations and therefore is probably not a precise determination, the fact remains that total body water remains constant and compartment determinations are reproducible when the same marker is used. Since water is freely movable between plasma, interstitial fluid, and cellular water, the composition of these fluids must be tightly controlled to prevent significant decreases or increases in cellular water.

COMPOSITION OF BODY FLUIDS

Although the individual constituents of extracellular and intracellular fluids are controlled within narrow limits, there are considerable differences in the composition of these different fluid compartments. The major cation in plasma is sodium, while the major anions are chloride, bicarbonate, and protein. Plasma protein occupies a volume out of proportion to the few milliequivalents of anion it represents. Interstitial fluid, on the other hand, has a much lower concentration of protein but similar electrolyte concentrations. The small differences in electrolyte concentrations between plasma and interstitial fluid can be explained by the Gibbs-Donnan rule, which is discussed later. The high concentration of sodium in the extracellular fluid appears to be directly related to the need for a sufficient volume to supply nutrients to the cell. The volume of this essential fluid space is directly dependent on the sodium concentration. Sodium salts are virtually restricted to the extracellular fluid and are the principal osmotically active component. Regulation of total body sodium content by the kidney is one mechanism that the body uses to maintain a normal extracellular fluid volume and therefore the transport system of cellular nutrients and ions necessary for optimal cell function. There are significant differences in the constituents of intracellular fluid compared with extracellular fluid. The major intracellular cation is potassium. Potassium plays a significant role in cell function. Several functions of potassium are crucial to cell integrity, including cell volume maintenance,[18] protein synthesis,[19] enzyme function,[20] and intracellular pH regulation.[21] Furthermore, the transcellular potassium concentration differences are responsible for many of the electrical properties of cells.[20]

Other ions present in greater concentrations in intracellular fluid compared with extracellular fluid are magnesium, phosphate, and sulfate. Magnesium serves as the cofactor for ATP-dependent cellular processes and activates a wide spectrum of enzymatic reactions. Phosphorus plays a major role in energy production. Intracellular fluid also contains very large amounts of protein, approximately four times as much as in plasma. Protein is essential for cell integrity and function. Thus the differences in composition of the various fluid compartments are best explained by the functions of each fluid space. Furthermore, the differences in ion and protein concentrations between intracellular and extracellular fluid compartments and those between plasma and interstitial fluid play a major role in the regulation of volume distribution between these compartments.

OSMOTIC PROPERTIES OF FLUID SPACES

To understand how the body maintains solute concentration differences across body fluid compartments without changes in volume distribution requires understanding of semipermeable membranes and the chemical laws that govern water and solute concentrations across these membranes. The body fluid compartments are separated by semipermeable membranes, the capillary endothelium and the cell membrane. The capillary endothelium, for example, is freely permeable to water and ions but relatively impermeable to larger molecules such as plasma proteins. This favors the movement of water from the interstitial space to plasma for the following reasons: If water is placed on either side of a membrane freely permeable to water, there will be continual movement of water molecules from one side to the other. The kinetic activity of the water molecules is equal on both sides, so the same number of molecules will strike the pores on both sides of the membrane. Thus an equal exchange of water from one side to the other will occur. If a permeable ion, such as sodium, is added to one side of the membrane, then there will be a change in kinetic activity on that side compared with the solute-free side. Sodium will displace water molecules, and fewer water molecules will strike the pores on that side. This will favor movement of water to the side of the membrane with solute. In addition, the sodium will strike the membrane pores and will diffuse to the other side until the concentrations of sodium and water are equal on either side of the membrane. If a nonpermeable ion, such as protein, is added to one side of the membrane, it will not diffuse. It will, however, reduce the kinetic activity of the water, and water will diffuse to the solute side until the kinetic activity of water is equal on both sides. This movement of water to the side of greater solute concentration is called *osmosis*. The movement of water molecules can be opposed by pressure applied across the semipermeable membrane in the opposite direction of the osmosis. The pressure required to prevent this flow is the *osmotic pressure.*

Osmotic pressure is determined by the number of particles or molecules to which the membrane is impermeable. Particles are equally osmotically active regardless of their size or valence. When a molecule dissociates into two or more ions, each ion exerts osmotic pressure if the membrane is impermeable to it. Thus one molecule of albumin with a molecular weight of 69,000 has the same osmotic effect as a molecule of sodium with a molecular weight of 23. Osmole (osmol) is the unit of measurement used to determine osmotic pressure. One mole (1 mol) of solute that dissociates into x number of particles is equal to x osmoles per liter of solution. One mole of sodium is equal to one osmole of sodium, while one mole of NaCl is equal to two osmoles, since NaCl dissociates into two osmotically active particles.

In the body, fluids are so dilute that milliosmoles per liter is the unit used for measuring osmotic activity. The terms *osmolarity* and *osmolality* also should be defined. *Osmolarity* refers to the measurement of osmoles per liter, while *osmolality* is the measurement of osmoles per kilogram of H_2O. Again, since the body fluids are quite dilute, the differences are so slight that the preceding terms are used almost interchangeably. Since it is easier to measure and express body fluids as per liter, most calculations are made using osmolarity.

Osmotic pressure is also a measurement that reflects osmotically active particles. The relationship between osmolality and osmotic pressure is expressed as follows:

$$\text{Osmotic pressure (mmHg)} = 19.3 \times \text{osmolality (osmol/kg } H_2O)$$

It is obvious that if significant changes in osmolality were to occur, significant fluid shifts between body fluid compartments would occur. In this regard, if cellular water osmotic activity remains constant, then cell volume changes will occur if extracellular osmolality changes. During health, homeostatic mechanisms keep the extracellular osmolality remarkably constant. Extracellular osmolality, indeed, does not vary by more than 1 percent from the norm.[22,23] Thus cell volume also remains constant.

GIBBS-DONNAN RULE

The Gibbs-Donnan rule was derived from thermodynamic principles and predicts under conditions of equilibrium that the product of any pair of diffusible ions on one side of a membrane will equal the product of the same pair on the opposite side. The distribution of Na^+ and Cl^- between plasma and interstitial fluid according to the Gibbs-Donnan relationship is

$$P_{Na} \times P_{Cl} = ISF_{Na} \times ISF_{Cl}$$

where P is plasma and ISF is the interstitial fluid. In addition, electrical neutrality must be maintained on both sides of the membrane. Since an impermeable anion, i.e., protein, occupies the interstitial space, an additional cation, i.e., sodium, is needed to maintain electrical neutrality. However, this upsets the Gibbs-Donnan principle for Na^+ and Cl^- in these two compartments. To reestablish equilibrium, redistribution of Na^+ and Cl^- occurs. Na^+ concentration is slightly higher in the protein-containing plasma compartment, and Cl^- is slightly higher in the interstitial fluid compartment. This reestablishes electrical equilibrium as well, since total cations equal total anions on each side of the capillary endothelium. However, the osmotic pressure in the plasma secondary to protein is slightly greater than the osmotic pressure in the interstitial fluid compartment. This favors transfer of fluid to the plasma. In the capillaries, net transfer of fluid is prevented by an outwardly directed hydrostatic pressure. Thus the relationship between plasma and interstitial fluid is a balance between osmotic, electrochemical, and hydrostatic forces.

The cell also has a high concentration of impermeable anions, namely, proteins. They exert an osmotic force via the Gibbs-Donnan effect that promotes the movement of water into cells (Fig. 2–1). However, the cells do not swell because the intracellular osmotic pressure is counteracted by the osmotic pressure exerted in the interstitial fluid by Na^+. This occurs despite the fact that Na^+ is freely diffusible from interstitial fluid into the cell. The active extrusion of Na^+ from the cell results in sufficient Na^+ and its accompanying anion Cl^- to maintain their concentrations in excess of the expected Gibbs-Donnan distribution. This is accomplished by the active transport of Na^+ out of the cell and accompanying K^+ transport into the cell in a ratio of 3:2. This is an energy-requiring process utilizing ATP and the enzyme Na^+, K^+-ATPase. The net result is an increased concentration of K^+ within the cell and an increased concentration of Na^+ in the interstitial fluid. Osmotic equilibrium is therefore maintained, since the passive flow of Na^+ into the cell and its active extrusion result in an osmotic equivalent of Na^+ being an impermeable ion.

In view of the preceding information, it appears that both the volume distribution and solute concentration in the various fluid compartments of the body have a teleologic function. Not only are the fluid compartments designed to deliver nutrients and oxygen, but the solute concentrations are such that volume

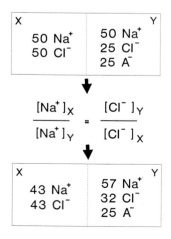

FIG. 2–1. The Gibbs-Donnan effect. The Gibbs-Donnan principle states that under conditions of equilibrium, the product of any pair of diffusible ions on one side of a membrane will equal the product of the same pair on the opposite side. However, an impermeable (e.g., protein) anion A^- upsets the Gibbs-Donnan principle and reestablishing equilibrium results in a slightly higher concentration of Na^+ on the side of the impermeable anion and a slightly higher concentration of Cl^- on the other side. Furthermore, osmotic pressure is slightly higher on the side of the impermeable anion, resulting in a shift of fluid away from that side.

necessary for transport is preserved and facilitates diffusion of nutrients to the cell.

FLUID EXCHANGE IN THE MICROCIRCULATION

The microcirculation is the site where the major body fluid compartments are physically and functionally interrelated. The number of blood vessels progressively increases in the arterial vessels so that the total cross-sectional area of the capillaries and venules is 250 times that of terminal arteries and 10 times that of the arterioles. The number of capillaries and their surface area are immense. Furthermore, capillaries are very close to cells. Indeed, cells in the body are separated from capillaries by no more than 20 to 30 μm. This space is occupied by the interstitial fluid, which is separated from the plasma by a unicellular endothelial layer, with a thickness of about 0.5 μm, and from cell water by the cell membrane, with a thickness of only 7.5 to 10 nm. It is in this close physical relationship that the maintenance of tissue homeostasis occurs. This includes the physical transport of blood in the microcirculation, i.e., capillaries, as well as the flow of fluid through the interstitial space. As has already been noted, this flow occurs without any net change in the fluid volumes of the individual compartments or net change in their composition. The actual distribution of nutrients and waste materials is accomplished by this extravascular flow system. To gain access to the interstitial space and thus the cell, nutrients must first move across the capillary endothelium, while waste substances from the cell must be returned from the interstitial fluid to the systemic circulation. The fluid exchange between these closely approximated fluid compartments is determined by hydrostatic and osmotic factors as formulated by the Starling equation, while nutrients and ions are transferred between plasma and interstitial fluid by diffusion.

E. H. Starling[24] developed an equation to describe fluid movement across the capillary bed. Starling's law states that

$$FM = K[(P_c - II_c) - (P_i - II_i)]$$

where FM is the volume flow per unit area of the capillary wall, P_c and P_i are the hydrostatic pressures in the capillary plasma and interstitial fluid, II_c and II_i are the protein osmotic pressures of the capillary plasma and interstitial fluid, and K is the filtration coefficient. The filtration coefficient is the hydraulic conductivity of the capillary wall, indicating the flow per minute through a given capillary area per millimeter of mercury (mmHg) of hydraulic pressure (Fig. 2–2). Capillary beds in various organs differ markedly in their filtration properties.[25,26] The unusually extensive and rapid transcapillary passage of water, including net filtration, into the interstitial fluid implies the existence of some fluid-filled pathway(s) directly connecting the vascular lumen with the interstitial space. The initial explanations of this fluid pathway centered on the pore theory. According to this theory, the capillary endothelium has two sets of pores with relatively stable size and density.[27,28] Smaller pores with a diameter of ~6 to 7 nm at a frequency of ~15 to 20 units/μm² and an aggregate area of ~0.1 percent are assumed to be the principal barrier to transport of larger molecules.[29] Larger pores were postulated as being less frequent, 1 per 20 μm², allowing fewer larger

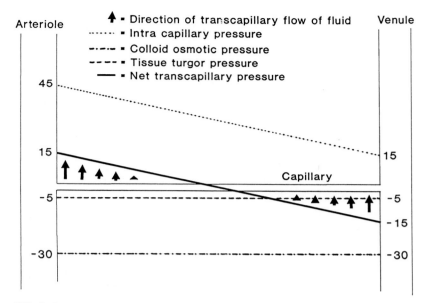

FIG. 2–2. Starling's principle of fluid distribution. The rate of filtration at any point along a capillary depends on a balance of the intracapillary hydrostatic pressure, the colloid osmotic pressure, and the tissue turgor pressure. This results in a net outflow of fluid from the capillary at the arteriolar end and a net inflow of fluid into the capillary at the venule end. However, capillary beds vary markedly in their filtration properties in different organs.

molecules to pass into the interstitial fluid. Although most recent evidence indicates that the cell membrane is permeated by pores with a radius of ~7 nm,[29] it has become evident that these structures do not fully explain the filtration of water and other molecules. Besides the physical properties of the endothelial layer, complex biochemical and electrochemical properties of the endothelium are involved in the passage of water. Thus two general routes of water movement have been identified (Fig. 2–3). The transmembranous route involves the cell membrane, cytoplasm, and opposite cell membrane and is assumed to be a passive-transport pathway. The contribution of the endothelial plasma membrane to hydraulic conductivity does not exceed 10 percent.[30,31] Accounting for 90 percent of the volume flow are the extramembranous routes for fluid movement. Transmembranous routes are transcellular (via vesicles, channels, and fenestrae) and intercellular (via endothelial junctions). These routes are not simple fluid pores but rather are complex structures that have dynamic, highly organized, complex molecular and electrochemical features.[30,32] Thus a highly complex structure determines the filtration coefficient for individual tissues and allows for the differing transcapillary flows necessary for the function of various organs. An example of this is that the filtration coefficient for the kidney is much greater than that of skeletal muscle. This facilitates glomerular filtration. Regardless of individual differences in filtration coefficients, it is the balance of hydrostatic and osmotic pressures that determines the net filtration rate across capillaries.

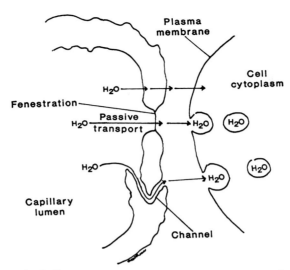

FIG. 2–3. Extra- and intramembranous routes of fluid movement. Two general routes of water transport have been described: transcellular and extracellular (through fenestrations and through intercellular channels).

Fluid movement across the capillary endothelium results from hydrostatic and osmotic pressure differences between the capillary and the interstitial fluid. The capillary hydrostatic pressure tends to force fluid outward through the capillary membrane. Again, the structure and function of the vasculature system, in particular the microcirculation (Fig. 2–4), determine capillary pressure. The contractile action of the heart is the force that creates pressure in the arterial system. Dissipation of the arterial pressure is due mainly to frictional losses during the movement of blood through progressively smaller vessels. The largest pressure drop occurs between the arterioles and capillaries.[30] The mean pressure of 85 mmHg in the aorta falls to 35 to 40 mmHg in the arterial ends of the capillaries. The increased resistance is due to constriction of the arterioles and precapillary sphincters. In the capillary system, vessel number, length, diameter, and branching characteristics are the primary factors involved in this dramatic reduction in pressure. In addition, the ratio of wall thickness to lumen size contributes to the overall reduction in pressure. Mean capillary pressure is about 25 mmHg. In several mammals, mean capillary pressures are consistently higher than plasma oncotic pressures by 4 to 6 mmHg.[33,34] Differences between the pressures in the arterial ends of capillaries and the venous ends have been observed.[28] Measurements have yielded pressures of 30 to 40 mmHg in the arterial ends of capillaries and 10 to 15 mmHg in the venous ends.[28] Possibly more important, a factor controlling the hydrostatic pressure in the capillaries of various tissues is the presence of vasomotion. Measurements of capillary pressure have shown spontaneous and relatively long periods of contraction or even closure of terminal arterioles or precapillary sphincters, producing a lower capillary hydrostatic pressure of 5 to 10 mmHg.[35] Furthermore, precapillary vessels have been ob-

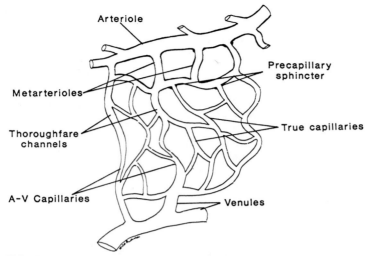

FIG. 2–4. Capillary structure and precapillary sphincters. Capillary bed flow and intracapillary pressure are regulated by precapillary sphincters.

served to spontaneously open widely, generating capillary pressures as high as 40 to 60 mmHg.[36] The basic feedback mechanism leading to vasomotion is presumed to be changes in the chemical composition of the tissue fluid accompanying either an excess or diminished flow.[35,37] Vasoactive agents of both the polypeptide and prostaglandin classes may be involved.[38] It is thus apparent that capillary hydrostatic pressure can vary remarkably over time and at different ends of the capillary. These increases or decreases in hydrostatic pressure will influence the filtration of water if other pressures influencing transcapillary flow are constant.

Plasma osmotic pressure opposes plasma hydrostatic pressure. Plasma proteins are the only dissolved substances that do not diffuse readily through the capillary membrane. There is, however, some movement throughout the endothelium, either by fenestrations or by vesicular transport. Fenestrated endothelial cells are found in the liver, kidney, and intestine, while other capillary beds, such as skeletal muscle and nervous tissue, do not have many of these cells. However, even in these capillary systems there is some movement of protein across the epithelium. Despite this movement, there is a concentration gradient of protein from plasma to interstitial fluid, since diffusion is quite small. Furthermore, the small quantities of protein that do diffuse into the interstitial fluid are removed by the lymph vessels.

The osmotic pressure of human plasma averages approximately 25 to 30 mmHg. Protein accounts for approximately 20 mmHg. As previously discussed, the Gibbs-Donnan effect accounts for the additional osmotic pressure. The extra cations in the plasma necessary to neutralize the electronegative charges of the proteins increase the number of osmotically active substances. Furthermore, as protein concentrations increase, the concentration of osmotically active ions increases progressively. Although this pressure is actually a weak osmotic force, it plays an important role in counteracting the hydrostatic pressure of the plasma. Since this force also increases when water is filtered out, there is an increase in colloid osmotic pressure in the venous ends of the capillaries, further favoring water movement into the capillaries.

Starling's equation also accounts for pressures in the interstitial compartment that influence the net fluid flow from capillaries to the interstitial space. Interstitial fluid pressure measurements have been made.[39] The level of hydrostatic pressure in the interstitial fluid is controversial, since both small positive and small negative values have been reported under normal conditions. Interstitial fluid pressures in loose subcutaneous fluid have been recorded as -1 to -3 mmHg compared with the atmosphere.[40] In internal organs, interstitial pressures are usually positive, but less than the pressure exerted by their capsule.[41] Thus interstitial fluid has little effect on fluid movement and may favor movement from the plasma to the interstitium.

Although protein does not pass through the endothelial cell pores, the endothelium is not totally impermeable to protein. Proteins are found in the interstitial fluid in a lower concentration than in plasma.[42] Movement of protein is probably through fenestrae or vesicles. The accumulation of protein in the interstitial fluid to levels that would upset the balance of pressures regulating fluid movement is prevented by the removal of protein via the lymphatics. It has been shown, depending on the organ, that 50 to 100 percent of plasma proteins escape across the capillary membrane and reenter the blood through the lymphatics each day.[42] The protein in the interstitial space exerts a colloid osmotic pressure of 8 to 10 mmHg, which promotes flow from the plasma into the interstitium.

Transcapillary exchange by filtration takes place almost continuously without any marked changes in circulating blood volume, interstitial fluid volume, or electrolyte balance. This is best explained by the balance of pressures favoring filtration (plasma hydrostatic pressure, interstitial hydrostatic pressure, and interstitial oncotic pressure) and those favoring flow into the plasma (plasma oncotic pressure). The amount of fluid filtered out from the capillaries almost equals the amount of fluid returned to the circulation by absorption through other capillaries. This is best explained by a mean capillary pressure which, in addition to the other pressures favoring filtration, is balanced by the plasma osmotic pressure. Obviously, this is an oversimplification. Significant differences in filtration are operative at different capillary levels. The greater hydrostatic pressure in the arterial ends of the capillaries (30 mmHg) tips this balance so that there is net filtration. In the venous ends, lower hydrostatic pressure (10 to 15 mmHg) increases the filtration coefficient and plasma osmotic pressure, causing reabsorption into the capillaries. Indeed, these pressures have been measured in skin and found to be $+7$ mmHg pressure at the arterial ends.[28] The normal pressure at the venous ends is a -9 mmHg.[28] Thus fluid is filtered from the arterial ends of the capillaries, where hydrostatic pressure exceeds the protein osmotic pressure, while at the venous ends hydrostatic pressure is less than osmotic pressure and fluid is reabsorbed into the circulation. This results in the reabsorption of 90 percent of the filtered volume. Therefore, the net filtration in the body is only 2 ml/min and is returned to the circulation via the lymphatic system. Finally, when vasomotion is operative, either filtration or absorption may take place across most of the capillary at any given time.

In addition to filtration, the exchange of water and small molecules between plasma and interstitial fluid occurs by diffusion. Unlike filtration, where pressure is the driving force, diffusion is regulated by a concentration gradient. This is by far the major process by which nutrients and ions and the water carrying them are exchanged across the capillary endothelium. Furthermore, diffusion occurs in both directions and does not result in net water exchange in one or the other direction, since there is no concentration difference for water. Water molecules are 20 times smaller than the 6- to 7-nm pores through which diffusion occurs. For nutrients, oxygen, waste products, and carbon dioxide there is a net diffusion to plasma or interstitial fluid. The rate of diffusion for most of these substances, although less rapid than water, is also so great that only slight concentration gradients cause more than adequate amounts to be transported to the interstitium or into the plasma. Thus extreme concentration differences do not occur, and transport of nutrients and waste products is efficient while maintaining constancy of the interstitial space.

INTERSTITIAL SPACE AND LYMPHATICS

The transport of nutrients from the plasma to the cell requires fluid movement in the interstitial space as well as lymphatic flow. However, the interstitium is not a homogeneous fluid. There is indeed both a solid, structural phase and a fluid phase, which provides water channels for transport of materials.[43,44] The solid phase contains a fixed collagen component and a "gel" of proteoglycans interspersed between this framework.[45] This gel consists of 5 to 15 percent proteoglycan fibers and water trapped within these fibers. This configuration allows fluid to flow through the gel slowly but also fixes the volume of the interstitial space under steady-state conditions. Water and nutrients are highly diffusible through this gel, however, thus facilitating their transfer without the need for large flow secondary to filtration. Movement of substrates through the interstitial fluid is dependent on hydraulic and osmotic conditions, similar to flow from plasma to the interstitium. Total flow from the interstitium involves reabsorption by the capillary and lymphatic flow. The majority of fluid flow through the interstitium involves reabsorption. The primary mechanisms are the increased plasma osmotic pressure and reduction in venous capillary pressure so that forces are inward to the plasma. Lymphatic flow accounts for only a small fraction of net fluid movement. The lymphatic flow, however, returns excess tissue fluid and proteins to the circulation, thus contributing significantly to maintenance of a constant interstitial volume. The establishment of hydraulic pressure differences between the interstitial fluid and lymph channels has not been fully explained. It requires some active process that would result in hydraulic pressure reduction in the lymph channels. One mechanism that has been suggested is that of an interstitial lymph pump. It has been noted that lymphatic channels are in close association with arterioles.[46] If contraction of the arteriole leads to expansion of the lymphatic channel, and dilation of the arteriole would compress these channels, the intermittent vasomotion could compress and expand these channels and thereby serve as a pump. Retrograde flow of lymph is prevented by valves. Furthermore, it has been shown that terminal lymphatic channels enter into larger ducts with contractile smooth muscle.[47] The progressive myogenic activity along the lymphatic channels facilitates the transfer of lymph into the circulation. Such a system could create a sump effect, facilitating flow from the interstitial space into the terminal lymphatic channels.

Having dealt with the structural and functional features of the capillary bed, interstitial fluid, and lymphatic channels, the negative feedback mechanisms that match the fluid movement and the microcirculation with the metabolic needs of the cell will be described.

CONTROL OF THE MICROCIRCULATION

Intrinsic to the homeostasis of the internal environment is the matching of the microcirculatory blood flow and thus fluid and nutrient exchange with the interstitial space and the changing metabolic needs of the cell. What becomes apparent in this regard is that the microcirculation has structural and functional characteristics that are responsive to the biochemical activities of the tissues. By a series of apparent negative-feedback systems, the control of blood flow and pressure is related not only to the delivery of oxygen and nutrients necessary for cell function but also to their utilization, since accumulation of the products of cell metabolism plays a major role in these feedback loops. Thus the microcirculatory portion of the circulation is unique because it is largely controlled by the metabolic activity of the local tissue. Indeed, tissues with greater metabolic needs have greater blood flow. Furthermore, this autoregulation maintains constancy of blood flow despite changes in systemic blood pressure. This allows the microcirculation to function as an independent entity. Its effective operation is essential in maintaining the extracellular environment within narrowly prescribed chemical and physical (fluid) ranges. In addition, the autoregulation of blood flow, the tendency for blood flow to remain constant despite changes in arterial pressure, stabilizes diffusion rates by maintaining constant flow. In this way, interstitial fluid composition of an organ can be stabilized as well.

The correlation of microcirculatory blood flow with metabolic rates in various organs suggests a chemical control. In this regard, it has been hypothesized that the concentration of metabolic substrates[48] or metabolic products[49] in the interstitial fluid controls the resistant vessels of the microcirculation. Indeed, metabolically active organs, such as the brain and myocardium, exhibit a high degree of autoregulation, and blood flow correlates closely with oxygen consumption.[50,51] Moreover, it has been proposed that tissue metabolites in these highly metabolic organs complete a negative-feedback loop that either increases or decreases blood flow for the support of metabolic processes.[52] A reduction in arterial blood flow would cause a buildup of vasodilator metabolites in the tissue, which, in turn, would reduce arteriolar resistance and increase flow. This increased flow would restore metabolic processes as well as reduce the buildup of metabolites, thus completing the negative-feedback loop. Although many substances have been proposed as the principal mediator of this process, no single agent can account for the in vivo observations. This has therefore led to the hypothesis that multiple agents are involved in the negative-feedback loop. Oxygen usually is suggested as a primary agent.[53] It appears that in the myocardium, blood flow is regulated to maintain a constant tissue PO_2.[54] These effects have been attributed to the vasodilator effects of oxygen by inhibiting contraction of arteriolar smooth muscle.[55] However, PO_2 levels at arteriolar surfaces do not correlate with changes evoked by decreased tissue oxygen.[56] Other substances that have been suggested include CO_2, hydrogen ion concentration, potassium, adenosine, lactate, prostaglandins, and vasoactive peptides.[51,52] Adenosine appears to play a major role in cardiac autoregulation.[57] The relaxation of precapillary sphincters appears to be the mechanism that restores adequate tissue blood flow. These structures are capillaries in which arteriolar smooth muscle continues along for a variable distance.[58] Their relaxation can increase the number of blood-perfused capillaries and increase flow in individual capillaries.[59] This appears to be a secondary line of defense that can compensate for flow changes and increase diffusion to the interstitial space.

In addition to the apparent metabolic control of local blood flow, the microcirculation appears to limit or prevent the changes in blood flow that might otherwise be produced by a change in arterial pressure. According to this hypothesis, the increase in intravascular pressure stretches arteriolar smooth muscle and causes constriction, thus reducing flow.[60] This action appears to be particularly pronounced in skeletal muscle and may contribute to basal vascular tone.[60] In addition, elevation in venous pressure increases resistance in some vascular beds.[61,62] The feedback mechanism of this response has been questioned,[63] since a complete feedback response is not provided for the control of blood flow. Moreover, the functional stimulus is local pressure, not flow. A model of myogenic autoregulation has been proposed in which arterioles at various levels of branching function independently in their response, and the microcirculation is not perceived as a single resistance.[64] In this model, dilation of the larger arterioles would initially increase flow and thus pressure in the smaller arterioles. Further reductions in systemic pressure would cause a decrease in pressure within the smaller arterioles, which would then dilate. A similar effect on pressure in the terminal arterioles would ensue, and pressure and flow would be maintained in the capillaries.

When blood flow is held constant by autoregulation, it is expected that capillary blood pressure will be constant as well. In several vascular beds, such as the kidney[65] and intestine,[66] capillary hydrostatic pressure appears to be nearly independent of arterial pressure. Obviously, there is much benefit to a system that maintains constant circulatory parameters in the microcirculation. A fluid system that controls its effective nutritional flow while maintaining constancy of volume is optimal. Autoregulation, therefore, appears to play a major role within the limits of change in systemic blood pressure and increasing or decreasing metabolic demand under normal circumstances.

HOMEOSTASIS OF FLUIDS UNDER NORMAL CONDITIONS

Under normal conditions, the constancy of total body water and, in particular, the extracellular fluid is maintained despite wide fluctuations in the intake of water and sodium, the principal ion of the extracellular space (Fig. 2–5). Indeed, the volume of the extracellular compartment is closely related to the amount of total body sodium. This is true for several reasons. Sodium is virtually confined

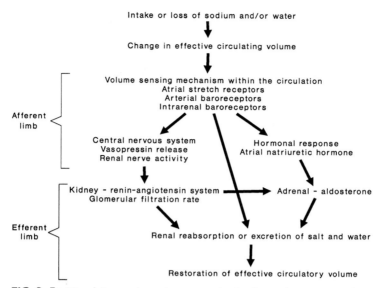

FIG. 2–5. Circulatory volume homeostasis. A schematic representation of the mechanisms involved in circulatory volume homeostasis under normal conditions.

to the extracellular space and is the primary osmotically active component of this fluid space. Thus an increase in sodium intake is accompanied by an increase in fluid volume. Furthermore, it is the excretion of sodium and water by the kidney that is the major control mechanism affecting extracellular fluid volume. The body has extensive feedback mechanisms that respond to alterations in extracellular volume and osmolality and which stimulate neural, endocrine, and circulatory systems to effect the renal response. It is apparent that under normal conditions the alterations in the extracellular fluid volume and sodium concentrations are quite small. Nevertheless, the body has remarkable control mechanisms that can regulate these changes such that total body fluid and sodium concentration of the extracellular space are kept within very narrow ranges.

AFFERENT LIMB OF NORMAL FLUID HOMEOSTASIS

The aim of extracellular fluid volume regulation is to preserve an optimal circulation. Although the circulation by itself does not have intrinsic value, it is the primary mechanism for the transport of water, ions, and nutrients from the environment to the cell. Indeed, maintenance of the circulatory volume appears to be the primary homeostatic mechanism, and when conflict between preservation of volume-related hemodynamic parameters and other homeostatic mechanisms occurs, those related to regulation of the cardiovascular system take priority. In this regard, the cardiac filling volume and the mean arterial pressure are the primary parameters that reflect optimal circulatory function. It is not surprising, therefore, that the measuring devices for extracellular volume ho-

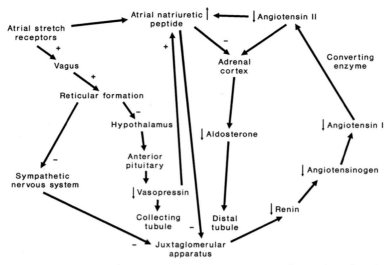

FIG. 2–6. The afferent limb of fluid homeostasis. Atrial stretch (volume) receptors play a central role in neural and hormonal control of fluid homeostasis. Atrial stretching inhibits vasopressin and renin release. Atrial natriuretic peptide also inhibits vasopressin and renin release as well as inhibiting aldosterone production (+ = stimulatory; − = inhibitory; ↑ = increased levels; ↓ = decreased levels).

meostasis are located within the circulation and respond to changes in these indices. It is the signals that emanate from these sites that cause the effector arm of this feedback process to modify salt and water excretion (Fig. 2–6 and Table 2–2).

An important concept in the understanding of the body's afferent sensing devices for the regulation of extracellular fluid volume is the concept of adequate functional volume. It is not necessarily the absolute volume of the circulating blood that evokes changes in renal excretion of sodium and water. For example, when the upright position is assumed, there is a sharp decrease in urinary sodium excretion. This occurs despite the fact that there is no absolute change in the circulating volume.[67] Conversely, when one sits immersed in water with the head and neck out,[68] there is a marked excretion of sodium despite the fact that volume is neither increased nor decreased. However, there is an increase in venous return to the heart, thoracic blood volume, cardiac output, and left atrial pressure.[69] Thus, although an absolute change in blood volume does not occur, the changes in "effective blood volume," increasing filling pressure and cardiac output, are interpreted as an increase in blood volume and affect renal excretion of sodium and water.

These observations of increased natriuresis when cardiac filling pressure is increased and the antinatriuretic effect in conditions that decrease cardiac preload and filling pressure, such as ligation of the superior vena cava,[70] standing,[67] or applying peripheral tourniquets,[71] suggest a volume-sensing receptor in the right side of the central circulation. The distensibility and compliance character-

TABLE 2–2. Afferent Limb of Volume Homeostasis: A Summary of the Affectors in Homeostasis and the Mechanisms and Consequences of Stimulation

Receptor	Stimulus	Mechanism	End-Organ Response
Atrial stretch receptor	Cardiac filling	Neural	CNS—inhibits vasopressin release Kidney—inhibits renin release
		Hormonal	CNS—inhibits vasopressin release Kidney—inhibits renin release Adrenal—inhibits aldosterone production
Arterial baroreceptors (carotid sinus)	Arterial pressure	Neural	CNS—inhibits vasopressin release Kidney—natriuresis
Renal baroreceptor	Renal perfusion pressure	Juxtaglomerular apparatus	Kidney—inhibits renin release
Hepatic volume receptor?	Hepatic congestion; portal sodium delivery	Neural	Kidney—natriuresis

istics of the atria suggested that mechanical stretching in this organ would be an ideal mechanism for detecting volume changes. Numerous investigators have demonstrated that when left atrial pressure is increased by balloon distension within the atrium, a prompt excretion of sodium occurs.[72,73] Similar responses were noted in a model of mitral stenosis that produced atrial distension in dogs.[74] In addition, increases in right-sided atrial pressure also increased renal excretion of sodium.[75]

Further evidence that changes in left atrial pressures were capable of influencing sodium excretion was the identification of neural mechanoreceptors whose electrical characteristics varied with atrial stretching.[76] Direct stimulation of these afferent fibers induced a natriuretic response.[77] Two distinct atrial neural mechanoreceptors have been identified.[78] Type A receptors discharge during atrial systole and are not responsive to volume changes, whereas type B fibers discharge during diastole and vary with atrial distension.[78] This further supports the concept of the cardiac filling pressure as a regulator of sodium excretion. These signals are believed to travel via cranial nerves X and XI to the medullary and hypothalamic centers.[79] The response to this central nerve stimulation includes alterations in pre- and postcapillary resistance,[80] inhibition of renal sympathetic discharge,[81] and suppression of vasopressin release.[82]

Despite these data in animals supporting the role of mechanoreceptors and neurologic reflexes in producing changes in the renal excretion of sodium, the importance of this mechanism in humans has been questioned. Interruption of afferent vagal nerves from the heart has produced a natriuretic response,[83] while others have not been able to detect any effect on renal sodium excretion.[84] More recently, it has been found that increases in left atrial pressure in nonhuman primates produced significantly less natriuresis than in dogs.[85] However, the changes in humans when standing,[67] after tourniquet application,[71] and when immersed in water[68] certainly suggest that such a mechanism may be operative.

ATRIAL NATRIURETIC HORMONE

Several studies have shown that the neural response to atrial distension cannot totally account for the observed changes in the renal excretion of sodium. Vagotomy does not entirely abolish renal sodium excretion secondary to atrial distension.[72] Also, vasopressin release is not totally abolished following isosmotic volume expansion.[86] Recently, a humoral signaling mechanism originating in the cardiac atria has been identified. An atrial natriuretic peptide (ANP) has been characterized and its peptide sequences determined.[87,88] Using sensitive immunoreactive assays, ANP reactivity in the plasma of rats occurred following volume expansion.[89] ANP has direct vasodilatory effects and natriuretic effects on the kidney.[90] In addition, it suppresses renin release by the kidney[91] and plasma aldosterone levels.[92] Thus ANP may provide an explanation for the effects of atrial distension that could not be explained by the neural response alone.

ARTERIAL BARORECEPTORS

In addition to the stretch receptors in these low-pressure areas of the circulation, there are other critical receptors that respond to changes in arterial pressure and play a role in the maintenance of optimal circulatory function. The purpose of these receptors is to optimize organ perfusion. Again, it appears that vessel wall stretching or changes in tension are the parameters monitored. Considerable evidence has accumulated implicating the carotid sinus as a receptor that influences renal sodium handling. Acute increases in carotid sinus pressure without renal perfusion increases cause sodium excretion.[93] Conversely, a decrease in baroreceptor activity decreases renal sodium excretion.[94] In an elaborate set of experiments it has been shown that the natriuresis that occurs after unilateral nephrectomy can be abolished by bilateral carotid sinus denervation,[95] and if perfusion pressure was maintained constant before and after nephrectomy, this excretion of sodium was similarly prevented.[96] These observations certainly suggest that the baroreceptors play a role in the renal control of body sodium excretion.

ORGAN-RELATED BARORECEPTORS

The kidney plays a primary role as the effector limb of the homeostatic mechanism to maintain volume. In addition, evidence has been presented that would implicate the kidney as part of the afferent limb. As such, the kidney also may participate in the volume-sensing mechanisms of the body. This capability of the kidney is intimately connected with the renin-secreting juxtaglomerular apparatus (Fig. 2–7). An inverse relationship between renal perfusion pressure and renin release has been reported.[97] This complex response involves several different mechanisms, including the baroreceptor of the afferent arterioles. A nonfil-

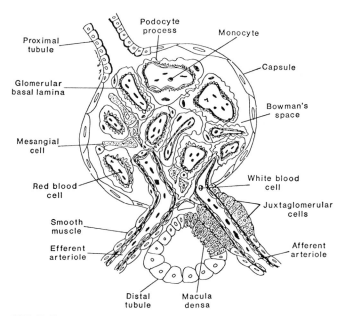

FIG. 2–7. The juxtaglomerular apparatus. A diagramatic representation of the juxtaglomerular apparatus and the macula densa.

tering kidney model in dogs in which the macula densa, another receptor that can cause renin release but should have been nonfunctional in this model, still released renin in response to hemorrhage or suprarenal aortic constriction.[98] In a similar nonfiltering preparation, renin levels were inversely correlated with renal perfusion pressure.[99] The administration of vasodilators blocked the renin response to thoracic vena caval constriction.[100] Thus it appears that baroreceptors provide the kidney with direct measurement of renal blood flow and participate in the renal control of sodium excretion.

Although not fully defined, there is evidence for an intrahepatic volume receptor that regulates sodium excretion. The liver, by virtue of the portal system, receives oral sodium loads, and from a teleologic point of view, it would make sense to have receptors that monitor sodium loads and produce rapid excretion. Investigators have reported that a greater natriuresis follows an oral load of sodium compared with intravenous administration.[101] Similar results have been reported with portal vein infusions.[102] Others have not been able to repeat these findings.[103] Intrahepatic venous congestion has been shown to elicit increased hepatic nervous afferent activity, as well as renal sympathetic efferent activity.[104] This supports the concept of receptors in the liver that respond to pressure changes, but this mechanism remains controversial.

The central nervous system also has been implicated as a volume-sensing mechanism that modifies renal sodium excretion. Changes in sodium concentration within the ventricles can increase or decrease renal sodium excretion,[105] modifying renal handling of sodium. The relationship of this to volume control comes from the observation that volume depletion reduces cerebrospinal fluid sodium concentration,[106] which should decrease sodium excretion. Furthermore, the administration of hypertonic salt into the carotid arteries causes a prompt natriuresis.[107] In addition, animals who have been decapitated have markedly blunted renal excretion after volume expansion.[108]

Besides receptors in the circulatory system, there is evidence that volume changes in the interstitial fluid also may contribute to volume control. In salt-depleted and salt-loaded dogs, expansion of the blood volume caused a natriuretic response that correlated with the state of sodium balance.[109] It was concluded that extravascular volume was the primary mechanism for renal salt excretion. Comparisons of the infusion of saline and red blood cells resulted in greater blood volume expansion in the blood cell group but greater sodium excretion in the saline group.[110] Furthermore, in hemorrhaged animals after a saline load there was persistence of the natriuretic response.[111] Thus the possibility exists that interstitial volume expansion may contribute to volume homeostasis. No evidence for receptor involvement in this respect has been presented.

EFFERENT LIMB OF SODIUM AND VOLUME HOMEOSTASIS

The afferent limb of extracellular volume regulation responds to changes in the intravascular volume. The effector mechanisms prevent increases or decreases in volume by appropriate changes in renal sodium excretion. Several mechanisms are operative in this portion of the feedback mechanism (Table 2–3). However, the primary mechanism for the control of blood volume and extracellular fluid links this control with the arterial blood pressure. This is essentially a mechanical effect of increased arterial pressure to cause increased sodium and volume loss by the kidney. Several investigators have correlated urinary sodium and volume output with arterial pressure.[112–114] An increase in blood pressure

TABLE 2–3. Efferent Limb and Its Effects: A Summary of the Effectors in Homeostasis and the Mechanisms and Consequences of Stimulation

Effector	Stimulus	Effect
Renin	Macula densa receptor Renal baroreceptor Sympathetic nerves	Converts angiotensinogen to angiotensin I in blood and kidney
Angiotensin II	Conversion of angiotensin I by converting enzyme in the lung	Causes intense systemic and renal arteriolar vasoconstriction; acts directly on kidney to retain salt and water; causes adrenal glands to secrete aldosterone; suppresses vasopressin release
Aldosterone	Angiotensin II Potassium ACTH	Stimulates sodium reabsorption by renal collecting tubules
Vasopressin	Osmolality	Increases reabsorption of water in renal tubules
Renal nerves	Atrial filling pressure and arterial pressure	Increases renin release; regulates renal blood flow and GFR; causes antinatriuretic effect

to 200 mmHg causes an eightfold increase in sodium and water loss. Conversely, reduction in arterial blood pressure to 50 mmHg essentially stops urine output.[114] This is a phenomenon that is observable to the clinician when resuscitating the hypotensive patient. The prompt increase in urinary output parallels the restoration of arterial blood pressure. The exact mechanisms responsible for the effects of arterial pressure on sodium and water excretion are still not completely understood. For many years it was thought that increased glomerular filtration accounted for this relationship of arterial pressure and sodium excretion. More recently, it has been necessary to postulate additional mechanisms to explain this phenomenon. Physical forces in the glomerular and peritubular capillaries as well as hormonal changes have been implicated.[114,115]

GLOMERULAR FILTRATION RATE

The factors affecting glomerular filtration rate (GFR) may be expressed as

$$GFR = LpA(P_{GC} - P_T - \pi_{GC})$$

where Lp is the glomerular capillary hydraulic conductivity, A is the glomerular capillary surface area, P_{GC} is the hydrostatic pressure within the glomerular capillary, P_T is the hydrostatic pressure opposing filtration in Bowman's capsule, and π is the mean colloid osmotic pressure.[116] Thus the major factors affecting GFR are changes in capillary permeability or surface area, changes in capillary hydrostatic pressure, and changes in plasma protein, the major determinant of osmotic pressure. Furthermore, the rate of filtration may determine the rate of rise in osmotic pressure, thus affecting the mean osmotic pressure.[116] Since increased extracellular volume results in increased cardiac output and therefore increased blood pressure, GFR could be increased by the increase in glomerular capillary pressure. In addition, an increase in blood flow without a change in perfusion pressure also will increase GFR, since osmotic pressure does not increase as much when blood flow is increased. Under normal conditions, both renal blood flow and GFR remain very constant. This has led investigators to question whether GFR plays a major role in normal regulation of extracellular volume in which changes are quite small following oral sodium or fluid intake. In this regard, de Wardener et al.[117] found that acute expansion of the extracellular volume was accompanied by a brisk natriuresis when GFR was reduced by inflation of a balloon catheter in the aorta just proximal to the renal arteries. Thus it appears that the renal excretion of sodium following volume expansion is in part independent of changes in GFR. However, increasing GFR by other means than volume expansion does not increase sodium excretion to the same extent.[118] The mechanism of glomerulotubular balance also argues against the GFR as a major determinant of sodium excretion. This phenomenon dictates that as GFR rises or falls, absolute tubular reabsorption changes in a similar direction.[119] However, since the filtered load of sodium is large, even a moderate increase in GFR and a corresponding increase in tubular reabsorption could still result in increased sodium excretion. At present, however, GFR cannot be implicated as the major efferent response for sodium excretion following volume expansion.

PHYSICAL FACTORS

Under conditions of a constant extracellular volume, a tight regulation exists between the GFR and tubular sodium reabsorption. This relationship exists because changes in glomerular filtration rate exert parallel changes in the peritubular capillaries that either increase or decrease sodium reabsorption. The physical factors that influence this process have been reviewed in detail[113] and are briefly stated here. Essentially, hydrostatic and osmotic pressures in the tubular fluid and the peritubular capillary determine exchange and reabsorption of fluid from the surrounding interstitial space. Thus a low peritubular oncotic pressure and/or increased hydrostatic pressure would be associated with a decreased rate of reabsorption of sodium and fluid. On the other hand, an increased tubular reabsorption would occur with an increase in peritubular osmotic pressure and a decrease in peritubular hydrostatic pressure. As stated above, the parallel changes in these physical factors and GFR prevent dramatic changes in sodium excretion. However, there is evidence that under conditions of volume expansion there is a significant increase in urinary sodium loss due to changes in the proximal and distal tubules.[113]

RENAL NERVES

Many investigators have shown that denervation of the kidney is associated with an increased excretion of sodium.[120,121] The stimulation of renal nerves decreased sodium excretion independently of changes in renal blood flow and GFR.[122] Furthermore, bilateral carotid ligation, which increases renal nerve activity, with constant renal perfusion also caused an antinatriuresis.[123] Direct effects of renal nerve activity on tubule water and sodium reabsorption have been demonstrated.[123] Thus there appears to be considerable evidence to indicate that renal nervous innervation plays a role in the maintenance of body sodium and volume regulation. However, the maintenance of normal volume in patients with denervated transplanted kidneys points out that several effector mechanisms can control sodium excretion. The precise role of renal nerves in this scheme will require further investigation.

RENIN-ANGIOTENSIN SYSTEM

Activation of the renin-angiotensin system is associated usually with decreased effective blood volume or arterial pressure. Therefore, investigation of the physiologic role of the renin-angiotensin system has focused primarily on its contribution to blood pressure homeostasis rather than on its involvement in regulating extracellular fluid homeostasis. However, it is apparent that maneuvers that lead to increased renin release generally involve a change in extracellular volume.[124] Several observations suggest that renin release plays a role in the regulation of total body sodium and effective blood volume. A close association between sodium intake, sodium excretion, and the renin-angiotensin system has been observed.[124] Furthermore, standing, which decreases atrial filling, results in a rapid release of renin. Conversely, water immersion, which increases atrial filling, suppresses renin release.[125] Further evidence for the regulation of renin release by sodium comes from the infusion of sodium directly into the kidney. The intrarenal infusion of sodium promptly decreases renin release.[124] However, in the day-to-day regulation of sodium, it is doubtful that direct effects of sodium concentration play a significant role in renin release.

The responses of renin to changes in atrial filling pressure are probably mediated by renal nerves. Direct stimulation of renal nerves increases renin release.[124] Although the stimulation of these nerves produces significant acute changes in volume, it is uncertain what role the kidney nervous innervation plays in the day-to-day maintenance of extracellular fluid volume and sodium excretion. It has been proposed that renal nerves may be essential for the control of renin release by the macula densa. Low levels of renal nerve stimulation potentiate the renin response to suprarenal aortic constriction in normal kidneys but have no effect in nonfunctioning kidneys.

Besides the control of renin release by the renal nerves, control by the macula densa may play a role in the homeostasis of the extracellular volume. These specialized cells of the proximal portion of the distal tubule are in close physical proximity to the renin-producing cells of the juxtaglomerular apparatus. The signal that stimulates macula densa activity has not been identified. It appears to be related to chloride transport.[126] Thus renin secretion appears to be elevated under circumstances in which there is reduced sodium chloride delivery from the loop of Henle. Conversely, increased transport of sodium chloride by the cells of the macula densa is associated with decreased renin release.[126] This relationship provides an explanation for the control of extracellular fluid and sodium excretion, but definitive evidence has not been presented.

In addition to the evidence suggesting that the sympathetic nervous system and the macula densa contribute to the homeostasis of extracellular volume regulation, the role of the intrarenal baroreceptor also may be important in this respect. Evidence was presented earlier in this chapter for the role of this receptor in the afferent limb of this process. Recently, studies have suggested that there is a correlation between arterial blood pressure and renin release. Indeed, there is a linear relationship between these two events below a blood pressure of 80 mmHg.[127] However, renin release was relatively unresponsive to the initial 10- to 20-mmHg reduction in pressure, and thus one must question the role of baroreceptors and renin in day-to-day volume regulation.

Although the importance of renin release by the sympathetic nervous system, intrarenal baroreceptors, and the macula densa is well established for the mediation of short-term renin responses, the role of this system in volume homeostasis is not established. Obviously, the involvement of this system must include the effects of aldosterone and angiotensin II.

ALDOSTERONE

Aldosterone, the principal sodium-retaining steroid hormone in humans, is regulated primarily by angiotensin II, potassium, and adrenocorticotropic hormone (ACTH).[128] Aldosterone is a potent stimulator of sodium reabsorption by the renal collecting tubules. Since sodium is the principal osmotically active substance, it is accompanied by water reabsorption. To maintain electrical neutrality, potassium or hydrogen ion is secreted into the tubules or chloride accompanies the sodium. Again, much of the evidence for aldosterone as a contributor to homeostatic control of extracellular volume comes from several observations.

An inverse correlation between sodium intake, and thus extracellular volume, and the secretion of aldosterone has provided the impetus for investigation of its role in volume homeostasis.[129] Observations in deficiency states, as well as excess states, have provided further information. The prolonged administration of aldosterone results in a significant reduction in sodium excretion and an increase in total body sodium and extracellular fluid.[130] However, after a period of time, the effect of aldosterone on the collecting tubules will be blunted, and excretion of sodium will match intake.[131] Accompanying this retention of sodium is an increase in extracellular volume and mean arterial pressure.[131] Thus renal excretion of sodium is restored via increases in pressure. This blunting phenomenon has been prevented experimentally by keeping the renal perfusion pressure at a normal level.[131] Of interest is the apparent inability of natriuretic substances, which would be expected to be released by volume expansion, to overcome the effects of aldosterone. The mechanism of pressure natriuresis thus assumes a primary role in reestablishing volume homeostasis. An aldosterone deficiency, on the other hand, is associated with increased urinary sodium loss of subsequent hyponatremia and hypovolemia.[132] These observations certainly suggest a major role of aldosterone in sodium natriuresis when extremes of aldosterone levels are present. Dogs with fixed levels of aldosterone and after adrenalectomy had greater extracellular volumes and weight gain compared with normal animals with similar low-salt intakes.[133] Since the inability to modulate mineralocorticoid levels resulted in sodium and water retention, it could be suggested that aldosterone also may play a role in normal volume homeostasis.

ANGIOTENSIN II

The regulation of sodium homeostasis by angiotensin II could occur at several different sites. Angiotensin II is a potent stimulator of aldosterone release. In addition, it is a potent vasoconstrictor in both the systemic and renal vasculatures. In the systemic circulation, it causes a marked increase in systemic resistance. In the kidney, its site of action appears to be the efferent arteriole, where vasoconstriction can modify peritubular physical factors that affect tubular reabsorption.[134] In addition, angiotensin II may directly stimulate proximal tubule sodium reabsorption.[135]

The role of aldosterone in regulating fluid homeostasis was discussed earlier. Although it has been assumed that the primary control of sodium and volume homeostasis by angiotensin II is by release of aldosterone, there is evidence that suggests that angiotensin II exerts an influence on salt and volume regulation at other sites. Adrenalectomized animals with a fixed mineralocorticoid replacement have a marked natriuresis after angiotensin II blockade.[136] Young[137] has concluded that aldosterone does not seem to be as important as angiotensin II and its other actions, particularly its direct effect on the kidney.

The two intrarenal effects of angiotensin II that occur at very low concentrations are constriction of renal efferent arterioles and increased sodium transport by the renal tubule. These effects occur at concentrations that are lower than those necessary to stimulate the release of aldosterone. In most conditions in which the renin-angiotensin system is activated, angiotensin helps stabilize the

GFR by increasing systemic pressure and constricting efferent arterioles.[138] Thus angiotensin II appears to prevent large fluctuations in GFR. In addition, the effect of angiotensin II on efferent arterioles appears to increase sodium and water reabsorption by the renal tubules.[139] Constriction of the efferent arteriole reduces peritubular capillary pressure, and the increase in GFR increases capillary osmotic pressure. Both these pressure changes favor the reabsorption of sodium and water.

In addition to these physical effects of angiotensin II on renal reabsorption, there is evidence that angiotensin II has a direct effect on sodium and water reabsorption as well. Angiotensin II can be formed locally in the kidney[140] and thus could be a local control for sodium reabsorption. In addition, marked increases in proximal tubular reabsorption of sodium occur with low levels of angiotensin II infusion.[141] However, in these studies, although the GFR did not change, there were increases in renal blood flow that could cause proximal tubular sodium reabsorption. In vitro microperfused proximal tubules exposed to low concentrations of angiotensin II also show increased sodium reabsorption.[142]

Thus it is evident that angiotensin II mediates the sodium- and water-retaining actions of the renin-angiotensin II system by both intrarenal and extrarenal mechanisms. The intrarenal effects include a direct effect on the renal tubules, as well as a potent constrictor action on efferent arterioles. This efferent arteriolar constriction increases tubular reabsorption by changing peritubular capillary hydrostatic and osmotic pressures, favoring reabsorption. The systemic vasoconstriction increases system pressure, preserving renal blood flow and GFR. Also, under certain conditions, the release of aldosterone further increases sodium retention.

VASOPRESSIN

Regulation of a constant extracellular volume also requires the antidiuretic hormone arginine vasopressin, which fine-tunes sodium concentrations by regulating free-water excretion. The release of vasopressin is osmotically regulated and prevents wide fluctuations in sodium concentrations. Thus, under normal conditions, this system maintains body fluid osmolality within a relatively narrow range and preserves efficient cell function.

Vasopressin is synthesized in the hypothalamus and is transported through axons for storage in the posterior pituitary.[143] The release of vasopressin from nerve terminals follows depolarization of the neurons. The initial studies that recognized plasma osmolality as an important factor in the regulation of vasopressin were done by Verney.[144] He demonstrated that the intracarotid infusion of hypertonic sodium chloride produced a decrease in urine output and hypothesized that an osmoreceptor was responsible for the regulation of vasopressin release from the posterior pituitary. Simultaneous measurements of plasma vasopressin and osmolality have identified the set point of this receptor. Vasopressin levels are very low or not detectable when plasma osmolality falls below approximately 280 mosmol/kg.[145] In the absence of vasopressin, hypotonic changes are rapidly corrected by free-water excretion. Increases in osmolality above the set point release vasopressin in a direct relationship to increases in osmolality.[146] The release of vasopressin is dependent on the rate of rise in osmolality as well as the absolute increase.[147] Thus the secretion of vasopressin is enhanced when rapid changes in osmolality occur. The type of solute also influences the osmoreceptor responsiveness. In humans, sodium accounts for 95 percent of the osmolality of plasma and extracellular fluid. In comparison with sodium, glucose and urea[148] have significantly fewer stimulatory effects.

The release of vasopressin is also responsive to lowering of the blood pressure. Unlike the linear relationship of vasopressin release to increases in osmolality, the release of vasopressin in response to hypotension is exponential.[149] Although vasopressin has been detected after a 5 percent decline in mean arterial blood pressure, an increase in vasopressin release is not consistent until the mean arterial pressure declines greater than 15 percent from normal.[149] Thus phlebotomy sufficient to decrease mean arterial pressure by 7 to 9 percent does not increase detectable vasopressin,[150] yet the upright posture, which reduces blood pressure by 10 to 15 percent, produces a small but significant increase in plasma vasopressin.[151] At these small levels, or even at levels that are not detectable, some degree of antidiuresis occurs, and maximal antidiuresis occurs at levels as low as 5 pg/ml.[150] This is in contrast to the pressor effects of vasopressin, which are not evident in animals until plasma levels exceed 30 pg/ml.[152] This results in a system that is highly effective in the control of water balance, since it tightly controls low circulating levels with a minimal stimulus and does not require large amounts for a maximal antidiuretic effect. Thus the regulation of extracellular osmolality is tightly regulated and prevents wide swings in osmotic pressure that could affect cell volume and thus function.

Thirst is defined as the craving for water. It should not be confused with the anticipatory and habitual drinking that characterizes normal humans. The stimulus for thirst is also an osmoreceptor that is in close proximity, but separate from, the receptor for vasopressin release. Similar to the osmoreceptor for vasopressin, the receptor for thirst also has a set point above which thirst is perceived. However, this set point is higher than that for vasopressin release. Thirst is not perceived usually until an osmolality of 290 mosmol/kg is exceeded.[148] Therefore, thirst is not a control mechanism until maximal efforts to reduce osmolality by renal conservation of water have failed. Moreover, thirst can result from hypotension but, similar to vasopressin release, requires a significant reduction in mean arterial blood pressure.[153]

The importance of vasopressin for controlling extracellular fluid osmolality and extracellular fluid sodium concentration is thus obvious. An increase in sodium concentration causes a parallel increase in osmolality, which, in turn, stimulates the osmoreceptors of the hypothalamus. This causes the release of vasopressin, which markedly increases the reabsorption of water in the renal tubules. Consequently, little water is lost in the urine, and water increases in extracellular fluid, restoring sodium concentration and osmolality toward normal. This is a potent mechanism for controlling both extracellular osmolality and sodium concentration.

HOMEOSTATIC RESPONSE TO HEMORRHAGE

During the day-to-day regulation of water and sodium, the homeostatic mechanisms are primarily responding to water and salt intake. Following hemorrhage, there is a decrease in effective blood volume, and cardiovascular changes occur that are much larger than those seen even if one was to limit oral water and sodium intake. Furthermore, the priority of the body appears to be the preservation of the integrity of the circulation, sometimes at the expense of the local tissue or organ. This section will review the systems activated by hemorrhage.

HOMEOSTASIS DURING HYPOTENSION

Under normal conditions, there is a delicate balance and interaction between the various mechanisms controlling total body fluid balance. In the wisdom of the body this results in constancy of the various regulatory components, as well as their integration. Thus, under normal conditions, the circulatory system responds to the metabolic needs of individual tissues while maintaining cardiac parameters necessary for optimal function. For example, the arterioles contribute to the maintenance of systemic blood pressure by adjusting peripheral resistance through the intervention of neurogenically mediated reflex stimuli. In addition, these vessels adjust the volume of blood flow in tissues through local environmental factors. In turn, cardiac output is controlled by blood flow in local tissues via venous return to the heart and cardiac filling pressure. Under normal conditions, the functions of arterioles, i.e., maintenance of systemic blood pressure and control of local nutrient and oxygen delivery, are met without conflict. Thus any perturbations, either in systemic blood pressure or local tissue perfusion, are usually transient. However, in situations where systemic blood pressure and/or blood volume are lowered substantially, as in hemorrhagic shock, the dual functions of the arteriolar vessels conflict. When intrinsic homeostatic mechanisms are forced to make a choice in the various regulatory mechanisms of body fluids under these circumstances, the preservation of circulatory volume is the first priority. Regulation of circulatory volume becomes the primary homeostatic response. Thus, in our example, constriction of arterioles in response to sympathetic nervous stimulation increases peripheral resistance in an attempt to restore arterial blood pressure. The autoregulation of tissue blood flow by the processes of metabolism is not operative. Unfortunately, this response, if prolonged, can compromise tissue perfusion and result in cellular injury and organ dysfunction. Many other homeostatic mechanisms for volume and sodium regulation are also operative in this primary homeostatic response during hypotension. Again, if the body has to make a choice between volume preservation and other homeostatic mechanisms such as solute content or fluid composition, volume regulatory systems prevail. Indeed, under these circumstances, significant nervous, endocrine, and circulatory homeostatic mechanisms are activated to preserve circulatory volume and function.

SYMPATHETIC NERVOUS SYSTEM

The sympathetic nervous system provides the body with a mechanism for the very rapid control of arterial blood pressure. Sympathetic adrenergic nerves supply smooth muscle cells of arteries and arterioles in all organs. The principal action is to stimulate contraction of vascular smooth muscle and to produce vasoconstriction. The transmitter released is norepinephrine, and contraction is mediated by the alpha receptors on the smooth muscle cells.[154] There is a resting sympathetic stimulation that causes smooth muscle contraction and the normal vasomotor tone.[155,156] However, sympathetic activity varies among the different organs. Although sympathetic adrenergic activity has been demonstrated in lung,[157] heart,[158] and adipose tissue,[159] it does not participate significantly in reflex control of blood pressure. In the brain, stimulation of cervical sympathetics leads to weak vasoconstriction.[160] Indeed, participation of the adrenergic system in the control of cerebral circulation is slight or absent.[161] However, in muscle,[162] skin,[162] and visceral organs,[163] sympathetic discharge is a powerful and important mechanism for the control of the circulation.

In addition to the innervation of arterioles, there is sympathetic innervation of the venules and veins by fibers following different routes from those to the arterial tree.[164] Furthermore, sympathetic nerves abundantly supply other areas of the heart beside the blood vessels.[165] Adrenergic stimulation of the heart can markedly increase the heart rate, increase the force with which the heart muscle contracts, and thus increase cardiac output and ejection pressure.[165] The relationship of the sympathetic nervous system to the adrenal medulla is also an important component of the sympathetic vasoconstrictor system. Sympathetic stimulation of the adrenal medulla occurs at the same time peripheral transmission to blood vessels occurs. This causes the adrenal medulla to secrete both epinephrine and norepinephrine into the circulating blood. Thus further stimulus for vasoconstriction is produced.

The control of the sympathetic vasoconstrictor system is the vasomotor center in the reticular substance of the medulla and lower pons.[166] Specific anatomic areas within this center can stimulate or inhibit vasoconstrictor neurons of the sympathetic nervous system. In addition, there is a sensory area that receives nerve signals mainly from cranial nerves X and XI. Further control of this center occurs centrally. The hypothalamus can exert powerful excretory or inhibitory effects on the motor center.[166] Many additional parts of the cerebral cortex can affect the vasomotor center as well.[166]

Following hemorrhage, there is a decrease in venous return and a reduction in the filling pressure of the heart, resulting in a decrease in cardiac output and a reduction in arterial blood pressure. Rapid hemorrhage over ½ h is tolerated up to a 10 percent loss of blood volume, but greater losses reduce cardiac output and arterial pressure. As previously discussed, baroreceptors located in the atrial and arterial system are sensitive to changes in filling pressure and arterial pressure changes.[167] Stimulation of the baroreceptors under normal conditions inhibits sympathetic activity by down-regulating the vasomotor center. With reduction in baroreceptor stimulation secondary to decreases in filling pressure and arterial blood pressure, the normal inhibitory effect by the baroreceptors is removed, and sympathetic activity is, in turn, increased. Indeed, the increased sympathetic activity in hemorrhagic shock, as manifested by elevated levels of plasma catecholamines, correlates best with the volume of blood loss.[168] Furthermore, in the absence of sympathetic activity, the tolerance to hemorrhage is impaired. Under normal conditions, 30 to 40 percent of the blood volume can be lost over ½ h before a person will die, while in the absence of sympathetic activity, only 10 to 15 percent of the blood volume can be lost.[169]

This intense sympathetic activity results in several effects that are designed to preserve functional circulating volume and restore normal hemodynamics. The increase in sympathetic activity causes a marked vasoconstriction, especially in the small arteries and arterioles. This results in a graded increase in vascular resistance which correlates with the level of sympathetic nerve activity.[170] Indeed, this vasoconstriction causes total occlusion of some of these vessels with cessation of flow in the capillaries supplied by these arterioles.[170] Furthermore, this intense vasoconstriction not only reduces flow but also lowers capillary pressure. Reduction in capillary pressure promotes the movement of fluid from the interstitium into the capillaries.[171,172] While capillary pressure is reduced in those vascular beds heavily innervated by sympathetic nerves, the increase in systemic arterial pressure preserves blood flow to organs that are not heavily innervated by sympathetic nerves and whose blood flow is not regulated by adrenergic stimulation. Thus, when arterial pressure is restored by sympathetic discharge, flow is better maintained in vital organs, such as the brain[173] and myocardium,[54] than in skin,[174] skeletal muscle,[175] liver,[62] gastrointestinal tract,[176] and kidney.[177] The redistribution of flow and restriction of flow to various organs reduce the vascular volume while preserving the functional blood volume for distribution to vital organs. Furthermore, the constriction of venular smooth muscle also reduces the capacitance of the vascular system.[178,179] Reduction in the venous capacitance is particularly effective, since under normal conditions approximately 60 percent of the blood volume is in the veins. Indeed, 30 to 40 percent of the blood volume can be displaced from the veins to the heart with a sustained maximal stimulation of the venous sympathetic nerves.[63] Thus not only is the capacitance of the vascular system reduced, but also increased venous return increases cardiac filling in an attempt to restore cardiac output. Although the increase in sympathetic tone can temporize the cardiovascular effects of hemorrhage and actually maintain cardiac output and arterial pressure when the blood volume lost is small, prolonged vasoconstriction is detrimental because ischemic conditions exist in capillary beds distal to arterioles that are constricted. In this regard, when the blood pressure is less than 50 mmHg, ischemic changes in the central nervous system trigger an intense sympathetic response that even further increases vasoconstriction and may cause a transient increase in blood pressure.[180,181] This appears to be the body's final attempt to increase arterial blood pressure and blood flow to the brain.

The increase in sympathetic activity following hemorrhage also has direct effects on the heart. Following moderate hemorrhage, cardiac output is maintained by the increase in heart rate and inotropic effect of the catecholamines.[182] Although the release of norepinephrine by nerves innervating the myocardium contributes significantly to these effects, the release of epinephrine from the adrenal medulla also has effects on the peripheral circulation and the cardiac response.

Plasma epinephrine concentrations are markedly elevated following hemorrhage. A 20-fold increase in plasma epinephrine concentrations following hemorrhage corresponds to a mean arterial blood pressure of 40 mmHg in dogs.[183] The blood levels of epinephrine also can be correlated with the severity of hemorrhage and the arterial pressure.[184] These elevations in catecholamine levels can be prevented by adrenalectomy, indicating that the adrenal medulla is the source of the increased plasma catecholamines.[184] Indeed, the rate of catecholamine secretion by the adrenal medulla is a function of the rate of hemorrhage.[185] In addition to the release of epinephrine from the adrenal medulla, the sympathetic nervous system is also a potent stimulator of the renin-angiotensin system. The role of this system in hypovolemia will be discussed in the next section.

RENIN-ANGIOTENSIN SYSTEM FOLLOWING HEMORRHAGE

Renin is a proteolytic enzyme released by the juxtaglomerular cells in the kidney. Renin cleaves angiotensin, a glycoprotein produced in the liver, to angiotensin I. Angiotensin I is acted on by angiotensin-converting enzyme, producing angiotensin II (Fig. 2–8). As previously discussed, angiotensin II plays a role in normal sodium reabsorption. In addition, however, angiotensin II is a potent vasoconstrictor that appears to play a role in the body's response to hemorrhage. As previously stated, the three factors believed to be the most important in the physiologic control of renin release include (1) a macula densa receptor, (2) an intrarenal baroreceptor, and (3) the sympathetic nervous system. As was discussed earlier, following hemorrhage there is an intense activation of the sympathetic nervous system, and one would expect the release of renin in hypotensive states. Indeed, increased plasma renin levels have been reported following hemorrhage.[186,187] Furthermore, the importance of the sympathetic nervous system in mediating renin secretion in response to hemorrhage is well established.[124] In this regard, renal denervation reduced renin secretion by 80 percent following hypotension.[98] The observation that a rapid hemorrhage produces a

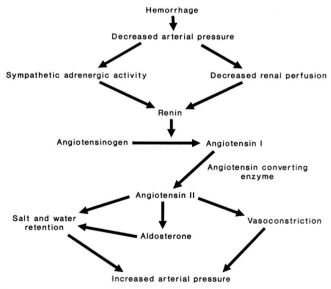

FIG. 2–8. The effect of hemorrhage on the renin-angiotensin system. Hemorrhage results in hypovolemic hypotension, which sets off the renin-angiotensin defense mechanism.

greater renin response[186] also suggests a role for the renal nerves, since sympathetic activity also correlates with the rate of hemorrhage and is rapidly activated. Furthermore, hemorrhage that did not lower arterial blood pressure also was effective in raising plasma renin levels.[188] In fact, denervation of the kidney in moderate hemorrhage abolished the renin response.[189]

Although renin release by sympathetic adrenergic activity via renal nerves plays a major role following hemorrhage, there is evidence that the other two primary stimulants of renin secretion are also operative following hemorrhage. After hemorrhage, renin secretion by normal kidneys was greater than that produced by ureteral-ligated kidneys.[98] The difference is presumably due to the loss of stimulation of the juxtaglomerular cells by the macula densa receptor. Infusing hypertonic saline into the renal artery also blunts renin release following hemorrhage,[190] further supporting the involvement of the macula densa receptor. In moderate hemorrhage, renal perfusion pressure is maintained, and release of renin by baroreceptor stimulation should be minimal. However, in more severe hemorrhage, one would expect renin release by this mechanism. Indeed, the infusion of papaverine to dilate the renal artery in a denervated nonfiltering renal model ablated renin release, indicating involvement of the baroreceptor.[191]

In the normal homeostatic mechanisms of volume and sodium regulation, angiotensin II can alter the basic pressure-induced sodium secretion by the kidney and promote sodium reabsorption by the renal tubules. Angiotensin II is also a potent stimulus of aldosterone secretion (Table 2–4). Its role in the regulation of sodium excretion is thus well established. However, angiotensin II is also one of the most powerful natural vasoconstrictors, particularly of the splanchnic and renal circulation. In addition, angiotensin II has been shown to stimulate the release of catecholamines from the adrenal medulla and peripheral

TABLE 2–4. Effects of Angiotensin II, Aldosterone, and Vasopressin: A Summary of the Effects and Mechanisms of Action

Hormone	Effect	Mechanism
Angiotensin II	Increased arterial pressure	Vasoconstriction; catecholamine release from adrenal medulla and sympathetic nerves; potentiation of sympathetic neurotransmission
	Redistribution of blood flow	Vasoconstriction—splanchnic and renal vasculature most sensitive
	Increased cardiac output	Inotropic and chronotropic effect on myocardium
	Restoration of extracellular fluid volume	Renal tubular reabsorption of sodium and water; aldosterone release
Aldosterone	Restoration of extracellular fluid volume	Tubular reabsorption of sodium and water
Vasopressin	Increased arterial pressure	Vasoconstriction; tubular reabsorption of water
	Restoration of extracellular fluid volume	

sympathetic nerve endings.[192] Furthermore, angiotensin II has a direct inhibitory effect on renin release by juxtaglomerular cells and by constriction of the efferent arterioles, thereby raising pressure in the capillaries. This provides an intrarenal feedback loop for the reduction of renin release. Thus the production of angiotensin II following hemorrhage has actions that can potentially restore blood pressure.

Angiotensin II levels are elevated following hemorrhage.[193,194] During slow hemorrhage, increases in angiotensin levels can be detected before hypotension occurs.[193] This suggests that angiotensin participates in the early homeostatic mechanisms to preserve arterial blood pressure. The vasoconstrictive action of angiotensin II is the most likely candidate to explain this effect. In dogs with denervation of the baroreceptor, thus blunting catecholamine release, there was significant vasoconstriction secondary to angiotensin increase.[194] Not only does angiotensin II have a direct vasoconstricting effect, but also angiotensin II may increase vasoconstriction by releasing catecholamines. Epinephrine release from the adrenal medulla is stimulated by angiotensin II following hemorrhage.[195] Furthermore, angiotensin appears to potentiate sympathetic neurotransmission, thus enhancing sympathetic vasoconstriction.[192] Angiotensin II also may participate in the redistribution of blood flow that occurs in severe hemorrhage. Although all vascular beds appear to be responsive to the vasoconstrictor effect, the intestinal and renal vasculatures are particularly sensitive.[196] Thus angiotensin II appears to be involved in the immediate response to hemorrhage by preserving systemic blood pressure and in the response to life-threatening hemorrhage by maximally stimulating vasoconstriction. This occurs both by its direct effects and by the release and potentiation of catecholamines. Indeed, following an acute decrease in arterial pressure after hemorrhage to 50 mmHg,[197] recovery to 80 mmHg within 30 min occurred in intact animals, but recovery to only 60 mmHg was observed when the angiotensin-renin system was blocked.[197]

Other actions of angiotensin II may be involved in the immediate response of the body to acute life-threatening hemorrhage. Angiotensin II has direct inotropic and chronotropic effects on the myocardium.[198] It also increases secretion of hormones that are known to be acutely elevated following hemorrhage. Angiotensin II increases vasopressin secretion[198] and ACTH secretion.[199] Furthermore, it potentiates ACTH-stimulated corticosteroid secretion by the adrenal cortex.[200]

In addition to the acute response to maintain arterial blood pressure in severe hemorrhage, a more potent effect of angiotensin II to restore the extracellular volume is its action on water and sodium excretion by the kidney. Angiotensin II causes increased conservation of water and salt by the kidney directly by its action on tubular reabsorption of sodium and indirectly by the release of aldosterone. This long-term effect of angiotensin II is therefore more effective in re-establishing effective arterial blood pressure because it restores the extracellular blood volume. Thus the renin-angiotensin II system plays a major role in the negative feedback control mechanisms of the circulation that return cardiac output and arterial pressure to normal by restoration of blood volume.

The marked vasoconstriction caused by angiotensin II has been implicated in the local tissue ischemic changes seen after severe hemorrhage.[196] Furthermore, studies have shown that the infusion of angiotensin-converting enzyme inhibitors prolonged survival and blunted the severe vasoconstriction of the splanchnic circulation.[201] Additionally, following severe hemorrhage and resuscitation, the infusion of these drugs maintained postinfusion blood pressure longer.[201,202]

A major role of the renin-angiotensin system has been identified in the regulation of extracellular volume. Both the day-to-day homeostatic regulation of sodium excretion and the homeostatic response to moderate hemorrhage have the renin-angiotensin system as an integral part. Furthermore, the body's attempt to preserve cardiovascular function with life-threatening hemorrhage evokes the potent vasoconstrictor response, which, if prolonged, has detrimental effects on cell and organ function.

ALDOSTERONE FOLLOWING HEMORRHAGE

Aldosterone is the principal mineralocorticoid in the body. It is synthesized and secreted by the adrenal zona glomerulosa. The most important function of aldosterone is to promote transport of sodium and water in the renal tubules, resulting in net absorption. Aldosterone can decrease the sodium loss in the urine to a few milligrams a day. The release of aldosterone is related to the homeostatic regulation of extracellular volume and sodium concentration and circulatory function. Simple restriction of water and salt will, over a few hours, stimulate the production of aldosterone. The most potent factors in the regulation of aldosterone secretion are potassium ion concentration and the renin-angiotensin system. In addition, sodium concentration and ACTH play important roles in aldosterone secretion. In response to hemorrhage, the renin-angiotensin system and ACTH are both activated and increase aldosterone secretion. The renin-angiotensin system appears to be the principal stimulus.

Aldosterone secretion is increased following hemorrhage. Increases up to three to four times normal have been found following hemorrhage in dogs.[203] Similar increases in aldosterone were produced in humans with graded hemorrhage.[204] These increases correlated with renin secretion.[204] Furthermore, rapid hemorrhage was a greater stimulus for aldosterone production than slow hemorrhage.[204]

The primary mechanisms for the release of aldosterone after hemorrhage are angiotensin II and ACTH. Nephrectomy reduced aldosterone secretion by greater than 50 percent after hemorrhage in dogs.[205] Adding hypophysectomy to nephrectomy eliminated the secretion of aldosterone.[205] A similar reduction in plasma aldosterone following endotoxin shock was prevented by angiotensin II infusion.[206] In this study, infusion rates were adjusted to maintain plasma angiotensin II levels in the range of those observed in shock.[206] This observation further supports the importance of the renin-angiotensin system following hemorrhage or shock in the regulation of aldosterone secretion. The correlation of the rate of hemorrhage and the amount of aldosterone and renin secretion, even when arterial pressure is maintained,[204] implicates the sympathetic nervous system as the initial stimulus. Alterations in potassium and sodium plasma concentrations, although stimuli for aldosterone secretion, were not involved in the increased aldosterone secretion in response to blood loss.[207]

The retention of sodium and water by the stimulation of sodium out of the fluid in the distal tubule and collecting duct by aldosterone is vital to the restoration of extracellular fluid following moderate hemorrhage. As in the complex regulating system of normal fluid homeostasis, aldosterone interacts with several neural, circulatory, and renal systems designed to optimize extracellular fluid volume restoration following hemorrhage.

ANTIDIURETIC HORMONE (VASOPRESSIN) FOLLOWING HEMORRHAGE

Although the primary physiologic role of vasopressin is that associated with conservation of water, it was its potent pressor effects that led to its identification.[208] At present, it is recognized that normal plasma levels of vasopressin are well below those necessary to appreciably affect blood pressure[152] and that only after severe hypotension do vasopressin levels increase sufficiently to produce the vasoconstricting effect.[209]

The primary stimulus to vasopressin release is via the osmoreceptor in the anterior hypothalamus (Fig. 2–9). However, during hemorrhagic shock, the plasma osmolality may not change. The relationship of vasopressin to central venous pressure and arterial pressure was first recognized by Gauer et al.[210] Subsequently, it was demonstrated that vasopressin release correlated in a linear fashion with decreasing atrial pressures.[211] Furthermore, arterial baroreceptors also regulate vasopressin release.[212]

The amount of blood loss necessary to stimulate vasopressin release also has been studied. When blood volume was reduced in animals, vasopressin was not detected in plasma until blood loss exceeded 10 percent.[149,213] In healthy recumbent adults, a 7 to 9 percent reduction in blood volume does not have any effect on plasma vasopressin levels.[214] However, upright posture, which decreases effective blood volume by 10 to 15 percent, produced small but significant in-

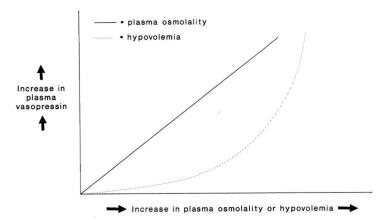

FIG. 2–9. Vasopressin correlation to hemorrhage. A diagramatic representation of the effect of increasing plasma osmolality and of reducing blood volume on plasma vasopressin levels. There is a direct relationship with osmolality, but hypovolemia results in an exponential increase in plasma vasopressin levels.

creases in plasma vasopressin.[151] Graded hemorrhage and orthostasis, however, resulted in much greater vasopressin secretion.[150]

Stimulus-response curves for vasopressin and its pressor effects provide further insight into the physiologic effects of vasopressin (Fig. 2–9). There is a high linear correlation between plasma vasopressin and osmolality.[147] However, plasma vasopressin increases exponentially as the degree of hypovolemia increases.[149,213] Furthermore, there is maximal antidiuresis when plasma vasopressin levels are as low as 5 pg/ml,[215] while the pressor effects of vasopressin are not evident in normal animals until plasma levels exceed 30 pg/ml.[152] In addition, the high levels of vasopressin have been shown to be necessary for hemodynamic recovery after significant hemorrhage.[216] It therefore appears that vasopressin is not regulated by the baroreceptors when small changes in volume occur, but when a significant stimulus arises, a large amount of vasopressin is released. Thus, in a life-threatening situation of significant blood loss, vasopressin increases arterial pressure by its vasoconstricting action. The body, in its wisdom, has established an arterial pressure-regulatory system whose receptors do not initiate a response to small-volume losses but release large amounts of hormone when cardiac output and arterial pressure are compromised.

HYPOTHALAMIC-PITUITARY-ADRENOCORTICAL AXIS

Throughout the various homeostatic mechanisms involved in normal fluid and electrolyte regulation and those involved following hypotension are examples of the integration and coordination of the nervous, endocrine, renal, and circulatory systems. In most instances, the variable is under the influence of several control systems. Furthermore, hormones involved are also stimulated by angiotensin II and ACTH. However, cortisol, one of the primary hormones released following hemorrhage, is controlled primarily by ACTH. Nevertheless, this system integrates the central nervous system in the homeostatic endocrine response.

Corticotropin-releasing factor (CRF), produced in the hypothalamus, is an important releasing factor in the control of ACTH secretion (Fig. 2–10). CRF is a peptide produced in the paraventricular nucleus of the hypothalamus. This nucleus receives nervous input from other portions of the nervous system, which, in turn, receive sensory input from peripheral nerves. ACTH can be secreted only in minimal amounts in the absence of CRF. CRF is secreted into the capillary system and carried to the anterior pituitary, where it induces ACTH secretion. ACTH, in turn, stimulates cortisol production and secretion by the adrenal cortex.

Almost any physical or mental stress can cause an instant secretion of ACTH and cortisol. Following hypotension, the sensory input to the hypothalamus originates in the atrial stretch receptors and vascular baroreceptors. Normally, these receptors exert a tonic inhibition preventing the release of CRF and ACTH.[217] When receptor activity is reduced by decreases in filling pressure or arterial blood pressure, this tonic inhibition is removed, and ACTH is secreted. In this regard, vagotomy prevents ACTH secretion after hemorrhage.[218] ACTH secretion following hemorrhage also can be prevented by maintaining intraarterial pressure using an intraarterial balloon.[219] Another stimulus to ACTH release is angiotensin II.[220] Furthermore, nephrectomy eliminated angiotensin

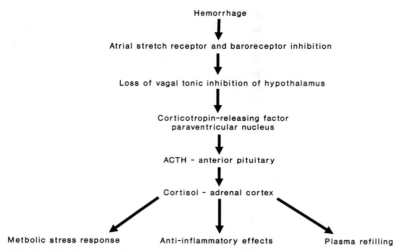

FIG. 2–10. The hypothalamic-pituitary axis following hemorrhage. Hemorrhage results in ACTH release from the anterior pituitary via the hypthalamic-pituitary axis. The ACTH stimulates cortisol release from the adrenal cortex with widespread consequences.

secretion and attenuated cortisol secretion in response to splanchnic hypotension.[221] Cortisol itself is an inhibitor of ACTH release, completing a feedback control.[222] However, repeated episodes of hemorrhage and the resultant stimulus to the hypothalamus can disrupt this inhibition.[223,224] Indeed, either normal or increased ACTH and cortisol may be secreted in response to the subsequent episodes of hemorrhage.[222,224]

The actions of cortisol are multiple and include metabolic activities, stimulation of hepatic gluconeogenesis, mobilization of amino acids and fats, and anti-inflammatory effects. However, it is not known specifically why cortisol is released in stressful conditions and why this is a significant benefit to the organism. Such a benefit can be presumed by studies that showed the beneficial effect of cortisol replacement in adrenalectomized animals. Significant alterations in metabolic processes, resistance to increased infection, and mortality in these animals could be corrected by exogenous administration of corticosteroids. Although the release of cortisol following hemorrhage can be considered one of many stressful stimuli for maintenance of body metabolic homeostasis, there is evidence that cortisol is involved in body fluid homeostasis as well, including responses to hemorrhage.

Studies in adrenalectomized animals were the first to suggest that corticosteroids were required for the regulation of fluid balance.[225,226] It was demonstrated that adrenal-deficient animals lost plasma volume somewhere within the body.[225,226] Subsequently, it was found that cells gained water during adrenal insufficiency.[227] Furthermore, this accumulation of cellular fluid could be prevented by corticosteroid replacement.[228] Cortisol also promotes the refill of plasma volume following hemorrhage.[229] Pirkle and Gann[230] have suggested that cortisol, in part, is responsible for the increase in extracellular osmolality after hemorrhage. If so, cortisol is involved in plasma refill by the mobilization of cell fluid to the plasma. Although the precise mechanism(s) by which cortisol prevents the increased mortality following severe stress and hemorrhage is unknown, it appears that cortisol secretion is necessary for many vital functions, including fluid homeostasis.

PLASMA REFILLING FOLLOWING HEMORRHAGE

In moderate amounts of hemorrhage, it is obvious that multiple systems are activated. These responses are initially directed at preserving cardiovascular function, in particular arterial blood pressure and cardiac output. Also, the neural and endocrine systems prevent further loss of fluid by the kidney. However, it has been shown that if cardiac output and arterial pressure are to return to normal after hemorrhagic shock, the volume loss must be restored.[231] In this regard, Moore[232] has shown that following a loss of 500 to 1000 ml of blood by slow venous hemorrhage, which does not produce hypotension, there is a net movement of water, salt, and protein into the plasma. In accordance with Starling's hypothesis,[24] the initial decrease in plasma hydrostatic pressure after hemorrhage causes movement from the interstitial fluid into the capillary. This flow is rapid (as high as 2 ml/min) and can restore 20 to 50 percent of the volume lost.[232] However, this rapid restoration of plasma volume does not persist. The fluid that moves from the interstitial space is protein-free and therefore reduces plasma osmotic pressure by dilution. This reduction in plasma osmotic pressure, as well as increases in plasma hydrostatic pressure secondary to improvement in cardiac output and arterial pressure as a result of the increased plasma volume, prevents further interstitial flow into the capillary. Nevertheless, plasma refilling continues until plasma volume is restored to normal in 20 to 40 h.[232]

This second phase of plasma volume restoration involves the movement of protein from the interstitial space and a shift of fluid from the cells into the interstitial fluid and finally into the plasma. Coincident with the restoration of the blood volume following moderate hemorrhage is the normalization of plasma protein concentrations.[233] Albumin is the protein that is primarily involved in this restitution. Since the synthesis of albumin takes several days to significantly raise plasma levels,[234] the increase in plasma albumin must come from the interstitial space, which is the only other source.[234] As previously discussed, the two major mechanisms for the return of protein to the plasma are via the lymphatic system and by limited diffusion through the capillary. Both these routes require an increase in interstitial fluid pressure to move fluid into the lymphatics and/or protein into the capillaries. An increase in interstitial pressure requires an increase in interstitial volume. Since the interstitial space's physical characteristics are quite rigid, the compliance of this space is fixed. An increase in interstitial fluid, therefore, raises interstitial hydrostatic pressure. The source of this fluid following hemorrhage appears to be cellular water. Since water movement between the cell and the interstitium is dependent on an osmotic gradient, an increase in interstitial osmolarity must occur to initiate this process.

Following hemorrhage, an increase in plasma osmolality has been found in both animals[235] and humans.[236] This increase in osmolality appears to correlate with the degree and rate of hemorrhage.[237,238] The solutes responsible for the increase in plasma osmolality are readily diffusible across the capillary endothelium. Solutes that are increased following hemorrhage include glucose, phosphate, lactate, pyruvate, amino acids, and electrolytes.[239,240] Diffusion of these substances across the capillary endothelium raises the interstitial osmolarity. Since these substances are not freely diffusible across the cell membrane, an osmotic pressure gradient is created. The movement of cell water into the interstitium causes an increase in interstitial hydrostatic pressure, which increases water and protein flow into the capillaries[241] and the lymphatics.[233]

The mechanism of the increase in solutes following hemorrhage is not fully known. The liver appears to be the major source of these solutes.[241] Presumably, these are the products of the increased metabolic response to hemorrhage and trauma. The counterregulatory hormones play a central role in this response.[242] Indeed, an increase in cortisol is necessary to produce hyperosmolarity.[243,244] Additional agents, however, appear to be necessary to produce the levels of hyperosmolarity that occur following hemorrhage. Evidence has been presented that an additional adrenal factor,[233] a pituitary factor,[245] and glucagon[231] are required. Thus it appears that the mobilization of substrates following hemorrhage occurs not only to support the increased metabolic needs of the body but also to restore the plasma volume. It should be noted, however, that the movement of water from the cell into the plasma does not correlate with the severity of hemorrhage. The blood-volume restoration following a hemorrhage of 25 percent is no greater than that following a 10 percent loss.[246] Furthermore, it has been shown that the infusion of lactated Ringer's solution in addition to the replacement of shed blood in hemorrhagic shock greatly improves survival compared with replacement of blood alone.[247] The infused crystalloid may substitute for the fluid shift from the cells into the interstitial fluid for restoration of plasma volume.

KIDNEY AND HYPOTENSION

To meet the filtration needs necessary to excrete the waste products of metabolism, the kidney receives a large blood supply. Approximately 25 percent of the cardiac output, or 1200 ml/min in adults, goes to the kidney. The kidney blood flow has a high degree of autoregulation. Over the range of blood pressure from 75 mmHg to as high as 160 mmHg, renal blood flow remains near its normal value.[248] Accompanying this autoregulation of blood flow is a simultaneous autoregulation of GFR. The GFR is approximately 125 ml/min under normal conditions and is unchanged over a similar blood pressure range within which autoregulation of renal blood flow occurs.[249] The constancy of GFR optimizes the fluid flow in the renal tubules so that waste products can be excreted and substances necessary for the body can be reabsorbed. Under normal conditions, the glomerular capillary hydrostatic pressure is 45 mmHg. The large drop in pressure that occurs in the afferent arterioles identifies these vessels as the major site of renal vascular resistance.[250] Any change in perfusion pressure must be accompanied by a change in resistance. Furthermore, since GFR is also unchanged, this change in resistance must occur without significantly altering glomerular capillary hydrostatic pressure. The mechanism responsible for autoregulation is the perfusion pressure, which appears to have a direct effect on the arteriolar smooth muscle and the juxtaglomerular apparatus. These were discussed earlier in the section dealing with the homeostatic mechanisms regulating body fluid and sodium.

Despite this high degree of autoregulation, blood pressure that decreases below the autoregulatory range causes a marked decrease in renal blood flow. In dogs, a drop in arterial blood pressure to 50 mmHg reduces renal blood flow to 20 to 25 percent of normal.[177] Furthermore, a decrease in the mean arterial pressure to this level causes complete cessation of urine output.[114] The mechanism of this response is the marked increase in afferent arteriolar constriction in response to the increase in sympathetic nerve stimulation. With hemorrhage that does not drop the blood pressure to below the autoregulatory range for the kidney, it appears that both afferent and efferent arterioles are constricted, thus preserving glomerular capillary pressure and GFR. Because of this, GFR does not decrease as much as renal blood flow with moderate degrees of hemorrhage.[251] Following hemorrhage, the release of angiotensin II also can cause an increase in renal vasoconstriction.[252]

Another factor influencing the effect of hypotension on renal function is the distribution of blood flow within the kidney. Approximately 90 percent of the total renal blood flow perfuses the cortex, and only 10 percent goes to the medulla.[253] This appears to be secondary to a high resistance in the vasa recta of the renal medulla.[253] Hemorrhage causes a reduction in cortical flow, whereas medullary flow is less affected.[254] These effects appear to be mediated by alpha-adrenergic activity[255] and angiotensin II.[256]

Following hemorrhage that does not alter blood pressure beyond the limits of autoregulation, blood flow to the kidney and GFR are maintained. However, when excessive adrenergic activity is present, as occurs when the major homeostatic response is to protect the circulation, then the kidney participates in an attempt to maintain arterial blood pressure by increasing renal arteriolar resistance. Furthermore, redistribution of blood flow from the cortical areas of the kidney may be responsible for ischemic changes seen with severe hemorrhage.

INTESTINE

Autoregulation of the blood flow to the intestine has been documented.[176] The blood flow in the small intestine stays fairly constant with changes of perfusion pressure between 80 and 160 mmHg.[176] Autoregulation in the intestine is usually considered to be less than in the kidney or brain but greater than in muscle.[176] The autoregulatory response is located primarily in the precapillary arterial vessels.[257] These precapillary sphincters relax with low perfusion pressures.[258] The villous blood flow appears to be a major site for autoregulation,[259] and blood flow to the villi can be maintained with perfusion pressures of 30 mmHg.[259] A possible explanation for the preservation of villous blood flow is the autoregulatory escape from the influence of sympathetic vasoconstrictive fibers.[260] Following activation of splanchnic nerves to the intestine, a decreased blood flow ensues, which is followed within minutes by an increase in flow.[261] This increase appears to occur primarily in the mucosa[262] due to redistribution of blood flow. Villous blood flow, if anything, slightly increases above the steady state.[263]

An additional effect of the sympathetic nervous system is vasoconstriction in the capacitance vessels of the intestine. Under normal stimulation, the intestinal resting blood volume can be reduced 40 percent.[261] Thus the intestine appears to play a major role in reestablishing a functional blood volume following hypotension. It should be noted, however, that autoregulatory escape appears to be operative only for norepinephrine released from nerve endings and not for epinephrine, which is released with greater degrees of hypotension. Thus, with more severe hemorrhage, marked decreases in intestinal flow support circulating homeostasis rather than intestinal mucosal flow.

BRAIN

The brain exhibits the most efficient autoregulation over the widest pressure range. It has been reported that brain blood flow remains unchanged even at perfusion pressures as low as 30 to 40 mmHg.[264] The mechanism of autoregulation in the brain is primarily metabolic. Primary factors involved are tissue levels of oxygen, pH, and carbon dioxide.[265] Thus any decrease in perfusion pressure and the resultant decrease in oxygen delivery produce changes that relax cerebral arterioles, thereby increasing flow. The cerebral circulation has sympathetic innervation along the cerebral arteries. However, neither transection of these sympathetic nerves nor removal of baroreceptor tonic inhibition affected blood flow.[266] Although autoregulation protects the brain during moderate degrees of hypotension, sustained decreases in perfusion pressure result in ischemic changes. When hypoxia is present, a severe sympathetic response is initiated by the brain which may be manifested peripherally by a transient increase in blood pressure.

LIVER

The hepatic circulation is unique in several ways. The blood supply to the liver comprises both portal venous blood from the intestine and arterial blood through the hepatic artery. The terminal portal venules and hepatic arterioles reach the portal triads, and both supply blood to the sinusoids, while the hepatic venules drain the sinusoids. The hepatic venules, the outflow vessels, are never positioned adjacent to the inflow vessels.[267] This physical relationship may explain why the portal vein and hepatic artery do not exhibit classic autoregulation. Since outflow metabolites are not physically close to the inflow vessels, one might expect that they do not play a significant role in inflow regulation. Indeed, outflow metabolite concentrations do not have any effect on blood flow in the liver.[268] Furthermore, there is no pressure-flow autoregulation or hyperemia in the portal venous bed.[269]

The hepatic artery does not exhibit the usual autoregulation either. A linear relation between pressure and flow has been found in most studies.[269] However, it appears that hepatic artery flow is controlled so that total hepatic flow can remain constant.[270] Reduction in oxygen delivery to the gut by hemodilution caused an increase in portal vein flow and a concomitant reduction in hepatic artery flow.[268] When oxidative phosphorylation was uncoupled, an increase in portal vein flow occurred secondary to gut vasculature dilation. However, hepatic artery flow decreased, while there was an increased oxygen uptake by the liver.[270] In humans during halothane anesthesia, portal venous flow decreased by 57 percent, while arterial flow increased by 30 percent.[271] However, the compensation was not adequate, since total hepatic blood flow decreased by 40 percent.[271] Also, clamping the superior mesenteric artery increased hepatic artery flow.[272] Thus the liver circulation under normal conditions maintains a constant flow. However, when hypotension occurs, the liver is susceptible to injury because the normal autoregulatory mechanisms to increase flow are not present.

The liver also has a large vascular capacitance. Stimulation of the hepatic sympathetic nerves decreases hepatic volume. Isolation of the carotid baroreceptors facilitated sympathetic stimulation. Reduction of carotid pressure to 40 mmHg caused a rapid decrease in liver circulating volume by 16 percent.[273] Conversely, an increase in pressure to 240 mmHg caused an increase in liver volume by 20 percent.[273] Thus the liver has the capability of mobilizing up to 400 ml of blood rapidly into the circulation, thereby increasing effective volume following shock.[274]

The hepatic circulation appears to be adapted to allow exchange of many substrates from the blood. This feature is useful to a highly metabolic organ such as the liver. Indeed, the hepatic capillaries are very permeable, even to protein, which also facilitates exchange. The increase in protein exchange across the capillaries also increases lymph protein concentration. The liver is a major source for thoracic duct flow. Although the microcirculation facilitates exchange, the lack of normal autoregulation makes this organ susceptible to ischemic changes during hypotension.

SUMMARY

The structural and functional features of the capillary bed, interstitial fluid, and lymphatic channels all ultimately contribute to a highly complex exchange of fluid, nutrients, and waste products necessary for optimal cell function. Tremendous fluxes of fluid occur between plasma and interstitial fluid, yet the net movement from plasma to the interstitial fluid is quite small. Lymphatic flow prohibits the accumulation of this fluid within the interstitium. In addition, the selective permeability of the endothelial cell to protein allows further filtration from plasma to interstitial fluid at the arteriole end of the capillary and reverses this flow at the venule end when hydrostatic pressure is reduced. The pores in the endothelial cells not only limit protein flow but also facilitate diffusion so that the availability of nutrients and removal of wastes under normal conditions are not limited. Furthermore, vasomotion appears to control these processes in response to the need of the tissues.

The maintenance of a nearly constant extracellular fluid volume involves the regulation of sodium balance. Sodium, in turn, is the major determinant of extracellular volume. An increased intake in sodium results in an increased release of antidiuretic hormone, which causes an increase in water. The increase in sodium and water expands the extracellular volume. This results in increased venous return and filling pressures of the heart. Cardiac output also increases, causing an increase in mean arterial pressure. The increase in arterial pressure has a direct effect on the excretion of sodium by the kidney. Indeed, this relationship appears to be the primary determinant of sodium excretion. However, the expected increase in GFR cannot account for the natriuretic effect observed under these circumstances. Additional mechanisms have been implicated, including peritubular physical factors and decreased renal nerve activity. In addition, the renin release will be reduced, and therefore, aldosterone and angiotensin II also will be reduced, minimizing their effects on sodium reabsorption. Thus the sum of these changes will be an appropriate increase in urinary sodium excretion and maintenance of the extracellular volume. The body has a complex feedback mechanism for the control of extracellular volume and sodium balance. It connects the afferent sensory devices that are primarily in the blood, the fluid space that shows dynamic change, with the effector organ that modifies the blood volume by the excretion of water and sodium.

Following hemorrhage, the same homeostatic mechanisms that regulate sodium and water balance under normal conditions are activated. However, when the blood volume is reduced to the extent that the blood pressure falls, the body is faced with an additional problem. Not only is there the necessity to restore blood volume, but the initial dilemma is survival. The immediate response is activation of the sympathetic nervous system. Vasoconstriction and redistribution of blood flow to vital organs appear to be a teleologic response designed for survival. In addition, if hemorrhage is limited, the changes effected by the sympathetic nervous system also help to restore volume. The immediate response of this system both to the loss of effective blood volume and to its restoration allows the physician to judge the effectiveness of volume resuscitation by physical examination and monitoring of systemic blood pressure and urine output.

In addition to the marked sympathetic response to hemorrhage, the hormonal responses are also altered. The release of renin in response to hemorrhage stimulates angiotensin II production to levels that cause marked vasoconstriction in the gut and kidney. Likewise, the release of vasopressin following hemorrhage increases plasma levels of vasopressin to those necessary for its vasoconstrictive action. Thus the body releases large amounts of these hormones following hemorrhage in an attempt to restore cardiac output and arterial pressure. The secretion of aldosterone also correlates with the severity of hemorrhage. However, aldosterone appears to play a more significant role in the restoration of blood volume after moderate hemorrhage.

The stimulation of ACTH release and the resulting increases in plasma cortisol levels are also necessary for the survival of the organism following hemorrhage. The specific mechanism by which cortisol exerts its beneficial effect is not fully defined. Nonetheless, its metabolic and anti-inflammatory effects are involved in this aspect. Moreover, cortisol appears to play a significant role in the restoration of plasma volume after hemorrhage by increasing interstitial osmotic pressure and the movement of cell water into the plasma.

Certainly one has to marvel at the wisdom of the body in its ability to maintain normal fluid and electrolyte homeostasis and allow the organism to live and function in various external environments. Furthermore, the body's ability to respond to large-volume losses using the same mechanisms that fine-tune normal fluid balance is truly remarkable. This provides the organism with a mechanism for survival until normal blood volume can be restored. Understanding the homeostatic mechanisms involved provides a rational basis for the resuscitation of patients following hemorrhage and other shock states.

ACKNOWLEDGMENTS

The authors wish to express their sincere thanks and appreciation to Gurdev Singh, F.R.C.S., and M. Waheed Rana, Ph.D., for their assistance and skill in the design and preparation of the figures in this chapter, along with Renee Ziobron and Sharon Waite for their assistance in the preparation of this manuscript and for editorial assistance. This work was supported in part by Department of Surgery funds and by NIH Grant 5 R01 39519.

REFERENCES

1. Bernard C: *Lecons sur les phénomènes de la vie communs aux animaux et aux végétaux.* Paris, J-B Bailliere et fils, 1878.
2. Cannon WB: Organization for physiologic homeostasis. *Physiol Rev* 9:399, 1929.
3. Guyton AC: Functional organization of the human body and control of the "internal environment," in Guyton AC (ed): *Textbook of Medical Physiology.* Philadelphia, Saunders, 1991, pp 2–8.
4. McFarland D: *Animal Behaviour.* Bath, England, Pitman Press, 1985.
5. Mrosovsky N: *Rheostasis: The Physiology of Change.* New York, Oxford University Press, 1990.
6. Garner MG, Phippard AF, Fletcher JM, et al: Effect of angiotensin II on baroreceptor reflex control of heart rate in conscious baboons. *Hypertension* 10:628, 1987.
7. Manery J: Water and electrolyte metabolism. *Physiol Rev* 34:334, 1954.
8. Robinson JR: Metabolism of intracellular water. *Physiol Rev* 40:112, 1960.
9. Skelton H: The storage of water by various tissues of the body. *Arch Intern Med* 40:140, 1927.
10. Schloerb PR, Friis-Hansen BJ, Edelman IS, et al: The measurement of total body water in the human subject by deuterium oxide dilution with the dynamics of deuterium distribution. *J Clin Invest* 29:1296, 1950.
11. Pace N, Rathbun EN: Studies on body composition: III. The body water and chemically combined nitrogen content in relation to fat content. *J Biol Chem* 158:685, 1945.
12. Guyton AC: The body fluid compartments. Extracellular and intracellular fluids: Interstitial fluid and edema, in Guyton AC (ed): *Textbook of Medical Physiology.* Philadelphia, Saunders, 1991, pp 274–284.
13. Pinson EA: Water exchanges and barriers as studied by the use of hydrogen isotopes. *Physiol Rev* 32:123, 1952.
14. Edelman IS, Liebman J: Anatomy of body water and electrolytes. *Am J Med* 27:256, 1959.
15. Swan RC, Madisso H, Pitts RF: Measurement of extracellular fluid volume in nephrectomized dogs. *J Clin Invest* 33:1447, 1954.
16. Yasumura S, Cohn SH, Ellis KJ: Measurement of extracellular space by total body neutron activation. *Am J Physiol* 244:R36, 1983.
17. Hays RM: Dynamics of body water and electrolytes, in Maxwell MH, Kleeman CR (eds): *Clinical Disorders of Fluid and Electrolyte Metabolism,* 3d ed. New York, McGraw-Hill, 1980, pp 1–43.

18. Macknight ADC, Leaf A: Regulation of cellular volume, in Andreoli TA, Hoffman JF, Fanestel DD (eds): *Physiology of Membrane Disorders*. New York, Plenum Press, 1978, pp 315–334.

19. Bygrave FL: The ionic environment and metabolic control. *Nature* 214:667, 1967.

20. Ussing HH: The alkali metal ions in isolated systems and tissues, in Deane HW, Rubin BL (eds): *Handbuch der Experimentellen Pharmakologie*. Heidelberg, Springer-Verlag, 1960, p 1.

21. Adler S, Fraley D: Potassium and intracellular pH. *Kidney Int* 11:433, 1977.

22. Robertson GL, Athar S: The interaction of blood osmolality and blood volume in regulating vasopressin secretion in man. *J Clin Endocrinol Metab* 42:613, 1976.

23. Macknight ADC: Cellular volume under physiologic conditions, in Staub NC, Taylor AE (eds): *Edema*. New York, Raven Press, 1984, pp 81–93.

24. Starling EH: The Aris and Gale lectures on the physiological factors involved in the causation of dropsy. *Lancet* 1:1267, 1896.

25. Krogh AE, Landis EM, Turner AH: The movement of fluid through the human capillary wall in relation to venous pressure and to the colloid osmotic pressure of the blood. *J Clin Invest* 11:63, 1932.

26. Zweifach BW, Lipowsky HH: Pressure flow relationships in blood and lymph microcirculation, in Renkin EM, Michel CC (eds): *Handbook of Physiology*, Section 2: *The Cardiovascular System*. Bethesda, Maryland, American Physiologic Society, 1984, pp 251–306.

27. Grotte G: Passage of dextran molecules across the blood-lymph barrier. *Acta Chir Scand Suppl* 211:1, 1956.

28. Landis EM, Pappenheimer JR: Exchange of substances through capillary walls, in Hamilton WF (ed): *Handbook of Physiology: Circulation*. Washington, American Physiological Society, 1963, pp 961–1034.

29. Solomon AK: Characterization of biological membranes by equivalent pores. *J Gen Physiol* 51:3555, 1968.

30. Renkin EM: Multiple pathways of capillary permeability. *Circ Res* 41:735, 1977.

31. Johnson P: Autoregulation of blood flow. *Circ Res* 59:483, 1986.

32. Crone C, Christensen O: Transcapillary transport of small solutes and water, in Guyton AC, Young DB (eds): *Cardiovascular Physiology III*. Baltimore, University Park Press, 1978, pp 149–213.

33. Zweifach BW, Fronck A: The interplay of central and peripheral factors in irreversible shock. *Prog Cardiovasc Dis* 18:147, 1975.

34. Zweifach BW, Richardson DR: Microcirculatory adjustments of pressure in the mesentery, in Ditzel J, Lewis DH (eds): *Proceedings of the European Conference on Microcirculation*. Basel, Karger, 1971, pp 248–253.

35. Johnson PC, Wayland H: Oscillatory flow pattern in single mesenteric capillaries. *Bibl Anat* 9:164, 1967.

36. Colantuoni A, Bertuglia S, Intaglietta M: Quantication of rhythmic diameter changes in arterial microcirculation. *Am J Physiol* 246:H508, 1984.

37. Zweifach BW: *Functional Behavior of the Microcirculation*. Springfield, Illinois, Charles C Thomas, 1961, pp 51–61.

38. Messina EJ, Rodenburg BL, Slomeany AM, et al: Microcirculatory effects of arachidonic acid and a prostaglandin endoperoxide (PGH_2). *Microvasc Res* 19:288, 1980.

39. Katz MA: Validity of interstitial fluid hydrostatic pressure measurements in hollow porous polyethylene capsules. *Microvasc Res* 16:316, 1978.

40. Zweifach BW, Silberberg A: The interstitial-lymphatic flow system, in Guyton AC, Young DB (eds): *Cardiovascular Physiology III*, Baltimore, University Park Press, 1979, pp 216–260.

41. Guyton AC, Granger HJ, Taylor AE: Interstitial fluid pressure. *Physiol Rev* 51:527, 1971.

42. Yoffey JM, Courtice FC: *Lymphatics, Lymph and Lymphoid Tissue*. Cambridge, Harvard University Press, 1956, pp 112–145.

43. Haljamäe H, Linde A, Amundson B: Comparative analyses of capsular fluid and interstitial fluid. *Am J Physiol* 227:1199, 1974.

44. Hargens AR, Zweifach BW: Transport between blood and peripheral lymph in intestine. *Microvasc Res* 11:89, 1976.

45. Wierderhelm CA: The interstitial space, in Fung YC, Perrone N, Anliher M (eds): *Biomechanics: Its Foundations and Objectives*. Englewood Cliffs, New Jersey, Prentice-Hall, 1972, pp 273–286.

46. Shalak TC, Schmid-Schönbein GW, Zweifach BW: New morphologic evidence for a mechanism of lymph formation in skeletal muscle. *Microvasc Res* 28:95, 1984.

47. Nicoll PA, Cortese TA Jr.: The physiology of the skin. *Annu Rev Physiol* 34:177, 1972.

48. Johnson PC: Autoregulation of blood flow. *Circ Res* 59:483, 1986.

49. Guyton AC, Ross JM, Carrier O, et al: Evidence for tissue oxygen demand as the major factor causing autoregulation. *Circ Res* 14/15(suppl):60, 1964.

50. Eckenhoff JE, Hafkenschiel JH, Landmesser CM, et al: Cardiac oxygen metabolism and control of the coronary circulation. *Am J Physiol* 149:634, 1947.

51. Eklof B, Lassen NA, Nilsson L, et al: Blood flow and metabolic rate for oxygen in the cerebral cortex of the rat. *Acta Physiol Scand* 88:587, 1973.

52. Haddy FJ, Scott JB: Metabolically linked vasoactive chemicals in local regulation of blood flow. *Physiol Rev* 48:688, 1968.

53. Fairchild HM, Ross J, Guyton AC: Failure of recovery from reactive hyperemia in the absence of oxygen. *Am J Physiol* 210:490, 1966.

54. Berne RM: Regulation of coronary blood flow. *Physiol Rev* 44:1, 1964.

55. Detar R, Bohr DF: Oxygen and vascular smooth muscle contraction. *Am J Physiol* 214:241, 1968.

56. Gorczynski RJ, Duling BR: Role of oxygen in arteriolar functional vasodilation in hamster striated muscle. *Am J Physiol* 235:H505, 1978.

57. Schrader J, Haddy FJ, Gerlach E: Release of adenosine, inosine and hypoxanthine from the isolated guinea pig heart during hypoxia, flow autoregulation and reactive hyperemia. *Pflugers Arch* 369:1, 1977.

58. Rhodin JAG: The ultrastructure of mammalian arterioles and precapillary sphincters. *J Ultrastruct Res* 18:181, 1967.

59. Vetterlein F, Schmidt G: Functional capillary density in skeletal muscle during vasodilation induced by isoprenatine and muscular exercise. *Microvasc Res* 20:156, 1980.

60. Grande P-O, Lundvall J, Mellander S: Evidence for a rate-sensitive regulatory mechanism in myogenic microvascular control. *Acta Physiol Scand* 99:432, 1977.

61. Johnson PC: Myogenic nature of increase in intestinal vascular resistance with venous pressure elevation. *Circ Res* 6:992, 1959.

62. Hanson KM, Johnson PC: Local control of hepatic arterial and portal venous flow in the dog. *Am J Physiol* 211:712, 1966.

63. Renkin EM, Michel CC, Geiger SR: Control of microcirculation and blood-tissue exchange, in Renkin EM (ed): *Handbook of Physiology*, Section 2: *The Cardiovascular System*. Bethesda, Maryland, American Physiologic Society, 1984, pp 627–687.

64. Oien AH, Aukland K: A mathematical analysis of the myogenic hypothesis with special reference to autoregulation of renal blood flow. *Circ Res* 52:241, 1983.

65. Thurau KWA: Autoregulation of renal blood flow and glomerular filtration rate, including data on tubular and peritubular capillary pressures and vessel wall tension circulation. *Circ Res* 15(suppl):1132, 1964.

66. Jarhult J, Mellander S: Autoregulation of capillary hydrostatic pressure in skeletal muscle during regional arterial hypo- and hypertension. *Acta Physiol Scand* 91:32, 1974.

67. Epstein FH, Goodyer AVN, Lawrason FD, et al: Studies of the antidiuresis of quiet standing, the importance of changes in plasma volume in glomerular filtration rate. *J Clin Invest* 30:63, 1951.

68. Epstein FH, Duncan DC, Fishman LM: Characterization of the natriuresis caused in normal man by immersion in water. *Clin Sci* 43:275, 1972.

69. Gauer OH, Henry JP: Neurohormonal control of plasma volume, in Guyton AC, Cowley AW (eds): *Cardiovascular Physiology II: International Review of Physiology.* Baltimore, University Park Press, 1976, pp 146–190.

70. Davis JO, Howell DS: Mechanisms of fluid and electrolyte retention in experimental preparations in dogs: II. Thoracic inferior vena cava obstruction. *Circ Res* 1:171, 1953.

71. Fitzhugh FW, McWhorter RL, Estes EH Jr, et al: The effect of application of tourniquet to the legs on cardiac output and renal function in normal human subjects. *J Clin Invest* 32:1163, 1953.

72. Linden RJ: Atrial reflexes and renal function. *Am J Cardiol* 44:879, 1979.

73. Gupta BN, Linden RJ, Mary DASG, et al: The diuretic and natriuretic responses to stimulation of left atrial receptors in dogs with different blood volumes. *Q J Exp Physiol* 67:235, 1982.

74. Kaczmarczyk C, Drake A, Eisele R, et al: The role of the cardiac nerves in the regulation of sodium excretion in conscious dogs. *Pflugers Arch* 390:125, 1981.

75. Kappagoda CT, Linden RJ, Snow HM: Effect of stimulating right atrial receptors on urine flow in the dog. *J Physiol* 235:493, 1973.

76. Coleridge HM, Coleridge JCG, Kidd C: Cardiac receptors in the dog, with particular reference to two types of apparent endings in the ventricular wall. *J Physiol* 174:323, 1964.

77. Wennergen G, Henriksson B-A, Weiss L-G, et al: Effects of stimulation of non-medullated cardiac afferents on renal water and sodium excretion. *Acta Physiol Scand* 97:261, 1976.

78. Parntal AS: Vagal sensory receptors and their reflex effects. *Physiol Rev* 53:159, 1973.

79. Baertshi AJ, Munzner RF, Ward DA, et al: The right and left atrial B-fiber input to the medulla of the cat. *Brain Res* 98:189, 1975.

80. Mellander S, Oberg B: Transcapillary fluid absorption and other vascular reactions in the human forearm during reduction of the circulating blood volume. *Acta Physiol Scand* 71:37, 1967.

81. Schad H, Seller H: Reduction of renal nerve activity by volume expansion in conscious cats. *Pflugers Arch* 363:155, 1976.

82. DeTorrente A, Robertson G, McDonald KM, et al: Mechanism of diuretic response to increased left atrial pressure in the anesthetized dog. *Kidney Int* 8:355, 1975.

83. Atkins EL, Pearce JW: Mechanisms of the renal response to plasma volume expansion. *Can J Biochem Physiol* 37:91, 1959.

84. Pearse JW: The effect of vagotomy and dennervation of the choroid sinus on diuresis following plasma volume expansion. *Can J Biochem Physiol* 37:81, 1959.

85. Gilmore JP, Zucker IH: Contribution of vagal pathways to the renal response to head out immersion in the non-human primate. *Circ Res* 42:263, 1978.

86. Fater DC, Schultz HD, Sundet WD, et al: Effects of left atrial stretch in cardiac-denervated and intact conscious dogs. *Am J Physiol* 242:H1056, 1982.

87. Misono KS, Fukumi H, Grammer RT, et al: Rat atrial natriuretic factor: complete amino acid sequence and disulfide linkage essential for biological activity. *Biochem Biophys Res Commun* 119:524, 1984.

88. Cantin M, Genest J: The heart and atrial natriuretic factor. *Endocrinol Rev* 6:107, 1985.

89. Lang RE, Tholken H, Ganten D, et al: Atrial natriuretic factor: A circulating hormone stimulated by volume loading. *Nature* 314:264, 1985.

90. Ballerman BJ: Role of atrial natriuretic peptide in volume homeostasis, in Brenner BM, Stein JH (eds): *Body Fluid Homeostasis.* New York, Churchill Livingstone, 1987, pp 221–244.

91. Maack T, Carmago MJF, Kleinert HD, et al: Atrial natriuretic factor: Structure and functional properties. *Kidney Int* 27:607, 1985.

92. Shenker Y, Sider RS, Ostalin EA, et al: Plasma levels of immunoreactive atrial natriuretic factor in healthy subjects and in patients with edema. *J Clin Invest* 76:1684, 1985.

93. Keeler R: Natriuresis after unilateral stimulation of carotid receptors in unanesthetized rats. *Am J Physiol* 226:507, 1974.

94. DiBona GF: Neurogenic regulation of renal tubular sodium reabsorption. *Am J Physiol* 233:F73, 1977.

95. Humphreys MH, Ayus JC, Stanton J Jr: Prevention by vagotomy or atropine administration of the hemodynamic changes occurring after acute unilateral nephrectomy in the dog. *Circ Res* 46:575, 1980.

96. Ayus JC, Humphreys MH: Hemodynamic and renal functional changes after acute unilateral nephrectomy in the dog: role of carotid sinus baroreceptors. *Am J Physiol* 242:F181, 1982.

97. Tobian L, Tomboulian A, Janeck J: The effect of high perfusion pressure on the granulation of juxtaglomerular cells in an isolated kidney. *J Clin Invest* 38:605, 1959.

98. Blaine EH, Davis JO: Evidence for a renal vascular mechanism in renin release: New observations with graded stimulation by aortic constriction. *Circ Res* 28/29(suppl 2):118, 1971.

99. Kaloyanides GJ, Bastron RD, DiBona GF: Effect of ureteral clamping and increased renal arterial pressure on renin release. *Am J Physiol* 225:95, 1973.

100. Witty RT, Davis JO, Shade RE, et al: Mechanisms regulating renin release in dogs with thoracic caval constriction. *Circ Res* 31:339, 1973.

101. Carey RM: Evidence for a splanchnic sodium input monitor regulating renal sodium excretion in man: Lack of dependence upon aldosterone. *Circ Res* 43:19, 1978.

102. Daly JJ, Roe JW, Horrocks P: A comparison of sodium excretion following the infusion of saline into systemic and portal veins in the dog: Evidence for a hepatic role in the control of sodium excretion. *Clin Sci* 33:481, 1967.

103. Schneider EG, Davis JO, Robb CA, et al: Lack of evidence for a hepatic osmoreceptor in conscious dogs. *Am J Physiol* 218:42, 1970.

104. Kostreva DR, Castaner A, Kampine JP: Reflex effects of hepatic baroreceptors on renal and cardiac sympathetic nerve activity. *Am J Physiol* 238:R390, 1980.

105. Corn J, Porter JC: Diencephalic involvement in sodium excretion in the rat. *Endocrinology* 86:1112, 1970.

106. Mouw DR, Abraham JR, Blair-West JR, et al: Brain receptors, renin secretion and renal sodium retention in conscious sheep. *Am J Physiol* 226:56, 1974.

107. Blaine EH, Denton DA, McKinley MJ, et al: A central osmosensitive receptor for renal sodium excretion. *J Physiol* 244:497, 1975.

108. Kaloyamides GJ, Balabanian MB, Bowman RL: Evidence that the brain participates in humoral natriuretic mechanism of blood volume expansion in the dog. *J Clin Invest* 62:1288, 1978.

109. Sonneberg H, Pearce JW: Renal response to measured blood volume expansion in differently hydrated dogs. *Am J Physiol* 203:344, 1962.

110. Wright FS, Davis JO, Johnston CI, et al: Renal sodium excretion after volume expansion with saline and blood. *Proc Soc Exp Biol Med* 128:1044, 1968.

111. Coehlo JD, Bradley SE: Persistence of the natriuretic response to isotonic saline load during hemorrhagic hypotension in the dog. *Proc Soc Exp Biol Med* 131:265, 1969.

112. Selkurt EE, Hall PW, Spencer MD: Effect of graded arterial pressure decrement on renal clearance of creatinine, p-amino-hippurate and sodium. *Am J Physiol* 159:369, 1949.

113. Thompson JMA, Dickinson CJ: The relation between the excretion of sodium and water and the perfusion pressure in the isolated, blood perfused, rabbit kidney, with special reference to changes in clip hypertension. *Clin Sci Mol Med* 50:223, 1976.

114. Guyton AC: Formation of urine by the kidney: I. Renal blood flow, glomerular filtration,

and their control, in Guyton AC (ed): *Textbook of Medical Physiology,* 8th ed. Philadelphia, Saunders, 1991, pp 286–297.

115. Knox FG, Mertz JI, Burnett JC Jr, et al: Role of hydrostatic and oncotic pressures in renal sodium reabsorption. *Circ Res* 52:491, 1983.

116. Raymond KH, Stein JH: Efferent limb of volume homeostasis, in Brenner BM, Stein JH (eds): *Body Fluid Homeostasis.* New York, Churchill Livingstone, 1987, pp 33–68.

117. de Wardener HE, Mills IH, Clapham WF, et al: Studies on the efferent mechanisms of the sodium diuresis which follows the administration of intravenous saline in the dog. *Clin Sci* 21:249, 1961.

118. Lindheimer MD, Lalone RC, Levinsky WB: Evidence that an increase in glomerular filtration has little effect on sodium excretion in the dog unless extracellular volume is expanded. *J Clin Invest* 46:256, 1967.

119. Haberle DA, von Bayer H: Characteristics of glomerulotubular balance. *Am J Physiol* 244:F355, 1983.

120. Kaplan SA, Rappaport S: Urinary excretion of sodium and chloride after splanchnicotomy: Effect on sodium reabsorption. *J Lab Clin Med* 83:263, 1974.

121. Bencsath P, Asztalos B, Szalay L: Renal handling of sodium after chronic renal sympathectomy in the anesthetized rat. *Am J Physiol* 236:F513, 1979.

122. Bello-Reuss E, Trevino DL, Gottschalk CW: Effect of renal sympathetic nerve stimulation on proximal water and sodium reabsorption. *J Clin Invest* 57:1104, 1976.

123. Bencsath P, Szenasi G, Takacs L: Water and electrolyte transport in Henle's loop and distal tubule after renal sympathectomy in the rat. *Am J Physiol* 249:F308, 1985.

124. Davis JO, Freeman RH: Mechanisms regulating renin release. *Physiol Rev* 56:1, 1976.

125. Epstein M: Studies of volume homeostasis in man utilizing the model of head out water immersion. *Nephron* 22:9, 1978.

126. Kotchan TA, Welch WJ, Lorenz JN, et al: Renal tubular chloride and renin release. *J Lab Clin Med* 110:533, 1987.

127. Farhi ER, Cant JR, Barger AC: Interactions between intrarenal epinephrine receptors and the renal baroreceptors in the control of PRA in conscious dogs. *Circ Res* 50:477, 1982.

128. Laragh JH, Sealy JE: The renin-angiotensin-aldosterone hormonal system and regulation of sodium, potassium and blood pressure homeostasis, in Orloff J, Berliner BW (eds): *Handbook of Physiology,* Section 8: *Renal Physiology.* Washington, American Physiological Society, 1973, pp 831–908.

129. Coghlan JP, Denton DA, Gogling JR: The control of aldosterone secretion. *Postgrad Med J* 36:76, 1960.

130. Mills JN, Thomas S, Williamson KS: The acute effect of hydrocortisone deoxycorticosterone and aldosterone upon the excretion of sodium, potassium and acid by the human kidney. *J Physiol* 151:312, 1960.

131. Hall JE, Granger JP, Smith MJ, et al: Role of renal hemodynamics and arterial pressure in aldosterone "escape." *Hypertension* 6(suppl):I183, 1984.

132. Hulter HS, Ilnicki LP, Harbottle JA, et al: Impaired renal H^+ secretion and NH_3 production in mineralocorticoid-deficient glucocorticoid replete dogs. *Am J Physiol* 232:F136, 1977.

133. Samuels AI, Miller ED, Fray JCS, et al: Renin-angiotensin antagonists and the regulation of blood pressure. *Fed Proc* 35:2512, 1976.

134. Edwards RM: Segmental effects of norepinephrine and angiotensin II in isolated renal microvessels. *Am J Physiol* 24:F526, 1983.

135. Schaster VL, Kokks JP, Jacobson HR: Angiotensin II directly stimulates sodium transport in rabbit proximal tubules. *J Clin Invest* 73:507, 1984.

136. Lohmeier TE, Cowley AW Jr, Treppodo NC, et al: Effects of endogenous angiotensin II on renal sodium excretion and renal hemodynamics. *Am J Physiol* 233:F388, 1977.

137. Young DB: Analysis of long term potassium regulation. *Endocrinol Rev* 6:24, 1985.

138. Hall JE: Regulation of renal hemodynamics, in Guyton AC, Hall JE (eds): *International Review of Physiology: Cardiovascular Physiology IV.* Baltimore, University Park Press, 1982, pp 243–322.

139. Ichebawa I, Brenner BM: Importance of efferent arteriolar vascular tone in regulation of proximal tubular reabsorption and glomerulotubular balance in the rat. *J Clin Invest* 65:1192, 1980.

140. Mendelsohn FAO: Angiotensin II: Evidence for its role as an intrarenal hormone. *Kidney Int* 22(suppl 12):578, 1982.

141. Olsen ME, Hall JE, Montani J-P, et al: Mechanisms of angiotensin II natriuresis and anti-natriuresis. *Am J Physiol* 249:F299, 1985.

142. Harris PJ, Young JA: Dose-dependent stimulation and inhibition of proximal tubular sodium reabsorption by angiotensin II in the rat kidney. *Pflugers Arch* 367:295, 1977.

143. Barker JL, Crayton JW, Nicoll RA: Supraoptic neurosecretory cells: Adrenergic and cholinergic sensitivity. *Science* 171:208, 1971.

144. Verney EB: The antidiuretic hormone and the factors which determine its release. *Proc R Soc Lond* 135:25, 1947.

145. Robertson GL, Aycinena P, Zerbe RL: Neurogenic disorders of osmoregulation. *Am J Med* 72:339, 1982.

146. Hammer M, Ladefoged J, Olgaaro K: Relationship between plasma osmolality and plasma vasopressin in human subjects. *Am J Physiol* 238:E313, 1979.

147. Robertson GL, Shelton RL, Athar S: The osmoregulation of vasopressin. *Kidney Int* 10:25, 1976.

148. Zerbe RL, Robertson GL: Osmoregulation of thirst and vasopressin secretion in man: The effect of various solutes. *Am J Physiol* 244:E607, 1983.

149. Dunn FL, Brennan TJ, Nelson AE, et al: The role of blood osmolality and volume in regulating vasopressin secretion in the rat. *J Clin Invest* 52:3212, 1973.

150. Robertson GL, Mahr EA, Athar S, et al: Development and clinical application of a new method for the radioimmunoassay of arginine vasopressin in human plasma. *J Clin Invest* 52:2340, 1973.

151. Segar WE, Moore WW: The regulation of antidiuretic hormone release in man: I. The effects of change in position and ambient temperature on blood ADH levels. *J Clin Invest* 47:2143, 1968.

152. Malayan S, Ramsay DS, Keil LC, et al: Effects of increases in plasma vasopressin concentration on plasma renin activity, blood pressure, heart rate and plasma corticosteroid concentration in conscious dogs. *Endocrinology* 107:1899, 1980.

153. Larsson B, Olsson K, Fyhrquist F: Vasopressin release induced by hemorrhage in the goat. *Acta Physiol Scand* 104:309, 1978.

154. Youmans PL, Green HD, Denison AB Jr: Nature of the vasodilator and constrictor receptors in skeletal muscle in the dog. *Circ Res* 3:171, 1955.

155. DeMey JG, Vanhoutte PM: Role of the intima in cholinergic and purinergic relaxation of isolated canine femoral arteries. *J Physiol* 316:347, 1981.

156. Baey S, Kopman AF, Orkin LR: Microvascular hypersensitivity subsequent to chemical denervation. *Circ Res* 20:328, 1967.

157. Daley I, De B, Ramsay DJ, et al: The site of action of nerves in the pulmonary vascular bed in the dog. *J Physiol* 209:317, 1970.

158. Berne RM, Rubio R: Coronary circulation, in Berne RM, Sperelakis N (eds): *Handbook of Physiology: The Cardiovascular System. The Heart.* Bethesda, Maryland, American Physiological Society, 1979, pp 873–952.

159. Ballard K, Malmfors T, Rosell S: Adrenergic innervation and vascular patterns in canine adipose tissue. *Microvasc Res* 8:164, 1974.

160. D'Alecy LE, Fergl EO: Sympathetic control of cerebral blood flow in dogs. *Circ Res* 31:267, 1972.

161. Hersted DD, Busija DW, Marcus JL: Neural effects on cerebral vessels: alterations of pressure-flow relationship. *Fed Proc* 40:2317, 1981.

162. Celander O, Folkow B: A comparison of the sympathetic vasomotor fibre control of the vessels of the skin and the muscles. *Acta Physiol Scand* 29:241, 1953.

163. Folkow B: Regional adjustments of intestinal blood flow. *Gastroenterology* 52:423, 1967.

164. Zimmerman BG: Separation of responses of arteries and veins to sympathetic stimulation. *Circ Res* 18:429, 1966.

165. Hoffman BB, Lefkowtiz RJ: Adrenergic receptors in the heart. *Annu Rev Physiol* 44:475, 1982.

166. Hilton SM, Spyer KM: Central nervous regulation of vascular resistance. *Annu Rev Physiol* 42:399, 1980.

167. Bishop VS, Mallani A, Thoren P: Cardiac mechanoreceptors, in Shepherd JT, Aboud FM (eds): *Handbook of Physiology*, Sec. 2, Vol. 3. Bethesda, Maryland, American Physiological Society, 1983, pp 917–951.

168. Anderson WP, Ludbrook J: Effects of the sympathetic nervous system and the adrenal medullary hormones on dog hindlimb flow after hemorrhage. *Aust J Exp Biol Med Sci* 54:169, 1976.

169. Guyton AC: Circulatory shock and physiology of its treatment, in Guyton AC (ed): *Textbook of Medical Physiology*. Philadelphia, Saunders, 1991, pp 263–271.

170. Eriksson E, Lisanler B: Changes in precapillary resistance in skeletal muscle vessels studied by intravital microscopy. *Acta Physiol Scand* 84:295, 1972.

171. Hollenberg NK, Nickerson M: Changes in pre- and postcapillary resistance in pathogenesis of hemorrhagic shock. *Am J Physiol* 219:1483, 1970.

172. Mellander S, Lewis DH: Effect of hemorrhagic shock on the reactivity of resistance and capacitance vessels and on capillary filtration transfer in cat skeletal muscle. *Circ Res* 13:105, 1963.

173. Rapela CE, Green HD: Autoregulation of cerebral blood flow. *Circ Res* 14/15(suppl):I205, 1964.

174. Green HD, Rapela CE: Blood flow in passive vascular beds. *Circ Res* 14/15(suppl):I11, 1964.

175. Jones RD, Berne RM: Evidence for a metabolic mechanism in autoregulation of blood flow in skeletal muscle. *Circ Res* 17:540, 1965.

176. Johnson PC: Autoregulation of intestinal blood flow. *Am J Physiol* 199:311, 1960.

177. Passmore JC, Barker CH: Intrarenal flow distribution in irreversible hemorrhagic shock in dogs. *J Trauma* 13:1066, 1973.

178. Appelgren KL: Effect of perfusion pressure and hematocrit on capillary flow and transport in hyperemic skeletal muscle of the dog. *Microvasc Res* 4:231, 1972.

179. Shadle OW, Zutof M, Diana J: Translocation of blood from the isolated dog's hindlimb during levarterenol infusion and sciatic nerve stimulation. *Circ Res* 6:326, 1958.

180. Guyton AC: Nervous regulation of the circulation and rapid control of arterial pressure, in Guyton AC (ed): *Textbook of Medical Physiology*. Philadelphia, Saunders, 1991, pp 194–204.

181. Sagawa K, Ross J, Guyton AC: Quantitation of the cerebral ischemic pressor response in dogs. *Am J Physiol* 200:1164, 1961.

182. Chien S: Role of the sympathetic nervous system in hemorrhage. *Physiol Rev* 47:214, 1967.

183. Watts DT: Arterial blood epinephrine levels during hemorrhagic hypotension in dogs. *Am J Physiol* 184:271, 1955.

184. Watts DT: Adrenergic mechanisms in hypovolemic shock, in Mills LC, Moyer JH (eds): *Shock and Hypotension*. New York, Grune & Stratton, 1965, pp 385–391.

185. Carey LD, Sapira JD, Curtin RA: Hemorrhage as a stimulus to adrenal epinephrine secretion. *Bull Soc Intern Chir* 5:393, 1972.

186. Wang BC, Sundet WD, Hakumaki OK, et al: Vasopressin and renin responses to hemorrhage in conscious, cardiac denervated dogs. *Am J Physiol* 245:H399, 1983.

187. Clayburgh JR, Share L: Vasopressin, renin and cardiovascular responses to continuous slow hemorrhage. *Am J Physiol* 224:519, 1973.

188. Errington ML, Rocha e Silva M: On the role of vasopressin and angiotensin in the development of irreversible hemorrhagic shock. *J Physiol* 242:119, 1974.

189. Bunag RD, Page IH, McCubbin JW: Neural stimulation of release of renin. *Circ Res* 19:851, 1966.

190. Finkielman S, Worcel M, Massani ZM, et al: Angiotensin blood levels in hypovolemic shock during osmotic diuresis. *Am J Physiol* 215:308, 1968.

191. Witty RT, Davis JO, Johnson JA, et al: Effects of papaverine and hemorrhage on renin secretion in the non-filtering kidney. *Am J Physiol* 221:1666, 1971.

192. Kairallah PA: Action of angiotensin on adrenergic nerve endings: Inhibition of norepinephrine uptake. *Fed Proc* 31:1351, 1972.

193. Hall RC, Hodge RL: Changes in catecholamine and angiotensin levels in the cat and dog during hemorrhage. *Am J Physiol* 221:1305, 1971.

194. Averill DB, Scher AM, Feigl ED: Angiotensin causes vasoconstriction during hemorrhage in baroreceptor-denervated dogs. *Am J Physiol* 245:H667, 1983.

195. Feuerstein G, Boonyavioj P, Gutman Y: Renin-angiotensin mediation of adrenal catecholamine secretion induced by hemorrhage. *Eur J Pharmacol* 44:131, 1977.

196. Trachte GJ, Lefer AM: Shock potentiating actions of angiotensin II in cats. *Circ Shock* 7:343, 1980.

197. Guyton AC: Role of the kidney in regulation of arterial pressure and hypertension, in Guyton AC (ed): *Textbook of Medical Physiology.* Philadelphia, Saunders, 1991, pp 194–220.

198. Peach MJ: Renin-angiotensin system: Biochemistry and mechanisms of action. *Physiol Rev* 57:313, 1977.

199. Gann DS: Cortisol secretion after hemorrhage: Multiple mechanisms. *Nephron* 23:119, 1979.

200. Maran JW, Yates FE: Cortisol secretion during intrapituitary infusion of angiotensin II in conscious dogs. *Am J Physiol* 233:E273, 1977.

201. Freeman JE, Hock CE, Edmondo JS, et al: Anti-shock actions of a new converting enzyme inhibitor, nalaprilic acid, in hemorrhagic shock in cats. *J Pharmacol Exp Ther* 231:610, 1984.

202. Bitterman H, Phillips GR III, Gragon G, et al: Potentiation of the protecting effects of a converting enzyme inhibitor and a thromboxane synthetase inhibitor in hemorrhagic shock. *J Pharmacol Exp Ther* 242:8, 1987.

203. Mulrow PJ, Ganong WF: The effect of hemorrhage upon aldosterone secretion in normal and hypophysectomized dogs. *J Clin Invest* 40:579, 1961.

204. Skillman JJ, Lawler DP, Hickler RB, et al: Hemorrhage in normal man: Effect on renin, cortisol, aldosterone, and urine composition. *Ann Surg* 166:865, 1967.

205. Ganong WF, Mulrow PJ: Role of the kidney in the adrenocortical responses to hemorrhage in hypophysectomized dogs. *Endocrinology* 70:182, 1962.

206. White FN, Gold EM, Vaughn DL: Renin-aldosterone system in endotoxin shock in the dog. *Am J Physiol* 212:1195, 1967.

207. Farrell GL, Rosnagle RS, Rauschkolb EW: Increased aldosterone secretion in response to blood loss. *Circ Res* 4:606, 1956.

208. Oliver G, Shafer EA: On the physiologic actions of extracts of pituitary body. *J Physiol* 18:227, 1895.

209. Zerbe RL, Feuerstein G, Meyer DK, et al: Cardiovascular, sympathetic and renin-angiotensin system responses to hemorrhage in vasopressin deficient rats. *Endocrinology* 111:608, 1982.

210. Gauer OH, Henry JP, Behn C: The regulation of extracellular fluid volume. *Annu Rev Physiol* 32:547, 1971.

211. Goetz KL, Bond GC, Hermreck AS, et al: Plasma ADH levels following a decrease in mean atrial transmural pressure in dogs. *Am J Physiol* 219:1424, 1970.

212. Share L: Control of plasma ADH titer in hemorrhage: Role of atrial and arterial receptors. *Am J Physiol* 215:1384, 1968.

213. Johnson JA, Zehr JE, Moore WW: Effects of separate and concurrent osmotic and volume stimuli on plasma ADH in sheep. *Am J Physiol* 218:1273, 1970.

214. Goetz KL, Bond GC, Smith WE: Effect of moderate hemorrhage in humans on plasma AVP and renin. *Proc Soc Exp Biol Med* 145:277, 1974.

215. Robertson GL: The role of osmotic and hemodynamic variables in regulation vasopressin, in James VHT (ed): *Proceedings of the Fifth International Congress of Endocrinology, Hamburg, July 1976* (Exerpta Medica Congress, Series No. 402). Amsterdam, Exerpta Medica, 1977, pp 126–130.

216. Zerbe RL, Bayorh MA, Feuerstein G: Vasopressin: An essential pressor factor for blood pressure recovery following hemorrhage. *Peptides* 3:509, 1982.

217. Gann DS, Ward DG, Carlson DE: Neural control of ACTH: A hemostatic reflex. *Recent Prog Horm Res* 34:357, 1978.

218. Gann DS: Parameters of the stimulus initiating the adrenocorticol response to hemorrhage. *Ann NY Acad Sci* 156:740, 1969.

219. Cryer GL, Gann DS: Right atrial receptors mediate the adrenocorticol response to small hemorrhage. *Am J Physiol* 227:325, 1974.

220. Donzalex-Lugue A, L'Age M, Dharimal APS, et al: Stimulation of corticotropin release by corticotropin-releasing factor or by vasopressin following intrapituitary infusions in unanesthetized dogs: Inhibition of responses by dexamethasone. *Endocrinology* 86:1134, 1970.

221. Ganong WF, Mulrow PJ: Responses of adrenal corticosteroid secretion to hypotension and hypovolemia. *J Clin Invest* 44:1, 1965.

222. Keller-Wood ME, Dallman MF: Corticosteroid inhibition of ACTH secretion. *Endocrinol Rev* 5:1, 1984.

223. Lilly MP, Engeland WC, Gann DS: Adrenal response to repeated hemorrhage: Implications for studies of trauma. *J Trauma* 22:809, 1982.

224. Gann DS, Cryer GL, Pirkle JC Jr: Physiologic inhibition and facilitation of adrenocorticol response to hemorrhage. *Am J Physiol* 232:R5, 1977.

225. Banting FG, Gairns S: Suprarenal insufficiency. *Am J Physiol* 77:100, 1926.

226. Rogoff JM, Stewart GN: Studies on adrenal insufficiency. *Am J Physiol* 84:649, 1928.

227. Gaudino M, Levitt MF: Influences of the adrenal cortex on body water distribution and renal function. *J Clin Invest* 28:1487, 1949.

228. Swingle WW, DaVango JP, Crossfield HC, et al: Glucocorticoids and maintenance of blood pressure and plasma volume of adrenalectomized dogs subjected to stress. *Proc Soc Exp Biol Med* 100:617, 1959.

229. Marks LJ, King DW, Kingsbury PF, et al: Physiologic role of the adrenal cortex in the maintenance of plasma volume following hemorrhage or surgical operations. *Surgery* 58:510, 1965.

230. Pirkle JC Jr, Gann DS: Restitution of blood volume after hemorrhage: Role of the adrenal cortex. *Am J Physiol* 230:1683, 1976.

231. Byrnes GT, Pirkle JC Jr, Gann DS: Cardiovascular stabilization after hemorrhage depends upon restitution of blood volume. *J Trauma* 18:623, 1978.

232. Moore FD: The effects of hemorrhage on body composition. *N Engl J Med* 273:567, 1965.

233. Cope O, Litwin SB: Contribution of the lymphatic system to the replenishment of plasma volume following a hemorrhage. *Ann Surg* 156:655, 1962.

234. Malt RA, Wang C, Yamazaki Z, et al: Stimulation of albumin synthesis by hemorrhage. *Surgery* 66:65, 1969.

235. Brooks DK, Williams WG, Manley RW, et al: Osmolar and electrolyte changes in hemorrhagic shock. *Lancet* 1:521, 1963.

236. Boyd DR, Mansberger AR: Serum water and osmolal changes in hemorrhagic shock. *Ann Surg* 34:744, 1968.

237. Farhült J, Holmberg J, Lundvall J, et al: Hyperglycemic and hyperosmolar responses to graded hemorrhage. *Acta Physiol Scand* 97:470, 1976.

238. Gann DS: Carotid vascular receptors and control of adrenal corticosteroid secretion. *Am J Physiol* 211:193, 1966.

239. Friedman SG, Pearce FJ, Drucker WR: The role of blood glucose in defense of plasma volume during hemorrhage. *J Trauma* 22:86, 1982.

240. Gann DS: Endocrine control of plasma protein and volume. *Surg Clin North Am* 56:1135, 1976.

241. Gann DS, Carlson DE, Byrnes GJ, et al: Role of solute in the early restitution of blood volume after hemorrhage. *Surgery* 94:439, 1983.

242. Gelfand RA, Mathews DE, Bier DM, et al: Role of the counterregulatory hormones in the catabolic response to stress. *J Clin Invest* 74:2238, 1984.

243. Gann DS, Pirkle JC Jr: Role of cortisol in the restitution of blood volume after hemorrhage. *Am J Surg* 130:565, 1975.

244. Pirkle JC Jr, Gann DS: Restitution of blood volume after hemorrhage: Role of the adrenal cortex. *Am J Physiol* 230:1683, 1976.

245. Pirkle JC Jr, Gann DS, Allen-Rowlands CF: Role of the pituitary in restoration of blood volume after hemorrhage. *Endocrinology* 110:7, 1982.

246. Gann DS, Carlson DE, Byrnes GJ, et al: Impaired restitution of blood volume after large hemorrhage. *J Trauma* 21:598, 1981.

247. Shires T, Coln D, Carrico J, et al: Fluid therapy in hemorrhagic shock. *Arch Surg* 88:688, 1964.

248. Thurau K: Renal hemodynamics. *Am J Med* 36:698, 1964.

249. Shipley RE, Study RS: Changes in renal blood flow, extraction of inulin, GFR, tissue pressure, and urine flow with acute alterations of renal artery pressure. *Am J Physiol* 167:676, 1951.

250. Blantz RC: Segmental renal vascular resistance: a single nephron. *Annu Rev Physiol* 42:573, 1980.

251. Laiken ND, Fanestil DD: Filtration and blood flow, in West JB (ed): *Physiologic Basis of Medical Practice,* 12th ed. Baltimore, Williams & Wilkins, 1991, pp 419–439.

252. McGiff JC, Fasy TM: The relationship of renal vascular activity of angiotensin II to the autonomic system. *J Clin Invest* 44:1911, 1965.

253. Barger AC, Herd JH: The renal circulation. *N Engl J Med* 284:482, 1971.

254. Carriere S, Friborg J: Intrarenal blood flow and PAH extraction during angiotensin infusion. *Am J Physiol* 217:1708, 1969.

255. Passmore JC, Strauss HL, Kolozsi WZ: Intrarenal blood flow in carotid sinus nerve stimulation and hemorrhage in dogs. *Kidney Int* 8:135, 1975.

256. Hock CE, Passmore JC, Levin JI, et al: Angiotensin II and alpha-adrenergic control of intrarenal circulation in hemorrhage. *Circ Shock* 9:81, 1982.

257. Johnson PC, Hansom KM: Effect of arterial pressure on arterial and venous resistance of intestine. *J Appl Physiol* 17:503, 1962.

258. Haglund U, Lundgren O: Reactions within consecutive vascular sections of the small intestine of the cat during prolonged hypotension. *Acta Physiol Scand* 84:151, 1972.

259. Lundgren O, Svanvik J: Mucosal hemodynamics in the small intestine of the cat during reduced perfusion pressure. *Acta Physiol Scand* 88:551, 1973.

260. Dressel PB, Folkow B, Wallentin I: Rubidium[86] clearance during neurogenic redistribution of intestinal blood flow. *Acta Physiol Scand* 67:173, 1966.

261. Folkow B, Lewis DH, Lundgren O, et al: The effect of graded vasoconstriction fibre stimulation on the intestinal resistance and capacitance vessels. *Acta Physiol Scand* 61:445, 1964.

262. Hultèn L, Lindhagen J, Lundgren O, et al: Sympathetic nervous control of intramural blood flow in feline and human intestines. *Gastroenterology* 72:41, 1977.

263. Svanvik J: The effect of reduced perfusion pressure and regional sympathetic vasoconstrictor activation on the rate of absorption of ^{85}Kr from the small intestine of the cat. *Acta Physiol Scand* 89:239, 1973.

264. Rapela CE, Green HD: Autoregulation of canine cerebral blood flow. *Circ Res* 15(suppl 1): I205, 1964.

265. Slater G, Vladeck BC, Bassen R, et al: Sequential changes in cerebral blood flow and distribution of flow within the brain during hemorrhagic shock. *Ann Surg* 181:1, 1975.

266. Rapela CE, Green HD, Denison AB Jr: Baroreceptor reflexes and autoregulation of cerebral blood flow in the dog. *Circ Res* 21:559, 1967.

267. Girsham JW, Nopanetaya W: Scanning electron microscopy of hepatic microvessels: review of methods and results, in Lautt WW (ed): *The Circulation of the Liver in Health and Disease*. New York, Plenum Press, 1981, pp 87–109.

268. Lautt WW: Control of hepatic and intestinal blood flow: Effect of isovolemic haemodilution on blood flow and oxygen uptake in the intact liver and intestines. *J Physiol* 265:313, 1977.

269. Richardson PDI, Withrington PG: Liver blood flow: I. Intrinsic and nervous control of liver blood flow. *Gastroenterology* 81:159, 1981.

270. Lautt WW: Control of hepatic arterial flow: independence from liver metabolic activity. *Am J Physiol* 239:H559, 1980.

271. Gelman SI: The effect of enteral oxygen administration on the hepatic circulation during halothane anesthesia: Experimental investigations. *Br J Anaesth* 47:1253, 1975.

272. Lautt WW: Role and control of the hepatic artery, in Lautt WW (ed): *The Circulation of the Liver in Health and Disease*. New York, Plenum Press, 1981, pp 203–226.

273. Greenway CV, Stark RD, Lautt WW: Capacitance responses and fluid exchange in the cat liver during stimulation of the hepatic nerves. *Circ Res* 25:277, 1969.

274. Cowley RA, Hankins JR, Jones RT, et al: Pathology and pathophysiology of the liver, in Crowley RA, Trump BF (eds): *Pathophysiology of Shock, Anoxia and Ischemia*. Baltimore, Williams & Wilkins, 1982, pp 285–301.

3

PHYSIOLOGY OF SHOCK AND INJURY

Arthur E. Baue

Shock is a manifestation of the rude unhinging of the machinery of life.

Samuel Gross, 1862[1]

Accidental injury, interpersonal violence, planned or emergency operations, and many acute illnesses produce demands on the circulatory system while contributing to its failure. An inadequate circulation or failure of the circulation with shock is one of the most common problems in injured patients or in those undergoing operation. Support of the circulation has been a major achievement of modern medicine. The treatment of shock has become second nature to surgeons, emergency physicians, and intensivists.

For many years, traumatic or wound shock was thought to be a mysterious process produced by toxins, humors, or the neuroendocrine system. Beginning in the 1930s, Blalock[2] and others developed the concept of hypovolemia and provided evidence that the major circulatory problem after injury was loss of blood volume. This concept led to the treatment of traumatic shock by replacement of losses of blood and extracellular fluid volume. As recently as the beginning of World War II, however, shock or an inadequate circulation was a common cause of death in otherwise normal individuals after injury. At the beginning of World War II, shock was the single limiting disease recognized to cause morbidity and mortality after injury. During the war, the concepts of hypovolemia, volume replacement, and blood transfusions became better understood and accepted. Blood and plasma were made available for resuscitation, and hemodynamic studies eliminated the mystique of wound shock. Thus the treatment of the injured and of shock improved[3-5] so greatly that shock was no longer the limiting morbidity following injury.

Problems with the kidneys and the lungs soon followed.[6] Today, rapidly resuscitating injured patients by restoring and maintaining vascular and extracellular fluid volumes after an operation produce excellent support for the circulation. The association of circulatory failure with infection, cardiac disease, and central nervous system injury led to improved treatment of these problems as well. These definitions and concepts seem simple in retrospect, but recognizing them was difficult. Complexities that now confront us will seem simple to coming generations. Shock, although common and well understood by many, remains a critical factor in survival after injury or operation. In the recent experiences of the Regional Trauma Center at Yale–New Haven Hospital and in our reviews of multiple organ failure (MOF) after injury, the most important factors that predicted increased morbidity and mortality were the severity and duration of shock after injury or during operation. Thus shock remains a problem, particularly if it persists or is not treated expeditiously or adequately. Many of the effects of decreased blood flow on various organs are known. Information on systems such as the immune system, coagulation, and metabolism are being described. Among the concerns now facing us are the stresses that metabolic failure, sepsis, inflammation, and tissue necrosis place on the circulation and that further reduce blood flow to individual organs and alter intraorgan distribution of blood flow. The mediators of these changes are complex and interrelated. The world of cytokines, eicosanoids, complement activation, immune complexes, kinins, coagulation factors, white cells with proteases and superoxide radicals, adhesion molecules, endothelial factors, and intracellular factors such as heat shock proteins is now upon us. There is great excitement about this information and the potential it may have for patient care, but there is also great confusion. Much has been learned, and much remains to be learned.

Sepsis, cardiac depression, multiple systems disease, and multiple systems injury continue to present problems for adequate and complete circulatory support. Support of the circulation remains the most critical factor in preventing MOF.[7] Reduced blood flow to various organs with ischemia and its affects on cell function seems to underlie much of this syndrome. Therefore, both overall blood flow with an adequate circulation and blood flow to each of the various organ systems become important.

HISTORICAL NOTES

Recognition of a depression of vital processes after injury began in antiquity. Homer, Hippocrates, and writers of the Old Testament clearly recognized the problem of blood loss after injury. As with other knowledge in the arts and sciences, the fundamental importance of hypovolemia after injury and operation was forgotten for centuries. During the Renaissance, the problems with injury were ascribed to mystical relationships. Even though Ambroise Paré[8] wrote in the sixteenth century that "the cause of swooning that happens to those who are wounded is—bleeding"; he and others practiced blood letting. Paré wrote that phlebotomy is "required in great wounds when there is fear of deflexion, pain, delirium, raving, and unquietness." Later, Le Dran,[9] in his description of shock, wrote that "this coldness may likewise be occasioned by a loss of blood." Clarke,[9] in his translation of Le Dran's treatise, used the word *shock* to convey the impression of a blow or jolt (a *comonotio*, "commotion," or concussion with an injury leading to deterioration, loss of consciousness, and death). Le Dran had used the word *secousse* or *saisissement*. The word *shock* was next used by John Latta[10] in 1795 to describe the clinical picture after injury. Thomas Latta[11] first used saline in 1831 for the treatment of hypovolemic shock due to cholera. Despite this knowledge, shock was treated by strychnine and stimulants as late as the Boer War (1899–1902). Often the injury or insult seemed small in relationship to the profound effect of shock on the patient. Sir Astley Cooper,[12] in his "Commentary on War Injuries," described the enigma of soldiers dying without significant blood loss, severe pain, or gross injury. The best clinical description of this dilemma was provided by John Collins Warren[13] in 1895:

> A patient is brought into the hospital with a compound comminuted fracture or with a dislocation of the hip joint added to other injuries where the bleeding has been slight. As the litter is gently deposited on the floor, he makes no effort to move or look about him. He lies staring at the surgeon with an expression of complete indifference as to his condition. There is no movement of the muscles of the face; the eyes, which are deeply sunken in their sockets, have a weird, uncanny look. The features are pinched and the face shrunken. A cold, clammy sweat exudes from the pores of the skin, which has an appearance of anemia. The lips are bloodless, and the fingers and nails are blue. The pulse is almost imperceptible; a weak, thread-like stream may, however, be detected in the radial artery. The thermometer, placed in the rectum, registers 96 or 97°F. The muscles are not paralyzed anywhere, but the patient seems disinclined to make any muscular effort. Even respiratory movements seem, for the time, to be reduced to a minimum. Occasionally, the patient may feebly throw about one of his limbs and give vent to a hoarse, weak groan. There is no insensibility (coma is not observed in cases of shock), but he is strangely apathetic and seems to realize but imperfectly the full meaning of the questions put to him. It is of no use to attempt an operation until appropriate remedies have brought about a reaction. The pulse, however, does not respond; it grows feebler and finally disappears and, "this momentary pause in the act of death" is soon followed by the grim reality. A postmortem examination reveals no visible changes in the internal organs.

Early studies of the circulation and its control during the beginnings of experimental physiology by Claude Bernard, Brown-Sequard, and Charcot led to the concept that shock was the result of inhibition of the vasomotor center, producing weakening of the heartbeat and peripheral pooling of blood. In 1889, George W. Crile,[14] who worked originally with Victor Horseley in London, published a series of pioneering experimental studies of shock. He defined the importance of venous pressures and failure of venous return in hemorrhagic shock, of fluid loss in shock, and of saline therapy. Nine years later, Yendel Henderson[15] wrote that "venous pressure is, so to speak, the fulcrum of circulation. Shock, as physicians use the word, is due to failure of the fulcrum."

The first systematic observations of clinical shock came during World War I, when Cannon and Bayliss[16] led a team of physiologists and clinicians who provided descriptions in the injured of a fall in blood volume, reduction in alkali reserve, accumulation of fixed acids, loss of vasomotor tone, cardiac failure, and stagnation in venous reservoirs. Keith[17] used dye dilution methods to show that the severity of shock correlated with reductions in blood volume. Archibald and McLean[18] recognized the differences between blood flow and blood pressure in shock and emphasized the importance of decreased blood flow. However, shock from injury without external blood loss or with crush injury and in patients who did not respond to blood, gum acacia, or saline solutions was a problem. This was not understood as hypovolemia per se, but rather as a problem of blood vessels holding fluid in the circulation. The problem was called *wound shock* or *secondary shock.* Toxins were sought as an explanation, and from the work of Dale and Richards[19] at that time, histamine was implicated in producing "traumatic toxemia."

In 1930, Blalock[20] and Parsons and Phemister,[21] working independently, documented that shock after trauma was due to blood and plasma loss in and around the wounds and not due to a toxin. Blalock further documented the importance of blood transfusion for such injuries and showed that histamine was not a factor. Despite this, until the middle of World War II, the definition of shock by the National Research Conference was "the clinical condition characterized by progressive reduction in the circulatory blood volume due to increased capillary permeability." During World War II, further contributions were made by trauma research units such as the one headed by Henry K. Beecher[22] in the Mediterranean theater. Their studies indicated that the major cause of shock was hemorrhage and fluid loss that leads to acidosis. Cournand and associates[23] first measured cardiac output in patients in shock in 1943 and ascribed traumatic shock to an inadequate return of blood flow to the heart. Surgical research units during the Korean War documented the importance of triage, early resuscitation, and evaluation.[24] Posttraumatic renal insufficiency was described as occurring when fluid resuscitation was not as rapid or as extensive as required for renal function. During the Vietnam conflict, shock and renal failure were no longer major clinical problems, but infection and posttraumatic pulmonary insufficiency were identified as frequent limitations after injury or operation. Head injury, infection, and MOF are now the major limitations after trauma. The development of knowledge about septic and cardiogenic shock will be described later.

DEFINITIONS OF SHOCK

Shock was first used as a medical term in 1743 in Clarke's English translation of French surgeon Henri Francois Le Dran's *A Treatise, or Reflections, Drawn from Practice on Gun-Shot Wounds.*[9] Even though the term *shock* has been criticized for its vagueness, it is a valuable word because injury, whether accidental or produced by operation, frequently results in circulatory abnormalities. *Shock* is no more exact than *fever,* but it does describe a clinical abnormality that requires immediate attention to improve blood flow. An all-encompassing definition of shock—wherein shock becomes the final common pathway of many disease processes—is meaningless.

Definitions from the past reflect the emphasis and understanding of their times. In 1876, Samuel Gross[1] described shock as a "manifestation of the rude unhinging of the machinery of life." John Collins Warren,[13] in 1895, said that shock was a "momentary pause in the act of death." Blalock,[2] after extensive studies, wrote, "Shock is a peripheral circulatory failure resulting from a discrepancy in the size of the vascular bed and the volume of the intravascular fluid." In 1942, Wiggers[25] further emphasized the concept of an inadequate circulating blood volume. "Shock is a syndrome that results from a depression of many functions, but in which reduction of the effective circulating blood volume is of basic importance, and in which impairment of the circulation steadily progresses until it eventuates in a state of irreversible circulatory failure." The emphasis was on blood volume, which eventually led to the concept of hypovolemia after injury. Harkins and Long[26] provided a pathophysiologic definition, describing shock as "progressive vasoconstrictive oligemic anoxia." Simeone[27] gave a broad definition a few years ago: "[Shock is] a clinical condition characterized by signs and symptoms, which arise when the cardiac output is insufficient to fill the arterial tree with blood, under sufficient pressure to provide organs and tissues with adequate blood flow." Significant then are blood volume, the vascular system, the heart, and the distribution of blood flow, each of which can be abnormal. These are the major determinants of cardiac output.

Shock is not just a transient decrease in blood pressure, as in syncope or hypotension alone, since controlled hypotension produced by ganglionic block during anesthesia allows normal nutrient blood flow to tissues. Shock is also an acute generalized problem of the entire individual, even though it may later produce failure of a single organ system such as the kidney. The circulation conducts its affairs at the capillary level. The common thread in all forms of shock is an inadequate circulation with diminished blood flow to tissues. This produces organ and cell ischemia, hypoxia, and their sequelae.[7] Haldane described the final result of this process, saying that anoxia not only stops the machine but wrecks the machinery.

CLASSIFICATION

The classification of shock into hypovolemic, septic, cardiogenic, and neurogenic categories is well known and serves as an initial framework for discussion and therapy. Shock with injury is usually hypovolemic and introduces the complexities of the biologic response to injury. A classification is necessary not only for research but also for our clinical understanding to define the etiology and, particularly, to recognize the hemodynamic manifestations upon which treatment must be based. Thus shock can be classified according to etiology, or it can be classified according to the hemodynamic manifestations that we see in the patient in the operating room, emergency department, or intensive care unit. Both classifications must be considered, but they may or may not be similar, depending on the patient and the circumstances.

ETIOLOGY

The four components of the circulation that determine cardiac output or blood flow are preload (ventricular filling pressure and volume), afterload (peripheral vascular resistance), contractility (inotropic function of the myocardium), and heart rate (chronotropy). Abnormalities of any one of these components may produce shock. The etiology of shock can then be classified into these four general categories based on the abnormal circulatory component. Inadequate blood volume (low preload) is called *hypovolemic shock*. If the heart cannot provide an adequate cardiac output, the result is called *cardiogenic shock* (pump failure). The inability of the circulation to meet the need for increased blood flow and the decreased peripheral vascular resistance required or produced by infection is called *septic shock.* Many mediators are involved in this clinical problem. *Neurogenic shock* (low afterload) is inability of the nervous system or peripheral circulation to maintain vascular resistance. Many other problems, although associated with hypotension or circulatory failure, are not considered primary circulatory problems. These problems include various types of organ failure such as adrenal cortical insufficiency or hepatic failure; injuries such as traumatic tension pneumothorax, flail chest, vena caval obstruction or compression; and problems such as electrolyte abnormalities and increased intracranial pressure.

If shock is associated with or produced by tissue injury during or after an operation or with trauma, then additional factors are activated. An inflammatory response by various cells and mediators with tissue injury will produce additional changes in the circulation, the microcirculation, and cell and organ function. Thus the circulatory failure after injury may be primarily or initially a problem of hypovolemia, but other factors will be operational.

Hypovolemic shock may be further classified according to the type of fluid lost: blood loss alone from a bleeding duodenal ulcer; loss of fluid with a high protein content, as with a burn or perforated ulcer; extracellular fluid loss with intestinal obstructions; or water loss from fever and hyperventilation (Table 3–1). Synonyms for hypovolemic shock include *oligemic* or *hemorrhagic shock, traumatic shock, wound shock,* and *burn shock.* The location of the loss and the disease or injury producing the loss also may be part of such categorization.

Shock with tissue injury (traumatic or wound shock) is usually a combination of hemorrhagic or hypovolemic shock with tissue (organ or cell) injury. The tissue injury initiates a response by the patient, an inflammatory, reparative response that occurs through cell aggregation and activation and the activation of mediators. This response, when appropriate, promotes healing of the wounds and survival. If the inflammatory response is overwhelming, there is increasing evidence that it becomes deleterious and may contribute to organ damage remote to the injury. This chain of events is thought to be a major factor in the development of MOF. Localized inflammation at the site of injury is essential; if the inflammatory process becomes generalized (systemic), then the lungs, liver, kidneys, and other systems may be damaged and may fail.

The effects of hypovolemia alone and the additional effects of tissue injury and inflammation may be studied in experimental animals but may be impossible to separate in humans. Cardiogenic and septic shock also may occur with tissue injury, such as after a cardiac operation or an injury with colon perforation and peritonitis. Thus the initial etiology and hemodynamic characteristics of shock with tissue injury will be those of hypovolemia. Later, mediator cell effects will be evident.

Cardiogenic shock is classified according to primary intrinsic problems of the heart or myocardium or problems extrinsic to the heart that interfere with its ability to provide adequate blood flow (see Table 3–1). Although valvular heart disease and other forms of congestive heart failure may eventually produce acute circulatory failure, they are not usually considered forms of shock.

Any type of infection may produce septic shock. The complex demands of an infection on the circulation fall into two categories: (1) an increase in circulation required by fever and infection and (2) alterations of the circulation, heart, and

TABLE 3–1. Classification of Shock

I. Hypovolemic shock
  A. Etiology
    1. Bleeding
    2. Burns
    3. Intestinal obstruction
    4. Perforated ulcer (early)
    5. Crush injury
    6. Dehydration
    7. Gastrointestinal
  B. Type of fluid lost
    1. Blood
    2. Plasma
    3. Extracellular (ECF) and extra-vascular fluid (salt and water loss or deficiency)
    4. Gastric contents, *succus entericus*, colonic loss
    5. Exudate
    6. Water
  C. Location of loss
    1. External loss—blood, water by sweating, vomitus, stool, fistulas
    2. Internal loss
II. Shock with tissue injury
  A. Etiology
    1. Trauma and/or operation with volume loss and an inflammatory response and mediator activation
  B. Type of fluid lost
    1. Blood
    2. ECF
  C. Location of loss
    1. External
    2. The wound—sequestration of ECF, blood, plasma, and hematomas
    3. Body cavities

III. Cardiogenic shock
  A. Intrinsic
    1. Myocardial infarction, ventricular aneurysm
    2. Myocardial contractility failure, ischemia or depression from sepsis, pulmonary failure, or late hypovolemia
    3. Myocardiopathy
    4. Myocardial contusion
    5. Arrhythmias—slow or rapid rates
    6. Drugs, including anesthetic agents
  B. Extrinsic
    1. Pulmonary embolism
    2. Cardiac tamponade
    3. Respiratory failure and pulmonary hypertension
    4. High levels of positive end-expiratory pressure
IV. Septic shock—Infection with bacteremia or septicemia from any gram-negative or gram-positive organisms or fungi
  A. Peritonitis
  B. Late abscesses
  C. Genitourinary instrumentation
  D. Septic abortion
  E. Intravenous catheters
  F. Pulmonary or other infections
  G. Toxic shock syndrome
V. Vasogenic or neurogenic shock
  A. Spinal anesthesia
  B. Spinal cord injury
  C. Anaphylactic shock

vascular bed with peripheral vasodilatation, which is produced by the infection or its metabolic products and mediators.

Vasogenic and neurogenic shock is primarily a problem of loss of vascular tone or resistance of both the peripheral arterial and venous capacitance systems. Vasogenic shock may result from injuries to the central nervous system or from agents that block peripheral vascular tone, such as a spinal anesthetic.

HEMODYNAMIC MANIFESTATIONS

Generally, the five categories or causes of shock produce characteristic hemodynamic pictures that can be distinguished from one another. All, of course, have the manifestations of inadequate peripheral tissue and organ perfusion, but they differ in an inadequate cardiac filling pressure with hypovolemia, a high filling pressure with cardiogenic shock, and a hyperdynamic (albeit inadequate) circulation with early septic shock. However, clinical manifestations are frequently not so neatly categorized, and an abnormality may not occur in pure form. Clinical characteristics are determined not only by the cause of the abnormality but also by the patient's condition at the time shock develops and by the stage of disease or injury. One must therefore recognize not only the cause of shock but also the exact hemodynamic manifestations that are present in each patient. This is important because hypovolemia is frequently present, no matter what the cause of shock. Increasing the vascular volume by infusing fluids may be helpful in many patients with shock from causes other than hypovolemia. As an illustration of the importance of individual characteristics, an elderly patient with severe coronary artery disease with gastrointestinal bleeding and circulatory failure may be said to have hypovolemic shock based on the cause of the problem. However, the presence of coronary artery disease would decrease myocardial blood flow, possibly producing ventricular failure. Thus the hemodynamic manifestation in such a patient may be that of cardiogenic shock with a high central venous pressure. In contrast, a patient whose circulatory failure results from an acute myocardial infarction may previously have had a salt restriction program and diuretic therapy that decreased extracellular blood vol-

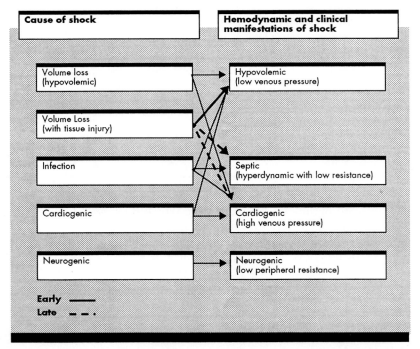

FIG. 3–1. The interrelationships of the cause or etiology of shock and the hemodynamic manifestations will vary depending on the previous health and complexities that occur in an injury.

ume. The hemodynamic manifestations in this patient may be those of hypovolemic shock (decreased filling pressures). The same may be true in a patient with sepsis. Sepsis often produces peripheral vasodilatation and a hyperdynamic circulation that requires a high cardiac output. The central venous pressure may be extremely low, indicating the need for volume replacement and, therefore, simulating the hemodynamic picture of hypovolemic shock. Cardiac failure also may be produced by sepsis, or the vasodilatation of sepsis in itself may be excessive. The etiology of shock after injury is hypovolemic initially, but later, with an inflammatory response, there may be sepsis (septic shock) or cardiac depression and failure. The interrelationships of these are shown in Fig. 3–1.

EVALUATION

Rapidly assessing the circulation and the patient shows the magnitude and urgency of the problem, the cause, and the hemodynamic manifestations. Assessment is followed by insertion of venous and arterial conduits for therapy and monitoring and by institution of other methods of support as required. The manifestations of shock vary with the severity, stage, and cause of the problem. In early circulatory failure, the various causes of shock may produce strikingly different clinical characteristics. In late shock or the terminal stages, however, the clinical picture is similar, no matter what the cause. Patients may have evidence

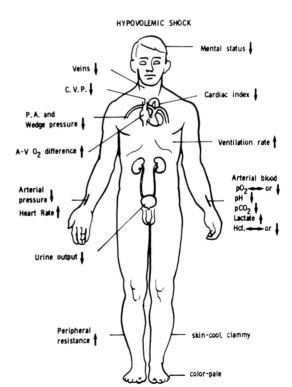

FIG. 3–2. The clinical and hemodynamic characteristics of hypovolemic shock.

of both decreased blood flow to all organs and tissues and sympathoadrenal stimulation (cold, clammy, cyanotic).[7]

In severely wounded soldiers, Beecher et al.[22] defined three grades of hypovolemic shock that are still accurate. With *slight shock* (i.e., acute loss of less than 20 percent of blood volume), blood pressure is normal or even increases slightly and pulse is normal or increased, but the skin is cool and pale. The skin and nails blanch with pressure, and a somewhat distressed mental state develops. *Moderate shock* is defined as a 20 to 40 percent reduction in blood volume, characterized by a decrease in pulse volume and blood pressure, an increase in pulse rate, and a thready pulse with cool and pale skin, prolonged blanching, thirst, and apathy. *Severe shock* is defined as a blood volume decrease of 40 percent or more and a blood pressure that is not recordable, with a pulse that is weak or imperceptible. The skin is cold, ashen, and cyanotic. Capillary filling is sluggish. A patient in severe shock is apathetic, stuporous, or comatose. If the patient is awake, he or she may have severe thirst. As shock progresses, the patient be-

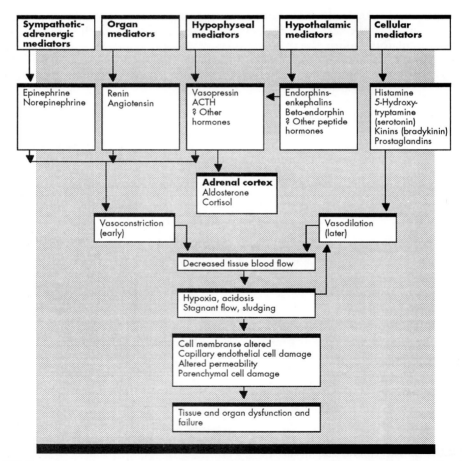

FIG. 3–3. The responses to injury and shock are protective initially, but eventually cell and organ failure occur.

comes fatigued and anxious, with restlessness that may progress to unrespon-
siveness. Patients who are not recumbent will have faintness, vertigo, and postural hypotension. The patient may be diaphoretic and have clammy skin. A
decrease in blood pressure and blood flow produces hyperventilation and tachycardia. Veins in the neck and extremities collapse. Muscles are weak, and the
body temperature is somewhat reduced. The clinical characteristics of hypovolemic shock are shown in Fig. 3–2. Some of the central nervous system depression that occurs with shock may be due to reduced blood flow and endorphin
secretion from the hypothalamus. Sympathoadrenal, hypothalamic, and hypo-
physeal reflexes affect the response to injury of an otherwise normal individual
(Fig. 3–3).

In the late phases of cardiogenic or septic shock, the patient's clinical appearance may be similar to that in hypovolemic shock. However, in the early stage
of cardiogenic shock, the patient has the manifestation of distended neck veins
and may have more difficulty breathing and less anxiety than seen following
injury (Fig. 3–4). The clinical manifestations of a patient in early septic shock
depend on the insult (Fig. 3–5). The patient commonly has had a shaking chill
with temperature elevation and is warm and dry, with a bounding pulse and
evidence of a hyperdynamic circulation and high cardiac output. MacLean[28,29]
described a prodrome of septic shock that includes hyperventilation, respiratory
alkalosis, and mental aberrations in a patient with sepsis. This prodrome may
occur before the blood pressure begins to fall and before other evidence of cir-

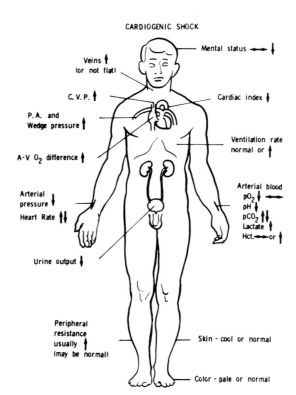

FIG. 3–4. The clinical and hemodynamic manifestations of cardiogenic shock.

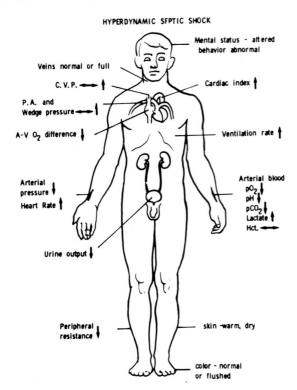

FIG. 3–5. The clinical and hemo-dynamic characteristics of early and hyperdynamic septic shock.

culatory failure arises. Sepsis requires a hyperdynamic circulation (increased cardiac output). As septic shock develops, the circulation may continue to be hyperdynamic in the early phases, provided the patient has an adequate extra-cellular and vascular volume. If the patient in early septic shock has an inadequate blood volume or myocardial compromise, an immediate hypodynamic circulation may occur, with low cardiac output and a constricted state similar to hypovolemic or cardiogenic shock. In all forms of shock the final or terminal phase is similar: reduced temperature, hypotension, decreased organ function, and apathy progressing to coma.

PATHOPHYSIOLOGY OF CIRCULATORY INADEQUACY

Although there are some similarities among the various forms of shock, particularly in the late or preterminal stages, the differences in mechanisms, manifestations, and pathologic physiology are so great that separate discussions of each are required. Decreased or inadequate blood flow brings about a complex homeostatic response to try to protect the individual and maintain perfusion of vital organs. A decrease in blood flow, whether due to decreased venous return or decreased cardiac output secondary to myocardial failure, will have similar compensatory mechanisms. These mechanisms will differ from the increased circulatory demands and vasodilatation of sepsis. Only in the end stage—the cold, clammy vasoconstrictive state—are these various shock states similar.

HYPOVOLEMIC SHOCK

ADAPTATION OF THE VASCULAR SYSTEM

With an altered circulation due to blood or fluid loss and a subsequent decrease in cardiac output, two things happen: First, there is cardiovascular system compensation for this alteration by neuroendocrine changes and transcapillary refilling.[30-32] Second, there are the effects of such changes in the circulation, including those on organ function, metabolism, the microcirculation, and cellular alterations. With loss of circulating volume, the major responses are to decrease the size of the vascular bed, maintain the circulation to the heart and brain, and mobilize body fluids to replace the loss.

When blood volume is lost, venous return to the heart is decreased and cardiac output is lessened. The medullary vasomotor center and the aortic arch and carotid baroreceptors sense the change in pressure and flow. This produces arterial and venous vasoconstriction, increased heart rate, and an inotropic effect on the ventricles due to sympathetic nervous system stimulation and decreased vagal tone. Arterial vasoconstriction in precapillary arterioles has the effect of maintaining central arterial blood pressure and redistributing flow to vital organs while decreasing flow to other organs and tissues. Since the arterial system is a small part of the overall vascular system, arterial vasoconstriction does little to decrease the size of the vascular bed or to shift blood volume to the central circulation. The decrease in volume of the circulatory bed occurs primarily through vasoconstriction of capacitance vessels existing in the venous system. This effect shifts more blood to the central circulation and tends to maintain venous pressure and return. There are endothelium-derived factors that play a role in vascular reactivity. The endothelins have potent vasoconstrictor properties. Endothelium-derived relaxing factors may be involved with reactive hyperemia.

The splanchnic bed in humans is the primary capacitance region, and 500 to 1000 ml of blood may be made available by venoconstriction in this area. Depending on the volume of loss, the initial compensatory mechanisms may be able to maintain a reasonable blood pressure, cardiac output, and venous return. Thus a loss of 350 to 400 ml of blood (as in a blood donation) may produce no particular hemodynamic effect, especially if the patient remains recumbent. Homeostatic mechanisms compensate for moderate blood or extracellular fluid (ECF) loss. However, syncope may occur even after giving a unit of blood as a blood donor. Donors are given juice to drink and kept recumbent for a period of time, until the circulation adjusts to this modest loss. A feeling of light-headedness, syncope, or postural hypotension may occur if an individual sits up rapidly in such a circumstance. If an individual loses 800 to 1000 ml of blood over a few minutes, the effect may be profound. If the loss occurs slowly over hours, compensatory mechanisms may allow replenishment with only postural hypotension. A fairly rapid loss of 1000 to 1500 ml of blood will produce evidence of circulatory inadequacy with hypotension, reduced organ flow, and beginning signs of shock. Losses larger than this produce severe shock and will not allow survival unless treatment is provided.

After circulatory adjustments to maximize central blood flow and pressure to vital organs for survival, mechanisms begin to refill the circulation. Volume is restored to the circulation by two mechanisms: transcapillary refilling of the circulation from extravascular and extracellular fluid and restoration of protein to the circulation leading to increased oncotic pressure. The first phase of restoration of fluid volume occurs because of Starling forces resulting from a fall in capillary hydrostatic pressure due to arteriolar vasoconstriction. Fluid moves from the extravascular (extracellular) space into the capillaries (Fig. 3–6). This phenomenon has been studied by Skillman and coworkers,[30] who found that after the loss of 500 to 1000 ml of blood, plasma volume refilling in the capillary bed was usually quite rapid—as high as 2 ml/min initially and then decreasing with time. Plasma volume was restored to normal in 24 to 48 h. These workers found that albumin entered the circulation rapidly, at rates up to 4 g/h initially. Synthesis of protein also increased, along with a decreased rate of protein degradation. The return of protein to the circulation seems to depend initially on interstitial fluid that is then restored by oral ingestion or by intravenous injection. Participation of cells and cell water in this phenomenon has been studied by Gann and colleagues,[32] who believe that an extracellular increase in solute occurring with shock, particularly by glucose and, perhaps, other osmotically active solutes, draws water out of cells and into the interstitial space. A number of factors may influence this effect, including solute concentration in the splanchnic bed, glucose, cortisol, and, perhaps, epinephrine, along with adequate nutrition and prior hydration.

If an individual suffers from malnutrition or dehydration before injury or operation, compensation may not be possible. In severe or late hypovolemic shock, a number of other factors may be involved in this failure of compensation, including impaired vasomotor activity and an alteration in the macromolecules and collagen in the interstitial space, leading to the uptake or binding of fluids. Cell swelling also may occur. With cell ischemia, sodium is taken up into the cell and potassium is lost. There is increased hydration of cells, which results in a further decrease in ECF volume. Shires and his group[33] used measurements of cell transmembrane potential and ECF volume measurements to show a greater decrease in ECF volume than could be explained by blood loss or injury alone.

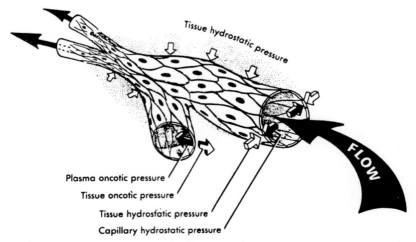

Tissue hydrostatic pressure

FLOW

Plasma oncotic pressure
Tissue oncotic pressure
Tissue hydrosfatic pressure
Capillary hydrostatic pressure

FIG. 3–6. The Starling forces in the capillary bed require a balance of oncotic and hydrostatic pressures, which allows capillary refilling with shock.

They introduced the concept of volume replacement of ECF, as well as blood, and replacement in a greater volume than might be predicted. In severe late shock, epinephrine, norepinephrine, and angiotensin may maintain high venous pressures. Such elevations in venous pressures may be deleterious because they prevent capillary refilling and increase capillary fluid loss.

NEUROENDOCRINE COMPENSATION

The metabolic and neuroendocrine response to injury is an important part of the stress reaction and teleologically provides a better opportunity for the biologic organism to survive under adverse circumstances or when injured. Shock, blood loss, and an inadequate circulation are powerful forces that initiate these changes. Thus the responses brought about by shock are similar to those occurring in patients with the stress of an injury. With starvation, bed rest, and a general anesthetic alone, the neuroendocrine response is minimal. With modest hemorrhage, there is an increase in adrenocorticotropic hormone (ACTH) secretion that stimulates cortisol release. Sympathetic activity is increased as an early response to hypovolemia, as is an increase in epinephrine from the adrenal medulla, when blood pressure and blood flow decrease. Additional stimuli include acidosis and hypercapnia. Peripheral release of norepinephrine contributes to the vasoconstriction.

Other effects of the stresses of hypovolemia or injury include the production of hyperglycemia due to glycogen breakdown from the liver, stimulation of glucagon production, decreased insulin production and depression of its peripheral actions, and stimulation of ACTH. Decreased renal blood flow and pulse pressure stimulate the juxtaglomerular apparatus to produce renin, which in turn stimulates the production of angiotensin. Angiotensin contributes its vasoconstrictor effect and stimulates the production of aldosterone. ACTH is released from the anterior pituitary and further increases aldosterone production, along with cortisol. The posterior pituitary secretes vasopressin or antidiuretic hormone (ADH) with its dual effect on the circulation and water retention by the kidney. Arginine vasopressin is a potent splanchnic bed vasoconstrictor, as is angiotensin II, but vasopressin also seems to help maintain blood pressure after shock is treated.[34]

The hypothalamus is activated with production of beta-endorphin, which increases vasopressin release and may have a morphine-like effect throughout the body. Central and peripheral opiate receptors are activated during blood loss and may contribute to hypotension.[35] The reason for this effect is not clear. The role, if any, of the other hypothalamic hormones such as somatostatin, thyrotropin-releasing factor, beta-lipoprotein, and other pituitary hormones such as prolactin, growth hormone, and thyroid-stimulating hormone (TSH) is not known. The gastrointestinal and metabolic hormones play a role after injury, but no specific activities of pancreatic polypeptide, vasoactive intestinal peptide, or secretin are recognized. The decrease in insulin and depression of its peripheral effects by epinephrine may be responsible for the diabetic-like state seen in the injured and shocked patient. Glucagon also may contribute.

Precise alterations and effects of cellular or tissue mediators such as the prostaglandin and kinin-kallikrein systems are not clear in humans. It seems likely that these systems may be an important factor in the deterioration seen in prolonged and severe shock. Studies in experimental animals suggest such a role. There is increasing evidence that while prolonged ischemia will result in tissue injury, with treatment there may be additional damage due to activation of circulating cells and mediators, a phenomenon termed *reperfusion injury* (see Ischemia-Reperfusion Problems, below).

CHANGES IN ORGAN AND SYSTEM FUNCTION WITH DECREASED BLOOD FLOW

Compensation for decreased vascular volume or for a decrease in cardiac output decreases blood flow to those areas which can tolerate ischemia for brief periods of time. These include the skin, muscle, the splanchnic bed, and the kidneys, where decreased flow also serves the purpose of fluid conservation. Compensation for a severe decrease in vascular volume, when carried out over a period of time, will eventually result in alterations in organ function. There is no particular stage or combination of hemodynamic variables in which shock is said to be present. Shock indicates an inadequate circulation with diminished blood pressure, cardiac output, and blood flow to organs so that compensation is either impossible or the compensation itself becomes deleterious. Many of the effects of decreased blood flow on various organs are known. Information on other systems, such as the immune system, coagulation, and metabolism, is being described.

When there is tissue injury from trauma, along with shock, the effects are additive. Many years ago, Overman and Wang[36] showed that stimulation of afferent nerve fibers from injured tissues reduced the survival time following hemorrhage. Little and Kirkman[37] and Anderson et al.[38] demonstrated that baroreflexes and heart rate responses to hemorrhage are depressed by peripheral tissue injury. Thus injury reduces the ability of a person to tolerate blood loss.

Kidney. As blood flow to the kidneys is decreased, there is an alteration in the intrarenal distribution of flow from the cortex to the medulla. This change is probably produced by aldosterone. There is also decreased renal function, with depression in glomerular filtration rate (GFR) and oliguria. Decreased free water clearance is one of the first measurements indicating reduced renal function. Medullary sodium is decreased, with loss of the medullary hyperosmolar zone and failure of the countercurrent concentrating system. If decreased blood flow continues, or if the kidney is presented large amounts of pigment (e.g., hemoglobin or myoglobin), eventually tubular necrosis and acute renal failure develop. If the injury is severe, total renal shutdown with anuria and rapid development of azotemia, hyperkalemia, and acidosis may develop. However, if the injury is not severe enough to produce oliguric or anuric renal failure, high output renal failure may result. This is a less severe injury that may be more difficult to recognize, since urine output may be normal or high despite the inability to excrete waste products and a progressive rise in blood urea nitrogen and creatinine.

Heart. With hypovolemia and decreased cardiac output, the central circulation is maintained initially, and coronary blood flow may be adequate, particularly if there is no occlusive disease of the coronary arteries. However, with further decreases in cardiac output, coronary flow may not keep pace. This may then contribute to a further decrease in cardiac output. Myocardial oxygen extraction is normally high, so increasing oxygen extraction is only of modest benefit, unless blood flow can be maintained or increased. The coronary circulation is subject to autoregulation and dilates as cardiac output decreases, but this may not be adequate if the decrease in cardiac output is extensive or if the patient has coronary artery disease. ECG changes of myocardial ischemia, premature ventricular contractions, and other arrhythmias may be seen. The ischemic heart produces lactate, rather than using it for metabolic needs. There is also altered utilization of free fatty acids. Myocardial depression is said to occur in late or severe septic shock. In any form of circulatory failure there may ultimately be depression of the myocardium that would be expressed clinically by low cardiac output and a high and rising venous pressure. Whether such changes in late shock in humans are due to toxic factors depressing the myocardium or are simply the late result of a prolonged decrease in blood flow has not been determined. Thus, no matter what the etiology of the shock, a careful search for adequacy of ventricular performance is necessary.

Liver. Although decreased splanchnic blood flow, including flow to the liver, occurs with any form of circulatory failure, the immediate acute manifestations of hepatic ischemia are difficult to recognize or describe. Certainly it is known that there is decreased ability to metabolize lactate and, perhaps, to detoxify other substances. Synthetic activities of the liver are probably depressed, such as the production of albumin and other acute phase proteins. With severe shock there may be elevation of certain enzymes suggesting hepatic injury. Alterations in Bromsulphalein (BSP) retention or an abnormal cephalin flocculation test also may accompany the shock state. However, the effects of ischemia on the liver may not be evident until later, when bilirubin increases and other aspects of hepatic function are altered. Depression of the reticuloendothelial system and, particularly, the Kupffer cells in the liver, may be of clinical importance. Much more study is required, especially in humans, on the acute effects of hepatic ischemia with shock.

Brain. Cerebral blood flow during circulatory failure is maintained at the expense of other organ systems. Blood flow to the brain remained stable up to a withdrawal of blood of 30 mg/kg of body weight in a study in dogs.[39] Despite this preservation of flow, there are often alterations in the sensorium; a distressed mental state, apathy, diminished responsiveness, fatigue, anxiety, and other manifestations may attend the shock state. Blood flow is preferentially protected in brain areas that control the cardiovascular system. Electroencephalographic activity may be depressed if circulatory failure and hypotension are severe. Clinical response is variable, however, since even with severe hypotension an individual may remain lucid. After cerebral ischemia, brain edema may be a manifestation of secondary brain damage.

Gastrointestinal Tract. The gastrointestinal tract has decreased activity with shock. Decreased blood flow to the gastric mucosa makes it more susceptible to injury. This, along with hydrochloric acid in the stomach, contributes eventually to stress ulceration and bleeding.

The splanchnic circulation is a major resistance and capacitance region for circulatory support. With decreased blood flow, blood is shunted to the mucosa of the bowel. This mechanism may involve the prostaglandin pathway, particularly prostacyclin.[40] However, prolonged shock decreases prostacyclin synthesis in the gut, which may allow the vasoconstrictor prostaglandin thromboxane to dominate.[41] The effects of vasopressin and angiotensin II also may contribute to bowel ischemia. It has been suggested that this ischemia may initiate the production of toxins such as myocardial depressant factor and proteolytic enzymes. With hemorrhage in experimental animals, loss of tight junctions in small intestinal mucosal cells, subepithelial edema, and mucosal erosions occur, and gut absorptive capacity is decreased.[42] After ischemia, bacterial translocation of organisms from the gut lumen to mesenteric lymph nodes has been found to occur.[43] However, Gelfand et al.[44] found no bacterial translocation after prolonged hypoperfusion and hypovolemia in pigs. Ferarro et al.[45] found increased survival after hemorrhagic shock in germ-free animals. Rush et al.[46,47] found that rats subjected to hemorrhagic shock commonly demonstrated bacteremia and endotoxemia. In patients admitted to a trauma unit with a blood pressure of less than 80 mmHg, 56 percent had positive blood cultures. Endotoxemia also was demonstrable in several of these patients. We are reminded of Jacob Fine's thesis on the importance of gut bacteria in problems of shock.[48] Thus ischemia of the splanchnic bed may be a factor with prolonged shock, but its role in humans is not completely understood. After shock with injury, the gut undergoes atrophy if it is not used. This also may contribute to bacterial translocation. Methods of prevention of stress ulceration that decrease hydrochloric acid may allow bacterial overgrowth in the upper gut. It would appear that the best approach to all these problems involves the earliest possible resumption of enteral nutrition after shock has been treated.

Lungs. A decrease in blood flow produces hyperventilation. This is a central effect related to increased P_{CO_2} in the respiratory center of the medulla rather than a direct effect on the lungs. This initial hyperventilation may produce respiratory alkalosis and contribute to a further decrease in cerebral blood flow as a result of the fall in arterial P_{CO_2}. In shock, increased ventilation occurs as a result of metabolic acidosis from increased lactate production. Decreased blood flow to the lungs may contribute to hypoxia and carbon dioxide retention. Pulmonary problems are frequent after injury and shock, with the development of posttraumatic pulmonary insufficiency and the need for ventilatory support. The lungs, however, are quite resistant to ischemia, and it is unlikely that hypovolemic or hemorrhagic shock per se produces significant damage to the lungs.[49] Not only do the lungs receive whatever cardiac output there is, albeit with shunting, but the lungs are exposed to whatever oxygen is breathed.

Studies during the Vietnam conflict indicated that hemorrhagic shock per se was not associated with a high incidence of pulmonary complications.[50] Pulmonary changes, however, occurred with severe tissue injuries, particularly crush injuries and injuries of the extremities, thorax, and abdomen. There was a high incidence of pulmonary dysfunction and failure with sepsis. Thus the term *posttraumatic pulmonary insufficiency* is more appropriate for pulmonary failure occurring after shock and injury than *shock lung.* There are many factors involved in the development of pulmonary problems with injury, shock being only one of them and probably not a major one. However, shock and decreased blood flow may make the lung more vulnerable to fluid overload and increase the likelihood of subsequent pulmonary capillary permeability alterations.

With tissue injury or ischemia, the lungs may be affected by mediators that are activated at the injury site and circulate to the lungs. For example, Goldman and his group[51] demonstrated in a series of experiments that hindlimb ischemia produces leukotrienes (LBT$_4$) that activate white cells. It is thought that these activated white cells in the lungs produce superoxide radicals and/or proteolytic enzymes; these, in turn, damage the pulmonary capillary endothelium, producing a "capillary leak syndrome," interstitial edema, and lung damage.[52] These investigators have documented this effect in patients undergoing abdominal aortic aneurysmectomy.[53] Protection is provided by mannitol, which has some antioxidant activity. With organ injuries and shock, the development of ventilatory failure is thought to be due to such mediator activation and damage to the lungs.

Coagulation System. In injured and operated patients, particularly with shock, coagulation changes are frequent. With massive injuries and external and internal bleeding, clotting of blood in the pleural and peritoneal cavities, in soft tissues, and in the retroperitoneal spaces is indeed a problem. Trauma, shock, and blood loss all activate the clotting cascade and subsequent thrombolytic activity. The possibility of intravascular coagulation is present. Available evidence suggests, however, that coagulation changes are not a major problem following brief periods of hypovolemic shock in humans. With treatment of hypovolemic shock, dilutional coagulopathy may occur, but in rabbits there is no impairment of clotting factor regeneration.[54] Hemorrhagic shock in injured patients is associated with a transient, short period of hypercoagulability, followed by a longer period of hypocoagulability.[55] Initially in the operating room, fibrinogen, factor V, and factor VIII levels are frequently low. These seem due to homeostatic demands, plasma dilution, and extravascular relocation. These levels return to normal quickly, as fibrinogen split products begin to increase.[55] With tissue injury, multiple operations, and multiple transfusions, abnormalities of coagulation are frequent. Even then, however, the coagulation change seems to follow the severity of the injury. At the present time, it is unclear how shock contributes to coagulopathy, to its severity, and to its outcome.

In experimental shock studies, anticoagulation with heparin is frequently employed, and this produces an aberration in the normal situation. Recently, Rana et al.[56] have found that this anticoagulation protects the animals from shock. Such protection is not provided for patients with injury. This group has now provided evidence that the protective effect of heparin is not through its anticoagulation action.[57] Microcirculatory blood flow may be improved in other ways.

Immune System. Both components of host defense—the nonspecific immune system of neutrophils, macrophages, opsonins, and complement and the specific system of lymphocytes and antibodies—are depressed with circulatory failure. There is decreased capacity for phagocytosis by white blood cells and macrophages of the reticuloendothelial system. Some injuries are associated with circulating immunosuppressive factors that may be related to activation of suppressor T cells. Hemorrhagic shock increases the release of PGE_2 from macrophages but depresses a number of other macrophage functions. This decreases interleukin 2 (IL-2) and subsequent lymphocyte production. Hemorrhage also increases IL-3, IL-6, and interferon-γ production. Experimental abscess size is increased after hemorrhage in animals,[58] and the ability to cope with peritonitis is greatly decreased.[59] In 1950, Miles and Niven[60] showed that experimental shock, regardless of its cause, increased the risk of infection. Decreased perfusion for 3 to 4 h increased the size of bacterial lesions. Decreased availability of leukocytes seemed to be involved. In a recent clinical study, Nichols et al.[61] found that the risk of infection increased in patients with injury who arrived at the hospital in shock. It is clear that the patient, in or after a period of shock, has increased susceptibility to infection.

Metabolic Alterations. Although certain specific metabolic abnormalities occur with shock per se, it may be difficult to separate these changes from the metabolic alterations that occur with injury and stress. The cardiovascular and endocrine responses to shock, along with decreased tissue blood flow, produce characteristic metabolic changes.[62]

Some changes are adaptive to provide energy during stress. Others are the direct effect of anoxia and ischemia. Hyperglycemia occurs early in shock despite increased glucose utilization. Epinephrine seems to be the major factor producing hepatic glycogenolysis, early hyperglycemia, and muscle glycogen breakdown into lactate. Both pyruvate and lactate increases in early shock are followed later by an increase in lactate production that leads to metabolic acidosis. With shock there is decreased oxygen consumption, increased oxygen extraction, and an oxygen debt. The tissue hypoxia that occurs has profound effects on cells, cell membranes, and organ function. Much of the increased lactate produced in shock has been thought to be due to anaerobic glycolysis that occurs when cellular hypoxia forces a shift from the aerobic Krebs cycle–electron transport system. Certainly this is part of it, but there are other mechanisms as well. In experimental animals, epinephrine induces muscle glycogenolysis. Also, elevations of lactate have not correlated with lack of oxygen, decreased production of carbon dioxide, or ultimate death of patients. Weil and Abdelmonen[63] provide evidence that when blood lactate increases to 8 mmol/liter in a patient, survival is unlikely. Thus the high lactate level in shock may indicate not only tissue and cell hypoxia but also decreased ability of the liver to clear organic acids and altered substrate metabolism produced by epinephrine. The base deficit also has been used as a guide to the severity of shock and to satisfactory treatment.[64,65] This value is calculated from the arterial pH and P_{CO_2} using the Sigaard-Anderson nomogram. The normal base deficit is between 2 and -2, with a severe deficit being -15.

In shock, protein synthesis is also decreased, and circulating amino acid levels increase, particularly alanine. Increased rates of urea production indicate greater breakdown of amino acids. The release of amino acids from muscle may result from pyruvate accepting amino groups through glycolysis. Alanine, so produced, would then be available to the liver for gluconeogenesis.

In humans, free fatty acids increase when there has been modest blood loss, but when shock occurs, fat mobilization shuts off. With glycogenolysis, there is also a tendency toward hyperkalemia and decreased serum sodium. Evidence of adrenal activation is also present, with eosinopenia, lymphocytopenia, and reduced platelets. Other changes, if they occur, would indicate impaired organ function due to decreased blood flow to the liver, kidneys, muscle, and other organs.

If tissue injury is predominant without shock, as with a major operation, the metabolic response to injury produces mobilization of carbohydrate reserves, increased breakdown of protein, and bypassing of fat stores. The excessive catabolism and alteration in glucose metabolism can be reproduced experimentally in humans by the simultaneous infusion of cortisol, epinephrine, and glucagon, with IL-1 as a major determinant of the degree of catabolism. Patients will have a diabetic glucose tolerance curve during and after injury and shock, particularly due to increased glycolysis, reduced insulin secretion, and some tissue insulin resistance as well. Later in shock, particularly shock due to sepsis, hypoglycemia may be present, which is probably related to the failure of glucose production by the liver and a severe and prolonged decrease in blood flow.

Late Sequelae of Experimental Hemorrhagic Shock. Most studies of shock in the experimental laboratory have been acute studies with resuscitation, therapy, and study of immediate survival over several days. Recently, Dunham et al.[66] studied dogs 4 to 7 days after hemorrhage and found evidence of hepatic insufficiency, catabolism, hypermetabolism, and a hyperdynamic circulation. This is a parallel pattern to patients with stress, injury, or sepsis.

ALTERATIONS IN THE MICROCIRCULATION WITH SHOCK

Alterations in the microcirculation, particularly in humans, are not well understood. The microvasculature is defined as all vessels of 100 μm or less in size. This segment of the circulation consists of precapillary arterioles, capillaries, and venules. Once decreased blood flow occurs, not only is there a shutdown of many capillaries with lack of perfusion of those regions in the circulation, but cell swelling and permeability changes also occur in the microcirculation, which may produce problems later. Clearly, the objective of treatment of shock is improvement in blood flow to this segment of the vascular bed to improve cell nutrition.

In a normal capillary bed, there is an ebb and flow of circulation so that capillaries open and close periodically. Blood is a viscid fluid due to the presence of red cells, platelets, white cells, and proteins, especially fibrinogen and globulins, and this quality becomes important in the microcirculation, when flow may be slow or halted temporarily. Thus blood is described as having a non-Newtonian behavior. It was observed many years ago that during shock, blood flow in capillary beds decreases and rouleaux of red cells form. Capillaries become plugged with such cell aggregates. This was called *sludging* of blood and was thought by some to be a pathologic event in itself, impairing the microcirculation with shock. Another explanation postulated that this is a transient phenomenon with low blood flow that is reversed as soon as blood flow is improved. Most observations of the microcirculation suggest that capillaries open up and red cell aggregates disappear if blood flow is improved, no matter what is used to improve the flow. This suggests that sludging of red cells is a nonspecific event.[67]

Platelet aggregates or microthrombi also have been described. Their importance has not been established. Bagge et al.[68] described plugging of skeletal muscle capillaries by white blood cells in cats with hemorrhagic shock. They found that nonperfused capillaries contained several leukocytes that were usually located at the site of bulging of endothelial cell nuclei. They did not observe platelet or erythrocyte aggregates. The adherence of leukocytes in capillaries may lead to their activation, with the production and release of proteolytic enzymes and superoxides. These compounds could damage the endothelium and increase capillary permeability. Kreis et al.[69] and others have observed endothelial cell swelling with shock that could impede the microcirculation. Again, the clinical significance of this is not established.

Messmer and his group[70] found local driving pressure, arteriolar vasomotion, and endothelial cells to be key factors in the microcirculation. With shock, the perfusion pattern became inhomogeneous owing to a lack of arteriolar vasomotion, changes of flow patterns of blood, endothelial cell swelling, and blood–cell endothelium interactions. Alpha receptor–mediated constriction is most pronounced in precapillary arterioles but occurs also in postcapillary venules. The number of perfused capillaries is thus reduced. The spatial and temporal distribution of alternating flow in various capillaries is lost. The relationship between blood flow and the capillary surface area available for exchange of nutrients and metabolites (the permeability surface area product) is greatly reduced. There are areas of stagnant flow and those perfused only with plasma. Later in shock, dilation of precapillary resistance vessels and constriction of postcapillary venules leads to fluid loss. As described earlier, most studies of experimental hemorrhagic shock were done with the animals heparinized. This treatment maintains microvascular patency and blood flow[71,72] in a manner not reflected in patients who are injured or lose blood.

A number of substances have been targeted as specific agents to improve microcirculatory blood flow. Low-molecular-weight dextran (average molecular weight 40,000) was thought to be an antisludging agent. Its effect, however, does not appear to be specific, and after considerable initial enthusiasm, it is no longer used for this purpose. It seems most likely that any fluid that decreases hematocrit by hemodilution will increase blood flow. Lactated Ringer's solution and saline are as effective as dextran in decreasing the cell aggregates and improving capillary flow. The critical factor is an adequate volume of Ringers lactate[73] or whatever crystalloid solution is used.[74,75]

Recently, hypertonic saline and hyperoncotic clinical dextran 70 (dextran with an average molecular weight of 70) have been studied in animals and patients. Hemodynamic depression has been improved with these substances. Kreimeier et al.[76] found that 7.2% saline/10% dextran 60 was particularly effective in improving nutritional blood flow after shock. The effects of heparin on the microcirculation were described earlier.

In some types of shock, such as septic shock, there may be an early increase in capillary permeability, particularly in the lung, which will produce pulmonary failure. In any form of shock with prolonged decrease in blood flow, there also may be a reversal of capillary fluid exchange with loss of fluid from the capillaries rather than capillary refilling. Some possible explanations for such changes include an alteration in interstitial collagen and other macromolecules

TABLE 3–2. Cell Adhesion Molecules—Receptors

1. Integrins—LFA-1, fibronectin, platelet glycoprotein
2. Ams of immunoglobulins
3. Cadherins
4. LEC-CAM—ELAM-1
5. Lymphocyte homing receptors

Note: LFA-1, leukocyte-associated molecule; Ams, adhesion molecules; LEC-CAM, lectin–epidermal growth factor complement-binding cell adhesion molecule; ELAM-1, endothelial-leukocyte adhesion molecule.

to form a "gel" that may trap water and sodium; a movement of water and sodium into the cells, as suggested by Shires and colleagues[77] and by Chaudry et al.[78]; or a failure of capillary refilling with major hemorrhage or persistence of increased postcapillary resistance. Late alterations in capillary membrane permeability also could be a factor.

There are two other important mechanisms operative in the microcirculation. These are cell adhesion molecules or receptors and endothelial factors.[79] There are five major groups of adhesion molecules that participate in cell-to-cell interactions and cell-to-matrix or endothelium adherence (Table 3–2). This system contributes to the adherence of white cells to endothelium. These receptors may contribute to the tissue damage that occurs with shock, but without them, fatal infections may occur. Endothelium-derived factors play a role in vascular reactivity. They include the endothelins—endothelium-derived peptides, which are potent vasoconstrictors. Endothelium-derived relaxing factor may be involved with reactive hyperemia. The clinical relevance of these factors has not been established.

Endothelial cells also synthesize eicosanoids such as prostacyclin and anticoagulant factors such as tissue plasminogen activator, thrombomodulin, and proteins S and C. After injury to vessel walls, procoagulant factors are produced by the endothelium, such as platelet-activating factor, von Willebrand's factor, and others.[80]

Thus the microcirculation occupies a central role in shock pathophysiology. There may be changes in late shock that are not reversed as rapidly. There is evidence that microvascular blood flow does not return to normal immediately, after what is thought to be adequate clinical treatment of shock.[72] Specific agents to improve microcirculatory flow may have certain advantages after prolonged ischemia.[81–83] The exact place for agents such as hypertonic solutions, however, has yet to be established, at least for clinical use. Hypertonic solutions have been used in smaller volumes in burn patients with good results. The edema of the burn is greatly reduced. Drugs such as adenosine triphosphate or pentoxyphylline may have a selective positive effect on the microcirculation.[79]

PROGRESSIVE ABNORMALITIES IN CELL FUNCTION WITH SHOCK

With severe or prolonged shock in humans, organ malfunction becomes evident, even if successful resuscitation of the circulation can be carried out. The effects of ischemia on the kidney, liver, lung, myocardium, and perhaps other systems is evident clinically, particularly with single or multiple organ failure after severe injury, along with shock. Organ injury must begin with progressive cell injury. It is well established that this occurs with shock and ischemia. Cell hypoxia clearly plays a major role in the pathophysiology of shock. It is difficult to separate, however, the effects of hypoxia per se from those of ischemia with decreased tissue oxygenation. Improvement in survival of experimental animals given supplementary oxygen after hemorrhagic shock provides evidence for a sizable oxygen debt.[84] The evidence for progressive cellular alterations with shock comes from studies primarily in experimental animals, although there is sufficient clinical correlation to indicate the importance of these phenomena. The altered hepatic function seen in patients after injury is clearly due to ischemic damage to hepatocytes. Shires and coworkers[33,77] have demonstrated changes in skeletal muscle membrane potential and decreased functional ECF in patients with severe shock. The tissue, organ, and cell swelling that occurs after injury, or with ischemia, are easily recognized. The major advance in cardiac surgery, the use of cold chemical cardioplegia intraoperatively for myocardial preservation, is an example of the use of this experimental information for practical clinical purposes. The same is true in the preservation of organs to be used for transplantation.

Extensive studies in our laboratory, with contributions from many other laboratories, have provided a sequence of events that begins with decreased blood flow or ischemia and leads to progressive cell injury and cell destruction.[85,86] These changes are shown in Fig. 3–7. The initial change with ischemia seems to be an intracellular one, with increases in lactate and hydrogen ions, so that intracellular acidosis becomes a major factor. Cell membrane changes soon follow, with alterations in membrane transport and function. Later, membrane potential decreases, sodium enters, and potassium leaves the cells. The Na^+, K^+-ATPase enzyme system is activated. Metabolic capability of the cell is altered so that ATP is used but not replenished. Mitochondria, although stimulated, are unable to keep up with the energy needs, and ATP and cyclic adenosine monophosphate levels decrease. Various changes in mitochondrial function, the Krebs cycle, and electron transport occur, such as a fall in cytochrome C oxidase, succinate dehydrogenase, and coenzyme Q10.[87] An important factor is an alteration in membrane regulation of calcium. Protein synthetic activities are depressed. Cell swelling occurs as progressive deterioration in the metabolic systems of the cell takes place. Lysosomes eventually leak, mitochondria are disrupted, and cell is gradually destroyed. There are many clinical examples of such altered cell and organ functions with ischemia and shock. They seem to play a critical role in the development of multiple systems or organ failure after injury. Treatment requires rapid restoration of adequate blood flow by initially providing fluid volume replacement of what has been lost. Additional benefits also may be achieved by biochemical support of these cell abnormalities.

During and after shock, there is enhancement of certain genes for the production of acute phase proteins by the liver and for heat shock proteins in all cells.[88,89] Heat shock proteins are important for intracellular homeostasis and protection from oxidants. A thorough review of the cell in shock has been provided by Schlag et al.[90]

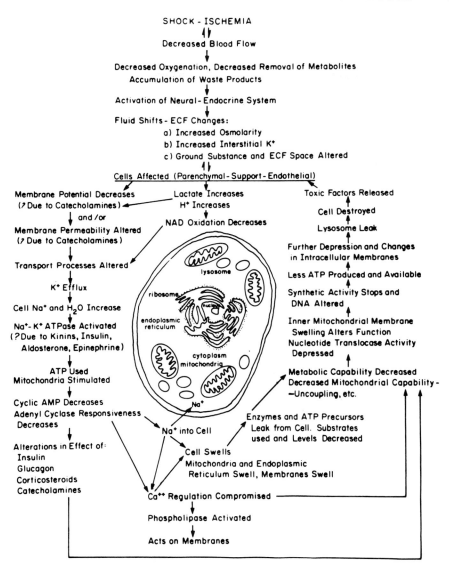

SHOCK - ISCHEMIA

Decreased Blood Flow

Decreased Oxygenation, Decreased Removal of Metabolites
Accumulation of Waste Products

Activation of Neural-Endocrine System

Fluid Shifts-ECF Changes:
a) Increased Osmolarity
b) Increased Interstitial K⁺
c) Ground Substance and ECF Space Altered

Cells Affected (Parenchymal-Support-Endothelial)

Membrane Potential Decreases
(? Due to Catecholamines)
and/or
Membrane Permeability Altered
(? Due to Catecholamines)

Transport Processes Altered

K⁺ Efflux

Cell Na⁺ and H₂O Increase

Na⁺-K⁺ ATPase Activated
(? Due to Kinins, Insulin,
Aldosterone, Epinephrine)

ATP Used
Mitochondria Stimulated

Cyclic AMP Decreases
Adenyl Cyclase Responsiveness
Decreases

Alterations in Effect of:
Insulin
Glucagon
Corticosteroids
Catecholamines

Lactate Increases
H⁺ Increases
NAD Oxidation Decreases

lysosome
ribosome
nucleus
endoplasmic reticulum
cytoplasm
mitochondria
Na⁺

Na⁺ into Cell

Toxic Factors Released

Cell Destroyed

Lysosome Leak

Further Depression and Changes
in Intracellular Membranes

Less ATP Produced and Available

Synthetic Activity Stops and
DNA Altered

Inner Mitochondrial Membrane
Swelling Alters Function
Nucleotide Translocase Activity
Depressed

Metabolic Capability Decreased
Decreased Mitochondrial Capability-
—Uncoupling, etc.

Enzymes and ATP Precursors
Leak from Cell. Substrates
used and Levels Decreased

Cell Swells
Mitochondria and Endoplasmic
Reticulum Swell, Membranes Swell

Ca⁺⁺ Regulation Compromised

Phospholipase Activated

Acts on Membranes

FIG. 3–7. The changes in cell function following shock or ischemia are depicted, with eventual destruction of the cell.

SHOCK WITH TISSUE INJURY

With trauma and/or operation, loss of blood and fluids combines with tissue injury (a wound). This may result in shock. The initial hemodynamic manifestation will be hypovolemic shock. However, tissue injury will initiate an inflammatory response that will add another component to hypovolemia. The word *wound* is used here in the singular as a generic expression of all areas of injury.

TABLE 3–3. Hormonal Changes with Injury and Fluid Loss

Hypothalamus (neural control)
Corticotropin-releasing factor (CRF): stimulates release of adreno-corticotropin
Thyrotropin-releasing hormone (TRH): no recognized role
Luteinizing hormone-releasing hormone (LHRH): no recognized role
Somatostatin [growth hormone (somato-tropin)-releasing inhibitory factor, SRIF]: uncertain role
Arginine vasopressin (ADH): increased production in hypothalamus and release from posterior pituitary gland
Adrenalin: secretion from adrenal medulla increased
Norepinephrine: secretion from sympathetic nerve endings increased

Pituitary (neural and hormonal control)
Corticotropin: increased
Endorphins: increased
Growth hormone (somatotropin): increased
Prolactin: increased, function obscure
Follicle-stimulating hormone–leutinizing hormone (FSH-LH): decreased
Alpha-melanocyte–stimulating hormone: unknown function
Beta-lipotropin hormone: unknown
Thyroid-stimulating hormone (TSH): no change or decrease
Arginine vasopressin: increased

Adrenal gland (hormonal control)
Cortex (hormonal control)
Cortisol: increased
Aldosterone: increased
Adrenal estrogens and androgens: no change or decrease

Medulla (automatic control)
Catecholamines: increased

Thyroid gland (hormonal control)
Thyroxine: no change
Triiodythronine: decreased
Reverse triiodythyronine: increased

Pancreas (autonomic, hormonal, and substrate control)
Glucagon: increased
Insulin: less increase than hyperglycemia would produce

Kidney (autonomic and local control)
Erythropoietin produced
Renin-angiotensin activation

Wound
Endogenous mediators, enzyme cascades
Prostaglandins (prostacyclins, thromboxane)
Leukotrienes
Histamine
Serotonin
Kallikreins (bradykinin)
Monokines (cytokines)
    Interleukin 1 from monocytes
    Hepatocyte-stimulating factor
    Cachectin (tumor necrosis factor) from macrophages
    Lymphotoxin (a tumorlytic protein derived from lymphocytes)
    Interferons [alpha (leukocyte), beta (fibroblast), gamma (T-lymphocyte)]
    Granulocyte-macrophage colony-stimulating factor
    Others

Thus scalp lacerations, a fracture of the humerus, chest wall and lung contusions, a ruptured spleen, a fractured pelvis, and open fractures of the tibia and fibula in a single individual after an automobile accident are collectively referred to as the *wound*. The wound, then, is a specific part of an individual—an organ, if you will, that is parasitic and which calls on all other organ systems for full support. The demands the wound makes on the circulation, lungs, liver, kidneys, and other organs can be overwhelming. The wound communicates with the body by a system of signals through mediators. Wound-host communication is an afferent system of nerves and wound hormones to the central nervous system, with stimulation of the counterregulatory hormones glucagon, cortisol, and catecholamines as part of the efferent system. The wound and its components also have many local effects in this complex system of immunocytokinendocrinology. The inflammatory response so necessary for survival and healing of the wound may, with massive injury or infection, become generalized and damage remote organs, resulting in MOF.

The distinctions between hypovolemic shock from a bleeding duodenal ulcer (relatively pure blood loss) and the response to tissue injury with inflammation become blurred in the patient with multiple systems injury. Such a patient may have internal and external blood loss, hematomas, and ECF fluid and plasma loss that may continue for some time after injury as a result of sequestration (third space) and other changes. The effects of reduced blood volume (hypovolemia) and a low cardiac output will produce additive changes due to ischemia of the injured tissue.

RESPONSE TO INJURY

Metabolic and Neuroendocrine Responses to Injury. These are important parts of the stress reaction and teleologically provide an individual with the best opportunity to survive under adverse circumstances. The phases after injury are four: (1) the injury phase, lasting 2 to 5 days (catabolism), (2) the turning point, when the neuroendocrine response turns off if convalescence is uncomplicated, (3) the anabolic phase, involving a gain in strength and positive nitrogen balance, and (4) late anabolism, with a positive caloric balance. The components of this neuroendocrine response are listed in Table 3–3. These contribute to cardiovascular compensation, salt and water retention, catabolism with negative nitrogen balance, fat mobilization, immunomodulation, and beginning wound healing. Catabolism is necessary to provide glucose for the wound from muscle protein, by way of alanine to the liver. A detailed review of these changes is available.[7,79]

THE INFLAMMATORY PROCESS AND ITS MEDIATORS

The basic biologic response to a tissue injury is similar, regardless of whether it is due to tissue trauma, operation, infection, or attack by foreign antigens or antibodies. The mediators of such changes may be local within the wound, or they may be generalized and stimulate systematic factors. These are listed in Table 3–4. The enzyme cascades include the renin-angiotension-aldosterone

TABLE 3–4. Mediators of Injury and Inflammation

Enzyme cascades
Histamine, serotonin, bradykinin
Cytokines—IL-1, IL-2, IL-6, etc.; cachectin (TNF); interferons
Complement activation
Neutrophil products (white cell activation)—proteases, oxygen free radicals
Autacoids (eicosanoids)—prostaglandins, leukotrienes
Reticuloendothelial opsonins
Immune complexes
Endothelial factors
Adhesion molecules

system, coagulation and fibrinolysis, the kallikrein-kinin system, the complement cascade, and the eicosanoids—prostaglandins, prostacyclin, thromboxane, and leukotrienes. Many of the mediators of the inflammatory response are produced by the monocyte phagocytic system. These mediators include the cytokines (the monokines) or lymphokines [the interleukins, cachectin (tumor necrosis factor, TNF), and the interferons].

The effects of the various inflammatory agents are shown in Table 3–5. These mediators of inflammation are numerous, fascinating, complex, and incompletely understood. An early event in acute inflammation is adherence of activated neutrophils, monocytes, and platelets to endothelial cells and basement membranes. This occurs through the expression of cell adhesion molecules or receptors (see Table 3–2). These receptors are necessary to control infection and for repair of injury. They are absent in patients with certain genetic abnormalities who have overwhelming infection.[91] The most important change with local inflammation is increased capillary permeability contributed by the kinin, serotonin, complement, and coagulation systems. These alterations promote inflammatory cells to adhere, enter the area of injury, and begin the process of repair. A coagulum forms, and injured tissue is broken down by plasma factors, phagocytic cells, and hydrolytic enzymes. This results in wound debridement and initial repair. The detailed effects and interrelationships of these mediators are described elsewhere.[7,79] These mediators, particularly the cytokines, are important in the pathophysiology of infection.

TABLE 3–5. Inflammatory Agents

Histamine
Released from mast cells during antigen-antibody reactions (hay fever, cutaneous inflammation, asthma, rheumatoid arthritis)
Inhibited by H_1 and H_2 antihistamines
Bradykinin (the kallikrein-kinin system)
Causes pain, vasodilation, and edema
From many cells, from kallikrein
Stimulates prostacyclin
No effective inhibitors
Inhibitors of activation are captopril and enalopril
Serotonin
5-Hydroxytryptamine
Bronchoconstriction
Platelet aggregation
Increases permeability
Leukotrienes
Vascular changes (increased permeability, wheal, and flare)
Inhibitor is piriprost
Interleukin 1 and cachectin
Inflammatory changes

Prostaglandins
Prostaglandin E_2
Vasodilation, erythema, hyperalgesia, edema
Prostaglandin F_{2a}
Vasoconstriction
Thromboxane A_2
Constricts vessels
Aggregates platelets
Causes lysosomal membranes to leak
Prostacyclin
From endothelial cells
Opposite of thromboxane
Dilates
Inhibits platelet aggregation
Protects gastric mucosa
Inhibitors of prostaglandins are aspirin, nonsteroidal anti-inflammatory agents, and steroids through lipocortin and calpactin
Platelet-activating factor
From most inflammatory cells, endothelium, and platelets
Asthma-like effects, hyperreactivity
Inhibitors are antagonists, glucocorticoids, and ginkolides

This response of a biologic organism to injury seems teleologically to have developed to survive the greatest possible injury without therapy. If the inflammatory response remains localized to the wound, it remains helpful. If, however, the response becomes a systemic or generalized reaction, then it can produce damage elsewhere. With multisystem injury, a massive inflammatory reaction, so necessary for survival, may become destructive to remote organs. There may be down-regulation of the inhibitors or feedback responses that ordinarily would keep inflammation under control. This can contribute to MOF (Fig. 3–8). This has been called a "severe, generalized autoinflammatory response" by Goris.[92] The sequence of events begins with a severe trauma or operation that produces hypovolemic shock and tissue injury. An inflammatory reaction, combined with ischemia-reperfusion injury, can proceed appropriately with healing and repair or instead to remote organ malfunction, MOF, and death. This sequence of events and the organ systems involved are shown in Fig. 3–9.

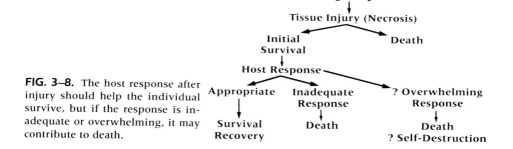

FIG. 3–8. The host response after injury should help the individual survive, but if the response is inadequate or overwhelming, it may contribute to death.

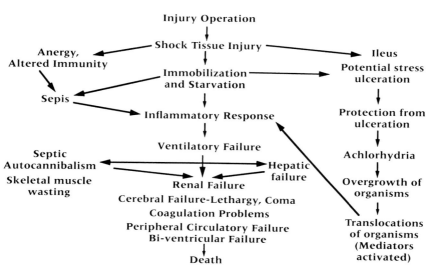

FIG. 3–9. The changes occurring with an injury and/or an operation that can lead to MOF and death.

CARDIOGENIC SHOCK

ETIOLOGY

Failure of the heart to provide an adequate circulation may be due to problems intrinsic to the heart itself or may be related to factors outside the heart. Specific intrinsic cardiac problems are those of myocardial infarction, ventricular ischemia, myocardial contusion, arrhythmias, and drug depression of the myocardium. More frequent in surgical patients, however, is a nonspecific problem in which there is myocardial failure due to depression of the myocardium. Whether this is caused by disease-related suppression of the myocardium from sepsis or general illness or is due to nonspecific stress is not known. It has been recognized, however, that after severe injury with significant infection or septicemia or in diseases that produce tissue necrosis (e.g., pancreatitis), the heart may quickly become the limiting factor in the circulation. This may occur in individuals who are young and have normal cardiac function prior to the injury or septic episode. Thus the definition of cardiogenic shock must be broad enough to include any circumstance in which the arterial circulation and perfusion of vital organs are less than adequate but with high filling pressures. There may be a specific extrinsic or intrinsic problem (see Table 3–1). In addition, the failure may be due initially to failure of the right ventricle as a primary problem or to primary left ventricular dysfunction. Right ventricular failure may lead to ventricular distension and shift of the septum, decreasing the filling capacity of the left ventricle and producing left ventricular failure as a consequence.

The definition of shock following myocardial infarction was developed by Fishberg and associates[93] in 1934. Classifications of circulatory failure in 1935 by Harrison[94] and in 1940 by Blalock[95] included, for the first time, the term *cardiogenic shock*. When cardiac output could first be measured in 1941, Grisham and Master[96] found that it was reduced after myocardial infarction in humans. Freis et al.,[97] in 1952, described the hemodynamic abnormalities of cardiogenic shock that developed after myocardial infarction. It is estimated that infarction of more than 40 percent of the left ventricle must occur before severe and progressive cardiogenic shock develops. Since that time, Crowell and Guyton,[98] Siegel and DelGuercio,[99] and others have described the importance and problems of the heart in all forms of shock. Goldberg et al.[100] have recently reported that neither the incidence nor the prognosis of cardiogenic shock due to acute myocardial infarction has improved over the 14 years from 1975 to 1988. The in-hospital and long-term survival rates are poor for patients who develop this complication. Recent interventional and thrombolytic therapy may improve this gloomy observation.

Extrinsic problems include those which increase afterload, including pulmonary embolism or high levels of positive end-expiratory pressure. Respiratory failure and pulmonary hypertension also can produce right ventricular failure. Cardiac tamponade, conversely, restricts the ability of the ventricles to fill and produces yet another type of cardiogenic shock.

HEMODYNAMIC CHARACTERISTICS

The measurements and observations found in a patient with cardiogenic shock are shown in Fig. 3–4. The patient may have normal or depressed mental status.

Veins in the neck and extremities, if the extremities are below the level of the right atrium, will be full. Ventilatory rate may be normal or increased. Pulse is normal or may be weak. The heart rate may be normal or increased. Color may be normal or pale, and the skin may be cool or normal in temperature. Central venous pressure or right atrial pressure will be elevated, as will pulmonary artery and wedge pressure, unless the failure is limited to the right ventricle initially. Cardiac index and arterial pressure will be decreased, as will urine output. The $a\text{-}vD_{O_2}$ difference will be widened, and the arterial P_{O_2} may be low or normal. pH will be decreased with the development of metabolic acidosis. P_{CO_2} may be increased or decreased. Lactate levels in the blood will be increased, and hematocrit will be unchanged. Peripheral resistance, if measured, may be normal or increased.

It is necessary to remember that a patient with a primary myocardial problem may manifest other forms of shock. For example, if a patient maintained on digitalis, diuretics, and salt restriction develops an acute myocardial infarction, the etiologic diagnosis is cardiogenic shock. However, the patient may additionally be volume deficient and respond to intravenous fluids to support the circulation and cardiac output. In the same way, an elderly patient with coronary artery disease and gastrointestinal bleeding would, by definition, have hypovolemic shock but may have the hemodynamic manifestations of cardiogenic shock (see Fig. 3–1). The major differential feature between cardiogenic shock and other circulatory problems is the high ventricular filling pressures. Septic shock may, of course, eventually result in cardiogenic shock as circulatory and myocardial depression occur. Thus the clinical features of cardiogenic shock are similar to those of hypovolemia, with the exception of increased venous pressure. This major differential point is critical in treatment.

PATHOPHYSIOLOGY

Cardiogenic shock may be produced by an abnormality of any of three of the determinants of cardiac output (Table 3–6). The first determinant of cardiac output is preload, or filling pressure of the ventricles during diastole. If inadequate, this is, by definition, hypovolemia that is to be corrected by volume expansion. A high volume or high preload, on the other hand, produces congestive heart failure rather than output failure initially. The Frank-Starling relationship is that increased ventricular filling pressure produces an increase in the length of myocardial fibers at the end of diastole. This alteration increases the force of ventricular contraction, which then increases cardiac output. However, if the optimal length of stretch of the fibers is exceeded, then contractions cannot increase and myocardial failure results. This is the so-called descending limb of the Starling curve.[101] Also, decreased ventricular filling by pericardial tamponade compresses the ventricles and does not allow them to fill. Positive end-expiratory pressure (PEEP), which decreases blood return to the thorax, will produce a form of extrinsic cardiogenic shock that is in actual fact a preload problem. The measurements needed to determine preload are the atrial pressures that are an indication of ventricular filling pressures. Although ventricular end-diastolic pressure is the most important measurement, it is impractical to measure this value directly other than during cardiac catheterization. Also, if ventricular function is depressed by injury, operation, infection, or other factors, a higher atrial pressure or preload may be necessary to obtain optimal ventricular muscle stretch and

TABLE 3–6. Determinants of Cardiac Output

Determinant	Definition	Effect on Cardiac Output	Measurement	Treatment
Preload	Length of myocardial fibers at end diastole, which is result of ventricular filling pressure	Direct, up to physiologic limit	End-diastolic volume and pressure of ventricles, pulmonary diastolic pressure, pulmonary capillary wedge pressure, direct left atrial pressure measurements, central venous (right atrial) pressure	Volume expansion, pericardiocentesis reduction in positive end-expiratory pressure
Contractility	Inotropic state of myocardium, length/tension/velocity relationship of myocardium independent of initial length and afterload	Direct	Ventricular function curves, ejection fraction, V_{max}, V_{CF}, $\dfrac{dP/dt}{iP}$	Dopamine, norepinephrine, epinephrine, isoproterenol, dobutamine, digitalis glucagon, glucose-potassium-insulin
Afterload	Systolic ventricular wall stress, which is produced by force against which myocardial fibers must contract	Inverse, as long as coronary flow is maintained	Aortic pressure for left ventricle, pulmonary artery pressure for right ventricle	Diuretics, phentolamine, sodium nitroprusside, nitroglycerin, intraaortic balloon pumping, external counterpulsation
Pulse rate	Number of cardiac systoles per minute	Direct, above 60 and below 180 beats per minute	Electrocardiogram, count pulse	Bradycardia: isoproterenol, pacemaker, tachycardia: digitalis, lidocaine, electroconversion

Note: V_{max}, maximum velocity; V_{CF}, velocity of circumferential fiber shortening; $(dP/dt)/iP$, time tension index.

force of contraction. For this reason, a trial of increased preload is always prudent, even with an acute myocardial infarction. Pulmonary edema should not occur until a wedge pressure of 20 to 25 cmH_2O is reached, unless colloid osmotic pressure has been reduced.

The second determinant of cardiac output is contractility, which reflects the health and vigor of the myocardium and can be affected by a number of primary and secondary problems. Its exact definition is the rate of myocardial fiber shortening, independent of the initial length or afterload. Alterations in contractility are the most common problems that produce cardiogenic shock. This can occur because of myocardial necrosis after a myocardial infarction, ischemia, anoxia, or depression of function by drugs or disease. Problems such as peritonitis or severe injury are also associated with decreased contractility. A commonly used measure to document such an abnormality is the ventricular function curve. Sarnoff et al.[101] developed a family of nesting ventricular function curves with changes in stroke work of the left ventricle and plotted over a range of end-diastolic volumes and/or pressures. The relationship of ventricular stroke work to a certain end-diastolic volume is the measure of contractility. In order to get an exact measurement of this, one would have to hold the other variables preload, afterload, and heart rate constant. This is obviously impossible in the clinical situation. Thus an approximation of contractility is generally used, such as measurement of left ventricular stroke work and the filling pressure (PCWP or left atrial pressure). Such points can then be plotted and compared with those obtained from normal individuals. This allows a determination as to whether contractility at a particular time is within the normal range or low. If the circulation is inadequate, filling pressures high, and contractility low by ventricular function curve measurement, then an inotropic agent is necessary, and the measurements can be repeated to determine if there is improvement. A ventricular function curve also can be constructed by using the shape of an indicator dilution curve in relation to ventricular work. Ventricular work is the product of stroke volume and arterial pressure. Ventricular contractility also can be expressed in terms of the ejection fraction. Contrast angiography, echocardiography, and gaited blood pool imaging with a scintillation camera will allow accurate measurement of ejection fraction. Acute changes in ejection fraction are most diagnostic of rapidly changing ventricular events and capabilities. The V_{max} is defined as the velocity of maximal shortening of the myocardial muscle; however, it is not independent of afterload and preload. V_{CF} is a velocity of circumferential muscle fiber shortening that can be analyzed from an electrocardiogram. Other measures of myocardial capability can be helpful, such as the dP/dt. This is the first derivative of the maximal rate of pressure rise in the left ventricle. It is divided by the intraventricular pressure, at the point of measurement. This is a good measure of contractility, but it requires a catheter-tip pressure transducer in the left ventricle. Currently, this is not suitable for intensive care monitoring. Ventricular function curves also can be developed for the right ventricle. The original concept of ventricular function curves and, particularly, the Frank-Starling mechanism related stroke work to diastolic volume. Since diastolic volume cannot be measured easily, the wedge or filling pressure has been substituted. This produces a problem, however, in interpretation of ventricular contractility because pressure measurements do not consider ventricular compliance or problems of how one ventricle may affect the other. Thus respiratory failure may be associated with reduced cardiac blood flow to the right ventricle and pulmonary hypertension; the failure of one ventricle can affect the other by septal shift and other dynamic influences.

The changes in contractility that occur with acute myocardial infarction, with various forms of myocardiopathy, with ventricular scarring, and with aneurysms are fairly well understood. Of particular importance for surgical patients, however, is the nonspecific depression of myocardial function that occurs with a number of problems of acute illness. Depression of the ventricles may occur with pancreatitis, peritonitis, septic abortion, severe multisystem injury, prolonged illness, and other problems of infection. A number of factors have been implicated in the production of such changes in the myocardium. Lefer[102,103] and others have identified a myocardial depressant factor (MDF) with experimental pancreatitis and other conditions, such as experimental burns. There have been a number of hypotheses and considerable experimental evidence indicating that with late hemorrhagic shock, gram-negative septicemia, and other problems, a circulating substance is produced that depresses the myocardium. Parillo et al.[104,105] found that plasma from patients in septic shock with a decreased left ventricular ejection fraction decreased the contractility of isolated myocardial cells. This provides further evidence for the presence of a myocardial depressant factor with infection. There is considerable difference of opinion, however, as to the nature and significance of such a substance. Lysosomal enzymes from ischemic cell materials produced by macrophages or leukocytes, plasma kinins such as bradykinin and endotoxin, as well as other substances have been implicated. It has not been possible to identify an exact etiologic agent in humans. Of particular importance is the fact that, at the present time, nothing can be done to reverse this factor other than to treat the septic or necrotic process and support the heart. It is most important to remember, however, that myocardial depression may occur or develop in many seriously ill patients, even those who are young and in otherwise good health with previously normal hearts. This must be treated appropriately by support of ventricular function.

Problems of heart rate can produce cardiogenic shock if tachycardia rises above 150 to 160 beats per minute. Diastolic filling time may be too short to allow satisfactory stroke volume and cardiac output. Thus uncontrolled atrial fibrillation with a rapid ventricular response or ventricular tachycardia can become life-threatening and require immediate therapy. Bradycardia, with a rate below 40 to 50 beats per minute, also may be associated with an inadequate cardiac output. This may be due to complete heart block, drug toxicity, or other problems.

The fourth component determining cardiac output is afterload. Problems of afterload may occur with either high or low peripheral or pulmonary vascular resistance. Low afterload is characteristic of both neurogenic and septic shock. It has been determined that certain patients with acute myocardial infarction have a lower peripheral vascular resistance than would be predicted from the decrease in cardiac output. Hypotension would be the result. Such a circumstance indicates the importance of measuring not only cardiac output and index but also peripheral vascular resistance. Acute increases in afterload, however, can quickly result in ventricular dilation and failure. This may occur with spontaneous aortic dissection, cross clamping of the aorta during surgery, or secondary to other hypertensive crises. Adjustment of afterload in such circumstances may be a critical factor in preserving myocardial function. If the ventricles are depressed or damaged, even normal resistance may not be tolerated. In such circumstances, a reduction in afterload may be necessary in order to maintain adequate ventricular performance. With ventricular injury, it may be necessary to provide a higher preload and lower afterload to maintain satisfactory cardiac output.

Cardiogenic shock will initiate a compensatory chain of events similar to those of hypovolemic shock. Eventually, the effects on organ function, metabolism, and particularly cellular events will be similar to those described previously.

PREVENTION OF CARDIOGENIC SHOCK

Many patients with cardiovascular disease, prior myocardial infarction, or arrhythmias require operation or sustain injury. In such surgical patients with urgent problems, or even in those requiring elective operations, study and support of the patient's circulation and cardiac reserve may prevent the development of cardiovascular embarrassment. Control of hypertension by reduction in afterload, improvement in ventricular performance by elective digitalization, reduction of high preload in congestive failure, control of rate and rhythm, and careful maintenance of oxygenation during operation may allow the patient with a very limited cardiovascular system or previous myocardial infarction to survive. Prospective consideration of these factors can be lifesaving. A patient with marginal cardiovascular status can be admitted to a surgical intensive care unit preoperatively, with measurement of cardiovascular parameters and treatment to provide maximum performance during and after operation.[105]

SEPTIC SHOCK

Circulatory failure occurring with infection was described by Laennec[106] in 1831. Boise,[107] in 1897, drew a clear distinction between shock due to hemorrhage and that due to sepsis. Bloodstream invasion by gram-negative organisms, particularly after urinary tract instrumentation, was recognized early in this century, but it was not a frequent occurrence. It remained for Waisbren,[108] in 1951, to provide a clear description of the hypotension and shock-like appearance that occurred with sepsis. He described two distinct clinical pictures with gram-negative bacteremia. In one, the patient appeared toxic. In the other, the patient was in a shock-like state. In the same year, Borden and Hall[109] described fulminant circulatory failure after transfusion of blood contaminated with gram-negative bacilli. In recent years, the focus of attention has been on septic shock due to gram-negative infection, because it has been the most frequent and devastating problem. It is important to recognize, however, that shock from infection may occur with any infecting agent, including viruses, rickettsiae, parasites, fungi, and gram-positive bacteria. It is now also recognized that the hemodynamic picture and characteristics of septic shock are similar regardless of the infecting organism.[110,111] Despite the availability of new information and the development of improved antimicrobial agents, septic shock remains a serious problem with a high mortality rate. Gram-negative bacteremia remains the most common problem, in part because of the widespread use of antibiotics. The occurrence of nosocomial infections, the emergence of resistant strains of organisms, the use of more extensive and complicated operations on elderly or poor-risk patients, and lowered patient resistance from trauma, chronic disease, steroid therapy, anticancer drugs, and immunosuppressive agents all contribute to this epidemic.

ETIOLOGY

The setting for septic shock is that of a hospitalized patient who has had an injury, an operation, or an underlying disease process that makes the patient susceptible to the growth of organisms, bloodstream invasion, and septicemia. The urinary tract is a frequent site of infection, with many cases preceded by instrumentation such as catheterization of the bladder, cystoscopy, passage of a urethral sound, or operations on the urogenital system. Recognition of this source of gram-negative septicemia and careful technique have decreased the frequency of this problem. The incidence of hospital-acquired urinary tract infections has been decreased by the routine use of closed catheter drainage systems. The respiratory tract is also a frequent source of such infections, often with an endotracheal tube in place or with a tracheostomy. The gastrointestinal tract may be involved when there has been an injury, perforation, anastomosis, or contamination of the peritoneal cavity. The biliary tract and the development of cholangitis may quickly produce septic shock. Burn wounds may be a source of sepsis. A large percentage of cases result from prolonged use of intravenous infusion sites. This has increased with the use of indwelling catheters in the central circulation for intravenous nutrition, infusion of chemotherapeutic agents, or prolonged antibiotic therapy. Septic abortion and postpartum infections account for a number of such problems. Recognition of many of these sites of invasive infection has decreased both the frequency and the severity of septic shock from many etiologies. Predisposing factors include advancing age, diabetes mellitus, cirrhosis, leukemia, lymphoma, disseminated carcinoma, chemotherapy, transplantation with its associated immunosuppressive therapy, and a variety of surgical procedures and injuries that may lead to peritoneal contamination and areas of infection or abscess.

It is now increasingly recognized that injury and operation produce immunosuppression. Shock is known to decrease the capability of neutrophils and both lung and liver macrophages. Protein-calorie malnutrition and prolonged catabolism with starvation are known to alter immunoglobin production and also depress T- and B-cell function. Such deficiencies are associated with decreased reactivity to skin test antigens and produce partial or complete anergy. Steroid secretion following injury and the administration of anesthetic agents also alter or depress host resistance. Finally, it has been recognized that there are circulating immunosuppressive factors with injury, particularly in the presence of tissue necrosis. This probably occurs through suppressor T-cell activation. It is clear that injury and operation depress host resistance and increase the possibility of invasive infection, even in a previously normal individual.

The most frequent single organism that produces septic shock has been *Escherichia coli*, followed by *Aerobacter aerogenes*, *Pseudomonas aeruginosa*, and *Kleb-*

siella pneumoniae. Bacteroides and *Proteus* organisms also have been implicated. Organisms that are not thought to be pathogens may produce shock with infection in immunosuppressed patients. *Staphylococcus aureus* and other gram-positive organisms also can produce septicemia with shock, as can pneumococcal and streptococcal infections. The widespread use of antibiotics, particularly in injured and operated patients, has decreased the incidence of these infections because of their general sensitivity to most broad-spectrum antibiotics. Fungal infections, particularly *Candida albicans,* occurring in patients on broad-spectrum antibiotics and with immunosuppression can be lethal. Viral infections also can produce septic shock. Because of the frequency of occurrence and the devastating effect, however, gram-negative organisms have been emphasized.

CLINICAL FEATURES AND HEMODYNAMIC CHARACTERISTICS

A septicemic episode usually begins with chills and is followed by elevation of the temperature above 101°F, with the temperature often going to 103 to 104°F. Initially, the circulation may be stable, particularly if the patient is otherwise in reasonable condition. A prodrome suggesting the development of septic shock has been suggested by MacLean[29,112] and others. This includes the triad of mental confusion or aberrations, hyperventilation, and metabolic alkalosis. This is one of the best indicators of the potential development of septic shock at a time before blood pressure has decreased. The most likely explanation for this prodrome is that there is a reduction in central nervous system blood flow, even though blood pressure still remains normal in such patients.

Shock may develop slowly or rapidly. Initially, the patient will be warm and dry, with hypotension but increased cardiac output. Vasodilatation and/or arteriovenous shunting, with warm, dry extremities, are typical of early septic shock; the classic picture of shock with vasoconstriction and hypotension is seen only later in the course. Heart rate may be slow rather than fast, and vomiting and diarrhea may occur initially, with blood in the stool later, depending on the infection. The individual's condition and response to the infection at the time that the septic process occurs largely determine the clinical picture of septic shock (see Fig. 3–1). Fever and sepsis require an increased circulation. There is a demand for a higher cardiac output. The patient is warm and manifests a hyperdynamic circulation. If the circulation can respond with adequate cardiac function in the presence of adequate vascular volume, then cardiac output increases, with bounding pulses and increased peripheral blood flow (even though blood pressure may be low). If, however, the circulation cannot meet this need or demand because of either decreased circulating vascular volume, decreased cardiac reserve, or excessive vasodilatation, then further circulatory inadequacy will develop, with further reduction in blood pressure. At this point, the patient may have one of the following hemodynamic manifestations:

1. Hypovolemic shock due to inadequate vascular volume
2. Cardiogenic shock due to inadequate cardiac reserve
3. A distributive problem with excess vasodilatation, in which even a high cardiac output cannot maintain flow

If circulatory inadequacy is prolonged and progressive, this will eventually lead to attempts at compensation and a cold, constricted, and hypodynamic circulation prior to death. Thus the two varieties—the cold, clammy, hypodynamic, hypotensive picture and the hyperdynamic, warm, dilated, but hypotensive picture—are not different responses to infection, but rather are determined by the condition of the patient at the time septicemia occurs, or the stage of septic shock.

Initially, in the septic patient, cardiac index is increased; pulmonary artery and wedge pressure may likewise be low or increased; central venous pressure may be low, normal, or increased; arterial pressure is decreased with a widened pulse pressure; urine output may initially be increased; $(a-v)D_{O_2}$ difference is decreased; and mixed venous oxygen content is increased. Arterial blood P_{O_2} may be decreased or normal; pH will be decreased with metabolic acidosis; P_{CO_2} will be decreased; lactate in arterial blood will be increased; and hematocrit may be normal. Peripheral resistance will be decreased initially, particularly total peripheral resistance. However, pulmonary vascular resistance may be increased, specifically if ventilatory failure is developing. Observation of the patient will show that mental status is altered. Behavior may be abnormal. Ventilatory rate is increased. Pulses will be full and bounding with an increased rate. Color of the patient may be normal or flushed, and the skin, initially, will be warm and dry. Although oxygen delivery increases, oxygen consumption remains the same or falls. The decrease in arteriovenous oxygen difference indicates that less oxygen is being taken up in the periphery of the body. Whether this is due to arteriovenous shunting, decreased utilization of oxygen by the tissues, or both is unknown.

The white blood cell count may be 15,000 to 20,000 cells per cubic milliliter or higher, but leukopenia may occur, particularly early in shock or with severe septic shock. There are no other characteristic laboratory findings other than the attendant features of the progressive development of circulatory failure.

In summary, with sepsis, cardiac output is increased, oxygen consumption is increased, $(a-v)D_{O_2}$ difference is decreased, total peripheral resistance is decreased, pulmonary vascular resistance is often increased, and oxygen delivery is increased. Oxygen consumption, however, either is the same or decreased. Eventually, left ventricular ejection fraction as well as right ventricular ejection fraction are decreased as progressive cardiac failure occurs. Seigel and his group[113] have described the entire spectrum of clinical severity in patients with trauma and sepsis as being in four pathophysiologic states. In state A there is a normal stress response that may be seen in compensated sepsis or after trauma or injury and is characterized by an increase in heart rate and cardiac index, with an improvement in contractility of the heart and an increase in oxygen consumption, without any overt metabolic abnormality. The B state represents increasing stages of severity and deterioration from the septic process. In the B state there is a hyperdynamic cardiovascular pattern that fails to supply peripheral needs adequately with reduced oxygen extraction, narrow $(a-v)D_{O_2}$ difference, and metabolic acidosis. The C state represents further deterioration, including respiratory failure on top of the unbalanced septic process, with the occurrence of profound metabolic and respiratory acidosis. This is characteristic of advanced septic shock with hypotension despite normal or increased cardiac output and a further fall in arterial vascular tone. The final state is the D state, or cardiogenic state, a pattern of primary myocardial rather than peripheral failure. There is a fall in cardiac output, a decline in myocardial contractility, prolonged mixing time, and a widening of the arteriovenous oxygen difference.

Extensive studies of patients in intensive care units with septic shock have now provided considerable information. Wiles et al.[110] found that there was no difference in any physiologic variable between infection and septic shock produced by either gram-positive or by gram-negative organisms or by fungi. There also were no differences between any specific organisms. After volume loading, all their patients exhibited a hyperdynamic cardiovascular response, with abnormally decreased vascular tone. Some degree of myocardial depression was seen in all forms of bacterial and fungal septicemia. Heart rate was the primary variable that produced the increased cardiac output in their patients. This study emphasizes that the primary defect with sepsis is decreased total peripheral resistance that is out of proportion to changes in cardiac output. This can be called a vascular tone abnormality. Vincent et al.[114] found that in patients who developed circulatory shock from purulent peritonitis, surviving patients had lower initial plasma and total blood volumes, and they improved with fluid replacement. Patients who died, however, failed to respond to infusion of equivalent volumes of fluid and had increases in both right- and left-sided cardiac filling pressures indicative of biventricular failure. This is further evidence that the outlook worsens as myocardial depression occurs. Myocardial depression may lead to dilation of both the right and left ventricles. Parillo et al.[105] found that this was a reversible state in patients who survived. Many nonsurvivors failed to develop ventricular dilation, which suggests a compensatory mechanism for dilation in surviving septic patients. Many patients treated for septic shock will respond to circulatory support, but will continue in a hyperdynamic septic state. This continued septic state progresses to MOF.[7,115]

PATHOPHYSIOLOGY: THE RESPONSE TO INFECTION

There is a characteristic sequence of alterations in the circulation, organ function, and metabolism with infection. The term *septic* is used generically to indicate a focus of infection having a systemic effect, such as generalized peritonitis, an abscess within the peritoneal cavity, a hepatic abscess, empyema of the lung, pulmonary infection, severe cellulitis, tissue ischemia with infection, or any other process with necrosis and invasion by pathogenic organisms. The similarity of the septic circulatory response to that of stable cirrhotic patients has been pointed out by Siegel et al.[113] and others. The septic process elevates temperature and increases metabolic demands.

Originally, *sepsis* meant bacterial infection. Now the term has been used by some to describe a clinical state, with or without bacteria present. This should more properly be called a *sepsis syndrome*—a clinical state of pyrexia, leukocytosis, and altered mentation with a hyperdynamic circulation and hypermetabolism. MOF in patients, although it frequently follows infection, may develop with inflammation without infection, as, for example, with pancreatitis, and it also may occur with inadequate blood flow, as with low cardiac output after cardiac operations. Organ malfunctions similar to sepsis and injury have been produced experimentally by Goris et al.[116–118] and others[119] through initiation of an inflammatory response with zymosan. Thus inflammation, if it becomes generalized rather than localized to the wound, presents real and potentially disastrous hazards to organs and tissues remote from the injury.

The phenomenon of local response to infection seems simple but is, in fact, complex. The throbbing pain, heat, redness, and swelling described originally by Celsus are due to local release of substances that produce vasodilatation and increased blood flow to the area, with altered capillary permeability, exudation, and swelling. Heat is produced by increased blood flow, pain from release of vasodilating peptides (histamine, bradykinin, and serotonin). These local effects may be caused by the bacterial organism itself, by endotoxin (a high-molecular-weight phospholipid-polysaccharide protein complex found in the wall of gram-negative organisms), or by exotoxins produced by gram-positive organisms. Interaction with white blood cells and macrophages liberates several compounds, particularly the cytokines, interleukin 1 (IL-1), IL-6, and tumor necrosis factor (TNF). These substances alter the temperature control center in the midbrain and produce other effects, particularly increased release of amino acids from muscle for protein synthesis and increased production of acute phase proteins in the liver. As temperature rises, the initial hemodynamic event is a fall in peripheral vascular resistance. This may be due to release of vasodilating substances, fever, or altered neurogenic control. An increase in cardiac output is required to accommodate these changes. Chills and shivering also increase heat production and heat loss.

In 1964, Albrecht and Clowes[120] described the increase in circulatory requirements of inflammation. Early studies by Albrecht and Clowes,[120] Border et al.,[121] and Siegel et al.,[122] demonstrated that with sepsis, the circulatory disorders are a high cardiac output, lower peripheral resistance, and decreased arteriovenous oxygen difference. Border et al.[121] suggested that arteriovenous shunts also play a role. Siegel and colleagues[122] found much the same thing and reported that myocardial contractility was reduced (myocardial failure), particularly in patients whose circulation went from hyperdynamic to hypodynamic. Clowes[120] found that patients with diffuse fulminant peritonitis initially had hypovolemia, electrolyte derangements, low cardiac output, metabolic acidosis, and lactic acidemia. If a patient responded to therapy, a high cardiac output ensued; if this high output was not maintained, however, the patient died. Metabolic rate and caloric expenditure were both elevated. Maintenance of a high cardiac output was associated with survival. MacLean[28] made similar observations in patients with septic shock and emphasized the high oxygen content of venous blood with a narrowed arteriovenous oxygen difference. Wilson et al.,[123] Rosoff et al.,[124] and Shoemaker[125] found similar results.

With infection, catecholamine output increases, protein catabolism begins, and oxygen consumption rises. Measurements of oxygen consumption in patients with sepsis and in animal models have shown, however, that for every 1°C rise in temperature, oxygen consumption increases only 12 percent. Thus the increase in cardiac output with infection is far in excess of the increase in oxygen demand. This is the hyperdynamic circulation of the septic state. Infection requires an increased circulation, both locally at the site of the process and generally to the entire organism. The initial decrease in total peripheral resistance could be mediated by such endogenous substances as histamine, beta-endorphin from the hypothalamus and pituitary gland, changes in components of the complement system (particularly C3 and C3 proactivator), and stimulation of the kallikrein system, particularly bradykinin and serotonin production.

With initial sepsis and septic shock, mixed venous oxygen increases. This situation contrasts with all other forms of shock, in which oxygen extraction increases in the peripheral circulation and venous oxygen levels are low. Several possible mechanisms may prompt this rising venous oxygen content of blood returning to the heart. First, an overall increase in peripheral blood flow may be a cause; however, whether extremely high peripheral blood flow alone can reduce oxygen extraction is unknown. Second, arteriovenous shunts may open because of high blood flow or diversion of blood from certain capillary beds. Shunts could dissipate heat in venous plexuses, through areas of inflammation, through pulmonary systemic artery (bronchial) shunts, or through peripheral arteriovenous shunts that are normally closed. Third, a direct cytotoxic effect on the cells of various organs may decrease their capability to utilize oxygen or the ability to move oxygen from the capillary bed into cells and mitochondria. Some evidence exists for the inability of cells to function and utilize oxygen with severe infection. The major mechanism for the increase in venous oxygen content seems to be increased blood flow with vasodilatation, rather than the other mechanisms. The hemodynamic situation does behave somewhat like an arteriovenous shunt by establishing a new steady state equilibrium with a very high blood flow and low resistance system. Total body oxygen consumption is not greatly increased, which suggests that peripheral oxygen insufficiency may not be the cause, at least initially. In early studies, Hermreck and Thal[126] found that neither the elevated energy requirement associated with sepsis and fever nor the increased flow through the area of sepsis could account for the extra cardiac output required and the general low peripheral resistance. They originally suggested a vasodilator from the septic region that increased blood flow to the area of sepsis, kidneys, splanchnic organs, and elsewhere. This substance, which could be an endothelial factor, remains to be identified—if it indeed exists. All these factors may play a role; a single explanation may not be found.

MEDIATORS

The mediators of inflammation, infection, and healing come from many cells and include the cytokines [interleukins 1, 2, 3, 4, 6, 8, 9, and 10, tumor necrosis factor (TNF) or cachectin, and interferons from lymphocytes (lymphokines), macrophages, other white cells, and probably other cells as well],[127,128] bradykinin from the kallikrein-kinin system, the eicosanoids (leukotrienes, thromboxane, and prostaglandins), complement activation (anaphylatoxins), histamine, serotonin, somatomedin, proteases and superoxides from white cells, platelet-activating factor, endothelial adherence molecules, growth factors, and many more yet to be identified. The complexities of these systems are illustrated by many overlapping actions of the various cytokines, synergistic effects, and the induction of one by another in certain situations. There is great redundancy in this system. The various T-cell subsets secrete different patterns of cytokines that may have mutually inhibitory actions.

The complexities of these systems are exemplified by Solbach et al.[129] in an article titled, "Lymphocytes Play the Music, but the Macrophages Call the Tune," where they state: "Dealing with a single cytokine on an isolated population of cells (or an organism) may be a gross oversimplification of events in vivo." Cytokines seem to produce some of their effects through an intermediate enzyme system called *phospholipase A$_2$.*[130]

Beeson,[131] in 1948, provided the first indication of an endogenous product with pyrogenic activity clearly distinct from endotoxin. This material, called *endogenous pyrogen,* was found in granulocytes. Injection of an extract produced a number of activities, including the release from bone marrow of neutrophils, granulopoiesis, synthesis of acute phase proteins, and flux of amino acids from the muscle to liver. Owing to its source and the multiplicity of host alterations produced, the active extract was called *leukocyte endogenous mediator.*[132] Evidence indicated that endogenous pyrogen and leukocyte endogenous mediator were the same or related proteins. In addition, it was determined that monocytes produced a larger quantity of endogenous pyrogen than did neutrophils. Activation of neutrophils or monocytes by bacteria, viruses, endotoxin, and other stimuli resulted in neutrophil release, granulopoiesis, lactoferrin production, stimulation of the reticuloendothelial system, and lowering of plasma iron. There was also increased iron storage in the liver, increased acute phase protein synthesis, increased release of amino acids from muscle, and a lymphokine was produced that stimulated lymphocytes. Subsequently, it was found that the lymphocyte-activating factor that stimulates T-lymphocyte proliferation and enhances immune responses was identical with endogenous pyrogen; it has now been called *interleukin 1* (IL-1).[133] The mitogenic action of IL-1 on T cells is mediated by the lymphocyte product or lymphokine called *interleukin 2* (IL-2). Endogenous pyrogen, leukocyte endogenous mediator, lymphocyte-activating factor, and IL-1 are functionally identical.[134]

The discovery of TNF resulted from earlier work that sought a factor that produced hemorrhagic necrosis of tumors in patients with infections.[136] Lipopolysaccharide (endotoxin) would induce this substance.[137] Early researchers also were looking for a substance that would explain the cachexia occurring with neoplasms and infections. Trypanosome infection in rabbits produced profound wasting and lipemia[138] and led to studies of endotoxin injection and identification of the mediator that was called *cachectin.* In 1985, Beutler et al.[139] purified cachectin. Cachectin, a monokine polypeptide produced primarily by macrophages, has many and profound effects on biologic organisms. It is now believed to be the major or proximal mediator of endotoxin.[135] After cachectin was isolated, it was found to be identical to TNF. Thus two lines of research—one on tumor necrosis and the other on cachexia—converged with the discovery of cachectin/TNF.

In a clinical trial, Warren et al.[140] injected recombinant human cachectin/TNF as a potential antineoplastic agent in patients with tumors. This agent increased C-reactive protein levels, reduced serum zinc levels, increased amino acid (alanine, glutamine) efflux from skeletal muscle, and decreased arterial levels of alanine, glutamine, and total amino acids. These effects are similar to those of IL-1. Cortisol levels also rose with the injections. Although endotoxin is the major stimulus for cachectin, virus particles and other biologic and infectious agents also may induce production.

Cachectin activates neutrophils by stimulating their adhesion to endothelial surfaces and enhancing their phagocytic activity via degranulation or superoxide production. Cachectin also stimulates IL-1 and stress hormone production, including epinephrine, norepinephrine, dopamine, cortisol, and glucagon. Other metabolic effects include loss of triglycerides from adipose tissue and decreased uptake and storage of fat as lipoprotein lipase is suppressed. When injected in rats, TNF increases peripheral muscle proteolysis, seemingly by activation of the hypothalamic-adrenal stress response.[141] TNF also produces liver hypertrophy, thus mediating interorgan substrate flux. Cachectin and IL-1, both of which are also endogenous pyrogens, have other similar effects. Antiviral and other protective effects against inflammation have been described.

The injection of larger amounts of cachectin in animals produces severe toxic reactions and death.[142,143] The effects are the same as those observed with endotoxin injections.[144] However, the lethal effects of endotoxin may require other mediators in addition to TNF.[145] Cortisol, given before the infectious insult or endotoxin injection, antagonized the effects of endotoxin.[146] Furthermore, cortisol completely inhibits cachectin biosynthesis if given before macrophage activation (being ineffective after activation). This explains in biochemical terms why steroids are not effective in the treatment of established septic shock.

Michie et al.[147] infused a bolus of *E. coli* endotoxin into normal, healthy male volunteers and found that TNF levels increased. The response peaked at 90 min and returned to normal by 4 h. Temperature and heart rate also increased, as did ACTH and epinephrine levels. The white blood cell count increased after the infusion, and no interferon-γ was detectable. The volunteers had chills, headaches, myalgia, and nausea with fever and tachycardia. Blood pressure did not decrease. Ibuprofen, given before the endotoxin infusion, did not alter the TNF levels but did eliminate the symptoms and attenuate the fever, tachycardia, and stress hormone responses. Thus a cyclooxygenase pathway seems to mediate the responses to TNF. Fromm et al.[148] reported a similar experiment in humans. Michie et al.[149] also gave TNF to a number of tumor-bearing patients and found that IL-1 levels did not change. The physiologic and metabolic changes they noted were the same as those after endotoxin infusions, which suggests that TNF may be the primary afferent signal that initiates many metabolic responses with sepsis. TNF also seems to be a major factor in producing the clinical features of infection. Waage et al.[150] have now found TNF in 10 of 11 patients who died of meningococcal disease but in only 8 of 68 who survived. *E. coli* endotoxin and TNF produced the same metabolic, hormonal, and clinical effects when given to patients or volunteers.

Michie and Wilmore[151] present evidence that Koch's postulates regarding the causes of infectious diseases have been fulfilled by TNF. In animal studies, an IL-1 receptor antagonist and monoclonal antibody to TNF will protect against their toxic effects. In another study, Michie et al.[152] found that TNF infusion for 5 days was associated with anorexia, fluid retention, acute phase responses, and negative nitrogen balance. The negative nitrogen balance was due to anorexia, however, and not to hypermetabolism or increased tissue breakdown. Thus TNF is not the entire answer.

Cachectin/TNF levels in monocytes studied from trauma and burned patients were elevated.[153] Levels were highest in patients who had sepsis and in those who ultimately died. These high levels occurred despite high levels of prostaglandin E_2 that should be immunosuppressive. The high degree of conservation of the gene for TNF in mammals led Cerami and Beutler[154] to hypothesize that the gene and TNF play an important role in host defense—in fact, they suggest some potential therapeutic benefits.

IL-4 down-regulates IL-1 and TNF gene expression and IL-1 production. IL-6 production is stimulated by IL-1 and TNF, and it may be the effector for many of the toxic effects of these cytokines. It is also important in acute phase protein production. IL-8 regulates endothelial cell and neutrophil interaction and may be inhibitory when it is intravascular or proinflammatory when extravascular. IL-10 inhibits cytokine synthesis. Other important cytokines include interferon-γ, platelet-activating factor, and the growth factors.

Metabolic changes produced by infection are initially similar to the stress response. Progressive alterations in glucose, fat, and protein metabolism develop with extensive catabolism. Abnormalities in peripheral muscle metabolism and liver metabolism may lead to metabolic failure and contribute to MOF. The mediators of injury, inflammation, and infection are similar. These relationships and mediators are shown in Fig. 3–10.

NEUROGENIC SHOCK

ETIOLOGY

Neurogenic shock also has been called *vasogenic shock* or *vasomotor collapse*. Syncope is a form of this problem. It also may occur with spinal anesthesia, spinal cord injury (also called *spinal shock*), or anaphylactic shock. Any etiology for decreased peripheral vascular resistance may result in hypotension and decreased blood flow. Thus a decrease in peripheral vascular resistance can occur from a number of insults. It can be a sudden and transient episode, such as syncope. It can result from the effects of an anesthetic agent—particularly a spinal anesthetic, which causes decreased vascular tone from the level of the anesthetic downward.

Decreased vascular resistance is also characteristic of early septic shock, since the patient's temperature is elevated with the infection. Vasodilatation occurs to attempt to increase heat loss and control the pyrogenic effect. This may resemble vasomotor collapse or vasogenic shock. The setting and the circumstances, however, are usually quite different. The septic patient with hypotension due to excessive vasodilatation will be warm and dry. Temperature, however, will be elevated, and pulse will be bounding but usually associated with tachycardia. The patient will appear quite ill. In patients with acute myocardial infarction, there also have been circumstances described in which peripheral vascular constriction does not occur as cardiac output fails. There may be a mismatch between cardiac output and the response by the peripheral circulation. This has been the rationale for the use of mild vasoconstrictors in some patients with early or mild cardiogenic shock. Here again, this situation would be associated with acute changes of chest pain and/or electrocardiographic changes and indicates something more than simply a vasogenic problem.

PATHOPHYSIOLOGY

A decrease in peripheral vascular resistance may not produce overt changes in a patient's hemodynamic status if there are adjustments elsewhere. Also, a modest decrease in blood pressure is well tolerated, if it occurs with vasodilatation. Most anesthetic agents are associated with some decrease in blood pressure.

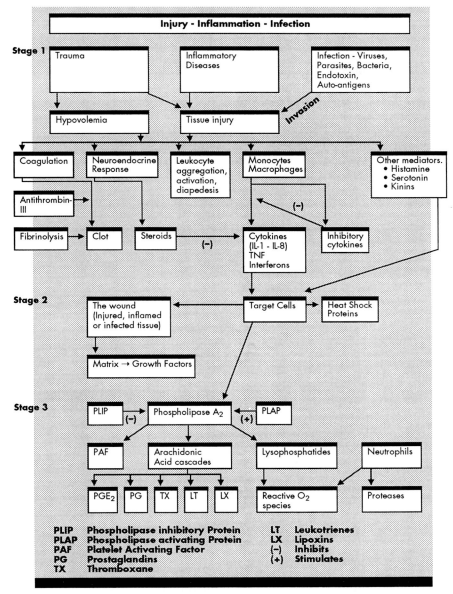

FIG. 3–10. The interrelationships and mediator sequences of the four stages of inflammation.

However, any alteration in cardiac output is probably due to a direct cardiac depressant effect.

At one time, ganglionic blocking agents were used to decrease peripheral resistance and blood flow, particularly with certain neurosurgical operations. An extremely low mean arterial blood pressure can be tolerated, as long as cardiac output is normal. With central nervous system injury—particularly to the spinal cord—reduced vascular tone from lost sympathetic innervation may lower blood pressure. If the individual cannot compensate for this, reduced tissue blood flow may occur as cardiac output fails. If neurogenic shock should persist and be associated with a significant decrease in cardiac output, the manifestation would be a reduction in blood flow to tissues and organs, with a response similar to that of hypovolemic or cardiogenic shock. Because of the low pressure, capillary refilling may occur; vasoconstriction would occur where vasomotor tone had not been eliminated. In most circumstances, however, the situation does not deteriorate to this point.

HEMODYNAMIC CHARACTERISTICS

By definition, in neurogenic shock, the blood pressure will be reduced. Usually, however, the heart rate is slow. Thus the characteristic picture of neurogenic shock is quite different from that of other types of shock. Initially, the pulse may be steady, although slow. If blood flow decreases, tachycardia may eventually occur, along with other changes, which suggests a prolonged decrease in blood flow. This would occur, of course, only if vascular volume and cardiac status were inadequate to deal with the loss of vasomotor tone.

TREATMENT

With mild forms of neurogenic shock, such as syncope, placing the patient in a supine position with legs elevated for a short period of time will probably be sufficient. If the decrease in resistance is excessive, such as with spinal shock or with a spinal anesthetic, then a mild vasoconstrictor agent would be helpful. The drug methoxamine (Vasoxyl) is effective in this regard, because it has a safe, mild alpha-adrenergic stimulating effect to increase peripheral vascular resistance without altering blood flow to vital organs. If neurogenic shock, such as with spinal cord injury, occurs with severe generalized trauma, then careful monitoring, resuscitation, and treatment are required. Blood and fluid loss, along with decreased vascular resistance and tone, may produce a complicated situation. In most such circumstances, increased vascular volume or overexpansion is much more appropriate than is the use of vasoconstrictor agents. In addition to methoxamine, the drug phenylephrine (Neo-Synephrine) also may be used safely and appropriately to produce a mild increase in peripheral vascular resistance without a reduction in blood flow to vital organs such as the kidneys and the myocardium.

Different problems, such as acute gastric dilation, have been described as producing a form of neurogenic shock. Acute gastric dilation, of course, indicates the insertion of a nasogastric tube on an emergent basis and decompression of the stomach. Acute gastric dilation can occur after injury and with air swallowing, such as with some forms of hysteria.

ISCHEMIA-REPERFUSION PROBLEMS

When the blood supply to an organ stops because of atherosclerosis and thrombosis, an embolus, vascular injury, or clamping (such as during heart surgery), there is an immediate progression of events. Function is altered, with progressive changes in energy availability, membrane function, and finally, cell damage and death. The rapidity of change and progression of damage are greatest in organs with the greatest metabolic activity (rate) and work and maximal normal oxygen extraction. Thus the heart and brain are first, with the kidneys and liver following and skeletal muscle later. If the blood supply to the organ is restored quickly, these events will be corrected. If restoring blood flow is delayed, the organ may not function adequately or survive. In between these extremes is a period where there will be organ damage. Some of this will occur during ischemia, but there also may be damage when blood flow is restored. This is called *reperfusion injury* and seems to involve the production of mediators such as leukotrienes and prostaglandins that, in turn, activate white blood cells to produce toxic products (proteases and oxygen free radicals). This process resembles the initiation of an inflammatory response. Inflammation produced by an inflammatory agent, a chemical agent, ischemia, or infection are similar and vary primarily in intensity.

These events have been described very well for the myocardium after occlusion of coronary arteries (myocardial infarction) and occlusion of the aorta during cardiac surgery. There is no doubt that there is a reperfusion injury, and many methods have been studied to eliminate or decrease its effects. The same seems to occur with the brain, kidney, liver, and skeletal muscle, but on a different scale. There is also evidence that ischemia of a region of the body will activate or produce mediators that can produce damage elsewhere. Thus ischemia of the legs, with clamping of the aorta during repair of an aortic aneurysm, may produce pulmonary changes and damage during reperfusion. This process has been studied extensively by Hechtman's group.[51-53] They implicate leukotriene B$_4$ from ischemic tissue that activates neutrophils. The activated neutrophils produce oxygen free radicals and release proteolytic enzymes that damage the pulmonary capillary endothelium. Whether or not there is an ischemia-reperfusion injury in injured humans has not been established. The evidence available for this will be reviewed later.

MYOCARDIAL ISCHEMIA

The most extensive studies of ischemia have been carried out with the heart. The cellular events are shown in detail in Table 3–7. In the myocardial circulation, the changes accompanying reperfusion resemble inflammation.[155] These changes are shown in Table 3–8. Other changes with ischemia, both in skeletal muscle and myocardium, include a reduction in superoxide dismutase (SOD), glutathione, and protein SH groups, but not glutathione peroxidase or reductase; production of oxygen free radicals in ischemic muscle by neutrophils; H$_2$O$_2$ inactivation of creatinine kinase, leading to inefficient phosphocreatine conversion to ATP; rapid decrease of intracellular pH and quick recovery with reperfusion; and a massive increase in oxygen consumption after "stunning." Mitochondria are not uncoupled, but ischemia induces inefficiency in ATP utilization. Global ischemia leads to extravascular compression of vessels and less adenine nucleotide translocase binding of fatty acyl-CoA to decrease amphipathic metabolites.

TABLE 3–7. Myocardial Ischemia

Seconds:	The ischemic myocardium switches from aerobic to anaerobic glycolysis.
Minutes:	Phosphocreatine and ATP reserves are severely depleted.
	Most creatine phosphate is lost within the first 3 min.
	ATP decreases over 30 min. more slowly.
	ATP is broken down to adenosine, inosine, hypoxanthine, and then xanthine.
	Contractility diminishes; ST segments are elevated.
	Potassium is lost; sodium is retained.
Within 30	There is glycogen depletion and proton accumulation.
Minutes:	The whole adenine nucleotide pool is destroyed; lower ATP levels are associated with depressed high-energy phosphate resynthesis and failed cell volume regulation before overt membrane damage. At 2 μmol ATP per gram, there is membrane damage.
	Protons, ammonium ions, and phosphate increase.
	Increased tissue osmolarity.
	Sarcoplasmic reticulum is swollen.
	Glycogen granules absent.
	Myofibrils, prominent I bands; nuclei, peripheral aggregation of chromatin and mitochondrial swelling.
	Endogenous norepinephrine mobilization.
	Calcium accumulation and the ability of the sacroplasmic reticulum is impaired.
	Phospholipase activation and altered phospholipid metabolism.
Beyond 30	Increased lysophosphoglycerides, increased membrane degradation,
Minutes:	xanthine oxidase activity increased.
	Endogenous free radical scavenger activity increases.
	This all leads to disruption of the sarcolemma by
	1. Physical stress due to tissue osmolarity.
	2. Phospholipid degradation.
	3. Lipid peroxidation.
	There is cell swelling of all elements. The plasmalemma has discontinuities. Hypoxia, of course, differs from ischemia, because the metabolic products are removed with hypoxia.

REPERFUSION INJURY

Jennings et al.,[156] in 1960, observed structural and electrophysiologic changes associated with coronary reperfusion and suggested reperfusion injury. In 1973, Bing et al.[157] found that acidosis during hypoxia reduced injury. In 1977, Greene and Weisfeld[158] found that reoxygenation produced contracture, which was prevented by acidosis. Hearse,[159] in 1977, popularized the concept of reperfusion injury with respect to the heart. In 1980, Powell et al.[160] and Powers et al.[161] found endothelial swelling with ischemia. In 1983, Shine and Douglas[162] found that ischemia with reperfusion with a low-calcium solution was protective, but this process was not affected by calcium channel blockers. Therefore, it was postulated to involve a different mechanism.

The changes that may contribute to an ischemia-reperfusion injury include

1. Ischemic cell swelling with loss of cell membrane integrity, occurring very early during postocclusion reflow. In skeletal muscle, there also may be interstitial edema that contributes to the compartment syndrome.

TABLE 3–8. Myocardial Ischemia

Resembles inflammation:
1. Accumulation of leukocytes
   A. Microvascular trapping of neutrophils
   B. Intercellular adhesion
2. Chemotactic factors
   A. Complement activation
   B. Lipid-derived chemotactic agents
3. Products of oxidative stress act as chemotactic agents in ischemia

The order of events seems to be:
1. The injured myocardial cell releases products that promote chemotaxis and increase surface expression of adherence molecules. White cells are then activated, releasing granular contents and producing oxygen free radicals.
2. Activated neutrophils adhere to the endothelium.
3. Additional adherence ligands help with this, such as expression of ICAM-1.
4. Complement is activated.
5. Other cells are activated.
6. Neutrophils migrate into the extracellular space.

2. A no-reflow phenomenon, which may be due to endothelial cell swelling, blebs, or plugging of the microvascular bed by leukocytes. There is also reperfusion-induced hemorrhage.

3. A "calcium paradox," described by Zimmerman and colleagues[163] in 1966. This is a condition in which the sudden readmission of calcium to the perfusate, after a brief period in which hearts are perfused with calcium-free media, causes massive tissue disruption, enzyme release, and the development of contracture and marked reductions in high-energy phosphate stores.

4. An "oxygen paradox." Reintroduction of oxygen to hypoxic or anoxic myocardium leads to excess liberation of cardiac enzymes and contracture.[164] Conceptually, when molecular oxygen is reintroduced, cells contain high concentrations of hypoxanthine and xanthine oxidase. This enzyme causes the release of O_2 and H_2O_2 and may be catalyzed by iron.[165] During the ischemic period, there has been loss of the enzymes superoxide dismutase, catalase, and glutathione peroxidase that protect the heart. Oxygen seems to be critical in this process of microvascular and parenchymal injury, since reperfusion with hypoxemic blood attenuates the injury.[166] The autooxidation of catecholamines, arachidonic acid metabolism, and mitochondria provide other sources of free radicals.

5. Leukocyte activation and migration with liberation of proteolytic enzymes and superoxide anions.

6. Complement activation.

7. High-energy phosphate depletion.

8. A "pH paradox," proposed by Lemasters et al.[167] and Currin et al.[168] They described the protection that acidosis provides for cells during anoxia/hypoxia. In addition, they found that in several organs a rapid increase in pH (correction of acidosis), rather than reoxygenation, accounted for the reperfusion injury. A rapid return from acidotic to physiologic pH initiates the onset of cell death.

9. A rewarming injury if an organ has been cooled for protection or preservation.[169]

Reperfusion then washes out intracellular enzymes, including creatine kinase. There is rapid accumulation of calcium. The tissue loses homeostasis with respect to calcium. Production of oxygen free radicals proceeds with marked changes in ultrastructure. Sixty minutes of ischemia, with 5 minutes of reperfusion, leads to sarcolemmal disruptions. Continued reperfusion produces release of contraction bands, and cell calcium increases fivefold.

IS THERE AN ISCHEMIA-REPERFUSION INJURY WITH SHOCK IN INJURED PATIENTS?

Ischemia-reperfusion injury may be a major contributing factor to morbidity and mortality with injury and/or operation. It is involved with the production of MOF along with sepsis. It may be produced by infection and the demands of a hyperdynamic circulation. Baker and Degutis[170] showed that after the age and injury severity score (ISS), the other important risk factors for death after injury were the level and duration of shock. The patients studied had been resuscitated, operated on, and taken to an intensive care unit, and days later developed infection and/or MOF. Why does an initial period of shock contribute to this sequence? Cell damage during ischemia (shock), with delay in providing complete or normal perfusion and reperfusion injury, may set the stage for late complications. Objective evidence for an ischemia-reperfusion injury in patients after shock has not been well established. In animals after hemorrhagic shock, elevation of the lipid peroxidation by-product malonyldialdehyde suggests the generation of oxygen free radicals.[171,172] Most of the evidence for this phenomenon comes from studies of protection of animals from the effects of hemorrhagic shock by pretreatment with allopurinol, SOD, leukocyte depletion, iron chelation with a deferoxamine conjugate, and other agents.[173–178] There is a decline in liver vitamin E (a free radical scavenger) content in rats with hemorrhagic shock that can be eliminated by inhibitors of lipid peroxidation but not by oxypurinol,[179] ibuprofen, or iron chelators. This suggests, but does not prove, that hypovolemic shock initiates cell and organ damage that may not be apparent initially. Girotti et al.,[180] however, failed to find evidence of early oxidative injury 2 to 6 h after major blunt trauma in patients. The ischemia-reperfusion debate remains unresolved at this juncture.[181–186]

PREVENTION OF ISCHEMIA-REPERFUSION INJURY

Numerous ways to prevent or treat this injury have been studied. Some agents must be given before the insult, which helps to define mechanisms of injury and could be helpful in planned events, such as cardiac surgery or organ preservation for transplantation. Others must be given at the time of the insult. Some may be helpful after the period of ischemia but before reperfusion. Examples of these are shown in Table 3–9. Most agents that are beneficial when used at the time of reperfusion have actions which control white blood cell activation and oxygen free radical production. Many are used in cardiac surgery to protect the myocardium during ischemia and to prevent reperfusion injury. Some are also being used in organ harvesting and preservation for transplantation. A few drugs, such as mannitol, are being used as mild antioxidant agents with abdom-

TABLE 3–9. Prevention of Ischemia-Reperfusion Injury

1. Beta-adrenergic blocking agents, before or at the onset of coronary occlusion, will decrease reperfusion injury.
2. Calcium channel antagonists, given before or at the time of the beginning of ischemia, will reduce reperfusion injury.
3. Substrates given before ischemia help protect cells:
   a. Adenosine
   b. Phosphocreatine
   c. Glucose and insulin
   d. Glutamine
4. Phosphodiesterase inhibitor (enoximone)
5. Adenosine deaminase inhibition
6. Agents that could be helpful when given at the time of reperfusion include:
   a. Hypertonic mannitol
   b. Allopurinol, oxypurinol, and deferoxamine
   c. Urokinase
   d. Fluorocarbons
   e. Free radical scavangers such as superoxide dismutase
   f. Agents which reduce leukocyte activation or adherence (monoclonal antibodies to adherence molecules)
   g. Leukocyte depletion
   h. Prostacyclin analogue

inal aortic surgery to decrease reperfusion injury. Whether any specific or general approach to reperfusion injury will be useful in the multiple system–injured patient who is brought to an emergency department in shock remains to be established.

SUMMARY

Patients with overwhelming injuries or blood loss may die quickly after injury. Many now arrive at an emergency department alive but die shortly thereafter from shock and injury despite attempts at resuscitation and emergency treatment. Others are resuscitated, treated, operated on, and cared for in an intensive care unit. The impact of the multisystem injury, a period of shock with possible ischemia-reperfusion problems, and an operation may initiate cell and organ failure. This may lead to progressive or sequential multiple systems or organ failures (MOF) and ultimate death. Infection (sepsis) either initiates this problem, occurs along with it, or represents another failed system (the host resistance immune system). Faist et al.[187] described an early and a late sequence of MOF. Early MOF occurs in the first few days after injury and is related to the severity of the injury and the number of organs involved. Late MOF occurs after 4 to 5 days or more and is due to or triggered by infection or inflammation.

The intricacies and interrelationships of injury, inflammation, and infection that contribute to this process are complex and incompletely understood. Four stages are shown in Fig. 3–9. The sequence of organ involvement after injury is shown in Fig. 3–10. The inflammatory response is the center of the influences on survival. The therapy of this process includes prevention of injury, early therapy, a zero-defect or no complication approach, and early organ support before organ failure develops.[1,7,182,184] Can we interfere with the inflammatory process and block or modulate it? Certainly the evidence for use of monoclonal antibodies for gram-negative infection and shock is impressive. An array of blocking and stimulating agents is being evaluated.[79] Advances in patient care should come from these.

REFERENCES

1. Gross SD: *A System of Surgery: Pathological, Diagnostic, Therapeutique, and Operative*, vol 1, 2d ed. Philadelphia, Blanchard and Lea, 1862, p 706.
2. Blalock A: Acute circulatory failure as exemplified by shock and hemorrhage. *Surg Gynecol Obstet* 58:551, 1934.
3. Churchill ED: Introduction, in HK Beecher (ed): *Surgery in World War II: The Physiologic Effects of Wounds*. Washington, Board for the Study of the Severely Wounded, Medical Department, U.S. Army, U.S. Government Printing Office, 1952, pp 1–20.
4. Churchill ED: *Surgeon to Soldiers: Diary and Records of the Surgical Consultant, Allied Force Headquarters, World War II*. Philadelphia, Lippincott, 1972.
5. Baue AE: Recent developments in the study and treatment of shock. *Surg Gynecol Obstet* 127:849, 1968.
6. Baue AE: Multiple, progressive or sequential systems failure: Syndrome of the 1970s. *Arch Surg* 110:779, 1975.
7. Baue AE: *Multiple Organ Failure: Patient Care and Prevention*. St. Louis, Mosby–Year Book, 1990.
8. Paré A: *Les oeuvres d'Ambroise Paré*. Paris, Daupauye, 1582, p 267.
9. Le Dran HF: *A Treatise, or Reflections, Drawn from Practice on Gun-Shot Wounds*. London, J Clarke, 1743.
10. Latta J: *A Practical System of Surgery*. Edinburgh, G Mudie & Son, 1795.
11. Latta T: Relative to the treatment of cholera by the copious injection of aqueous and saline fluids into the veins, letter to the Secretary of the Central Board of Health, London. *Lancet* 2:274, 1831–1832.
12. Cooper A: *A Dictionary of Practical Surgery*, 7th ed. London, Longman, 1838.
13. Warren JC: *Surgical Pathology and Therapeutics*. Philadelphia, Saunders, 1895.
14. Crile GW: *An Experimental Research into Surgical Shock*. Philadelphia, Lippincott, 1899.
15. Henderson Y: Fatal apnoea and the shock problem. *Johns Hopkins Hosp Bull* 21:235, 1910.
16. Cannon WB: *Traumatic Shock*. New York, D Appleton, 1923.
17. Keith NM: *Blood Volume Changes in Wound Shock and Primary Hemorrhage* (Special Report Series No. 27). London, Medical Research Council, 1919.
18. Archibald EW, McLean WS: Observations upon shock, with particular reference to the condition as seen in war surgery. *Trans Am Surg Assoc Phila* 35:522, 1917.
19. Dale HL, Richards AN: The vasodilator action of histamine and some other substances. *J Physiol* 52:110, 1918.
20. Blalock A: Experimental shock: Cause of low blood pressure produced by muscle injury. *Arch Surg* 20:959, 1930.
21. Parsons E, Phemister DB: Hemorrhage and "shock" in traumatized limbs: An experimental study. *Surg Gynecol Obstet* 51:196, 1930.
22. Beecher HK, Simeone FA, Burnett CH, et al: The internal state of the severely wounded man on entry to the most forward hospital. *Surgery* 22:672, 1947.

23. Cournand A, Riley RL, Bradley SE, et al: Studies of circulation in clinical shock. *Surgery* 13:964, 1943.

24. Howard JM (ed): *Battle Casualties in Korea* (Surgical Research Team in Korea), vol 1. Washington, Army Medical Service Graduate School, Walter Reed Army Medical Center, 1954.

25. Wiggers CJ: *Physiology of Shock.* Cambridge, Mass, Harvard University Press, 1950.

26. Harkins HN, Long CNH: Metabolic changes in shock after burns. *Am J Physiol* 144:661, 1945.

27. Simeone FA: Some issues in problems of shock. *Fed Proc* 20:3, 1961.

28. MacLean LD: Shock: Causes and management of circulatory collapse, in D Sabiston (ed): *Davis-Christopher Textbook of Surgery: The Biologic Basis of Modern Surgical Practice,* vol 1, 11th ed. Philadelphia, Saunders, 1977, pp 65–94.

29. MacLean LD, Mulligan WG, MacLean APH, et al: Patterns of septic shock in man: A detailed study of 56 patients. *Ann Surg* 166:543, 1967.

30. Skillman JJ, Awwad HK, Moore FD: Plasma protein kinetics of early transcapillary refill after hemorrhage in man. *Surg Gynecol Obstet* 125:983, 1967.

31. Drucker WR, Chadwick CDJ, Gann DS: Transcapillary refill in hemorrhage and shock. *Arch Surg* 116:1344, 1981.

32. Gann DS, Carlson DE, et al: Role of solute and the early restitution of blood volume after hemorrhage. *Surgery* 94:439, 1983.

33. Shires GT, Cunningham JN, Baker CRF, et al: Alterations in cellular membrane function during hemorrhagic shock in primates. *Ann Surg* 176:288, 1972.

34. Hock CE, Su JY, Lefer AM: Role of AVP in maintenance of circulatory homeostasis during hemorrhagic shock. *Am J Physiol* 246:H174, 1984.

35. van den Berg MH, van Giersbergen PLM, Cox-van Put J, de Jong W: Endogenous opioid peptides and blood pressure regulation during controlled, stepwise hemorrhagic hypotension. *Circ Shock* 35:102, 1991.

36. Overman RR, Wang SC: The contributory role of the afferent nervous factor in experimental shock: Sublethal hemorrhage and sciatic nerve stimulation. *Am J Physiol* 148:289, 1947.

37. Little RA, Kirkman E: Cardiovascular response to haemorrhage and injury. *Circ Shock* 34:7, 1991.

38. Anderson ID, Little RA, Irving MH: An effect of trauma on human cardiovascular control: Baroreflex suppression. *J Trauma* 30:974, 1990.

39. Baethmann A, Kempski O: The brain in shock: Secondary disturbances of cerebral function. *Chest* 100:205S, 1991.

40. Gosche JR, Garrison RN: Prostaglandins mediate the compensatory responses to hemorrhage in the small intestine of the rat. *J Surg Res* 50:584, 1991.

41. Myers SI, Small J: Prolonged hemorrhagic shock decreases splanchnic prostacyclin synthesis. *J Surg Res* 50:417, 1991.

42. Singh G, Chaudry KI, Chudler LC, Chaudry IH: Depressed gut absorptive capacity early after trauma-hemorrhagic shock. *Ann Surg* 214:712, 1991.

43. Deitch E, Winterton J, Berg R, et al: The gut as a portal of entry for bacteremia. *Ann Surg* 205:681, 1987.

44. Gelfand GAJ, Morales J, Jones RL, et al: Bacterial translocation after hemorrhagic shock in a swine model. *J Trauma* 31:867, 1991.

45. Ferraro FJ, Rush BF, McCullough J, et al. Histologic aspects of hemorrhagic shock in germ free vs conventional rats. *Circ Shock* 34:29, 1991.

46. Rush BF, Redan JA, Flanagan JJ, et al: Does the bacteremia observed in hemorrhagic shock have clinical significance? *Ann Surg* 210:342, 1989.

47. Rush BF Jr, Soki AJ, Murphy TF, et al: Endotoxemia and bacteremia during hemorrhagic shock. *Ann Surg* 207:549, 1988.

48. Fine J: Current status of problems of traumatic shock. *Surg Gynecol Obstet* 120:537, 1965.

49. Meyers JR, Meyer JS, Baue AE: Does hemorrhagic shock damage the lung? *J Trauma* 13:509, 1973.

50. Collins JA, James PM, Brendenberg CE, et al: The relationship between transfusion and hypoxemia in combat casualties. *Ann Surg* 188:513, 1978.

51. Goldman G, Welbourn R, Peterson IS, et al: Ischemia-induced neutrophil activation and diapedesis is lipoxygenase dependent. *Surgery* 107:428, 1990.

52. Paterson IS, Klausner JM, Goldman G, et al: Thromboxane mediates the ischemia-induced neutrophil oxidative burst. *Surgery* 106:224, 1989.

53. Paterson IS, Klausner JM, Pugatch R, et al: Noncardiogenic pulmonary edema after abdominal aortic aneurysm surgery. *Ann Surg* 209:231, 1989.

54. Hewson JR, Prodger D, Roberts RS, et al: Prolonged hemorrhagic shock does not impair regeneration of plasma coagulant masses in the rabbit. *Crit Care Med* 19:253, 1991.

55. Harrigan C, Lucas CE, Ledgerwood AM: The effect of hemorrhagic shock on the clotting cascade in injured patients. *J Trauma* 29:1416, 1989.

56. Rana MW, Singh G, Wang P, et al: Heparin administration before or after hemorrhagic shock protects microvascular patency. *Circ Shock* 31:59, 1990.

57. Wang P, Singh G, Rana MW, et al: Pre-heparinization improves cardiac output (CO), hepatocellular function (HF) and renal function (RF) after hemorrhage and resuscitation. *Circ Shock* 31:60, 1990.

58. Burke JF: The effective period of preventive antibiotic action in experimental incisions and dermal lesions. *Surgery* 50(1):161, 1961.

59. Stephan RN, Kupper TS, Geha AS, et al: Hemorrhage without tissue trauma produces immunosuppression and enhances susceptibility to sepsis. *Arch Surg* 122:62, 1987.

60. Miles AA, Niven JSF: The enhancement of infection during shock produced by bacterial toxins and other agents. *Br J Exp Pathol* 31:73, 1950.

61. Nichols RL, Smith JW, Klein DB, et al: Risk of infection after penetrating abdominal trauma. *N Engl J Med* 311:1065, 1984.

62. Baue AE: Metabolic abnormalities of shock. *Surg Clin North Am* 56:1059, 1976.

63. Weil MH, Abdelmonen AA: Experimental and clinical studies on lactate and pyruvate as indicators of severity of acute circulatory failure (shock). *Circulation* 41(6):989, 1970.

64. Davis JW, Shackford SR, Mackersie RC, Hoyt DB: Base deficit as a guide to volume resuscitation. *J Trauma* 28:1464, 1988.

65. Davis JW, Shackford SR, Holbrook TL: Base deficit as a sensitive indicator of compensated shock and tissue oxygen utilization. *Surg Gynecol Obstet* 173:473, 1991.

66. Dunham CM, Fabian M, Siegel JH, Gettings L: Hepatic insufficiency and increased proteolysis, cardiac output, and oxygen consumption following hemorrhage. *Circ Shock* 35:78, 1991.

67. Baue AE: Shock and cardiac arrest, in JD Hardy (ed): *Hardy's Textbook of Surgery*. Philadelphia, Lippincott, 1983, p 33.

68. Bagge U, Amundson B, Lauritzen C: White blood cell deformability and plugging of skeletal muscle capillaries in hemorrhagic shock. *Acta Physiol Scand* 108:159, 1980.

69. Kreis DJ Jr, Chaudry IH, Schleck SA, Baue AE: Red blood cell sodium, potassium and ATP levels during hemorrhagic shock. *J Surg Res* 31:225, 1981.

70. Messmer K, Kreimeier U: Microcirculatory therapy in shock. *Resuscitation* 18:S51, 1989.

71. Wang P, Singh G, Rana MW, et al: Preheparinization improves organ function after hemorrhage and resuscitation. *Am J Physiol* 259:R645, 1990.

72. Wang P, Hauptman JG, Chaudry IH: Hemorrhage produces depression in microvascular blood flow which persists despite fluid resuscitation. *Circ Shock* 32:307, 1990.

73. Canizaro PC, Prager MD, Shires GT: The infusion of Ringer's lactate solution during shock: Changes in lactate, excess lactate, and pH. *Am J Surg* 122:494, 1971.

74. Baue AE, Tragus ET, Parkins WM: A comparison of isotonic and hypertonic solutions and blood on blood flow and oxygen consumption in initial treatment of hemorrhagic shock. *J Trauma* 7:743, 1967.

75. Baue AE, Tragus ET, Parkins WM: The effects of increased osmolality and correction of acidosis on blood flow and oxygen consumption in hemorrhagic shock. *J Surg Res* 7:349, 1967.

76. Kreimeier U, Brueckner UB, Schmidt J, Messmer K: Instantaneous restoration of regional organ blood flow after severe hemorrhage: Effect of small-volume resuscitation with hypertonic-hyperoncotic solutions. *J Surg Res* 49:493, 1990.

77. Shires GT, Canizaro PC, Carrico CJ: Shock, in SI Schwartz (ed): *Textbook of Surgery,* 3d ed. New York, McGraw-Hill, 1979.

78. Chaudry IH, Clemens MG, Baue AE: Alterations in cell function with ischemia and shock and their correction. *Arch Surg* 116:1309, 1981.

79. Baue AE: The horror autotoxicus and multiple organ failure. *Arch Surg* 127:1451, 1992.

80. Palombo JD, Blackburn GL, Forse RA: Endothelial cell factors and response to injury. *Surg Gynecol Obstet* 173:505, 1991.

81. Chaudry IH, Sayeed MM, Baue AE: Effect of adenosine triphosphate-magnesium chloride administration in shock. *Surgery* 75:220, 1974.

82. Chaudry IH, Clemens MG, Ohkawa M, et al: Restoration of hepatocellular function and blood flow following hepatic ischemia with ATP-MgCl$_2$. *Adv Shock Res* 8:177, 1982.

83. Chaudry IH, Keefer JR, Barash P, et al: ATP-MgCl$_2$ infusion in man: Increased cardiac output without adverse systemic hemodynamic effects. *Surg Forum* 35:14, 1984.

84. Bitterman H, Reissman P, Bitterman N, et al: Oxygen therapy in hemorrhagic shock. *Circ Shock* 33:183, 1991.

85. Baue AE, Chaudry IH, Sayeed MM, et al: Cellular alterations with shock and ischemia. *Angiology* 25:31, 1974.

86. Chaudry IH: Cellular mechanisms in shock and ischemia and their correlation. *Am J Physiol* 245:117, 1983.

87. Corbucci GG, Gasparetto A, Antonelli M, et al: Aspects of the mitochondrial oxidative damage in human circulatory shock. *Circ Shock* 31:314, 1990.

88. Buchman TG, Cabin DE, Vickers S, et al: Molecular biology of circulatory shock: II. Expression of four groups of hepatic genes is enhanced after resuscitation from cardiogenic shock. *Surgery* 108:559, 1990.

89. Buchman TG, Cabin DE, Porter JM, Bulkley GB: Change in hepatic gene expression after shock/resuscitation. *Surgery* 106:283, 1989.

90. Schlag G, Redl H, Hallstrom S: The cell in shock: The origin of multiple organ failure. *Resuscitation* 21:137, 1991.

91. Hyers TM, Gee M, Andreadis NA: Cellular interactions in the multiple organ injury syndrome. *Am Rev Respir Dis* 135:952, 1987.

92. Goris RJA: Integral management of the multiple traumatized patient. *Circ Shock* 34:7, 1991.

93. Fishberg AM, Hitzig WM, King FH: Circulatory dynamics in myocardial infarction. *Arch Intern Med* 54:997, 1934.

94. Harrison TR: *Failure of the Circulation.* Baltimore, Williams & Wilkins, 1935.

95. Blalock A: *Principles of Surgical Care, Shock, and Other Problems.* St. Louis, Mosby, 1940.

96. Grishman A, Master AM: Cardiac output in coronary occlusion studied by the Wezler-Boeger physical method. *Proc Soc Exp Biol Med* 48:207, 1941.

97. Freis ED, Schnaper HW, Johnson RL, Schreiner GE: Hemodynamic alterations in acute myocardial infarction: I. Cardiac output, mean arterial pressure, total peripheral resistance, "central" and total blood volumes, venous pressure, and average circulation time. *J Clin Invest* 31:131, 1952.

98. Crowell JW, Guyton AC: Evidence favoring a cardiac mechanism in irreversible hemorrhagic shock. *Am J Physiol* 201:893, 1961.

99. Siegel JH, DelGeurcio LR: Hemodynamic assessment of the critically ill patient. *Cardiologia* 51:65, 1967.

100. Goldberg RJ, Gore JM, Alpert JS, et al: Cardiogenic shock after acute myocardial infarction: Incidence and mortality from a community-wide perspective, 1975 to 1988. *N Engl J Med* 325:1117, 1991.

101. Sarnoff SJ, et al: Homemetric autoregulation in the heart. *Circ Res* 8:1077, 1960.

102. Lefer AM: Blood-borne humoral-factors in the pathophysiology of circulatory shock. *Circ Res* 32:129, 1973.

103. Lefer AM: Properties of cardioinhibitory factors produced in shock. *Fed Proc* 37:2734, 1978.

104. Parillo JE, Burch C, Shelhamer JH, et al: A circulating myocardial depressant substance in humans with septic shock. *J Clin Invest* 76:1539, 1985.

105. Parillo JE, Parker MM, Natanson C, et al: Septic shock in humans: Advances in the understanding of pathogenesis, cardiovascular dysfunction, and therapy. *Ann Intern Med* 113:227, 1990.

106. Laennec RTH: *Traité de l'auscultation mediate at des maladies des poumons et du coeur.* Paris, JS Chaude, 1831.

107. Boise E: The differential diagnosis of shock, hemorrhage, and sepsis. *Trans Am Assoc Obstet Gynecol* 9:433, 1897.

108. Waisbren BA: Bacteremia due to gram-negative bacilli other than salmonella: A clinical and therapeutic study. *Arch Intern Med* 88:467, 1951.

109. Borden CW, Hall WH: Fatal transfusion reactions from massive bacterial contamination of blood. *N Engl J Med* 245:760, 1951.

110. Wiles JB, Cerra FB, Siegel JH, et al: The systemic septic response: Does the organism matter? *Crit Care Med* 8:55, 1980.

111. Deutschman CS, Konstantinides FN, Tsai M, Simmons RL, Cerra FB: Physiology and metabolism in isolated viral septicemia. *Arch Surg* 122:21, 1987.

112. MacLean LD: Shock: A century of progress. *Ann Surg* 201:407, 1985.

113. Siegel JH, Cerra FB, Coleman B, et al: Physiological and metabolic correlations in human sepsis. *Surgery* 86:163, 1979.

114. Vincent JL, et al: Circulatory shock associated with purulent peritonitis. *Am J Surg* 142:262, 1981.

115. Cerra FB: The systemic septic response: concepts of pathogenesis. *J Trauma* 30:S169, 1990.

116. Goris RJA, Teboekhorst TPA, Nuytinck JK, Gimbrere JSF: Multiple-organ failure: Generalized autodestructive inflammation. *Arch Surg* 120:1109, 1985.

117. Goris RJA, Boekholtz WKF, van Bebber IPT, et al: Multiple organ failure and sepsis without bacteria: An experimental model. *Arch Surg* 121:897, 1986.

118. Nuytinck HKS, Offermans XJMW, Kubat K, Goris RJA: Whole-body inflammation in trauma patients: An autopsy study. *Arch Surg* 123:1519, 1988.

119. Steinberg S, Flynn W, Kelley K, et al: Development of a bacteria-independent model of the multiple organ failure syndrome. *Arch Surg* 124:1390, 1989.

120. Albrecht M, Clowes GHA: The increase of circulatory requirements in the presence of inflammation. *Surgery* 56:158, 1964.

121. Border JR, Gallo E, Schenk WG: Systemic arteriovenous shunts in patients under severe stress: A common cause of high output cardiac failure? *Surgery* 60:225, 1966.

122. Siegel JH, Greenspan M, DelGuercio LRM: Abnormal vascular tone, defective oxygen transport, and myocardial failure in human septic shock. *Ann Surg* 165:504, 1967.

123. Wilson RF, Chiscano AD, Quadros E, et al: Some observations on 132 patients with septic shock. *Anesth Analg* 46:751, 1967.

124. Rosoff L, Weil M, Bradley EC, et al: Hemodynamic and metabolic changes associated with bacterial peritonitis. *Am J Surg* 114:180, 1967.

125. Shoemaker WC: Cardiorespiratory patterns in complicated and uncomplicated septic shock. *Ann Surg* 174:119, 1971.

126. Hermreck AS, Thal AP: Mechanisms for the high circulatory requirements in sepsis and septic shock. *Ann Surg* 170:677, 1969.

127. Fong Y, Moldawer LL, Shires GT, Lowry SF: The biologic characteristics of cytokines and their implication in surgical injury. *Surg Gynecol Obstet* 170:363, 1990.

128. Mizel SB: The interleukins. *FASEB J* 3:2379, 1989.

129. Solbach W, Moll H, Rollinghoff M: Lymphocytes play the music but the macrophage calls the tune. *Immunol Today* 12:4, 1991.

130. Pruzanski W, Vadas P: Phospholipase A_2: A mediator between proximal and distal effectors of inflammation. *Immunol Today* 12:143, 1991.

131. Beeson PB: Temperature-elevating effect of a substance obtained from polymorphonuclear leukocytes. *J Clin Invest* 27:524, 1948.

132. Kampschmidt RF, Upchurch HF, Eddington CL, et al: Multiple biological activities of a partially purified leukocytic endogenous mediator. *Am J Physiol* 224:530, 1973.

133. Mizel SB: Interleukin-1 and T-cell activation. *Immunol Today* 8:330, 1987.

134. Dinarello CA: Biology of interleukin 1. *FASEB J* 2:108, 1988.

135. Rock CS, Lowry SF: Tumor necrosis factor-α. *J Surg Res* 51:434, 1991.

136. Coley WB: The treatment of malignant tumors by repeated inoculations of erysipelas: With a report of original cases. *Am J Med Sci* 105:487, 1893.

137. O'Malley WE, Achinstein B, Shear MJ: Action of bacterial polysaccharide on tumors: II. Damage of sarcoma 37 by serum of mice treated with *Serratia marcescens* polysaccharide, and induced tolerance. *J Natl Cancer Inst* 29:1169, 1962.

138. Rouzer CA, Cerami A: Hypertriglyceridemia associated with *Trypanosoma brucei* infection in rabbits: Role of defective triglyceride removal. *Mol Biochem Parasitol* 2:31, 1980.

139. Beutler B, Mahoney J, Le Trang N, et al: Purification of cachectin, a lipoprotein lipase suppressing hormone secreted by endotoxin-induced RAW 264, 7 cells. *J Exp Med* 161:984, 1985.

140. Warren RS, Starnes F Jr, Gabrilove JL, et al: The acute metabolic effects of tumor necrosis factor administration in humans. *Arch Surg* 122:1396, 1987.

141. Mealy K, Van Lanschot JJB, et al: Are the catabolic effects of tumor necrosis factor mediated by glucocorticoids? *Arch Surg* 125:42, 1990.

142. Tracey KJ, Lowry SF, Fahey TJ III, et al: Cachectin/tumor necrosis factor induces lethal shock and stress hormone responses in the dog. *Surg Gynecol Obstet* 164:415, 1987.

143. Tracey KJ, Beutler B, Lowry SF, et al: Shock and tissue injury induced by recombinant human cachectin. *Science* 234:470, 1986.

144. Schirmer WJ, Schirmer JM, Fry DE: Recombinant human tumor necrosis factor produces hemodynamic changes characteristic of sepsis and endotoxemia. *Arch Surg* 124:445, 1989.

145. Cantu LS, Rode HN, Yun TJ, Christou NV: Tumor necrosis factor alone does not explain the lethal effect of lipopolysaccharide. *Arch Surg* 126:231, 1991.

146. Beutler BA, Milsark IW, Cerami A: Cachectin/tumor necrosis factor: Production, distribution, and metabolic fate in vivo. *J Immunol* 135:3972, 1985.

147. Michie HR, Manogue KR, Spriggs DR, et al: Detection of circulating tumor necrosis factor after endotoxin administration. *N Engl J Med* 318:1481, 1988.

148. Fromm RE, Suffredini AF, Kovacs JA, et al: Serum tumor necrosis factor response in humans receiving endotoxin. *Clin Res* 36:372A, 1988.

149. Michie HR, Spriggs DR, Manogue KR, et al: Tumor necrosis factor and endotoxin induce similar metabolic responses in human beings. *Surgery* 104:280, 1988.

150. Waage A, Halstensen A, Espevik T: Association between tumor necrosis factor in serum and fatal outcome in patients with meningococcal disease. *Lancet* 1:355, 1987.

151. Michie HR, Wilmore DW: Sepsis, signals and surgical sequelae: A hypothesis. *Arch Surg* 125:531, 1990.

152. Michie HR, Sherman ML, Spriggs DR, et al: Chronic TNF infusion causes anorexia but not accelerated nitrogen loss. *Ann Surg* 209:19, 1989.

153. Takayama TK, Miller C, Szabo G: Elevated tumor necrosis factor (TNF) alpha production concomitant to elevated PGE_2 production by trauma patients' monocytes (MO). *Arch Surg* 125:29, 1990.

154. Cerami A, Beutler B: The role of cachectin/TNF in endotoxic shock and cachexia. *Immunol Today* 9:28, 1988.

155. Entman ML, Michael L, Rossen RD, et al: Inflammation in the course of early myocardial ischemia. *FASEB J* 5:2529, 1991.

156. Jennings RB, Sommers HM, Smyth GA, et al: Myocardial necrosis induced by temporary occlusion of a coronary artery in the dog. *Arch Pathol* 70:68, 1960.

157. Bing OHL, Brooks WW, Messer JV: Heart muscle viability following hypoxia: Protective effect of acidosis. *Science* 180:1297, 1973.

158. Greene HL, Weisfeldt ML: Determinants of hypoxic and posthypoxic myocardial contracture. *Am J Physiol* 232:H526, 1977.

159. Hearse DJ: Reperfusion of the ischemic myocardium. *J Mol Cell Cardiol* 9:605, 1977.

160. Powell WJ Jr, Flores J, DiBona DR, Leaf A: The role of cell swelling in myocardial ischemia and the protective effect of hypertonic mannitol. *J Clin Invest* 52:66a, 1973.

161. Powers ER, DiBona DR, Powell WJ Jr: Myocardial cell volume and coronary resistance during diminished coronary perfusion. *Am J Physiol* 247:H467, 1984.

162. Shine KI, Douglas AM: Low calcium reperfusion of ischemic myocardium. *J Mol Cell Cardiol* 15:251, 1983.

163. Zimmerman AN, Hulsmann WC: Paradoxical influence of calcium ions on the permeability of the cell membranes of the isolated rat heart. *Nature* 211:646, 1966.

164. Hearse DJ, Crome R, Yellon DM, Wyse R: Metabolic and flow correlates of myocardial ischemia. *Cardiovasc Res* 17:452, 1983.

165. Linas SL, Whittenburg D, Repine JE: Role of xanthine oxidase in ischemia/reperfusion injury. *Am J Physiol* 258:F711, 1990.

166. Korthuis RJ, Smith JK, Carden DL: Hypoxic reperfusion attenuates postischemic microvascular injury. *Am J Physiol* 256:H315, 1989.

167. Lemasters JJ, Bond JM, Currin RC, et al: Role of pH in hypoxic ischemic and reperfusion injury. *Circ Shock* 31:32, 1990.

168. Currin RT, Gores GJ, Thurman RG, Lemasters JJ: Protection by acidotic pH against anoxic cell killing in perfused rat liver: evidence for a pH paradox. *FASEB J* 5:207, 1991.

169. Das DK: Rewarming injury: A novel concept in the pathogenesis of cold injury. *Circ Shock* 31:33, 1990.

170. Baker CC, Degutis LC: Predicting outcome in multiple trauma patients. *Infect Surg* 5:243, 1986.

171. Singh TP, Savino JA, Agarwal N, et al: Comparison of resuscitation fluids on lipid peroxidation in the liver and kidney after hemorrhagic shock. *Surg Forum* 41:59, 1990.

172. Strock LL, Singh H, Abdullah A, et al: The effect of insulin-like growth factor I on postburn hypermetabolism. *Surgery* 108:161, 1990.

173. Jacobs DM, Julsrud JM, Bubrick MP: Iron chelation with a deferoxamine conjugate in hemorrhagic shock. *J Surg Res* 51:484, 1991.

174. Dahn MS, Lange MP, Jacobs LA: Insulin-like growth factor 1 production is inhibited in human sepsis. *Arch Surg* 123:1409, 1988.

175. Bernard GR, Reines HD, Metz CA, et al: Effects of a short course of ibuprofen in patients with severe sepsis. *Am Rev Respir Dis* 137:138, 1988.

176. Reilly PM, Schiller HJ, Bulkley GB: Pharmacologic approach to tissue injury mediated by free radicals and other reactive oxygen metabolites. *Am J Surg* 161:488, 1991.

177. Zimmerman JJ: Therapeutic application of oxygen radical scavengers. *Chest* 100:189S, 1991.

178. Haglund U, Gerdin B: Oxygen free radicals (OFR) and circulatory shock. *Circ Shock* 34:405, 1991.

179. Fleckenstein AE, Smith SL, Linseman KL, et al: Comparison of the efficacy of mechanistically different antioxidants in the rat hemorrhagic shock model. *Circ Shock* 35:223, 1991.

180. Girotti MJ, Khan N, McLellan BA: Early measurement of systemic lipid peroxidation products in the plasma of major blunt trauma patients. *J Trauma* 31:32, 1991.

181. Weisfeldt ML: Reperfusion and reperfusion injury. *Clin Res* 35:13, 1987.

182. Baue AE: Multiple systems failure, in S Dudrick (ed): *ACS Manual of Preoperative and Postoperative Care*. Philadelphia, Saunders, 1983, pp 256–278.

183. Hearse DJ, Humphrey SM, Bullock GR: The oxygen paradox and the calcium paradox: Two faces of the same problem? *J Mol Chem Biol* 10:641, 1978.

184. Baue AE, Chaudry IH: Prevention of multiple systems failure. *Surg Clin North Am* 60:1167, 1980.

185. Braunwald E, Kloner RA: Myocardial reperfusion: A double-edged sword. *J Clin Invest* 76:1713, 1985.

186. Nayler WG, Elz JS: Reperfusion injury: Laboratory artifact or clinical dilemma? *Circulation* 74:215, 1986.

187. Faist E, Baue AE, Dittmer H, Heberer G: Multiple organ failure in polytrauma patients. *J Trauma* 23:775, 1983.

4

IMMUNOLOGY OF SHOCK AND INJURY

Carol L. Miller-Graziano

Shock and severe injury have a profound effect on the immune system. Derangement of immune cytokine production and immune cellular function resulting after injury and massive septic challenge are thought to be major contributors not only to septic shock but also to posttrauma immunopathology.[1-10] A number of investigators have described alterations in immune cell function or cytokine production during trauma-initiated shock, during hemorrhagic shock, and during experimental endotoxin-mediated shock. The aberrations observed in these three separate situations appear to be somewhat different, although complementary in their action on the immune system. These observed differences in the immune alterations detected under various shock conditions may reflect variations in the mediators generated in each case, they may reflect the different severity of the insult, or they may reflect the use of animal models versus human cells. It is essential to identify what alterations in immune cell and mediator function are most predictive of patients at risk of septic shock and which alterations are causal in the immunopathology. The relevant alterations can then be targeted for immunotherapy and/or monitored as indicators of the efficacy of different treatment protocols (Table 4–1).

NORMAL PHYSIOLOGY OF IMMUNOLOGIC RESPONSE

In the last 10 years, identification of the interactive effects of various cell types and their products in host defense has proliferated to include almost all the hemopoietic cell types (except erythrocytes) and vascular endothelial cells and epithelial cells as well.[11-14] The description of the immune interactions in the brain-adrenal-liver axis or the skin are beyond the scope of this review. However, those cytokines and other mediators produced and released by glia cells during head trauma or by skin keratinocytes after burns may be important modulators

TABLE 4–1. Mediator Changes after Various Shock States

Mediator in Serum	Direct Cell Production
Hemorrhagic Shock	
TNF-α ↑	Kupffer cell
IL-1 ↓	Mφ
IL-2 ↓	Th1
IFN-γ ↓	Th1
PGE$_2$ ↑	Mφ
IL-6 ↑	Mφ, Kupffer cell
IL-4 (?)	Th2
Trauma and Burns	
IL-2, IFN$_\gamma$ ↓	Th1, NK
IL-8 ↓	Mφ, endothelial cells
IL-6 ↑	Mφ, Th1
TNF-α ↑	Kupffer cells, Mφ
TGF-β ↑	Mφ
IL-1 ↑ ↓	B ↑ , Mφ ↓
PGE$_2$, LTB$_4$ ↑	Mφ, endothelial cells
Experimental Endotoxin	
IL-8 ↑	
IL-1 ↑	Mφ
IL-6 ↑	Mφ
TNF-α ↑	Mφ
PGE$_2$, LTB$_4$ ↑	Mφ
IFN-γ ↑	

of total circulating cytokine levels and therefore contributors to the final septic shock outcome.[15] Alterations in the cytokine microenvironment dramatically change the way T lymphocytes and macrophages (Mφ) are activated, the efficacy of polymorphonuclear leukocyte (PMN) function, and the balance between humoral and cellular immunity. The major change in our current view of immunologic interactions is the characterization of the roles of a variety of newly cloned protein factors called *cytokines* in the induction and regulation of immune function.[16–18] The immune response is channeled primarily toward cell-mediated cytotoxicity or antibody production (humoral immunity) by the activation of one or the other of the two CD4-positive T helper lymphocyte subsets. One T cell subset or the other is activated depending on what inflammatory cytokines are present in the microenvironment.[18–20] These T lymphocyte subsets, called *Th1* and *Th2,* secrete discrete lymphokines. Th1 lymphocytes secrete interferon-γ (IFN-γ) and interleukin 2 (IL-2), while Th2 lymphocytes secrete IL-4, IL-5, IL-6, and IL-10. Th1 and Th2 subsets, through their distinct secreted lymphokines, may either promote (Th1) or suppress (Th2) further monocyte/macrophage (Mφ) function. The Th2-produced cytokines IL-4 and IL-10, while stimulatory to some B lymphocyte functions, are inhibitory to a wide range of Mφ functions, while the Th1-produced growth factors IFN-γ and IL-2, are stimulatory to Mφ functions.[18–20]

Mφ are also producers of IL-10 after extensive activation and therefore can mediate autosuppression as well as suppression of other immune cells. Th1 activation, as well as natural killer cells (NK) and CD8 cytotoxic lymphocyte activities, is also indirectly inhibited by IL-10 through its direct action on Mϕ.[21] The Th1 and Th2 lymphocyte subsets are cross-regulatory in their interactions. Consequently, the degree of activation of either the Th1 or Th2 lymphocyte subset and the subsequent balance between humoral and cell-mediated immunity depends on the early cytokine milieu as secreted by the nonspecific inflammatory cells.[18–22] Mϕ secrete an enormous number of cytokines that both stimulate T lymphocytes, such as IL-1, IL-6, and tumor necrosis factor α (TNF-α), and inhibit T lymphocytes, such as transforming growth factor β (TGF-β) and IL-10.[3,17,23,24] Mast cells, PMN NK cells, and eosinophils are also potential producers of regulatory cytokines and can influence the eventual balance between Th1 and Th2 induction, as well as the cytokine milieu.[21,25–27] Changes in Mϕ function can alter the function and receptor expression of PMN and T lymphocytes, as well as alter receptor expression on lung and liver epithelia cells, resulting in the many organ pathologies associated with septic shock.[1–6] In fact, a new term *systemic inflammatory response syndrome* has been suggested as more appropriate to describe patients with a combination of immunologically mediated organ injury, hemorrhagic shock, and multitrauma.[28] Septic shock is suggested only in the subset of these cases where infection is clearly documented.[28] An even more appropriate term for the general syndrome might be *cytokine shock*.

Mϕ are also potent producers of a number of inflammatory mediators that can stimulate or suppress a variety of cell types and thereby profoundly influence the host-response outcome. For example, Mϕ produce eicosanoids, such as leukotriene B$_4$ (LTB$_4$) and prostaglandin E$_2$ (PGE$_2$), which can activate or suppress PMN, T lymphocytes, and B cells by altering their receptor expression and cyclic AMP (cAMP) levels.[3,29,30] Mϕ produce complement components, coagulation activation factors, plasminogen activators, plasminogen activator inhibitors, elastin, interferon-γ, GM-CSF, M-CSF, and a number of proteases, as well as nitric oxide (NO) and other oxygen-reactive species.[17,23,24,30] These mediators also augment some lymphocyte functions while inhibiting other lymphocyte functions. Monocytes produce a number of chemotactic factors for T cells, PMN, and Mϕ themselves.[31] These chemotactic factors include IL-8, macrophage-activating protein, and complement components.[31] In addition to producing many inflammatory factors, Mϕ also secrete inhibitors of these factors. For example, Mϕ secrete a natural inhibitor of IL-1α and β, the IL-1 receptor antagonist (IL-1RA).[8,32,33] Mϕ also up-regulate and shed their receptors for TNF-α during intense TNF-α induction.[34–36] The soluble shed TNF receptors can bind TNF-α + β, preventing action on other cell types.[34–37] Th1 cells secrete IFN-γ, which is inhibitory to some B lymphocytes and Th2 functions but stimulate Mϕ, NK cells, and cytotoxic T cell functions. Conversely, Th2 cells secrete IL-4 and IL-10, which negatively regulate Mϕ and Th1 lymphocytes.[18–21] Consequently, Mϕ and T cell regulation of cytokine production is important in maintaining the balance between excessive cytokine production with immune suppression and appropriate immune cell activation.

Characterization of immune dysfunctions now encompasses assessment of Th1 and Th2 function and lymphokine production; monitoring of receptor expression on T lymphocytes, Mϕ, and PMNs, and cytokine assessment in discrete cell populations and in patient sera. Since Mϕ have a pivotal role in excessive cytokine production, metabolic aberrations, and inducing T cell function, this laboratory and many others have focused on Mφ function as an indicator of, and major contributor to, immune alteration and organ failure in systemic inflammatory response syndrome.[3-6]

When investigators first started to define the physiologic alterations seen in immune function during shock, they focused on major rather than specific immune functional changes while grouping together patients who were experiencing septic shock, hemorrhagic shock, and tissue damage–induced alterations. Consequently, dysfunctions originally attributed to bacterial shock are now thought to result from hemorrhage or trauma. The contribution of hemorrhagic shock to immune aberrations in subsequent septic shock is considerable. Hemorrhage alone causes depression in T cell proliferation, in T cell IFN-γ production, and in B cell proliferation.[38,40,42,43] Hemorrhage also causes depression of Mφ antigen-presenting capacity, decreases major histocompatability class II expression, and increases Mφ PGE_2 production. Therefore, the subsequent T and B lymphocyte depression may be secondary to Mφ alterations.[38,40,42,43] In addition, experimental models have suggested that not all Mφ populations are equally affected by sepsis or hemorrhage.[38,44] In a murine model, peritoneal and splenic Mφ antigen-presenting function was depressed, but their cytokine levels were unaffected by hemorrhage.[38] In contrast, Kupffer cell production of TNF-α and IL-1 was dramatically increased after hemorrhage.[38] Consequently, measurements of alterations in a particular cell population may miss dysfunctions in other cells. Current data support that it is TNF-α and IL-1 acting in synergy that produce major pathologic effects associated with hemorrhagic as well as septic or cytokine shock.[1,8,45,46] The increased white blood cell adhesion within liver sinusoids after hemorrhagic shock can be prevented with anti-TNF-α antibodies.[47] These data indicate up-regulation of adhesion receptors in the liver after hemorrhage and suggest that hemorrhage-induced TNF-α was mediating this response.[47] Interestingly, simple surgical trauma also appears to increase IL-6 levels in serum, while simple trauma plus hemorrhage was necessary to induce the appearance of TNF-α in the serum.[43]

The contribution of hemorrhage to an early rise in IL-6 levels may play an important role in subsequent cytokine shock. The very early rise of IL-6 and its correlation with actual development of cytokine shock has been described by many investigators.[2,3,39,43,48,49] This early rise in IL-6 levels in the sera and a rapid onset of increased Mφ production of IL-6 occurs only following trauma and hemorrhage.[39,43,48] In experimental models of endotoxin-mediated shock, IL-6 levels increase only after the appearance of TNF-α and IL-1, leading investigators to suggest the IL-6 elevation is only secondarily induced after TNF-α and IL-1 and contributes little to the acute pathology of endotoxin-mediated shock.[8] However, in most septic patient populations, IL-6 appears early in serum, concomitant with or even before TNF-α.[8,48-52] This rapid appearance of IL-6 may reflect the contribution of other insults such as surgical trauma, injury, hemorrhage, or disease processes, as well as bacterial challenges, to the mediator changes in the patient population. The correlation of serum levels of IL-6 with mortality from septic shock has proven better than the correlation with serum TNF-α or IL-1 level.[48,50-52] We have suggested that an increase in IL-6 levels lead to polyclonal stimulation of B lymphocytes with the subsequent characteristic rise in circulating immunoglobulin levels of the IgG type seen in acute trauma patients.[3,4,49] These circulating IgG aggregates then stimulate Mϕ through their 72-kDa type 1 receptor for IgG (Fc$_\gamma$RI). Cross-linking stimulation of Mϕ through their Fc$_\gamma$RI has been demonstrated by our laboratory and others to induce massively increased cytokine and mediator production, including IL-6, TNF-α, PGE$_2$, and the immunosuppressive cytokine transforming growth factor β (TGF-β).[3,4,49,53–55] Consequently, elevated IL-6 production, as a result of hemorrhage, initiates a cycle of increased Mϕ production of TNF-α, PGE$_2$, and TGF-β by its activation, increasing circulating IgG levels that cross-link Fc$_\gamma$RI on Mϕ. Serum from toxoplasma patients containing high IgG levels induces TNF-α production in normal Mϕ, confirming the contribution of circulating IgG to TNF-α production.[56] In addition, IL-6 increases the expression of TNF-α receptors on hepatocytes, increasing their sensitivity to TNF-α.[57] IL-6 also induces acute phase protein production and is a major mediator of cachexia and liver metabolic changes.[58] One of the most detrimental effects of hemorrhage may be its induction of elevated IL-6 levels.

IMMUNOLOGY OF HEMORRHAGIC SHOCK

Hemorrhagic shock alone can lead to profound immunosuppression. Hemorrhage increases Mϕ secretion of PGE$_1$ and PGE$_2$, which mediate immunosuppression of Mϕ, T cells, B cells, NK cells, and PMN function by down-regulating surface receptors and raising intracellular cAMP levels.[2,29,40,55] The level of cytokines produced by Kupffer cells, alveolar macrophages, Mϕ, and T lymphocytes is also altered.[38–40,47] In addition, hemorrhagic shock in patients generates additional mediators which can either augment immune suppression or exacerbate excessive cytokine production. Complement split products and fibrin degradation products are examples of mediators produced by Mϕ which can both suppress and enhance immune response. Split products of C3 have been shown to increase immunosuppression, while split products of C5 greatly augment TNF-α and IL-1 production by Mϕ.[3,8,59,60] The production of toxic oxygen metabolites by TNF-α activated PMNs in the lung is greatly enhanced by concomitant stimulation by C5.[61,62] The mediator/cytokine microenvironment not only determines the ultimate balance between immunosuppressive and immunostimulatory functions of the immune cell system but also can initiate a cycle of unregulated inflammatory cell activation and organ pathology. By altering that microenvironment, hemorrhage has a major effect on the subsequent activation of the immune system and the production of the inflammatory mediators of systemic inflammatory response syndrome and septic shock outcome after bacterial challenge.

IMMUNOLOGY OF POSTTRAUMA SHOCK AND SEPSIS

The identification of the independent contributions of hemorrhage to septic shock is easier than separating the relative contributions of traumatic injury versus endotoxin release in subsequent septic shock. Severe trauma has been suggested as causing endotoxin leakage from the gut as a result of increasing gut permeability.[63] Consequently, endotoxin stimulation may be present in the absence of overt infectious challenge. In addition, injury, especially soft tissue damage and burns, causes release of complement split products, fibrin degradation products, and substance P from damaged nerves. Each of these mediators can augment the Mϕ cytokine response to endotoxin as well as mediate Mϕ and PMN oxygen metabolite activation and chemotaxis.[17] Endotoxin stimulation of Mϕ induces secretion of TNF-α, IL-1, PGE_2, IL-6, IL-8, IL-10, platelet-activating factor (PAF), and TGF-β.[16,17,23] As already discussed, increasing these mediators significantly alters immune responses to subsequent immune challenge. The contribution of endogenous intestinally released endotoxin to altered immune function after trauma may be profound in augmenting cytokine production. Nontoxic concentrations of IL-1 and TNF-α can become lethal in the presence of small lipopolysaccharide (LPS) concentrations.[1,52,61]

Bolus infusion of endotoxin or *E. coli* leads to increases in IL-1, IL-6, TNF-α, IL-8, and PGE_2.[1,8,48,64–67] Serum TNF-α levels increase rapidly but are only transiently elevated, while IL-1 levels rise slightly later and persist over the entire time of LPS infusion.[1,8,48,64–67] IL-8 and IL-6 serum levels rise after both IL-1 and TNF-α and persist over the entire infusion period.[8,48,64,65] IFN-γ levels are also increased.[48,68] PMNs are activated, as measured by elastase release, but are sequestered out of the circulation.[65,68,69] This PMN sequestering may reflect the increased expression of adhesion molecules in certain target organs and accumulation of PMNs in the lung or liver.[65,66]

The most commonly used endotoxin-mediated shock models include an acute lethal endotoxin-mediated shock in rodent models and induction of acute hypertension in primates or pigs.[8,65–68] Since all these models are acute, no longer-term effect on immune T cells has been described. Cyclooxygenase inhibitors block the hypertension generated in these endotoxin models, suggesting that PGE_2, induced by IL-1 and TNF-α, may be mediating some of the pathologic symptoms.[8,66] A rise in PAF and LTB_4 occurs only in survivors of endotoxin injection, and therefore, these mediators are not involved in the immediate pathology of these acute models.[66] However, the pathology of endotoxin-mediated shock in experimental models appears to differ from the patterns seen in septic shock patients.[48] There are a number of differences between septic patients and endotoxin models besides the difference in the appearance time of IL-6 (i.e., preceding TNF-α in patients but following TNF-α in endotoxin-mediated shock models). The rapid lethality of LPS infusion (within 30 min) is quite different from the more prolonged deterioration seen in septic shock patients.[1,48] Circulating TNF-α levels remain elevated in patients over many days, even when no evidence of bacterial challenge is present.[36,39,48,70] IFN-γ levels are increased after *E. coli* infusion, while they are typically depressed in septic shock patients.[5,48,65] Cyclooxygenase inhibitors do not correct posttrauma T cell defects or neutrophil depression but do ameliorate endotoxin-mediated shock pathology.[3,6,8,66] Septic shock mediated by TNF-α is also seen in meningococcemia and *Staphylococcus* infection, as well as in acute respiratory distress syndrome (ARDS) and after acid aspiration, indicating that endotoxin is not the primary mediator of septic shock.[48,59,72,73] A recent report indicates that patients' absolute serum endotoxin levels correlate poorly with actual susceptibility to endotoxin-mediated shock.[48,52,67] Rather, the serum levels of IL-6 as a measure of cytokine activation were indicative of which patients would progress to endotoxin-mediated shock.[52] These data imply that the level of endotoxin is less critical than the preactivation state of the patients' cell population. Trauma-mediated increases in PGE_2, complement split products, PAF, and other mediators will determine the preactivation state of the leukocytes when they meet an endotoxin challenge. IL-1 plays an important role in accelerating the negative cycle of increasing IL-6 production, which increases polyclonal memory B lymphocyte activation to secrete immunoglobulin, which then increases triggering of Mϕ Fc$_\gamma$RI to produce IL-1, TNF-α, IL-6, PGE_2, and TGF-β. It has been demonstrated recently that PMNs can secrete IL-1 and TNF-α after stimulation with endotoxin.[25] Endotoxin may therefore also amplify the total cytokine production by stimulating PMNs to also secrete cytokines.

The magnitude of the contribution of LPS to the pathology of septic shock may be overemphasized. Antibodies against LPS were not found to be particularly effective in preventing septic shock in clinical trials.[75] Antiendotoxin (J-chain) antibody also was unsuccessful in lowering plasma TNF-α levels.[74,75] In addition, septic shock in meningococcal infections and pathology in severe malaria, where no LPS is detectable, also are mediated by excessive cytokine production, particularly TNF-α.[16,36,48] It seems contradictory that small endotoxin doses lead to LPS tolerance and depressed cytokine production in animals by down-regulating their CD14 (LPS) receptor levels, while low-dose endotoxin leakage from the gut is proposed to sensitize cells for increased cytokine production.[63,76] In a recent study, the endotoxin-insensitive mouse line C3H/HeJ was subjected to cecal ligation and puncture. Mϕ from these septic mice produced elevated TNF-α and IL-6 levels in response to the injury even while maintaining their endotoxin insensitivity.[77] These data point to a role for altered Mϕ, PMNs, and lymphocyte cytokine response capacity in the crucial change that leads to excessive cytokine production in septic or systemic inflammatory shock rather than large amounts of circulating LPS.

The increased production of cytokines, concomitant with depressed specific immunity, reflects a loss of appropriate immune activation and regulation. The septic shock patient is often a trauma victim, a leukemia patient, or a patient with severe hemorrhagic shock as a result of gastrointestinal bleeding rather than a patient with overt bacteremia.[36,48,49,52] As has already been pointed out, hemorrhagic shock in and of itself causes altered T lymphocyte function and decreases the Mϕ ability to activate T helper lymphocytes of either the Th2 or Th1 type. The same T lymphocyte and Mϕ immune defects can be mediated by trauma and can characterize the leukemia patients.[49,52] Major histocompatibility antigen expression, which is necessary for proper T cell activation, is also decreased in these types of patients.[6] There is some evidence to suggest that T cell contact with foreign antigens, in the absence of proper accessory cell help, leads to T cell anergy.[12] The result of hemorrhage, trauma, or any derangement of lymphocyte function is a decreased ability of the immune system to properly activate Mϕ and PMNs to clear bacteria and a depressed ability to activate B lymphocytes to produce primary antibody response.[3–6,78,79] Proper regulatory interactions between Mϕ and T lymphocytes are also lost when T cells are not properly activated, leading to exaggerated cytokine production.[12,13,16] The lack of proper interaction between inflammatory cells and bacteria also may be one underlying cause of the increased susceptibility to infection concomitant with exaggerated cytokine production which characterizes the patient who proceeds to septic shock.

Mechanical trauma, in the absence of overt infection or hemorrhage, produces immune defects, while thermal trauma, with its intense mediator release, is massively immunosuppressive.[2-6] Mechanical trauma causes increases in Mφ PGE_2 production, which accounts for some, but not all, of the posttrauma immune dysfunction.[3,6] Besides the PGE_2-mediated depression of IFN-γ synthesis, an intrinsic depression in T cell IL-2 synthesis occurs independent of Mφ inhibitory activity in the trauma victim.[5,6,42] This posttrauma IL-2 depression is not a result of an overall decrease in T cell protein synthesis capacity, because T cell IL-6 production is concomitantly highly elevated.[6] In addition, IL-1 production by Mφ is initially decreased in trauma patients.[5,39-41,80] Those septic patients who express low posttrauma serum IL-1 levels have a poor prognosis.[5,39,80] There is a reduction in the number of CD4-positive helper T lymphocytes.[5] Only a small percentage of blunt trauma patients' T cells show reduced IL-2 receptor expression, while thermal trauma patients' T cells experience significant reduction in IL-2 receptor expression.[10] This loss of T cell IL-2 receptors means patients' T cells of both the Th1 and the Th2 type are unable to proliferate and expand properly.[12] In addition, there appears to be an elevation in the Mφ expression of CD14 (the LPS receptor), indicating that posttrauma Mφ may be more sensitized to subsequent LPS stimulation.[5]

Mφ IL-6 and TNF-α production is often increased as early as 3 days after injury. This increase in posttrauma cytokine production frequently occurs well before any infectious episode.[3,5] The Mφ alterations in cytokines after thermal trauma are even more dramatic. PGE_2 levels, TNF-α production, IL-6 production, and TGF-β production are massively increased in these patients' Mφ.[3,5] This increase in TNF-α levels concomitant with elevated PGE_2 and TGF-β is particularly aberrant and indicative of the loss of proper cytokine regulation in these patients' Mφ. Normal human Mφ production of TNF-α induced by IFN-γ and LPS is down-regulated transcriptionally by both PGE_2 and TGF-β.[1,3,8,70] However, severe trauma and burn patients' Mφ have become desensitized to this PGE_2 inhibition.[3,4,70] As can be seen in Table 4–2, addition of exogenous PGE_2 to these patients' Mφ fails to down-regulate their TNF-α levels. Interestingly, the Mφ-secreted TNF-α appears to be affected by PGE_2, while cell-associated TNF-α is less affected. The predominant production of cell-associated TNF-α versus secreted TNF-α is another indicator of aberrant activation of posttrauma and posthemorrhage Mφ.[3,4,38,70] The desensitization of human Mφ TNF-α production to PGE_2 regulation has been described under in vitro conditions where high PGE_2 levels are copresent with other inducers and may be attributable to decreased Mφ PGE_2 receptors.[81] The mechanism for PGE_2 desensitization of patient Mφ remains to be defined.

Trauma patients' Mφ also produced excessive amounts of the immunosuppressive peptide (TGF-β).[82,83] Elevated levels of TGF-β not only depress T cell activation and decrease Mφ PMN phagocytic function but also can profoundly affect Mφ TNF-α levels.[83] The inhibitory or stimulatory effect of TGF-β on Mφ TNF-α production appears to depend on the type of Mφ activation that has occurred previously.[83-85] We have indicated that TGF-β increases Mφ TNF-α levels in trauma patients.[3] However, TGF-β decreases IFN-γ and LPS-stimulated normal Mφ in their TNF-α production.[3,83,84] Similarly, Mφ IL-6 production has been

TABLE 4–2. Suppressed* Trauma Patients' Mϕ TNF-α Production Is Insensitive to PGE$_2$ Down-Regulation

		TNF-α[†] ng/10^6 Mϕ		PGE$_2$ ng/10^6 Mϕ	
		10γ + MDP[‡]	10γ + MDP + PGE$_2$	10γ + MDP	10γ + MDP + PGE$_2$
Suppressed	Pt	5.2/6.4	17.5/0	41.5	142.7
	Nor	0.0/6.3	0.0/0	8.2	118.3
Suppressed	Pt	16.1/.3	15.9/0	29.7	60.0
	Nor	0.0/0	0.0/0	9.1	—
Suppressed	Pt	4.1/14.6	15.8/.24	29.1	184.5
Immunocompetent	Pt	3.8/1.3	0.0/0	11.5	79.1
	Nor	0.0/2.4	0.0/0	12.9	89.6

*Suppressed trauma patients were those with PGE$_2$ levels >25 ng/10^6 Mϕ.
†TNF-α presented as cell-associated/secreted.
‡γ + MDP = 10 units of interferon-γ + muramyl dipeptide.

reported as both increased and decreased by TGF-β, depending on the stimulation regimen.[84,85] TGF-β appears to increase IL-6 production by trauma patients' Mϕ.[3] These data again illustrate that the posttrauma microenvironment uniquely activates Mϕ so that normal regulatory patterns are disrupted. Our laboratory has demonstrated that cytokine synthesis by trauma patients' Mϕ is more sensitive to augmentation by LTB$_4$, more responsive to a bacterial cell wall analogue (muramyl dipeptide), and more responsive to TGF-β augmentation.[3,4]

PMN function is also altered in trauma. After an initial activation, the PMNs lose their immunoglobulin receptors and become less able to affect immune phagocytosis.[79] Changes in intracellular killing also occur during the second postinjury week.[79] Decreases in PMN bacterial capacity follow a sequestering of PMNs in the lungs, which may result from TNF-α and IL-1 up-regulation of adhesion molecules on vascular endothelium with subsequent endothelial binding of both Mϕ and PMNs.[8,11,36,59,65,79] In addition, increased concentrations of IL-8 are produced and released by both alveolar Mϕ and PMNs sequestered in the lung.[64,86] Chemoattractants, such as IL-8, secreted by Mϕ and PMNs, call additional PMNs to the lungs, increasing sequestration and tissue damage.[36,61,64,65,86] These sequestered PMNs can be activated to produce TNF-α and IL-1, further exacerbating the local PMN activation and tissue damage.[25,86] In this immediate postinjury period, PMNs accumulate in the lungs, degranulate, and then release both TNF-α and toxic oxygen radicals, initiating tissue damage.[36] It appears that in the pathology of acute respiratory distress syndrome, PMNs and Mϕ mediate tissue damage both directly, through toxic oxygen radicals and nitric oxide, and indirectly, through TNF-α, IL-1, and IL-8 secretion.[1,8,36,48] The degranulation of accumulated PMNs not only releases toxic radicals but also removes these PMNs from the system, finally leading to the decreased bactericidal capacity seen later in the posttrauma period.[65]

Other granulocytes, notably eosinophils, also can produce toxic radicals and cytokines and can be involved in lung pathology.[27] Programmed cell death, or apoptosis of inflammatory cells, can be delayed by T lymphokines.[87] These dying cells release additional mediators. The immunosuppressed trauma or septic patient has decreased T lymphokine production.[5,10] Accelerated apoptosis of inflammatory cells in the lungs of these patients may therefore be contributing to the levels of toxic oxygen metabolite release. The patient with excessive Mφ production of TNF-α, IL-1, IL-8, and TGF-β, in the face of depressed T lymphocyte synthesis of IL-2, IFN-γ, IL-4, and other lymphokines, is at double risk of pathologic complications. As TNF-α and IL-1 up-regulate adhesion receptors, causing accumulation of Mφ, PMNs, and other inflammatory cells in susceptible organs, more Mφ and granulocytes are chemotactically attracted by increased concentrations of IL-8, complement split products, arachidonic acid metabolites, and PAF, incurring more tissue damage. Meanwhile, decreased specific immunity leads to improper regulation of inflammatory cell cytokine release, inappropriate control of programmed cell death, and decreased ability to handle bacterial challenge, with a consequent increased concentration of bacterial endotoxins and exotoxins. With the disruption of appropriate lymphocyte-Mφ interactions, unusual activation pathways, such as Fc$_\gamma$RI cross-linking, in the absence of Th1-derived IFN-γ, become dominant. As we and others have demonstrated, Mφ activated by cross-linking Fc$_\gamma$RI, in the absence of IFN-γ, leads to altered Mφ production of TNF-α (increased cell-associated TNF-α) and increased resistance to PGE$_2$ down-regulation.[3,4]

The critical role of TNF-α in mediating the pathology of systemic inflammatory response syndrome is clear. TNF-α can be histologically located in the lungs of patients dying from acute respiratory distress syndrome.[88] Infusion of TNF-α mimics the pathology of endotoxin injection, and anti-TNF-α antibodies can prevent or ameliorate fatal endotoxin-mediated shock.[1,8,89,90] However, the correlation between the appearance of TNF-α in serum and the peak of shock pathology is poor.[36,39,41,48,52,91] There may be several reasons for this inconsistency. First, several investigators have data demonstrating that cell-associated TNF-α is a better correlate with shock pathology than secreted TNF-α.[3,38,39] In addition, Mφ actively producing TNF-α also up-regulate their receptors for TNF-α.[92] These receptors bind TNF-α in serum, leading to inaccurate measurements of TNF-α production. There are two different receptors for TNF-α, a high-molecular-weight (75 to 80 kDa) and a low-molecular-weight (55 to 60 kDa) receptor, that both bind TNF-α.[34] Consequently, TNF-α and its interaction with the two TNF receptors has been a primary experimental focus for recent investigations. Mφ, the primary producers of excess TNF-α, primarily express the high-molecular-weight receptor, while other cell types express both types of receptors.[93] As Mφ increase their TNF-α production, they also increase their production of the 75-kDa receptor and increasingly shed this receptor off the cell surface.[35,37,48,94] This shedding of the receptors is a natural protective and regulatory mechanism for controlling TNF-α effects.[8,37,94] Both the soluble TNF receptors can bind to TNF-α and prevent its binding to receptors on other cells.[8,94] This inhibition by the two types of soluble TNF-α receptor protects surrounding cells from secreted TNF-α and limits the activating capacity of TNF-α. Increased levels of both the 55- and 75-kDa receptors have been demonstrated in septic patients' sera.[8,36,37,94] These data imply that the pathologic effect of TNF-α must be occurring even in the face of high concentrations of the soluble TNF receptors. LPS injection or injection of TNF-α mediates the release of soluble TNF receptors.[92] In fact, in severe meningococcal septicemia, the ratio of TNF-α to TNF receptors rises proportionally until very high TNF-α levels are reached (>500 pg/ml). At this point,

TABLE 4–3. TNFR Expression* on Patients' Mφ Is Persistently Down-Regulated by IFN-γ[†] When Their Initial TNFR Levels Are Close to Those of Normal Mφ and Is Not Down-Regulated by IFN-γ if Initial TNFR Levels Are Low

Patients			Normals		
Time 0	18 Hours		Time 0	18 Hours	
Unstim	10 U IFN-γ + MDP	100 U IFN-γ + MDP	Unstim	10 U IFN-γ + MDP	100 U IFN-γ + MDP
3.5	1.8	0.8	4.2	2.1	1.2
9.7	3.8	—	11.7	6.1	—
6.7	4.4	—	7.3	—	1.7
3.1	1.9	0.8	5.2	1.7	1.0
4.2	1.5	—	6.6	3.2	—
3.4	1.6	0.9	3.3	1.5	1.1
5.3	1.9	—	8.2	1.5	—
8.0	1.4	—	7.3	1.7	—
9.7	3.8	—	11.7	6.1	—
6.7	4.4	—	7.3	—	1.7
6.7	2.5	—	7.0	2.6	1.1

Patients		Normals	
Time 0	18 Hours	Time 0	18 Hours
Unstim	10 U IFN-γ + MDP	Unstim	10 U IFN-γ + MDP
1.1	4.8	5.8	3.9
1.5	7.9	5.1	1.4
1.5	1.6	3.5	2.5
1.4	2.6	3.9	1.7
1.1	1.9	4.4	3.0
1.0	1.6	3.5	2.5
0.8	2.6	3.7	2.5
0.2	0.7	5.0	4.4

*TNFR expression presented as mean fluorescence intensity of 10^4 Mφ labeled with TNF-α PE.

[†]Patient/ or normal Mφ were cultured on matrix-coated plates for 2 hours with 10 U or 100 U of IFN-γ/10^6 Mφ/ml; then MDP was added and cultures continued for 16 hours. TNFR were assessed before (time 0, unstimulated) and after 18 hours of stimulation and culture.

TNF-α levels continue to increase, but TNF receptor levels do not. These data have led investigators to suggest that an imbalance between TNF receptor and TNF-α levels leads to onset of septic shock.[37]

The appearance of large amounts of soluble TNF receptors also interferes with accurate measurement of TNF-α levels in serum, since both ELISA and biological assays fail to detect TNF-α bound to the TNF receptors.[48] In a recently developed modified ELISA that detects both receptor-bound and free TNF-α, TNF-α levels have been shown to persist over long periods in septic patients.[48] It is also important to point out that cell-associated TNF-α will not be inhibited by the soluble receptor. The soluble receptor binds only the trimeric TNF-α complex, not the monomeric cell–associated form.[34] Secreted TNF-α is only able to actively bind to cells in its trimer form, which is rapidly degraded (half-life 30 min).[1] Consequently, the importance of the soluble receptors may be in binding secreted TNF-α for a period that exceeds the trimer's half-life. The increased posttrauma appearance of cell-associated TNF-α also may be important in escaping the protective effect of soluble TNF receptors and contributing to systemic inflammatory response syndrome. The important Mφ contribution to the TNF-α/TNF receptor ratio is illustrated by data showing that levels of 75-kDa receptors are more elevated than those of the 55-kDa receptors both in patient septicemia and in experimental endotoxemia.[94] Since most cell types express both receptors, the preponderance of 75-kDa receptors in sepsis is most likely reflecting increased Mφ shedding. We have shown increased Mφ TNF receptor shedding in patients producing excessive TNF-α (Table 4–3).

Septic patients have been shown to have elevated soluble TNF-α receptors and IL-2 receptors. These patients also could be producing soluble IL-6 receptors, since the IL-6 receptor is shed during Mφ activation.[95] However, soluble IL-6 receptors actually trigger increased IL-6 production and activate cells.[95] Assessing patient serum for soluble IL-6 receptors would provide valuable information on possible mechanisms for their increased IL-6 production. As described earlier, the expression of a number of cellular receptors is altered in septic shock and systemic inflammatory response syndrome. The up-regulation and shedding of TNF-α receptors, the shedding of T cell IL-2 receptors, the down-regulation of neutrophil Fc$_\gamma$RIII and complement receptors, the up-regulation of Mφ Fc$_\gamma$RI, and the increase in endothelial cell adhesion molecules have all been described. Many additional receptor changes remain to be investigated. For example, do Mφ become insensitive to PGE$_2$ because PGE$_2$ receptors are down-regulated? The alterations in TNF-α receptors on posttrauma Mφ need to be better defined. Changes in the LPS receptor (CD14), as well as the receptors for other bacterial cell wall products, need to be evaluated for correlation with increased cytokine induction by bacterial stimulation. It has already been demonstrated that cytokine levels can alter Fc receptor expression, complement receptor expression, and CD14 expression on Mφ and PMNs, altering their subsequent response capacity.[96–98] Some of these alterations may hallmark functional changes in patients and indicate increased risk of septic shock.

OVERVIEW

Only a minority of the extensive data available implicating altered Mφ–T cell interactions and subsequent cytokine imbalances has been mentioned in this chapter. The major conclusion is that loss of proper immune cell triggering, particularly Mφ–T cell triggering, plays a pivotal role in the development of deranged cytokine production and the consequent pathology of septic shock. This is illustrated by our data showing that the Th2 lymphokine IL-4 will suppress excessive trauma patients' production of IL-6, TNF-α, PGE$_2$, and TGF-β.[3,99] This regulatory Th2 lymphokine is not properly activated in these patients. Possible IL-4 therapy has been suggested by a number of investigators.[3,100,101] The fully developed systemic inflammatory response syndrome consists of the release of multiple mediators which initiate many self-perpetuating cycles. For example,

TNF-α induced by low-dose endotoxin is augmented by complement split products and induces platelet-activating factor (PAF). PAF induces Mϕ LTB$_4$ production, which increases TNF-α production to induce more PAF. Complement is activated and toxic oxygen radicals are induced by PAF. Complement split products augment more production of TNF-α and more toxic oxygen radicals release, ever increasing phagocytic cell activation and tissue damage.[61] This is one of many autocrine cycles involved in the pathology of systemic inflammatory response syndrome. Failure of T cell activation, with lymphokine secretion, parallels decreased NK cell activation. This failure of proper lymphocyte activation depresses host resistance while allowing runaway monokine production, because T regulatory lymphokines are not properly induced. T cell anergy develops. Overactivation, adhesion removal, and degranulation of PMNs cause organ damage and deplete the available phagocytic pool for subsequent bacterial challenge control. Mϕ are preactivated and become more sensitive to cytokine induction by endotoxin, complement, leukotrienes, TGF-β1, and a variety of other mediators, as well as resistant to the down-regulatory effects of PGE$_2$ and TGF-β.

Treatment modalities currently being explored are primarily focused on preventing or ameliorating the aberrant cytokine responses of the patients in septic or cytokine shock. As already mentioned, anti-J-chain antibodies have proved less than totally successful, probably because endotoxin contributes to early mortality but is less important once aberrant cytokine cycles are established.[73,74,91] Since TNF-α is a primary contributor to tissue damage and immune pathology, a number of strategies have been tried to reduce excessive TNF-α levels. Antibody to TNF-α prevents septic shock and lethality in a baboon model, even in the face of continued bacterial challenge.[1] The anti-TNF-α antibodies were given 2 h before the bacteria.[1] Antibodies to TNF-α can prevent death when even given after bacterial infusion, if lower *E. coli* doses are administered to the baboons.[102] Anti-TNF-α antibodies also prevented septic death in rabbits and mice.[1,8,47,48] Anti-TNF-α antibodies block IL-8 increases in septic baboons in the face of unlimited bacteremia.[89] Anti-TNF-α antibodies prevented lung edema, PMN activation, and neutrophil accumulation in a PAF/LPS septic rat model.[69] Although a murine antibody to TNF-α gave temporary improvement in treating patients with graft-versus-host disease, only in combination with prednisone was a permanent abatement response gained.[103] Destruction of the anti-TNF-α antibody was seen due to the patients' antimouse antibody response. In septic patients, infusion of anti-TNF-α antibodies was inconclusive. Although 28-day lethality was 4 of 12 in treated patients versus 12 of 23 in untreated patients, hemodynamic changes at 4 days after injury were similar in treated and untreated groups.[104] Attempts to develop a hybrid antibody (human-murine) against TNF-α which would be more stable during in vivo injection are underway.[105] Soluble TNF receptors are also proposed as possible TNF-α antagonists for therapy in patients.[1,8,48] The soluble 55-kDa receptor, which can be purified from human urine, was shown to protect against TNF-α/IL-1- or LPS-induced lethality in mice.[106]

Inhibitors of TNF-α transcription by the drug pentoxifylline also have been investigated.[107] Pentoxifylline prevented TNF-α release in transplant patients receiving OKT3, restored intestinal microvascular flow in a hemorrhagic shock model, and reduced TNF-α levels in tuberculosis patients.[108,109] The beneficial effects of ATP-MgCl$_2$ administration also has been attributed to its ability to block TNF-α and IL-6 release.[2] Although IL-6 infusion does not initiate hemodynamic shock or lethality, anti-IL-6 antibodies protected against lethal *E. coli* challenge in the mouse.[110] IL-6 antibodies also protected against cancer cachexia.[58] However, since IL-6 increases the TNF-α receptor levels on liver and lung, the effects of IL-6 antibody may be indirect.[57] IL-6 antibody may produce its beneficial effects by depressing IL-6–mediated increases in sensitivity to TNF-α.

Infusion of IL-1, like infusion of IL-6, does not produce lethal shock by itself.[1] However, IL-1 is a potent augmentor of TNF-α–mediated lethality.[8,48] The newly described IL-1 receptor antagonist (IL-1RA) has received widespread attention as a possible modulator of endotoxin-mediated shock.[8] The IL-1RA is a naturally occurring protein closely related to IL-1α + β which is made by a variety of cells, including Mϕ.[32,33] IL-1RA is naturally induced during bacteremia and secreted in the urine of febrile patients.[8,32,33] Infusion of IL-1RA can reduce endotoxin-induced IL-8 synthesis, prevent hemodynamic changes in an *E. coli* shock model (rabbit), and inhibit Mϕ release of LTB$_4$ after Mϕ activation by a calcium ionophore.[8,32,45,64,68] These data imply that disruption of a TNF-α amplifying mechanism like IL-1 synergy also can ameliorate endotoxin-mediated shock pathology. Indeed, PAF antagonists also reduce endotoxin-mediated shock pathology in animal models by intervening with amplification mechanisms for TNF-α.[61] Cyclooxygenase inhibitors appear to reduce the acute hemodynamic changes in endotoxin models and to improve some immune dysfunctions following trauma.[5,8,40] Cyclooxygenase inhibitors are less effective in decreasing cytokine levels, protecting against endotoxin-mediated lung injuries, or reversing PMN or T cell defects in septic patients.[6,66,69,71] Other therapies which modulate Mϕ activity are also being examined. These include the use of glucans to correct inappropriate Mϕ activation or the use of IL-10 to correct Mϕ overactivation.[19,41] The major problem with many proposed therapies is that they must be administered either before or simultaneous with the bacterial challenge. It is also unclear whether the therapies tested in experimental endotoxin models would be equally effective against trauma- or hemorrhage-induced cytokine and immune aberrations. One encouraging finding is that the T cell lymphokine IL-4 produces some improvement even in the aberrant activities of Mϕ collected many days after injury.[3,99] These data imply that regulatory cytokine therapy might be useful in correcting excessive monokine production even late in the cytokine shock syndrome.

The complexity of the alterations in immune activation and cytokine production in systemic inflammatory response syndrome have yet to be completely elucidated. The role of IL-10 in trauma needs to be explored. If IL-10 is a product of intensely activated Mϕ, why do not trauma patients down-regulate their TNF-α, IL-6, and IL-8 production with Mϕ produced IL-10? Is there a role for IL-10 in septic patient therapy? How is the altered sensitivity of patients' Mϕ and T cells to stimulation and inhibition first induced? Can combination treatments with antagonists be developed for all patient groups, or will hemorrhagic shock, trauma, and bacteremic patients each need different prophylactic modulators? Potential therapies need to be evaluated to determine the time of initial administration and length of administration. Clearly, the increased adhesion molecule expression in the lung, liver, and kidney needs to be closely examined as a possible target for immunotherapy. The restoration of appropriate T cell–Mφ inter-actions appears to be the most important target for correcting both immune suppression and inappropriate cytokine activation. The loss of specific Mφ–T cell functions is now recognized as contributing not just to immunosuppression but also to the pathology of shock by allowing cytokine overproduction. Current investigations need to focus on how the early Mφ–T cell interactions can be restored to allow proper regulatory and immune activation.

REFERENCES

1. Tracey KJ: Trends in shock research: Tumor necrosis factor (cachectin) in the biology of septic shock syndrome. *Circ Shock* 35:123, 1991.
2. Wang P, Ba ZF, Morrison MH, et al: Mechanism of the beneficial effects of ATP-MgCl$_2$ following trauma-hemorrhage and resuscitation: Downregulation of inflammatory cyto-kine (TNF,IL-6) release. *J Surg Res* 52:364, 1992.
3. Miller-Graziano CL, Szabo G, Kodys K, Mehta B: The interactions of immunopathological mediators (TNF-alpha, TGF-beta, PGE$_2$) in traumatized individuals, in Faist E (ed): *The Immune Consequences of Trauma, Shock and Sepsis—Mechanisms and Therapeutic Approaches.* London, Springer-Verlag (in press).
4. Miller-Graziano CL, Szabo G, Kodys K, Griffey K: Aberrations in post-trauma monocyte (Mφ) subpopulation: Role in septic shock syndrome. *J Trauma* 30(12)S86, 1990.
5. Faist E, Ertel W, Mewes A, et al: Mediators and the trauma induced cascade of immuno-logic defects. *Prog Clin Biol Res* 308:495, 1989.
6. Ertel W, Faist E, Nestle C, et al: Kinetics of interleukin-2 and interleukin-6 synthesis fol-lowing major mechanical trauma. *J Surg Res* 48:622, 1990.
7. Piguet PF, Grau GE, Vassalli P: Tumor necrosis factor and immunopathology. *Immunol Res* 10:122, 1991.
8. Dinarello CA: The proinflammatory cytokines interleukin-1 and tumor necrosis factor and treatment of the septic shock syndrome. *J Infect Dis* 163:1177, 1991.
9. Pittner RA, Spitzer JA: Endotoxin and TNF$_\alpha$ directly stimulate nitric oxide formation in cultured rat hepatocytes from chronically endotoxemic rats. *Biochem Biophy Res Commun* 185(1):430, 1992.
10. Teodorczyk-Injeyan JA, McRitchie DI, Peters WJ, et al: Expression and secretion of IL-2 receptor in trauma patients. *Ann Surg* 212(2):202, 1990.
11. Shimizu Y, Newman W, Yoshiya T, Shaw S: Lymphocyte interactions with endothelial cells. *Immunol Today* 13(3):106, 1992.
12. Jenkins MK: Models of lymphocyte activation: The role of cell division in the induction of clonal anergy. *Immunol Today* 13(2):69, 1992.
13. Mosmann TR, Moore KW: The role of IL-10 in crossregulation of Th1 and Th2 responses. *Immunol Today* 12:A49, 1991.
14. Nawroth PP, Bank I, Handley D, et al: Tumor necrosis factor/cachectin interacts with en-dothelial cell receptor to induce release of interleukins. *J Exp Med* 163:1363, 1986.
15. Harbuz MS, Stephanou A, Sarlis N, Lightman SL: The effects of recombinant human inter-leukin (IL)-1α, IL-1β or IL-6 on hypothalamo-pituitary-adrenal axis activation. *J Endocri-nol* 133:349, 1992.
16. Möller G: *Immunological Reviews: Cytokines in Infectious Diseases.* Copenhagen, Munksgaard International, 1992, p 127.

17. Hamilton TA, Ohmori Y, Narumi S, Tannenbaum CS: *Regulation of Diversity in Macrophage Activation: Mononuclear Phagocytes in Cell Biology.* New York, CRC Press, 1992.

18. Mosmann TR, Coffman RL: Heterogeneity of cytokine secretion patterns and functions of helper T cells. *Adv Immun* 46:111, 1989.

19. Howard M, O'Garra A, Ishida H, et al: Biological properties of interleukin 10. *J Clin Immunol* 12(4):239, 1992.

20. de Waal Malefyt R, Abrams J, Bennet B, et al: Interleukin 10 (IL-10) inhibits cytokine synthesis by human monocytes: An autoregulatory role of IL-10 produced by monocytes. *J Exp Med* 174:1209, 1991.

21. Bancroft GJ, Webster G: Regulation of IFNγ synthesis by natural cells: Differential effects of Th1 (IL-2) and Th2 (IL-10) derived cytokines. *Cytokines* (in press).

22. Oswald IP, Gazzinelli RT, Sher A, James SL: IL-10 synergizes with IL-4 and transforming growth factor-β to inhibit macrophage cytotoxic activity. *J Immunol* 148(11):3578, 1992.

23. Johnson RB: Monocytes and macrophage. *N Engl J Med* 318:747, 1988.

24. Adams DO, Hamilton TA: Molecular basis of macrophage activation: Diversity and its origins, in Lewis C, McGhee J (eds): *The Natural Immune System.* Oxford, Oxford University Press (in press).

25. Dubravec DB, Spriggs DR, Mannic JA, Rodrick ML: Circulating human peripheral blood granulocytes synthesize and secrete tumor necrosis factor α. *Proc Natl Acad Sci USA* 87:6758, 1990.

26. Cassatella MA, Bazzoni F, Ceska M, et al: IL-8 production by human polymorphonuclear leukocytes: The chemoattractant formyl-methionyl-leucyl-phenylalanine induces the gene expression and release of IL-8 through a pertussis toxin-sensitive pathway. *J Immunol* 148(10):3216, 1992.

27. Ohno I, Lea RG, Flanders KC, et al: Eosinophils in chronically inflamed human upper airway tissues express transforming growth factor β1 gene (TGFβ1). *J Clin Invest* 89:1662, 1992.

28. Bone RC, Sprung CL, Sibbald WJ: Definitions for sepsis and organ failure. *Crit Care Med* 20(6):724, 1992.

29. Bjornson AB, Knippenberg RW, Bjornson HS: Bactericidal defect of neutrophils in a guinea pig model of thermal injury is related to elevation of intracellular cyclic-3′,5′-adenosine monophosphate. *J Immunol* 143(8):2609, 1989.

30. Nathan CF: Secretory products of macrophages. *J Clin Invest* 79:319, 1987.

31. Oppenheim JJ, Zachariae COC, Mukaida N, Matsushima K: Properties of the novel proinflammatory supergene "intercrine" cytokine family. *Annu Rev Immunol* 9:617, 1991.

32. Conti P, Panara MR, Barbacane RC, et al: Inhibition of leukotriene B₄ (LTB₄) by recombinant interleukin-1 receptor antagonist (IL-1RA) on human monocytes. *Agents Actions* C93, 1992.

33. Arend WP, Welgus HG, Thompson RC, Eisenberg SP: Biological properties of recombinant human monocyte-derived interleukin-1 receptor antagonist. *J Clin Invest* 85:1694, 1990.

34. Tartaglia LA, Goeddel DV: Two TNF receptors. *Immunol Today* 13(5):151, 1992.

35. Lantz M, Malik S, Slevin ML, Olsson I: Infusion of tumor necrosis factor (TNF) causes an increase in circulating TNF-binding protein in humans. *Cytokines* 2(6):402, 1990.

36. Suter PM, Suter S, Girardin E, et al: High bronchoalveolar levels of tumor necrosis factor and its inhibitors, interleukin-1, interferon, and elastase, in patients with adult respiratory distress syndrome after trauma, shock, or sepsis. *Am Rev Respir Dis* 145:1016, 1992.

37. Girardin E, Roux-Lombard P, Grau GE, et al: Imbalance between tumour necrosis factor-alpha and soluble TNF receptor concentrations in severe meningococcaemia. *Immunol* 76:20, 1992.

38. Ayala A, Perrin MM, Wang P, et al: Hemorrhage induces enhanced Kupffer cell cytotoxicity while decreasing peritoneal or splenic macrophage capacity: Involvement of cell-associated tumor necrosis factor and reactive nitrogen. *J Immunol* 147:4147, 1991.

39. Munoz C, Misset B, Fitting C, et al: Dissociation between plasma and monocyte-associated cytokines during sepsis. *Eur J Immunol* 21:2177, 1991.

40. Ertel W, Morrison MH, Ayala A, et al: Blockade of prostaglandin production increases cachectin synthesis and prevents depression of macrophage functions after hemorrhagic shock. *Ann Surg* 213(3):265, 1991.

41. Browder W, Williams D, Pretus H, et al: Beneficial effects of enhanced macrophage function in the trauma patient. *Ann Surg* 211(5):605, 1990.

42. Abraham E, Regan RF: The effects of hemorrhage and trauma on interleukin 2 production. *Arch Surg* 120:1341, 1985.

43. Ayala A, Wang P, Ba ZF, et al: Hemorrhage-trauma alters plasma TNF and IL-6: Differential alterations in plasma IL-6 and TNF levels after trauma and hemorrhage. *Am J Physiol* 260:R167, 1991.

44. Xing XY, Hua SX, Jun MX: TNF and IL-6 production in different macrophages during sepsis (abstract). *Eur Cytokine Net* 3:250, 1992.

45. Wolchok JD, Vilcek J: There is more to hemorrhagic necrosis than tumor necrosis factor. *J Natl Can Inst* 83(12):807, 1991.

46. Sharma SA, Olchowy TWJ, Yang Z, Breider MA: Tumor necrosis factor α and interleukin 1α enhance lipopolysaccharide-mediated bovine endothelial cell injury. *J Leukoc Biol* 51:579, 1992.

47. Marzi I, Bauer M, Secchi A, et al: Influence of anti-TNF$_\alpha$ antibody on hepatic leukocyte adhesion after hemorrhagic shock in the rat (abstract). *Eur Cytokine Net* 3:266, 1992.

48. Waage A, Aasen AO: Different role of cytokine mediators in septic shock related to meningococcal disease and surgery/polytrauma. *Immunol Rev* 127:221, 1992.

49. Szabo G, Kodys K, Miller-Graziano CL: Elevated monocyte IL-6 production in immunosuppressed trauma patients: I. Role of Fc$_\gamma$RI crosslinking stimulation. *J Clin Immunol* 11(6):326, 1991.

50. Pullicino EA, Carli F, Poole S, et al: The relationship between the circulating concentrations of interleukin 6 (IL-6), tumor necrosis factor (TNF) and the acute phase response to elective surgery and accidental injury. *Lymphokine Res* 9(2):231, 1990.

51. Hack CE, De Groot ER, Felt-Bersma RJF, et al: Increased plasma levels of interleukin-6 in sepsis. *Blood* 74(5):1704, 1989.

52. Yoshimoto T, Nakanishi K, Hirose S, et al: High serum IL-6 level reflects susceptible status of the host to endotoxin and IL-1/tumor necrosis factor. *J Immunol* 148:3596, 1992.

53. Depets JMH, Van De Winkel JGJ, Ceuppens JL: Cross-linking of both Fc$_\gamma$RI and Fc$_\gamma$RII induces secretion of tumor necrosis factor by human monocytes, requiring high affinity Fc-Fc$_\gamma$R interactions. *J Immunol* 144:1304, 1990.

54. Krutmann J, Kirnbauer R, Köck A, et al: Cross-linking Fc receptors on monocytes triggers IL-6 production. *J Immunol* 145:1337, 1990.

55. Miller-Graziano CL, Fink M, Wu JY, et al: Mechanisms of altered monocyte prostaglandin E$_2$ production in severely injured patients. *Arch Surg* 123:293, 1988.

56. Pelloux H, Chumpitazi BFF, Santoro F, et al: Sera of patients with high titers of immunoglobulin G against *Toxoplasma gondii* induce secretion of tumor necrosis factor alpha by human monocytes. *Infect Immun* 60(7):2672, 1992.

57. Van Bladel S, Libert C, Fiers W: Interleukin-6 enhances the expression of tumor necrosis factor receptors on hepatoma cells and hepatocytes. *Cytokines* 3(2):149, 1991.

58. Strassmann G, Jacob CO, Evans R, et al: Mechanisms of experimental cancer cachexia: Interaction between mononuclear phagocytes and colon-26 carcinoma and its relevance to IL-6-mediated cancer cachexia. *J Immunol* 148(11):3674, 1992.

59. Wakabayashi G, Gelfand JA, Jung WK, et al: *Staphylococcus epidermidis* induces complement activation, tumor necrosis factor and interleukin-1. *J Clin Invest* 87:1925, 1991.

60. Gallinaro R, Cheadle WG, Applegate K, Polk HC Jr: The role of the complement system in trauma and infection. *Surg Gynecol Obstet* 174:435, 1992.

61. Sun X, Hsueh W: Platelet-activating factor produces shock, in vivo complement activation, and tissue injury in mice. *J Immunol* 147(2):509, 1991.

62. Ward P: Complement, cytokines and tissue injury, in Faist E (ed): *The Immune Consequences of Trauma*. Heidelberg, Springer-Verlag (in press).

63. Deitch EA: Bacterial translocation of the gut flora, in Faist E (ed): *The Immune Consequences of Trauma*. Heidelberg, Springer-Verlag (in press).

64. Porat R, Poutsiaka DD, Miller LC, et al: Interleukin (IL-1) receptor blockade reduces endotoxin and *Borellia burgdorferi*-stimulated IL-8 synthesis in human mononuclear cells. *FASEB J* 6:2482, 1992.

65. Redl H, Schlag G, Bahrami S, et al: Plasma neutrophil-activating peptide-1/interleukin-8 and neutrophil elastase in a primate bacteremia model. *J Infec Dis* 164:383, 1991.

66. Mozes T, Zijlstra FJ, Heiligers JPC, et al: Sequential release of tumour necrosis factor, platelet activating factor and eicosanoids during endotoxin shock in anaesthetized pigs: Protective effects of indomethacin. *Br J Pharmacol* 104:691, 1991.

67. Mozes T, Ben-Efraim S, Tak CJAM, et al: Serum levels of tumor necrosis factor determine the fatal or nonfatal course of endotoxic shock. *Immunol Lett* 27:157, 1991.

68. Wakabayashi G, Gelfand JA, Burke JF, et al: A specific receptor antagonist for interleukin 1 prevents *Escherichia coli*–induced shock in rabbits. *FASEB J* 5(3):338, 1991.

69. Rabinovici R, Esser KM, Hillegass LM, et al: TNF_α mediates endotoxin/PAF-induced microvascular lung injury (abstract). *Eur Cytokine Net* 3:250, 1992.

70. Takayama TK, Miller C, Szabo G: Elevated tumor necrosis factor α production concomitant to elevated prostaglandin E_2 production by trauma patients' monocytes. *Arch Surg* 125:29, 1990.

71. Gadd MA, Hansbrough JF: Postburn suppression of murine lymphocyte and neutrophil functions is not reversed by prostaglandin blockade. *J Surg Res* 48:84, 1990.

72. Waage A, Halstensen A, Shalaby R, et al: Local production of tumor necrosis factor α, interleukin 1, and interleukin 6 in meningococcal meningitis: Relation to the inflammatory response. *J Exp Med* 170:1859, 1989.

73. Goldman G, Welbourn R, Kobzik L, et al: Tumor necrosis factor-α mediates acid aspiration-induced systemic organ injury. *Ann Surg* 212(4):513, 1990.

74. Calandra T, Glauser MP, Schellekens J, et al: Treatment of gram-negative septic shock with IgG antibody to *Escherichia coli* J5: A prospective, double-blind, randomized trial. *J Infect Dis* 158:312, 1988.

75. Calandra T, Baumgartner J-D, Grau GE, et al: Prognostic values of tumor necrosis factor/cachectin, interleukin-1, interferon-α and interferon-γ in the serum of patients with septic shock. *J Infect Dis* 161:982, 1990.

76. Fantuzzi G, Mengozzi M, Sironi M, et al: Preexposure to LPS differentially regulates cytokine production in human monocytes: Involvement of CD14 (abstract). *Eur Cytokine Net* 3:150, 1992.

77. Ayala A, Kisala JM, Felt JA, et al: Does endotoxin tolerance prevent the release of inflammatory monokines (IL-1, IL-6 or TNF) during sepsis? Monokine release by septic endotoxin-tolerant mice. *Arch Surg* 127(2):191, 1992.

78. Ochoa JB, Udekwu AO, Billiar TR, et al: Nitrogen oxide levels in patients after trauma and during sepsis. *Ann Surg* 214(5):621, 1991.

79. Bjerknes R, Vindenes H, Laerum OD: Altered neutrophil functions in patients with large burns. *Blood Cells* 16:127, 1990.

80. Cannon JG, Tompkins RG, Gelfand JA, et al: Circulating interleukin-1 and tumor necrosis factor in septic shock and experimental endotoxin fever. *J Infect Dis* 161:79, 1990.

81. Kunkel SL, Scales WE, Spengler R, et al: Dynamics and regulation of macrophage tumor necrosis factor-α (TNF-α), interleukin-1α (IL-1α) and interleukin-1β (IL-1β) gene expression by arachidonate metabolites, in Powanda MC, Oppenheim JJ, Kluger MJ, Dinarello

CA (eds): *Monokines and Other Nonlymphocytic Cytokines.* New York, Alan R Liss, 1988, pp 61–66.

82. Miller-Graziano CL, Szabo G, Griffey K, et al: Role of elevated monocyte transforming growth factor β (TGF$_β$) production in posttrauma immunosuppression. *J Clin Immunol* 11(2):95, 1991.

83. Wahl SM: Transforming growth factor beta (TGF-β) in inflammation: A cause and a cure. *J Clin Immunol* 12(2):61, 1992.

84. Turner M, Chantry D, Katsikis P, et al: Induction of the interleukin 1 receptor antagonist protein by transforming growth factor-β. *Eur J Immunol* 21:1635, 1991.

85. Musso T, Espinoza-Delgado I, Pulkki K, et al: IL-2 induces IL-6 production in human monocytes. *J Immunol* 148(3):795, 1992.

86. Zhu D, Zhu JQ, Ye SM, Liang XF: Human rTNF-α stimulates polymorphonuclear granulocytes (PMN) production of cytokine IL-8 (abstract). *Eur Cytokine Net* 3:186, 1992.

87. Stern M, Meagher L, Savill J, Haslett C: Apoptosis in human eosinophils: Programmed cell death in the eosinophil leads to phagocytosis by macrophages and is modulated by IL-5. *J Immunol* 148(11):3543, 1992.

88. Nash JRG, McLaughlin PJ, Hoyle C, Roberts D: Immunolocalization of tumour necrosis factor α in lung tissue from patients dying with adult respiratory distress syndrome. *Histopathology* 19:395, 1991.

89. Redl H, Schlag G, Ceska M, et al: TNF dependent IL-8 release in baboon septicemia (abstract). *Eur Cytokine Net* 3:180, 1992.

90. Remick DG, McCurry KR, Colletti LM, et al: TNF represents the major mediator of organ injury following hepatic ischemia/reperfusion (I/R) (abstract). *Eur Cytokine Net* 3:249, 1992.

91. de Groote MA, Martin MA, Densen P, et al: Plasma tumor necrosis factor levels in patients with presumed sepsis. *JAMA* 262(2):249, 1989.

92. van der Poll T, Jansen J, van Leenen D, et al: Tumor necrosis factor (TNF) is involved in the release of its own soluble receptors (sTNFR) in experimental endotoxemia (abstract). *Eur Cytokine Net* 3:214, 1992.

93. Winzen R, Wallach D, Engelmann H, et al: Selective decrease in cell surface expression and mRNA level of the 55-kDa tumor necrosis factor receptor during differentiation of HL-60 cells into macrophage-like but not granulocyte-like cells. *J Immunol* 148(11):3454, 1992.

94. Gallati H, Brockhaus M: Detection of human soluble TNF receptors in biological fluids (abstract). *Eur Cytokine Net* 3:264, 1992.

95. Dower SK, Smith CA, Park LS: Human cytokine receptors. *J Clin Immunol* 10(6):289, 1990.

96. Te Velde AA, Huijbens RJF, De Vries JE, Figdor CG: IL-4 decreases Fc$_γ$R membrane expression and Fc$_γ$R-mediated cytotoxic activity of human monocytes. *J Immunol* 144(8):3046, 1990.

97. Te Velde AA, Rousset F, Peronne C, et al: IFN-α and IFN-γ have different regulatory effects on IL-4 induced membrane expression of Fc$_ε$RIIb and release of soluble Fc$_ε$RIIb by human monocytes. *J Immunol* 144(8):3052, 1990.

98. Wong HL, Lotze MT, Wahl LM, Wahl SM: Administration of recombinant IL-4 to humans regulates gene expression, phenotype, and function in circulating monocytes. *J Immunol* 148(7):2118, 1992.

99. Szabo G, Kodys K, Miller-Graziano CL: Elevated monocyte IL-6 production in immunosuppressed trauma patients: II. Downregulation by IL-4. *J Clin Immunol* 11(6):336, 1991.

100. Mangan DF, Robertson B, Wahl SM: IL-4 enhances programmed cell death (apoptosis) in stimulated human monocytes. *J Immunol* 148(6):1812, 1992.

101. Standiford TJ, Streiter RM, Chensue SW, et al: IL-4 inhibits the expression of IL-8 from stimulated human monocytes. *J Immunol* 145(4):1435, 1990.

102. Hinshaw L, Olson P, Kuo G: Efficacy of post-treatment with anti-TNF monoclonal antibody

in preventing the pathophysiology and lethality of sepsis in the baboon. *Circ Shock* 27:362, 1989.

103. Holler E, Kolb HJ, Kempeni J, et al: TNF alpha for treatment of acute graft-versus-host disease a pilot study (abstract). *Eur Cytokine Net* 3:255, 1992.

104. Boekstegers P, Weidenhöfer ST, Pilz G, et al: Response to TNF-antibody therapy (Mak 195F) in patients with severe sepsis: Comparison to polyvalent IgG-therapy (abstract). *Eur Cytokine Net* 3:215, 1992.

105. Bodmer M: The generation and preclinical testing of CDP571: A humanised anti-TNFα antibody for therapeutic use (abstract). *Eur Cytokine Net* 3:248, 1992.

106. Faggioni R, Bertini R, Gascon MP, et al: Urinary TNF-binding protein (TNF soluble receptor) protects mice against the lethal effects of TNF and endotoxic shock (abstract). *Eur Cytokine Net* 3:151, 1992.

107. Schandene L, Vandenbussche P, Crusiaux A, et al: Differential effects of pentoxifylline on the production of tumour necrosis factor-alpha (TNF-α) and interleukin-6 (IL-6) by monocytes and T cells. *Immunol* 76:30, 1992.

108. Flynn WJ, Cryer HG, Garrison RN: Pentoxifylline restores intestinal microvascular blood flow during resuscitated hemorrhagic shock. *Surgery* 110:350, 1991.

109. Zabel P, Greinert U, Entzian P, Schlaak M: Effects of pentoxifylline on circulating cytokines (TNF and IL-6) in severe pulmonary tuberculosis (abstract). *Eur Cytokine Net* 3:248, 1992.

110. Starnes HF Jr, Pearce MK, Tewari A, et al: Anti-IL-6 monoclonal antibodies protect against lethal *Escherichia coli* infection and lethal tumor necrosis factor-α challenge in mice. *J Immunol* 145:4185, 1990.

5

PRINCIPLES OF RESUSCITATION

Jonathan M. Saxe
Anna M. Ledgerwood
Charles E. Lucas

The term *resuscitation* is derived from the Latin word *resuscitatus,* which, literally, means "to stir up again or to put in motion." The intent of physicians caring for injured patients is to stir them up and to place their organs back into proper motion. One's ability to successfully resuscitate the injured patient with hypo-volemic shock is often hampered by ignorance of normal physiology and the manner in which the body responds to both hemorrhage and subsequent resuscitation. Just as each organ performs specific but well-defined vital functions in health, so does successful resuscitation require that therapy be designed to consider the needs of all organs in disease. Successful restoration of function in one organ at the expense of another organ will likely lead to failure or death, since the body is only as healthy as its sickest organ.

The emergency room or prehospital care of injured patients has been presented as an empiric systemic approach highlighting those critical functions which must be maintained or augmented on a priority basis. Consequently, one identifies various cardiopulmonary and ventilatory functions which take initial priority, followed closely by the need to control internal and external bleeding while correcting the intravascular volume deficit. The objectives herein are to examine the priorities in the initial resuscitation, to identify the homeostasis associated with shock and resuscitation, and to make recommendations for therapy throughout the period of insult until the patient is discharged from hospital.

CARDIOPULMONARY RESUSCITATION

The initial assessment of the injured patient upon arrival to the emergency department often focuses on determining whether the patient has cardiac activity. The severely injured patient with massive exsanguination may have no apparent

147

TABLE 5–1. Priorities in Resuscitation

1. Institute cardiopulmonary resuscitation
2. Provide ventilatory support
   a. Airway clearance
   b. Breathing or ventilation augmentation
3. Control external hemorrhage
4. Correct circulatory deficit
5. Identify and control internal bleeding
6. Obtain appropriate consultation

movement, very distant and quiet heart tones, and fixed dilated pupils which, to even the experienced observer, mimic the appearance of a patient arriving dead on arrival (DOA). When the first 10- to 15-second examination does not resolve the question of cardiac activity, immediate cardiopulmonary resuscitation (CPR) must be initiated (Table 5–1). When the patient has obvious cardiac activity, the priorities of resuscitation and treatment should be implemented. While implementing these priorities of treatment, further careful examination should identify the status of the skin color or capillary perfusion; the status of the neurologic deficit, including the assessment of the Glasgow coma scale; the status of the injury severity score; and the identification of any localized neurologic deficit indicative of central nervous system (CNS) injury.

Once the presence of cardiac activity and the status of the Glasgow coma scale and injury severity score are determined, the priorities identify the need for rapid assessment of the airway, breathing, and circulation, the ABCs of resuscitation. The Basic and Advanced Cardiac Life Support Courses of the American Heart Association and the Advanced Trauma Life Support Course of the American College of Surgeons highlight these priority objectives in great detail. This primary survey of the injured patient is crucial in establishing priorities of care, and within these priorities the ABCs are most critical.[1,2] The examining team may provide initial protection of the airway by means of an oral airway, which allows one to assist with ventilation by means of an ambu-bag while the presence of cardiac activity is being assessed. When there is question concerning the presence of life as judged by the presence of cardiac activity, immediate CPR with endotracheal intubation is mandated.[3] The technique of closed CPR has been widely promulgated by many organizations and needs no further discussion as to technique. In the patient whose injury has resulted from blunt torso trauma, there is little indication to escalate from closed CPR to the open technique of CPR. Most major or large-scale reviews of open cardiac massage following blunt torso trauma show that the survival rate is less than 1 percent.[4–6] In contrast, when the patient arrives after having sustained a penetrating chest injury with absent or impaired cardiac function, open cardiac massage with CPR is often lifesaving.

VENTILATORY SUPPORT

The next priority in resuscitation of the severely injured patient with hemorrhagic shock deals with the recognition and treatment of inadequate ventilation.

This phenomenon may be characterized by increased respiratory effort, fear or panic, cyanosis, nasal flaring, intercostal retraction with respiratory effort, or incontinence. The emergency department team must recognize agitation and combativeness as signs of ventilatory embarrassment and not treat the patient with restraints and sedation lest the patient suffer irreversible cardiac arrest and death. The emergency medical service team that identifies ventilatory difficulty in a prehospital setting needs to provide some type of assistance at the scene prior to transport to the closest hospital facility. Often support can be adequately provided in this setting by means of ambu-bag and mask–assisted ventilation while the patient's neck is held in slight extension and the jaw and tongue are kept in a forward position, thereby keeping the hypopharynx patent. An oral airway may assist in this maneuver. The use of the esophageal airway is no longer considered optimal therapy in this setting. Nasotracheal or oral tracheal intubation may be necessary on the scene if skilled personnel are available, but one of these procedures can usually be deferred until someone with more expertise sees the patient upon arrival at the emergency department or happens upon the scene in the prehospital setting. When the unfortunate circumstance occurs where a patient requires ventilatory support and no equipment including the ambu-bag is available, mouth-to-mouth or mouth-to-nose resuscitation will often provide temporizing support until equipment and skilled personnel are available. Most important throughout all this frustrating and challenging encounter is to remain calm, since panic will inevitably lead to inappropriate decision making.[7]

Certain conditions mitigate against the successful use of ambu-bag/mask ventilatory support in the acutely injured patient. Three such conditions include the presence of ongoing hyperpharyngeal or oral bleeding, upper airway blockage, or gastric distension, which sets the stage for vomiting and aspiration in patients receiving ambu-bag/mask ventilatory support.[8,9] Laryngeal injury should be suspected in any patient who is injured while riding in the front passenger seat of a vehicle that is involved in a head-on collision. When a patient with laryngeal injury presents to the emergency department, one expects to identify respiratory distress with or without stridor and cervical swelling. A patient with these findings may develop increasing respiratory distress during efforts to augment ventilation with the ambu-bag/mask technique. Such patients are candidates for rapid endotracheal intubation by means of the nasal, oral, or percutaneous cricothyroidotomy route.[9]

Other causes of upper airway obstruction include foreign bodies such as dentures, chewing gum, peanuts, or ingested portions of food that were eaten shortly prior to injury. Larger foreign bodies can be identified and extracted with a quick but careful digital examination of the mouth and hypopharynx. Smaller foreign bodies may gain access to the trachea and be more difficult to extract digitally. Such foreign bodies more often than not will become lodged near the glottis so that a cricothyroidotomy may be successful in bypassing the point of obstruction.

Gastric distension is not only a complication to the ambu-bag/mask ventilation technique but also makes this technique of ventilation more hazardous due to the threat of vomiting and aspiration. This complication can often be prevented by early insertion of a nasogastric tube in those patients without suspected fractures of the cribriform plate. Although the nasogastric tube will not successfully remove the recently ingested food particles, the tube will often provide a means for escape of swallowed air, thereby reducing the intraluminal gastric pressure and decreasing the likelihood of regurgitation. When blood, vomitus, or other ingested materials impair ventilation by the ambu-bag/mask technique in a patient requiring immediate establishment of an airway, a nasotracheal tube can often be passed blindly into the trachea while listening for airway movement as the tube negotiates the hypopharynx and then enters into the trachea.[10] Otherwise, the patient must be resuscitated by means of a cricothyroidotomy with placement of a tracheostomy tube through this incision. When a cricothyroidotomy is used to establish immediate airway control, conversion of this incision to a formal tracheostomy within the first 24 hours after the patient has been stabilized decreases the likelihood for irreversible or even temporary injury to the glottis.[11] Another cause of potential upper airway obstruction following penetrating cervical wounds is a peritracheal hematoma. For this reason, a tracheostomy tray should be near at hand in all patients being anesthetized for exploration of neck wounds in case the intraoperative attempts at intubation produce an acute obstruction. When one is unable to successfully perform a cricothyroidotomy in the patient in extremis, a 12- or 14-gauge intracath can be rapidly inserted into the trachea and then attached to a Y-connector for the rapid insufflation of oxygen through the connector at rates up to 15 liters/min. This may provide temporary oxygenation while steps are being taken to implement a more satisfactory airway.[12] The more frequent causes of lower airway obstruction in seriously injured patients are hemothorax, pneumothorax, and flail chest. The most threatening lower airway problem is a tension pneumothorax. This may be suspected in the acutely injured patient who displays evidence of anxiety, fear, and agitation along with the triad of hypotension, distant heart tones, and neck vein distension. This latter triad is similar to that seen with patients presenting with acute cardiac tamponade from penetrating injury; the difference between the two entities can be rapidly identified by the position of the trachea, which is midline in the patient with cardiac tamponade and shifted to the contralateral side in a patient with tension pneumothorax.[13] Intubation and assisted ventilation in the patient with tension pneumothorax may be fatal in that it may worsen the pneumothorax and cause further contralateral shift of the mediastinum, thus impeding cardiac return. Tension pneumothorax should be suspected in any patient with rapidly deteriorating vital signs. Any question about the presence of tension pneumothorax requires immediate diagnostic thoracentesis to relieve intrapleural tension. When this procedure serves as a lifesaving treatment, the rush of air can be heard escaping from the thoracentesis needle. Once confirmed clinically, a tube thoracostomy should be performed following the diagnostic thoracentesis without waiting for roentgenographic confirmation.

Patients with hemothorax, even a very large hemothorax filling most of one side of the chest, seldom have inadequate ventilation as the primary cause for threatened survival. When the hemothorax is extensive, the major threat to survival is the associated circulatory deficit. Consequently, such patients, when stable, usually can have roentgenographic confirmation of the hemothorax made prior to insertion of a therapeutic chest tube. When a patient with a suspected hemothorax is unstable, the immediate diagnosis of hemothorax can be verified, in most instances, by rapid thoracentesis, which is followed by tube thoracostomy when hemothorax was confirmed; this is all done prior to roentgeno-graphic confirmation in the unstable patient. Rapid transport of the unstable patient to the operating room for suspected hemothorax without confirmatory thoracentesis is not advocated because the performance of an unnecessary tho-racotomy in an already unstable patient adds significantly to the challenge of overcoming the hemorrhagic shock insult. Consequently, the use of needle tho-racentesis to confirm hemothorax is advocated.[14]

Flail chest may be a major cause of inadequate ventilation. This entity, how-ever, does not usually present a diagnostic dilemma. The flail segment is always associated with fracture of two or more ribs, often in more than one segment, thereby allowing for the paradoxical movement of this unstabilized portion of the chest wall. When the flail segment is located anteriorly, the diagnosis is read-ily apparent upon initial inspection of the chest. When the flail segment is lo-cated posterolaterally, a more careful observation may be required to identify the paradoxical movement under the scapula and attached muscles. Paradoxical movement, tenderness overlying fractured ribs, and chest wall crepitus due to the extrapleural air dissection provide important diagnostic clues for a flail chest. When such a patient has acute respiratory distress, the urgency of intubation cannot be overemphasized, since attempts at ambu-bag/mask ventilation may aggravate the underlying condition.

Occasionally, a patient with rib fractures involving multiple ribs at more than one site will not display the paradoxical movement during the initial emergency department examination. Subsequently, as the respiratory distress progresses, pulmonary compliance will decrease and the obvious paradoxical movement will ensue during the initial 48 hours of hospitalization.[15] Patients with multiple associated injuries such as injuries to the brain or profound hypovolemic shock will require long-term ventilatory support in order to successfully treat the flail chest. When such injuries are present, early tracheostomy performed when the patient is stabilized will provide the best means of ventilation with the least hazard of airway sepsis. Often the presence of a flail chest will obscure an as-sociated pneumothorax which is not apparent on the routine chest roentgeno-grams because of significant subcutaneous air within the chest wall structures. The presence of chest wall emphysema indicates that the visceral and parietal pleurae have been ruptured, thereby allowing air under tension to dissect into the chest wall. The performance of a tracheostomy within 1 week of serious multiple organ injuries in a patient requiring long-term ventilatory support gives a much better prognosis than continued long-term ventilation with an orotra-cheal or nasotracheal tube.[16,17] Consequently, all such patients are candidates for tube thoracostomy to control the lung leak and circumvent the need for the extravasated air to find its way to the chest wall.

Diaphragmatic rupture following blunt torso trauma is another important cause of impaired ventilation. This entity, which is seen more commonly on the left side, is associated with progressive respiratory distress as the intestinal viscera move further into the thorax. Whenever a patient with inadequate ventilation responds poorly to assisted ventilation with the ambu-bag/mask technique, diaphragmatic rupture should be considered. This worsening of symptoms occurs because the ambu-bag/mask ventilatory technique is associ-ated with air movement into the stomach, which further pushes the abdominal organs into the thorax. Consequently, gastric decompression and endotracheal intubation with controlled positive-pressure ventilation may be needed to provide satisfactory relief of the compressed lung in preparation for operative intervention.

CONTROL OF CIRCULATORY DEFICIT

Once successful cardiopulmonary resuscitation and adequate ventilatory support have been implemented, attention must be directed toward the control of bleeding and correction of the plasma volume deficit.[18] The activities necessary to achieve these ends are performed simultaneously as many members of the resuscitation team work in unison. Most external bleeding is optimally controlled by means of direct external pressure or digital pressure over sites of arterial bleeding.

Internal bleeding often can only be controlled by means of operative intervention. The more common sites of serious internal bleeding include fractures, hemothorax, hemoperitoneum, and large soft tissue trauma (Table 5–2). The most common cause of major bleeding after blunt trauma is fractures of long bones or the pelvis. Approximately 80 percent of the total bleeding from such fracture sites occurs within the first 6 h; the remaining 20 percent represents slower bleeding which occurs over the next 48 h. Consequently, a patient with multiple fractures should be identified as having significant bleeding during that first 6 h so that the treating team is not surprised by the sudden onset of hypotension 2 to 6 h after arrival in the emergency facility. When a laissez-faire attitude toward ongoing fracture bleeding is taken, the patient's condition may suddenly deteriorate, and the resuscitation team may suspect that there is a sudden onset of internal bleeding within the chest or within the abdomen. Once this panic mentality arises, the unfortunate patient may be rushed to the operating room for an unnecessary thoracotomy or laparotomy to explain this sudden onset of hypotension. Methods to prevent this inappropriate decision making are discussed later.

HEMORRHAGE FROM PELVIC FRACTURES

The potential for life-threatening hemorrhage from major pelvic fractures is so great that special attention should be directed toward recognition and treatment of such hemorrhage.[19] The extent of bleeding varies with the severity of pelvic fracture, which can be classified by the extent of disruption of the pelvic ring (Table 5–3). Patients presenting with class I pelvic fractures, which do not in-

TABLE 5–2. Blood Loss from Fracture Sites

Pelvis	1500–2000 ml
Stable fractures	500–1000 ml
Unstable fractures	2000–8000 ml
Femur	800–1200 ml
Tibia	350–650 ml
Smaller fracture sites	100–500 ml

TABLE 5–3. Severity of Pelvic Fracture

Class I	Nonring fractures, unilateral anterior fractures
Class II	Bilateral anterior ring fractures
Class III	Ipsilateral anterior and posterior ring fractures
Class IV	Unilateral anterior with bilateral posterior ring fractures
Class V	Bilateral anterior and posterior ring fractures

volve the ring or which involve only a unilateral anterior portion of the pelvic ring, will have minimal bleeding and little likelihood for circulatory volume embarrassment. Contrarily, patients with class IV pelvic ring fractures, in which there are bilateral anterior and posterior disruptions of the pelvic ring, have major bleeding from the pelvis and may be expected to have an acute circulatory embarrassment. The more severe pelvic fractures are associated with diapedesis of red cells into the peritoneal cavity, with the result that most of these patients will have a positive diagnostic peritoneal lavage (DPL). The decision to operate on all patients who have a positive DPL, defined as a lavage fluid that has a hematocrit of 1 percent or greater, will lead to unnecessary laparotomy, which further endangers the patient and compromises the patient's ability to recover from multiple injuries. Consequently, the decision to operate should be based on a DPL that yields a hematocrit of 3 percent rather than the traditional 1 percent. The patient with a badly fractured pelvis also will have recurrent bleeding whenever movement takes place for positioning on the roentgenographic table or for various other tests which are being performed. Consequently, the treating team must recognize that movement is to be avoided, if possible, and that support of the pelvis by either a sling or, more recently, early institution of external skeletal fixation will markedly reduce the amount of recurrent bleeding during the multiple patient movements that must occur in order to evaluate injuries to other organs.[20] The early institution of external fixation has markedly reduced the need for exploratory laparotomy in patients with major pelvic fractures. The frustrations associated with laparotomy and the exploration of retroperitoneal pelvic hematomas, ligation of the internal hypogastric arteries, and packing of the retroperitoneum are legend. The role of this approach has been markedly reduced to the extent that it is almost never required. Furthermore, the use of selective embolization of arteriographically defined bleeding sites in patients with major pelvic fractures should be deferred until the patient has had external skeletal fixation, which will circumvent the need for small vessel embolization in most patients. These other procedures are still available in the patient who does not respond to external skeletal fixation. Likewise, the very rare but lifesaving circumstance of performing hemipelvectomy in patients who are refractory to all other types of treatment is still present but rarely indicated following the more recent use of external skeletal fixation.[20]

INTERNAL BLEEDING FROM HEMOTHORAX

Blood sequestered within the pleural cavity is not only a potential cause for ventilatory insufficiency but also may be an important site of hidden blood loss.

Patients who have hemothorax with complete opacification of a hemithorax have up to 3 liters of internal blood loss. Such patients should be taken directly to surgery for tube thoracostomy, anticipating that the patient may soon need an open thoracotomy for control of bleeding. The extent of blood evacuated at the time of tube thoracostomy and the subsequent bleeding that ensues following evacuation identify those patients who require open thoracotomy in order to control bleeding while the resuscitation effort is continuing. When the initial evacuation of blood exceeds 1500 ml, thoracotomy will almost certainly be indicated for control of continuing bleeding. When the initial evacuation exceeds 1000 ml and the patient remains stable or even improves as the lung is able to better expand, observation is acceptable, but appropriate preparations should be made for any change in vital signs or any continuance or recurrence of drainage from the chest tube. Once the initial evacuation has been completed, further bleeding that exceeds 400 ml in the first hour or exceeds 200 ml per hour from hours 2 through 6 indicates significant ongoing bleeding which requires open thoracotomy for control. When a patient does not meet the criteria for open thoracotomy during the first 6 h but then continues to bleed more than 100 ml/h thereafter, open thoracotomy is indicated. Occasionally patients will have rapid bleeding of more than 200 ml/10 min after the initial evacuation of the hemothorax; such patients need immediate open thoracotomy for control of internal bleeding.[21] The most common sites for life-threatening bleeding into the hemithorax after blunt trauma include fractured ribs, ruptured intercostal vessels, and rupture of the thoracic aorta. The more common sites of active bleeding following gunshot wounds to the chest include the lung, great vessels, and heart. The more common sources of continued bleeding following stab wounds to the chest include the intercostal vessels, the internal mammary vessels, the great vessels, and the heart.

The abdomen is a common site for internal or hidden blood loss after both blunt and penetrating injury. Life-threatening hemoperitoneum should be suspected in any patient who has inappropriate deterioration in vital signs when other sites of both internal and external blood loss have been excluded. Intraabdominal bleeding is not apparent on routine roentgenographic examinations and may be present despite the absence of significant physical findings.[22] The decision to continue resuscitation or take a patient directly to the operating room may be based on the suspicion of hidden intraabdominal bleeding. Whenever question exists about the presence of massive hemoperitoneum following a penetrating abdominal wound, diagnostic paracentesis performed along the lateral border of each rectus muscle will almost always yield some blood if indeed massive hemoperitoneum is present. In this setting, a negative paracentesis should lead the surgeon to perform a DPL before doing an unnecessary operation for suspected hemoperitoneum. Both the paracentesis and DPL may be negative following retroperitoneal penetrating wounds, but the presence of a negative DPL indicates that massive hemorrhage, and therefore hypotension, is not due to hemoperitoneum.

Controversy exists about the relative merits of abdominal computed tomographic (CT) scan versus DPL in patients presenting after blunt trauma. Actually, these two examinations can be complementary, with each test having specific objectives. When the patient presents with stable vital signs, a DPL rules out hemoperitoneum and identifies whether there is any evidence for hollow viscus rupture. The DPL, however, gives little or no information regarding the retroperitoneal space. Consequently, patients with blunt rupture of the pancreas, duodenum, or genitourinary system with significant bleeding might have a negative DPL. Such patients are candidates for follow-up examination with an abdominal CT scan for assuming that there is no trunk injury. Adherence to this approach will allow the surgeon to avoid an unnecessary operation in a patient who has significant retroperitoneal bleeding and allow early identification of those patients who require operation for intraperitoneal hemorrhage. This knowledge can then be incorporated into the ongoing resuscitation for hemorrhagic shock.

HIDDEN RETROPERITONEAL HEMORRHAGE

The retroperitoneal organs, when injured, can be the source of significant bleeding which is not readily apparent on physical examination or on routine roentgenographic studies of the abdomen. Major bleeding from the kidney or bladder can be suspected on the basis of hematuria, which may be either gross or microscopic. Consequently, any degree of hematuria following major torso trauma mandates an emergency assessment of the urologic system in the stable patient. This assessment may include a drip-infusion pyelogram or a contrast CT scan to assess the kidneys and ureters and a cystogram to assess the integrity of the bladder. Based on these studies, one can estimate the severity of organ injury and consequent bleeding. Other organs in the retroperitoneum which may be associated with significant bleeding following both blunt and penetrating trauma are the adrenal glands and the pancreas. Pancreatic injury usually does not cause massive bleeding but may cause localized sepsis, which, if it goes on unrecognized, will complicate resuscitation efforts for bleeding from other organs. A suspicion of pancreatic injury exists whenever a patient has mild abdominal tenderness in association with a rising serum amylase level. Whenever there is a question of pancreatic injury, an abdominal CT scan will define such injury in most patients. When questions about the integrity of the pancreatic ductal system continue after abdominal CT scan, endoscopic retrograde cholangiopancreatography will define the state of the ductal system and help guide therapy.[24]

CORRECTION OF CIRCULATION

Although hemorrhagic shock has been well defined as a clinical entity for more than a century, the philosophies on management remain controversial and enigmatic. A prime essential in defining the optimal treatment of hemorrhagic shock is understanding of the natural history of this circulatory state. All injured patients subjected to a hypovolemic shock insult will pass through three distinct phases during recovery from this insult (Table 5–4). Phase I is the period of active bleeding. This phase extends from the time of injury through the cessation of bleeding, which is often accomplished at the time of operative intervention and repair or removal of injured organs. Phase II is the period of obligatory extravascular fluid sequestration. This phase extends from the point of cessation

TABLE 5–4. Treatment Phases for Hemorrhagic Shock

Phase I	Period of active bleeding, from injury to cessation of bleeding (often operative)
Phase II	Extravascular fluid sequestration, from cessation of bleeding to point of maximal weight gain
Phase III	Intravascular refilling and diuresis, from maximal weight gain to maximal weight loss

of bleeding until the time of maximal weight gain, reflecting the accumulation of fluid in extravascular spaces. Phase III is the period of intravascular refilling and diuresis. This phase extends from the time of maximal weight gain until the time of subsequent maximal weight loss, reflecting the renal excretion of fluid that has been returned to the intravascular compartment.[25]

HEMORRHAGIC SHOCK: A HISTORICAL PERSPECTIVE

Hypovolemic or hemorrhagic shock has been the most intensely studied type of shock. Many decades ago, surgeons recognized that patients responded better to treatment when parenteral salt and water solutions were used following major surgical operations. The recognition of many of the devastating consequences of the hemorrhagic shock insult date back to the nineteenth century and some of the early writings of Samuel Gross.[26] Further breakthroughs in the understanding of this entity occurred during the treatment of severely injured soldiers during and after World War I; many of these observations were summarized by Blalock in a dissertation on the pathophysiology of all types of shock.[27] Blalock suggested that shock was the end stage of a process that was initiated by many different clinical entities, including hemorrhage. Subsequently, Wiggers[28] developed some of the early experimental models of hemorrhagic shock in a canine model. Wiggers was able to demonstrate that animals bled to lethal levels of hypotension could not be successfully resuscitated by the return of the shed blood without additional resuscitation with balanced salt solution. Subsequently, Moore[29] published a series of reports which eventually led to a full treatise on the metabolic responses in the surgical patient. This treatise highlighted the importance of salt and water relocation in response to surgical intervention. Although this classic treatise identified the obligatory nature of this salt and water retention, the therapeutic adaptation was to withhold excessive salt and water replacement in order to adjust to the so-called inevitable release of antidiuretic hormone and aldosterone in response to surgical stress.[29] Subsequent studies have shown that this surgery-induced release of antidiuretic hormone and aldosterone reflects a compromised circulatory volume rather than being some ill-defined nonspecific response to surgical stress, but this treatise did provide a stimulus for elevating the treatment of the surgical patient to a level of physiologically based principles rather than simple conjecture.

The problem of identifying optimal fluid resuscitation during hemorrhagic shock insult remains a significant enigma. Although fluid replacement in the form of plasma was utilized during World War II, the level of understanding and subsequent implementation of total body resuscitation were woefully inadequate. During the Korean conflict, the pathophysiology of hypovolemic shock was better understood and managed. During this conflict, better appreciation of the significance of prerenal azotemia and renal failure evolved.[30] During this time, dialysis was first introduced into the treatment of injured soldiers, and better definitions of end points of resuscitation became defined. Concomitantly, Shires and coworkers[31] began studying the total pathophysiology of hypovolemic shock in animal models. Using a modified Wiggers hemorrhagic shock preparation, Shires and associates monitored the different fluid compartments with radioactive isotopes. These authors used chromium 51–tagged red blood cells and both iodine 125– and iodine 131–labeled albumin to estimate plasma volume and sulfate 35–labeled sodium sulfate to estimate the extracellular water space.[32] Volume of each space was determined by the dilution principle using multiple sampling techniques. These studies were really the first of a series of scientific models that eventually led to our modern understanding of the hemorrhagic shock insult for which logical resuscitation can be implemented.

The early studies by Shires and coworkers showed that the sublethal hypovolemic insult without shock was associated with fluid loss primarily from the plasma volume compartment. When animals were bled into hypotension, however, there was an associated reduction in the functional extracellular fluid volume. Subsequent studies showed that this loss in the extracellular compartment, including the interstitial fluid space, was most likely due to a redistribution or relocation of fluid into the intracellular space. When animals were subjected to severe hemorrhage with profound hypotension, the extracellular or interstitial fluid space was markedly reduced and led to a fatal outcome unless resuscitation in the form of "added" fluid was provided.[33] These observations in the controlled hemorrhagic shock canine model were substantiated during the Vietnam conflict when patients treated by additional salt and water replacement after severe hemorrhagic shock were found to have a much better outcome.

The injuries sustained during the Vietnam conflict were treated in settings which often allowed for the scientific observation of response to treatment. Doty and coworkers[34] confirmed the experimental studies of Shires and coworkers that the extracellular fluid compartment was severely depleted as a result of the hypovolemic shock insult in these injured soldiers. These studies highlighted cognizance of the now accepted principle that the movement of plasma volume into the extravascular space was insufficient to explain all the fluid loss and need for fluid replacement. These observations have since been documented by subsequent studies that show that there was a tremendous loss of interstitial fluid into, presumably, the intracellular space. The Shires' team further rejected the hypothesis proposed by Gann and coworkers[35] and Friedman and coworkers[36] that hyperosmolarity from hyperglycemia would draw major fluid volumes from the interstitial space into the plasma compartment.[37,38] In contrast, the Shires' team believed that the hemorrhagic shock insult caused fluid to move from the interstitial space into the intracellular space. Subsequent studies supported these conclusions by demonstrating that the hemorrhagic shock insult in baboons produced predictable changes in cell membrane potential, reflecting the results of salt and water sequestration within the cells.[39] The principle that the hemorrhagic shock insult led to intracellular swelling was supported by DePalma and coworkers,[40] who confirmed that muscle and liver cells became swollen during the hemorrhagic shock insult. These studies helped promulgate the conclusion that interstitial fluid moves into both the plasma compartment and the intracellular space in response to the hemorrhagic shock insult.

Although the classic studies by Shires and coworkers provide a compelling logic for the acute responses to the hemorrhagic shock insult, they do not fully explain Shires' own observation that resuscitation from hemorrhagic shock requires excess fluid replacement in order to maintain circulatory volume effectively following the period of hypotension. The volume of balanced salt solution needed to maintain circulation, vital signs, and life itself in the period immediately following control of bleeding far exceeds that which can be explained by the movement of interstitial fluid into the cellular compartment. Consequently, other physiologic events in the interstitial compartment must be operative. Studies of such events have helped provide a more complete understanding of the total homeostatic response to hemorrhagic shock.

PATHOPHYSIOLOGY OF HEMORRHAGIC SHOCK

When the injured patient presents to the emergency department with severe life-threatening hemorrhagic shock, one can predict that the patient has suffered an acute 40 to 50 percent reduction of the circulatory blood volume. These estimates correspond to those predicted in controlled animal model studies conducted by Wiggers many years ago.[28] This severe acute plasma volume reduction leads to the release of many hormones, including beta-endorphins, growth hormone, adrenal corticoids, catecholamines, antidiuretic hormone (ADH), renin, and aldosterone.[41] These humerol responses are highly integrated with the nervous system response to the hemorrhagic shock insult. Such responses have been confirmed in both human and animal studies.[42] Afferent signals from baroreceptors and stretch receptors lead to an increased production and release of pituitary hormones, which, in turn, cause the release of vasoactive peptides. This results in a reduction in cardiac output and an increase in peripheral vascular resistance. The renal response to these vascular events includes a reduction in renal blood flow due to a combination of preglomerular and postglomerular arteriolar vasoconstriction, decreased glomerular filtration, and a consequent reduction in the clearance of sodium osmoles and free water.[43] At the capillary level, systemically, there is a net reduction in hydrostatic pressure, which leads to a reduced tendency for protein-free filtrate to leave the plasma compartment for the interstitial compartment. Simultaneously, there is a net increase in the intravascular/interstitial oncotic ratio, which encourages the relocation of interstitial fluid into the intravascular space.[44] These two events encourage the refilling of the plasma compartment during the initial hemorrhagic shock insult prior to the institution of resuscitative fluids. The sympathetic discharge leads to vasoconstriction of large arterioles (90 to 150 μm); this is associated with the early dilation of smaller arterioles (20 to 50 μm). This dilation of the smaller arterioles provides the mechanism for the reduced hydrostatic pressure within the small capillaries, thus encouraging a net movement of water into the plasma compartment.[44] This flux of salt and water from the interstitial space to the plasma compartment by necessity leads to a contraction of the interstitial space matrix.

THE INTERSTITIAL FLUID SPACE AND HEMORRHAGIC SHOCK

The interstitium is the least understood component of the response to hemorrhagic shock and resuscitation. The interstitial fluid space matrix provides the intervening structure and space that lies between the capillaries and the cellular membranes. The interstitial fluid space is composed of both a structural segment and a fluid component, which are closely intertwined. The structural portion of the interstitial fluid compartment is known as the *interstitial matrix* and is made up of coarse collagen fibers and the finer hyaluronic acid moieties; the ultrafine structures are the proteoglycans. These matrix structures are closely intertwined with water and its contained ions, primarily the sodium ion. Such is the environmental milieu that allows for optimal cellular homeostasis in response to health and disease, including hemorrhagic shock. The interstitial space matrix of various organ systems is distinguished by the type, concentration, and organization of the materials within the matrix. Thus the interstitial matrix of the liver is far different from that of the kidney. Both are uniquely designed to best serve the needs of the particular cellular environment of each organ. The skin and muscle mass contain the largest reservoir of interstitial matrix fluid in the body. The vast majority of the interactions or exchanges between cellular water, interstitial space water, and plasma water through the capillary bed occur within these two vast organ systems. The interstitial space fluid of the skin represents the ideal organ for studying the contribution of interstitial space water to the homeostatic response to hemorrhagic shock, since the skin is a relatively acellular organ.[45] Consequently, the interstitial space relationship with the capillary bed and the dynamics across the capillary membrane are best studied by using prenodal skin lymph to monitor what is happening on the interstitial space side of the capillary in response to hemorrhagic shock and resuscitation. The interstitial matrix of the skin is composed predominantly of type IV collagen and elastin embedded in a ground substance of mucopolysaccharides and proteoglycans.[55] Elastin and collagen provide the tensile strength, and the proteoglycans serve to bind water and contribute to the optimal hydration of the interstitial space matrix.[45] The mucopolysaccharides include hyaluronate, chondroitin, the chondroitin sulfates, keratosulfates, dermatosulfates, and heparin sulfates.[46] Hyaluronate is the prototype mucopolysaccharide and is characteristically between 10^6 and 10^9 Da.[47] The mucopolysaccharide carries one anionic site for each disaccharide unit. For the hyaluronate molecule (10^7 Da), 25,000 anionic sites can be identified.[47] At physiologic pH and normal anionic strength, most of the anionic sites are neutralized.[48] In solution, the hyaluronate molecule assumes a three-dimensional coiled configuration. This configuration allows for various solvent domains to exist on the hyaluronate moiety and to interact with other elements of the matrix. At neutral pH, the anionic sites are neutralized, thus reducing ionization, which causes a reduction in conformational size and increased coiling.[47,49] An increase in the polyelectrical ionization, as is seen in severe hemorrhagic shock, will lead to increased anionic sites and consequent contraction of the matrix coil. The proteoglycans are molecules that contain a polysaccharide moiety which is covalently linked to protein.[50] These molecules are predominantly composed of protein, and the polysaccharide portion is relatively small and covalently linked to the protein framework. The proteoglycans, sometimes referred to as *glycoproteins,* are not well understood but constitute a wide spectrum of proteins. These proteins include the phosphate proteins, acid glycoproteins, fibronectin, link glycoprotein, and others.[45] Structural studies on these proteins have confirmed their extraordinarily elaborate three-dimensional structures with molecular weights ranging from a few hundred thousand to over 4 million.[51]

The interstitial space matrix and fluid are closely intertwined into an elastic gel–like substance, with the interrelationship between matrix, water, and ions being dependent on covalent, ionic, and associative binding.[47] Normally, the fluid within the interstitial space compartment is rather evenly divided between the matrix fluid and the free fluid. The free fluid forms the channels or rivers that extend from the capillary wall to the cell membranes and to the lymphatic orifices through which both balanced salt solution and proteins can return to the plasma compartment at a remote site. The structural macromolecules of the interstitial matrix vary in their ability to exclude solute molecules. This is related to the different spaces of solute distribution within the matrix.[52,53] A given solute will first determine its space of distribution on the basis of size. Consequently, the matrix will exclude solute molecules from those portions of the matrix which have dimensions smaller than the solute molecule. Thus the degree of solute exclusion from any portion of the matrix is determined by solute size and the mass density of the matrix elements at any given time. For a given solute, the extent of exclusion will be greatest in a dehydrated matrix and lowest in an overhydrated matrix. Furthermore, the ability of different portions of the matrix to exclude solutes also varies, with much of our understanding in this area of matrix function still evolving. Collagen can exclude albumin from about 4 ml of water per gram.[53] Mucopolysaccharides, however, can exclude up to 40 ml of water per gram, or 10 times that of collagen.[54] Collagen makes up the greatest portion of the interstitial space matrix and thus exerts a considerable effect on the extent of protein exclusion. The interrelationship between collagen, mucopolysaccharides, and proteoglycans is not always constant in that the interrelationships change in different sites of the matrix and with different matrix configurations. Stearic forces are not the only factor that affects the restriction of solute from the matrix. Electrostatic forces play an important role in the relationship between the matrix and solutes.[49] Albumin and the mucopolysaccharides are negatively charged. The charge between the mucopolysaccharides and albumin may augment the extent of albumin exclusion from the matrix.[53,55] The degree of matrix ionization also affects the extent of protein exclusion so that when the matrix becomes more ionized, the excluded volume of albumin also will increase. This phenomenon of increased albumin exclusion by as much as 25 percent with increased ionization occurs in the absence of changes in the matrix water content.[49] Increased exclusion of proteins from the interstitial matrix by force enhances colloid oncotic activity. This relationship is usually represented by the equation

$$\pi_{IP} = \frac{RTQp}{[(1 - f_E) \cdot V_I]}$$

where π_{IP} = oncotic pressure of plasma proteins
     R = universal gas constant
     T = absolute temperature
     Q_p = the quantity of protein in the matrix
     V_I = the interstitial fluid space volume
     f_E = the protein exclusion factor

which relates the oncotic pressure of plasma proteins to the total interstitial fluid space volume.[56] This equation shows that the volume of the interstitial matrix, under constant conditions, is inversely related to the interstitial space oncotic pressure. The result of decreasing interstitial space volume will be a conformational change within the helix. These conformational changes will increase the ionization of the matrix and thereby increase the exclusion of albumin and other charged plasma proteins. Hemorrhagic shock, by leading to a decrease in interstitial space volume, will likewise produce a profound conformational change in the matrix. This change in the helix configuration will lead to increased exclusion of albumin.[57] Prior studies from our laboratory have confirmed this phenomenon of increased albumin exclusion by identifying an increase in the prenodal skin lymphatic protein concentration during hemorrhagic shock.[58] The lymph-to-plasma ratios of albumin and globulin rise during the hemorrhagic shock insult. Thus the lymphatic system appears to be a major route for albumin relocation in response to the shock insult. That albumin which does return through the lymphatic system into the plasma volume enhances the plasma oncotic pressure and is part of the homeostatic protective mechanism.[59] These observations on the effects of shock on lymphatic dynamics confirm the studies by Shires and coworkers that interstitial space matrix contraction is part of the protective homeostatic response. During the hemorrhagic shock insult, the pattern of protein redistribution supports this concept of matrix contraction in response to hemorrhage.[60]

The mechanism for matrix contraction during shock and reexpansion to greater than normal degrees with resuscitation remains obscure. These structural alterations are likely the cause of the oncotic and osmotic shifts rather than the result of these changes. The concept that oncotic forces at the capillary level bring about these matrix changes is not supported by studies on lymph-to-plasma protein ratios, which suggest that some other factor, however cryptic, controls the matrix configuration. Likewise, studies on the prenodal skin lymph–to–plasma glucose ratios suggest that a pure osmotic force is not leading to these stearic changes within the matrix during shock and resuscitation.[61] Possibly these changes in matrix configuration are influenced or controlled by a cryptic hormone. Various humoral agents are known to exhibit a tremendous effect on the total homeostatic mechanism and the local capillary environment.[42] The recent explosion in the field of cytokines has identified complex relationships at the cellular level in response to a variety of insults.[62] Possibly a humoral agent or cytokine exerts a local effect on the interstitial matrix, thereby controlling matrix configuration in response to various insults. All these very complicated factors affect the resuscitation regimen, since adaptation of treatment must be made according to ongoing changes in both the circulatory volume and the extravascular spaces. Greater knowledge of these changes, therefore, can only enhance the success of our various resuscitation regimens.

CLASSIFICATION OF SHOCK INSULT

The severity of the hemorrhagic shock insult varies with the extent and duration of hemorrhage. Normally, a 70-kg individual has a red cell mass of about 2 liters and a plasma volume of about 3 liters. This leaves a total blood volume of 5 liters which circulates each minute. The extravascular space consists of the interstitial fluid space, which is about 11 liters, and the intracellular space of muscles, organs, and bones, which comes to about 26 liters. The total blood volume of 5 liters is the compartment that is lost first during the process of active bleeding. The severity of the acute loss and the ability of the extravascular compartments to compensate for this loss determine the later organ dysfunction.

CLASS I HEMORRHAGE

When a patient has a mild hemorrhage of 10 to 15 percent of the blood volume (750 ml), this will typically lead to tachycardia with little change in blood pressure or respiratory rate (Table 5–5).

The rapid infusion of 2000 ml of balanced salt solution effectively restores circulatory volume and cardiac output. The mild, or class I, hemorrhage causes little change in renal perfusion and seldom leads to significant oliguria. The peripheral vascular resistance and renal vascular resistance remain close to normal.

CLASS II HEMORRHAGE

A patient with a moderately severe hemorrhage resulting from a 20 to 25 percent acute reduction in the blood volume (1000 to 1250 ml) will likely present with tachycardia, a narrowing of the pulse pressure, and a decrease in the systolic blood pressure. Patients with this type of moderate, or class II, hemorrhage will have increased renovascular resistance with decreased filtration and a decrease in the excretion of urine, osmoles, and sodium. There will be some degree of autoregulation, as reflected by the fact that the reduction in renal blood flow will be due to the combination of both preglomerular and postglomerular vasoconstriction, resulting in a less significant reduction in glomerular filtration rate. Such patients are candidates for the rapid infusion of 3 to 4 liters of balanced salt solution during the early phase of resuscitation in order to reexpand not only the plasma volume but also the interstitial volume, which became depleted

TABLE 5–5. Homeostasis after Acute Hemorrhage

Severity of Bleeding	Blood Pressure (mmHg)	Plasma Volume (liters)	Interstitial Space (liters)	Urine Output (ml/min)	Acute Fluid Needs (liters)
Class I	120/80	4600	11	1.0	2
Class II	115/80	3800	9	0.3	4
Class III	90/70	3200	7	0.1	7
Class IV	60/40	2500	5–6	0	10

as part of the compensation for the acute plasma volume deficit. The restoration of renal perfusion and glomerular filtration usually occurs within 24 h. Prior to that time, the urine output will be restored to normal levels as long as the patient has no further bleeding.

CLASS III HEMORRHAGE

A severe, or class III, hemorrhagic insult is associated with a rapid depletion of 30 to 35 percent (1500 to 1750 ml) of the circulating blood volume. This severe type of insult will be associated with tachycardia, reduced peripheral perfusion with acidosis, tachypnea, a reduction in pulse pressure, hypotension, and oliguria. The systemic and renovascular resistance will be markedly elevated, and the renal blood flow will be markedly reduced, as will the glomerular filtration rate. Such patients require the rapid infusion of 4000 to 6000 ml of balanced salt solution during the early resuscitation phase while blood is being prepared for early transfusion. When the patient does not respond rapidly to the balanced salt replacement, the blood transfusion is begun as soon as the type and cross-match are completed. The increase in renovascular resistance will typically last for 48 to 96 h, although glomerular filtration and excretion of urine osmoles and electrolytes will usually be restored within 24 h.

CLASS IV HEMORRHAGE

Patients presenting in a moribund state with life-threatening acute hypovolemia will have an anticipated blood volume deficit of 40 to 45 percent (2000 to 2500 ml) and may have an impending cardiac arrest from hypovolemic shock if rapid resuscitation is not instituted. These critically ill moribund patients have a marked increase in peripheral and renovascular resistance. Consequently, the patients are cold and clammy and anuric, representing a lack of renal perfusion and filtration. Such patients require rapid replacement with balanced salt solution and type-specific whole blood during the early resuscitation within the emergency department. Patients with impending cardiac arrest may respond to the infusion of O-negative blood in order to restore circulatory volume and oxygen delivery potential. The increase in renovascular resistance in such patients persists for 4 to 7 days after resuscitation, and often it takes 48 to 72 h before the glomerular filtration rate is restored to normal.[63]

TREATMENT OF THE HEMORRHAGIC SHOCK INSULT

Resuscitation of the severely injured patient with hemorrhagic shock must be tailored to the severity or classification of the shock insult. Whereas a patient presenting with mild hypovolemia typical of a class I hypovolemic insult will require little intervention, the patient with a class IV hypovolemic insult will die rapidly unless major intervention is provided immediately. Likewise, treatment of the patient should be tailored to the sequential, predictable phase of homeostasis to hypovolemic shock and resuscitation.

PHASE I INTERVENTION

The treatment plan for resuscitation during the acute bleeding phase of hemor-rhagic shock must dovetail with ongoing efforts to identify and control active bleeding. The initial resuscitative efforts should be designed to rapidly establish two or more large-bore intravenous lines to allow for the rapid replenishment of plasma volume deficits. Such lines can be established by way of peripheral vein catheterization, basilic vein cut-downs, greater saphenous vein cut-downs, or percutaneous subclavian venipunctures. Although much controversy exists regarding the relative merits of the different access techniques, we support the use of percutaneous subclavian venipuncture, which, in the hands of experi-enced house officers and practicing surgeons, can be instituted within seconds with a complication rate below 1 percent. Once appropriate intravenous lines are established, correction of the plasma volume deficit is best achieved by the rapid infusion of at least 2 liters of balanced salt solution. This rapid infusion will restore compromised vital signs in most severely injured patients except those who have class III or class IV hypovolemic shock.[63] While the intravenous lines are being established, appropriate blood is drawn for determination of hemoglobin, hematocrit, electrolytes, and other blood studies depending on sus-pected organ injuries and for type and cross-matching of blood and, possibly, plasma. The rapidity of balanced salt solution infusion is judged by the clinical response of vital signs, primarily blood pressure, pulse pressure, pulse rate, and urine output. The decision to supplement the balanced salt solution with blood is based on the response of vital signs and urine output to the balanced salt solution replacement and the serial changes in hematocrit.[63] When the balanced salt solution replacement does not effectively restore vital signs and functions, packed red blood cell replacement becomes essential. Although, in theory, the clinical syndrome of hypovolemic shock brought about by whole blood loss would be best treated with whole blood replacement, the blood banking indus-try has obviated this option from the armamentarium of most resuscitation teams. Consequently, one must rely on the effectiveness of packed red blood cell replacement with the option of restoring plasma factors by means of fresh frozen plasma supplementation. During this early resuscitation period, indwelling blad-der catheter drainage is essential to monitor the urinary response to treatment, and nasogastric decompression of the stomach helps reduce the likelihood of vomiting with aspiration. The use of central pulmonary artery catheters to mon-itor pulmonary artery pressure and pulmonary capillary wedge pressure or the use of radial artery catheters to monitor mean arterial pressure is rarely indicated because the serial changes in clinical signs, peripheral pressures, and urine out-put will correctly guide ongoing therapy in the overwhelming majority of pa-tients with hypovolemic shock.

The need to supplement the resuscitation effort with fresh frozen plasma is related to the underlying condition of the patient and the extent of red blood cell replacement needed to maintain vital signs and hemoglobin.[64] Patients with known liver dysfunction due to prior hepatitis or cirrhosis and patients with a known clotting disorder due to a coagulation factor deficiency are candidates for early plasma supplementation to help achieve control of bleeding. The vast majority of patients will not have such concomitant diseases, so fresh frozen plasma replacement can be avoided unless there is evidence of factor deficiency based on examination of the prothrombin time or the partial thromboplastin time or in those patients who require close to 10 blood transfusions and the hemorrhagic shock insult has not yet been contained. Patients who require less than 10 transfusions can readily replace their coagulation factor losses by relocation of coagulation stores to the plasma volume from the interstitial fluid space.[64] When the hemorrhagic shock insult necessitates more than 10 units of blood and the insult is continuing, one may predict with high probability that a coagulopathy due to dilution and loss of procoagulants will ensue. Thus fresh frozen plasma replacement at this time is strongly encouraged in order to ameliorate or even abate the coagulopathy which is about to occur, even though the prothrombin time and partial thromboplastin time at that moment are still within normal limits.[65]

The greatest controversy regarding phase I treatment of hypovolemic shock over the past many years revolves around the addition of colloid supplementation to a resuscitation regimen. The most frequently recommended colloids for this purpose are albumin, dextran, or hydroxyethyl starch. The early administration of colloid has been proposed as a means of reducing the amount of fluid loss from the plasma compartment during the early hypovolemic shock insult. A clear understanding of the homeostatic mechanisms already operative shows that reduced movement from the vascular compartment brought about by relocation of interstitial fluid into the vascular compartment has already occurred and continues to occur in the patient with hypovolemic shock prior to resuscitation.[66] A better appreciation of the homeostasis of hemorrhagic shock mitigates against the concept of early phase I colloid supplementation in the resuscitation regimen. A more detailed discussion of colloid resuscitation, particularly albumin supplementation, will be presented later. As indicated, most hypotensive patients respond within 15 min to the rapid infusion of 2000 ml of balanced salt solution. Lack of response is indicative of a major life-threatening bleed and is an indication for red cell addition to the resuscitation regimen. Most patients can be maintained on balanced salt solution replacement during the initial 30 min required to have red blood cells typed and cross-matched for proper replacement. Occasionally, the severity of the hemorrhagic shock is so great that the patient needs to be transfused with blood within 10 or 15 min of arrival so that the use of type-specific but non-cross-matched blood must be implemented. The need to give type O blood, the universal donor, to the severely injured hypovolemic patient who is unresponsive to balanced salt solution is rarely indicated. The role of calcium supplementation in the phase I resuscitation regimen is controversial. Most patients who respond to the preceding resuscitation regimen do not require calcium supplementation, which will be discussed in more detail subsequently. Likewise, the use of sodium bicarbonate to supplement the patient with severe hemorrhagic shock is somewhat controversial but is recommended in patients who show persistence of hypotension and evidence that the resuscitation regimen has not restored arterial pH to normal levels. Corticosteroid supplementation in the resuscitation regimen is not indicated.

RESUSCITATION THROUGH THE OBLIGATORY EXTRAVASCULAR SEQUESTRATION PHASE

The hallmarks of phase II, which is the phase of obligatory extracellular fluid expansion, are decreased blood pressure, decreased pulse pressure, tachycardia, oliguria, and weight gain. The concomitant findings of impaired vital signs in conjunction with weight gain identify the phenomenon of obligatory extravascular fluid sequestration. Attempts to prevent the fluid sequestration and prevent weight gain by withholding fluid or the administration of colloid-supplemented balanced salt solution will lead to a serious plasma volume deficit, which, if not ultimately corrected, will lead to renal failure, multiple organ failure, and death.[66] Consequently, the severely injured patient with major hemorrhagic shock often requires invasive monitoring of central pressures, such as the central venous pressure or pulmonary artery pressure, in order to accommodate ongoing fluid therapy. Thus the treatment challenges of phase II are the greatest and the complexities of the physiologic homeostatic mechanisms are the most complex of the hemorrhagic shock insult. Since the extravascular fluid sequestration is obligatory, a regimen of forced diuresis, like that of colloid supplementation, prevents this expansion and aggravates the already existing plasma volume deficiency.[67] Shires and coworkers[39] demonstrated that a portion of this third space expansion in response to the resuscitation for hemorrhagic shock is intracellular fluid accumulation, as demonstrated by membrane depolarization. As noted during the phase I insult, this intracellular expansion of salt and water represents fluxes from the interstitial fluid space. During the resuscitation through the bleeding phase and on into the extravascular fluid sequestration phase, there is a marked expansion of the interstitial fluid space, reflecting an uncoiling of the interstitial space matrix and a reduction in the amount of solute and protein exclusion from the interstitial fluid space.[68] Intracellular expansion after the hemorrhagic shock insult is caused by reductions in the activity of the sodium–potassium–adenosine triphosphatase pump, which becomes compromised due to a deficiency in adenosine triphosphate, the energy source for this cell membrane pump.[39] Concomitantly, there is a postresuscitation expansion of the interstitial fluid space associated with a reduction in the intravascular colloid oncotic pressure and matrix expansion due to the stearic alterations in the interstitial space matrix.[69] Consequently, there is a total lack of correlation between the reduced plasma colloid oncotic pressure and the interstitial space expansion during phase II, suggesting that the reduced intravascular colloid oncotic factor occurs independently and is not a prime force in the interstitial space expansion.[70]

Prior views of capillary fluxes after resuscitation from hemorrhagic shock suggested that the reduction in colloid oncotic pressure seen during phase II is the result of decreased capillary integrity (increased permeability) causing a leakage of colloid, particularly albumin, into the interstitial compartment, where a reverse oncotic force is then exerted.[70,71] Such fluxes, by definition, must display selectivity, as reflected by the extravascular movement of small molecules occurring more efficiently than that of larger moieties such as proteins. Likewise, the smaller proteins, such as albumin, would move across the capillary more efficiently than the larger globulins. The purported pathways for such fluxes include transcellular diffusion, vesicular shuttling, transmembrane diffusion, intercellular junctional small pore diffusion, intercellular junctional large pore diffusion, and plasmalemmal vesicular diffusion.[72] Regardless of the route of protein and fluid flux, the concept that the plasma colloid oncotic pressure controls interstitial space expansion during the extravascular fluid sequestration phase after resuscitation presupposes a passive interstitial space matrix that accommodates this fluid and protein influx without significant structural change. The lack of a significant inverse correlation between colloid oncotic pressure and interstitial space expansion seen in patients resuscitated from severe hemorrhagic shock suggests that some other control factor for matrix expansion during phase II is operative.[70]

Attempts to define specific interstitial matrix changes responsible for the lack of correlation between interstitial space expansion and the colloid oncotic pressure are hampered by the relative inaccessibility of interstitial fluid for study. Consequently, the prenodal skin lymph has been used to mirror the sol or fluid portion of the interstitial space. By extrapolation from prenodal skin lymph studies, one can demonstrate that 55 percent of the extracellular albumin is located within the interstitial space.[73] Furthermore, albumin that enters the interstitial space by way of the capillary bed passes unidirectionally through the interstitial space channels into the lymphatic space, from which reentry into the plasma compartment occurs at a remote site. Studies of prenodal lymph-to-plasma ratios of proteins in a canine model of hemorrhagic shock and resuscitation suggest that reduced albumin exclusion is a prime force in the interstitial matrix expansion of phase II and thus the obligatory nature of this consequent fluid sequestration. These studies highlight the illogic of colloid, particularly albumin, supplementation to try to abort this obligatory fluid sequestration during phase II therapy.[74] The mechanism by which reduced albumin exclusion leads to this obligatory expansion is not entirely clear but presumably relates to structural alterations or stearic changes of the matrix. Such stearic changes would preclude reentry of albumin into the lymphatic system and thus the plasma volume. This would explain the lack of correlation between colloid oncotic pressure and interstitial space expansion during the phase II resuscitation period.

An important colloid during the phase II resuscitation is the red blood cell. Patient studies have demonstrated that there is a very clear and significant direct correlation between the colloid oncotic pressure and the red cell volume during phase II of resuscitation from hemorrhagic shock.[70] These positive and significant direct correlations suggest that the capillary membrane retains functional integrity and is responsive to the intravascular colloid oncotic pressure. Consequently, the lack of such correlation between interstitial fluid volume and colloid oncotic pressure further points to other forces that control the stearic configuration of the interstitial space during phase II. These changes suggesting capillary integrity following resuscitation from hemorrhagic shock are different from those changes in capillary integrity seen after septic shock.[70] Consequently, the principles of therapy outlined during phase II resuscitation from hemorrhagic shock cannot be automatically applied to the patient being treated during the extravascular expansion phase of septic shock.

The volume of obligatory extravascular fluid sequestration within the interstitial space is directly related to the degree of the hemorrhagic shock insult and can be correlated with the duration of shock and the severity of hypotension.[66] The most effective way to maintain the cardiovascular status during phase II is to restore the plasma volume with balanced salt solution in order to maintain vital signs and urine output and to provide appropriate red cell replacement to maintain the hemoglobin level at approximately 10 g%. The extent of interstitial space expansion, as judged by weight gain and total body swelling, will likewise correlate with the severity of the prior shock insult.[66] When the total fluid administration threatens other organs, particularly the heart and lungs, central lines to monitor central venous pressure and pulmonary artery pressure along with cardiac output will assist in determining ongoing fluid needs. One must remember, however, that during phase II the hyperdynamic state of resuscitation is normal, so patients with low central filling pressures will have elevated cardiac outputs. Consequently, one must be careful when monitoring the patient with excessive fluid retention and recognize that ongoing fluid therapy, as judged by the ratio of the pulmonary capillary wedge pressure to cardiac index in response to a bolus infusion of balanced salt solution, will help define the inotropic state of the heart. This is judged by the slope of the cardiac output curve in response to a fluid bolus based on the normal slope on the Frank-Starling curve. When the volume expansion achieved by balanced salt and red cell replacement restores vital signs, the renal blood flow will improve to the extent that glomerular filtration is restored and the spontaneous excretion of sodium, osmoles, and water returns. As indicated previously, the effect of hypovolemic shock on the renal circulation persists for a number of days after resuscitation, but the successful restoration of plasma volume will permit the kidneys to no longer be subject to excess antidiuretic hormone and aldosterone. Consequently, the kidneys serve as an excellent index of adequate plasma volume expansion and organ perfusion.[69]

One problem with resuscitation during phase II is that the volume of blood and fluid required to maintain cardiovascular and renal function often causes respiratory embarrassment and has led to the inappropriate term *fluid overload syndrome*.[66] This concept, unfortunately, has had adverse therapeutic implications, since the uninformed treatment team might conclude that this condition represents a plasma volume overload; the consequent restriction of fluids during phase II resuscitation would lead to oliguria, renal failure, and often death.[74] Interestingly, when advocates of fluid restriction during phase II are frustrated by the death of the patient, this demise is often ascribed to multiple organ failure and not to the decision to restrict fluids and the subsequent development of acute oliguric renal failure. Such conclusions are derived on the basis of dialysis efforts which maintain the creatinine and blood urine nitrogen levels within acceptable range, but then the patient dies of multiple organ failure. We ascribe this death from multiple organ failure to the inadequate plasma volume restoration, which is evidenced by the most sensitive cardiovascular organ, namely the kidney, which fails due to the inadequate resuscitation. Consequently, therapeutic efforts during this extravascular fluid sequestration phase are best directed at simultaneously maintaining effective inotropic support, ventilatory support, renal perfusion, and accommodation of the large volume extravascular fluid sequestration. Inotropic support can be provided by a multitude of pharmacologic agents, including the digitalis preparations and the vasoactive amines. Ventilatory support is provided by ongoing intubation with ventilation, which often is no longer needed when the patient mobilizes this excess fluid.

THERAPEUTIC ADJUSTMENTS DURING PHASE III

After the fluid sequestration has peaked, usually within 18 to 36 h following the control of bleeding, the patient will have "filled the tank" and will begin the reverse movement from the extracellular compartments to the plasma volume. The efflux of cellular salt and water has been well defined in experimental models that show a normalization of membrane potential and reestablishment of the sodium pump. This results in a reduction of the intracellular sodium and water toward normal levels as this fluid moves into the interstitial space and then into the plasma compartment. The simultaneous contraction of the interstitial space leads to an increase in solute and albumin exclusion from the matrix, which promotes salt and water reentry into the plasma compartment at the venular end of the capillary and protein reentry into the plasma compartment by way of the lymphatic system.[73] The mechanism for this interstitial space matrix contraction with plasma reentry remains cryptic but may be influenced by cellular mediators that are released in response to cellular needs. Such a mediator would allow for the interstitial space matrix to expand during phase II and then return toward the preshock state during phase III. Since there has been no identification of any such mediator, this concept is highly conjectural and warrants further study. During the late portions of phase II and the early portions of phase III, the treatment team recognizes that less intravenous fluids are needed to maintain vital signs as the blood pressure rises and the pulse pressure begins to expand. This expansion of pulse pressure is an early warning that massive plasma refilling is about to occur. Therefore, when the expansion of pulse pressure occurs, the rate of intravenous fluid administration should be rapidly slowed, the number of intravenous lines should be reduced to one, and the composition of the fluid should be changed from balanced salt solution to dextrose and water with little or no sodium added. Lack of attention to this refilling may lead to rapid acute hypervolemia with hypertension and cardiorespiratory failure. This acute hypertension with cardiorespiratory failure is due to the massive flux of this previously sequestered balanced salt solution at a time when the kidneys are not quite prepared to meet diuretic needs. This phenomenon should be anticipated and treated aggressively. Lack of appreciation of the pulse pressure expansion will unfortunately lead to a picture of postresuscitative hypertension with a sustained systolic and diastolic blood pressure response that exceeds 150 and 100 mmHg, respectively.[67] This syndrome is associated with respiratory failure and a persistence of the increased renal vascular resistance and decreased renal blood flow. Indeed, this syndrome in some part may be related to the fact that the effect of the hemorrhagic shock insult on the kidneys is a persistent rise in renovascular resistance which somehow mitigates against the normal diuretic response that should be seen in patients with acute plasma volume expansion.

Although diuresis with exogenous agents such as mannitol or furosemide will aggravate the resuscitation effort during phase II extravascular expansion, the reverse is true during the acute hypervolemic state seen with early phase III refilling. Exogenous diuresis is a most effective way to manage this sudden massive autoinfusion of balanced salt solution into the plasma compartment. The addition of small doses of furosemide to the sharp reduction in intravenous fluid replacement is usually all that is needed to carry the patient through the acute hypervolemic state of phase III. Indeed, a single intravenous infusion of 10 mg furosemide often serves as a stimulus to the kidney, which subsequently responds with a tremendous and sustained diuresis to the ongoing autoinfusion. As this spontaneous diuresis persists, the pulmonary state rapidly improves, and the total body edema is gradually mobilized over a several-day interval. One can project that the patient with severe hemorrhagic shock will continue this fluid mobilization for 3 or 4 days and sometimes as long as 10 days when there has been massive extravascular fluid sequestration during phase II.

THE COLLOID CONTROVERSY

Starling, a century ago, reported that the efflux of water out of the plasma volume correlates directly with capillary conductivity (often misappropriately thought of as permeability) multiplied by the capillary surface area, while the capillary is also influenced by plasma hydrostatic pressure, interstitial hydrostatic pressure, plasma oncotic pressure, and interstitial oncotic pressure. The equation on capillary fluxes states that the flux of water out of the plasma volume will be inversely related to the capillary oncotic pressure if all the preceding factors remain constant.[75] One should note that Starling's original thesis highlighted the inadequacies of this equation in its application to humans, since this is a two-compartment equation; in contrast, humans have a third fluid system, the lymphatic system, which exits from the interstitial space and carries solute and water back to the plasma volume at a remote location. Starling highlighted other reasons, including the presence of an intracellular compartment, as to why this formula did not apply to humans. Despite these many disclaimers by Starling in his original publication, many modern intensivists make reference to the Starling equation to justify the use of supplemental albumin in the resuscitation regimen for hemorrhagic shock. When early nonrandomized studies from our unit showed increased pulmonary dysfunction following albumin supplementation for hemorrhagic shock, several observers criticized our observations and conclusions.[76] This criticism stimulated the performance of a prospective, randomized analysis of albumin supplementation for hemorrhagic shock. During a 2-year interval, 94 patients with severe hemorrhagic shock were randomized to receive albumin or no albumin supplementation as part of their resuscitation. These patients were subjected to an average shock insult that exceeded 30 min, during which time the systolic blood pressure was less than 80 mmHg. During the emergency room and operating room resuscitation efforts, the patients received an average of 15 blood transfusions. The control patients received the blood transfusions, balanced salt solution, and some fresh frozen plasma to assist with the correction of coagulation abnormalities. The patients randomized to receive supplemental albumin received a comparable resuscitation regimen with the exception that albumin was started in the phase I resuscitation and continued for 3 to 5 days following operation, during which time prior studies had demonstrated that the serum albumin level was markedly reduced.[77]

In response to the albumin supplementation, the albumin-treated patients had a significant increase in capillary oncotic pressure, which averaged 19.7 mmHg compared with 14.8 mmHg in the control patients not receiving albumin supplementation; the normal capillary oncotic pressure is 22 to 24 mmHg. Consequent to the albumin supplementation, the albumin-treated patients had a marked increase in serum albumin levels, plasma volume, and effective renal plasma flow, as measured by *para*-aminohippurate clearance, when compared with the non-albumin-treated control patients. Despite the increase in renal plasma flow, the albumin-supplemented patients had a fall in glomerular filtration rate, sodium clearance, and urine output. These seemingly paradoxical results, whereby the albumin supplementation caused an increase in renal plasma flow but a reduction in filtration and the excretion of salt and water, are due to the albumin-induced increase in both the oncotic and osmotic pressures within the glomerular tuft.[67] This increase in the oncotic and osmotic pressures leads to salt and water retention within the glomerulus as well as to an increase in the oncotic pressure within the peritubular vessels which are perfusing the inner medulla of the kidney. Controversy exists among renal physiologists regarding the mechanism by which human serum albumin causes sodium retention. The findings in our albumin-supplemented patients support those renal physiologists who have concluded that the sodium retention after human serum albumin therapy is due to a sodium-potassium exchange at the distal tubular level. Consequently, the patients receiving albumin supplementation have increased sodium reabsorption associated with increased potassium excretion. These renal effects of albumin supplementation mitigate against the main purpose for which human serum albumin therapy has been recommended.[67] Ideally, the albumin supplementation would increase the capillary oncotic pressure of the pulmonary capillary bed and thereby bring about a reduction in the extravascular pulmonary fluid from the pulmonary interstices and deliver this fluid to the kidney for excretion. Unfortunately, the renal effects of serum albumin therapy lead to salt and water retention, with increased rather than decreased extravascular pulmonary water. This salt and water retention leads to an increased need for diuretic therapy, a higher incidence of renal failure, and worsening pulmonary function (as evidenced by higher central filling pressures, increased physiologic shunting in the lungs, and a prolonged need for ventilatory support). Part of the increased central filling pressure is due to a reduction in inotropic efficacy as monitored by the ratios of left ventricular stroke work index to pulmonary capillary wedge pressure. Part of this inotropic dysfunction may be due to the albumin-induced binding of calcium, which results in a reduction in the ionized calcium in the albumin-supplemented patients. Finally, the death rate after human albumin supplementation for hemorrhagic shock was significantly increased compared with those patients not receiving albumin supplementation.

PROTEIN KINETICS

The albumin-supplemented patients had a significant reduction in the serum globulin level.[69] This reduction in the globulin fraction was associated with a reduction in various immunoglobulins. Furthermore, the reduction in the immunoglobulins was associated with a decreased immunoglobulin activity in response to tetanus toxoid.[77] This observation raises the question as to whether albumin supplementation alters the immune response to various insults following resuscitation from hemorrhagic shock.

The albumin-treated patients also required more blood transfusions during the first 5 postoperative days. This increased need for blood therapy in the albumin-supplemented patients was associated with a significant decrease in fibrinogen activity and a significant prolongation in the prothrombin time. Frozen plasma samples from the two groups of patients were then analyzed, and these showed that the fibrinogen and prothrombin content in the albumin patients was significantly less than that seen in the control patients.[78] These results of supplemental albumin therapy for hemorrhagic shock have been reproduced in canine studies of hemorrhagic shock and resuscitation,[73] which have demonstrated that the animals receiving albumin supplementation for hemorrhagic shock have the same reduction in the globulin concentrations that were seen in the patients randomized for albumin supplementation. Likewise, the animal studies confirmed that the coagulation protein factors and the coagulation activity were decreased following albumin supplementation and that these changes were dose-related, being increased in those animals receiving the greater amount of albumin. Studies on thoracic duct and prenodal skin lymphatics have demonstrated that the albumin-supplemented animals have an increase in the amount of albumin and globulin present in the lymphatics, which presumably reflects a similar increase in the interstitial fluid space.[79] Thus it appears that albumin supplementation causes a relocation of the intravascular proteins to the interstitial space. Such a relocation could be explained as an attempt by the body to maintain a specific oncotic balance between the plasma volume and the interstitial fluid space. These conclusions regarding the maintenance of a specific plasma volume-to-interstitial fluid oncotic ratio have been supported by subsequent studies in which Hespan or fluorocarbons have been used to supplement the resuscitation in canine shock models.[80] The driving force of the extravascular relocation of colloid appears to be dependent on the degree of increased colloid oncotic pressure. As the intravascular oncotic pressure increases, the amount of albumin and globulin leaving the plasma and entering the prenodal and skin lymphatics also increases. These results suggest that the retention of fluid for prolonged periods following resuscitation with albumin supplementation is due to a reverse oncotic effect resulting from the slow removal of these albumin and globulin moieties within the interstitial space.

STEROID SUPPLEMENTATION DURING RESUSCITATION

The response of the lungs to various types of insults appears similar. Patients presenting with acute hemorrhagic shock are candidates for the development of subsequent respiratory distress, reflecting the combination of both alveolar collapse and pulmonary edema. Specific events that lead to either alveolar collapse or pulmonary edema after hemorrhagic shock are multiple and include (1) platelet aggregation within the pulmonary capillary bed, (2) consequent humoral release of vasoactive substances, (3) a reduction in fibronectin or other cytokines, (4) pulmonary white cell entrapment, which is associated with the further release of vasoactive substances, (5) lysosomal membrane dysfunction with release of vasoactive enzymes, (6) kinin activation independent of cellular aggregation, and (7) arachidonic product release within the capillaries.[81] All these factors are thought to be altered, to some degree, by adrenocortical hormones. Thus massive steroid infusions have been proposed to reduce the pulmonary insult of hemorrhagic shock by reducing the increase in pulmonary vascular resistance, reducing platelet entrapment, enhancing fibronectin activity, stabilizing lysosomal membranes, decreasing the overall inflammatory response, and facilitating the maturation of alveolar type II pneumocytes.[82] The potential for corticosteroids to achieve this goal was assessed prospectively in a group of 114 severely injured patients who received an average of 13 blood transfusions and 11.7 liters of crystalloid solution during their emergency and operating room resuscitation.[83] By random selection, 54 of these patients received massive doses of methylprednisolone, whereas the other patients were resuscitated in the same manner but without corticosteroids. The patients receiving the massive corticosteroids had a significant increase in the central venous pressure and a significant decrease in the average arterial oxygen tension compared with those patients not receiving steroid supplementation. The ratio of the inspired oxygen to the arterial oxygen tension was significantly decreased in the steroid-treated patients, and this was reflected by a significant increase in the percentage of pulmonary shunting. The number of days spent on a volume ventilator for on-going respiratory distress was not significantly different, averaging 5.1 days in the steroid-treated patients compared with 3.0 days in the non-steroid-treated patients. There were 7 deaths in the steroid-supplemented patients compared with 2 deaths in the patients not supplemented by steroids. These differences were not statistically significant ($p < 0.10$, $p > 0.05$). Consequently, it was established that the steroids neither prevented nor improved the sequelae of alveolar collapse following hemorrhagic shock, as evidenced by ongoing monitoring of the efficacy of oxygenation.[83] These findings indicate that the purported benefits of massive steroids seen in various animal shock lung models does not apply to humans.[84] Lack of benefit, either prophylactically or therapeutically, was the most striking result of this large prospective, randomized study. Consequently, steroids are no longer advocated for treatment of posthemorrhagic shock respiratory dysfunction.

THYROID AND PARATHYROID RESPONSE TO HEMORRHAGIC SHOCK AND RESUSCITATION

Those humoral responses which typically come to mind in the patient with hemorrhagic shock include the catecholamine response, the pituitary response with antidiuretic hormone release, the renal response to the catecholamine profusion and the consequent release of renin, and the adrenocortical response with release of aldosterone. Other humoral responses are also critical to the homeostatic adaptation to a hemorrhagic shock insult. Probably future studies will demonstrate that almost all the body's hormones undergo some adaptation to the hemorrhagic shock insult.

PANCREATIC RESPONSE

The hemorrhagic shock insult and the consequent release of catecholamines leads to an increase in the circulating glucose levels. Part of this increase is brought about by hepatic gluconeogenesis, whereas some of the increase in the blood sugar is due to the peripheral release of carbohydrate. Concomitant with the rise in circulating glucose levels, there is an increase in the pancreatic release of glucagon, which further stimulates the breakdown of glycogen from the liver and augments the hyperglycemic response. The beta cells within the pancreas respond to the hyperglycemia with an increase in insulin levels. This increase in the insulin level, however, is associated with an insulin resistance so that there is a reduced efficiency for the insulin to drive the glucose into the cell. Consequently, the glucose-to-insulin ratio is elevated during the period of acute hemorrhage. This response, in part, may serve to increase serum osmolality and thereby provide a temporary buffer to plasma volume expansion.[41]

PARATHYROID RESPONSE

Hypocalcemia has been defined as an end product of hemorrhagic shock for many years. Early studies demonstrated that this hypocalcemia was due to a reduction in the total serum calcium and was attributed to the concomitant reduction in serum proteins and to the binding to citrate which is present in the transfused blood. More recent studies have shown that the reductions in calcium also include predictable reductions in the ionized calcium independent of serum protein levels.[85] Since calcium is important in myocardial performance, a policy of routine calcium supplementation evolved during the post–World War II years. This policy of routine calcium supplementation to massive blood transfusions was challenged when it was determined that the simultaneous rise in the intracellular calcium concentrations may lead to altered intracellular metabolism, which is detrimental to brain cells during and following resuscitation for severe hemorrhagic shock.[86] Consequently, the use of calcium blockers became popular as part of the treatment for the hemorrhagic shock insult. More recent studies in humans and controlled animal models suggest that calcium channel blockers are detrimental during the acute resuscitation period and that calcium supplementation should be provided in those patients who show evidence of cardiac dysfunction during resuscitation.[87]

During the hypovolemic shock insult, the hypocalcemic response is associated with an increase in the parathyroid gland release of parathyroid hormone (PTH). The severity of hypocalcemia in these patients correlates directly with the shock insult, as determined by the degree of hypotension and the duration of hypotension. The increases in PTH during the resuscitation and postresuscitation periods are directly related to the reductions in ionized calcium, thus indicating an intact PTH-calcium axis.[88] No other cause for the elevated levels of PTH could be seen in patients prospectively studied after resuscitation from hemorrhagic shock. This parathyroid response in humans stimulated controlled studies in a hypovolemic shock canine model. These studies demonstrated that hypoparathyroid dogs respond more slowly to resuscitation from hemorrhagic shock than do normal parathyroid animals. Likewise, the acute response of the normal animals to hemorrhagic shock and resuscitation was uniformly associated with a rise in PTH, which, of course, was precluded in those animals who had had previous parathyroidectomy.[88] Consequently, it appears that the acute rise in PTH is not only a predictable response to the hypocalcemia following resuscitation from hemorrhagic shock but is also an important acute phase homeostatic response leading to improved cardiovascular dynamics during the resuscitation phase of hemorrhagic shock. Based on the parathyroid response to hemorrhagic shock, we advocate calcium supplementation during the emergency room and operating room phases of resuscitation in any patient who has any question of cardiac efficacy. When calcium supplementation is deemed necessary, a good cardiac response can be seen with the administration of 10 mg calcium chloride infused slowly during the resuscitation effort.

THYROID RESPONSE

The thyroid gland is also an acute responder to the hemorrhagic shock insult. Shatney and coworkers[89] previously demonstrated that recent thyroidectomy actually leads to an improvement in resuscitation from hemorrhagic shock. These authors, however, used a reservoir shock model, which leads to an inappropriately greater degree of hemorrhage in the control animals that had homeostatic protection against the shock by way of continued release of thyroid hormones. Subsequent studies performed in our laboratory showed that the thyroidectomy reduces the preshock mean arterial pressure so that the control animals have to sustain a greater hemorrhage in order to be brought down to a predetermined shock level.[90] Later studies utilizing a shock model determined by percentage of blood volume showed that the animals undergoing thyroidectomy with parathyroid preservation had an impaired cardiovascular response to the resuscitation regimen.[88] The euthyroid animals had an increased cardiac output and a concomitant reduction in pulmonary capillary wedge pressure, indicating that the thyroid is an important homeostatic organ in the compensatory response to hemorrhagic shock. The mechanism by which an intact pituitary-thyroid axis functions to benefit the animals subjected to hemorrhagic shock remains unclear but may be related to increased release of thyrotropin-releasing hormone (TRH) and to the circulating thyroid hormones. TRH has significant cardiovascular effects.[91] These include a predicted increase in mean arterial pressure, cardiac index, stroke index, and both right and left ventricular stroke work in disease. TRH also may augment the catecholamine response to hemorrhagic shock and modulate calcium homeostasis. Clearly, the secondary endocrine responses related to the pancreas, parathyroid, thyroid, and possibly other endocrine glands are important in the homeostatic response to hemorrhagic shock.

REFERENCES

1. Standards and guidelines for cardiopulmonary resuscitation (CPR) and emergency cardiac care (ECC). *JAMA* 255:2905, 1986 (published erratum appears in *JAMA* 256:1727, 1986).
2. *Advanced Trauma Life Support Instructor Manual.* Chicago, American College of Surgeons, 1989, p 11.
3. Phillips T, Goldstein AS: Airway management, in Mattox KL, Moore EE, Feliciano DV (eds): *Trauma.* Norwalk, Conn, Appleton & Lange, 1988, p 125.
4. Shimazu S, Shatney CH: Outcomes of trauma patients with no vital signs on hospital admission. *J Trauma* 23:213, 1983.

5. Bodai BI, Smith JP, Blaisdell FW: The role of thoracotomy in blunt trauma. *J Trauma* 22:487, 1982.

6. Vij D, Simoni E, Smith RF, et al: Resuscitative thoracotomy for patients with traumatic injury. *Surgery* 94:554, 1983.

7. *Advanced Trauma Life Support Instructor Manual.* Chicago, American College of Surgeons, 1989, p 33.

8. Ledgerwood AM, Lucas CE: Postresuscitation hypertension: Etiology, morbidity, and treatment. *Arch Surg* 108:531, 1974.

9. Lucas CE: Evaluation and resuscitation of critically injured patients. *S Afr J Surg* 14:3, 1976.

10. Iserson KV: Blind nasotracheal intubation. *Ann Emerg Med* 10:468, 1986.

11. Kress TD: Cricothyroidotomy. *Ann Emerg Med* 11:192, 1982.

12. Emergency percutaneous and transtracheal ventilation. *J Am Coll Emerg Phys* 8(10):396, 1979.

13. Rutherford RB, Campbell DN: Thoracic injuries, in Zuidema GD, Rutherford RB, Ballinger WF (eds): *The Management of Trauma.* Philadelphia, Saunders, 1985.

14. Ledgerwood AM, Goldstein M, Lucas CE: *Priorities in Care of Critically Injured Patients.* Detroit, Wayne State University Press, 1972.

15. Pate JW: Chest wall injuries. *Surg Clin North Am* 69(1):59, 1989.

16. Colice GL: Prolonged intubation versus tracheostomy in adults. *J Intensive Care Med* 2:85, 1987.

17. Berlauk JF: Prolonged endotracheal intubation versus tracheostomy. *Crit Care Med* 14:742, 1987.

18. Moore FA, Moore EE: Trauma resuscitation, in Wilmore DW, Brennan MF, Harken AH, et al (eds): *Care of the Surgical Patient.* New York, Scientific American Press, 1989.

19. Latenser BA, Gentilello LM, Tarver AA, et al: Improved outcome with early fixation of skeletally unstable pelvic fractures. *J Trauma* 31:28, 1991.

20. Bone LB, Johnson KD, Weigelt J, et al: Early versus delayed stabilization of femoral fractures: A prospective randomized study. *J Bone Joint Surg* 71A:336, 1989.

21. Mattox KL: Indications for thoracotomy: Deciding to operate. *Surg Clin North Am* 69(1):47, 1989.

22. Sorkey AJ, Farnell MB, Williams HJ Jr, et al: The complementary roles of diagnostic peritoneal lavage and computed tomography in the evaluation of blunt abdominal trauma. *Surgery* 106:794, 1989.

23. Lucas CE: Splenic trauma: Choice of management. *Ann Surg* 231(2):98, 1991.

24. Hayward SR, Lucas CE, Sugawa C, Ledgerwood AM: Emergent endoscopic retrograde cholangiopancreatography (brief clinical note). *Arch Surg* 124(6):745, 1989.

25. Ledgerwood AM, Lucas CE: Postresuscitation hypertension: Etiology, morbidity, treatment. *Arch Surg* 108:531, 1974.

26. Gross S: *A System of Surgery: Pathologic, Diagnostic, Therapeutic, and Operative.* Philadelphia, Lea & Febiger, 1972.

27. Blalock A: *Principles of Surgical Care: Shock and Other Problems.* St. Louis, Mosby, 1940.

28. Wiggers CJ: Present status of the shock problem. *Physiol Rev* 22:74, 1942.

29. Moore FD: *Metabolic Care of the Surgical Patient.* Philadelphia, Saunders, 1959.

30. Holcroft JW, Blaisdell FW: Shock: Causes and management of circulatory collapse, in Sabiston DC (ed): *Textbook of Surgery: The Modern Biological Basis of Modern Surgical Practice.* Philadelphia, Saunders, 1991.

31. Shires GT, Brown FT, Canizaro PC, et al: Distributional changes in the extracellular fluid during acute hemorrhagic shock. *Surg Forum* 11:115, 1960.

32. Middleton ES, Mathews R, Shires GT: Radiosulphate as a measure of extracellular fluid in acute hemorrhagic shock. *Ann Surg* 170:174, 1969.

33. Shires GT, Coln D, Carrico CJ, et al: Fluid therapy in hemorrhagic shock. *Arch Surg* 88:688, 1964.
34. Doty DB, Hufnagel HV, Moseley RV: The distribution of body fluid following hemorrhage and resuscitation in combat casualties. *Surg Gynecol Obstet* 130(3):453, 1970.
35. Gann DS, Carlson DE, Byrnes GJ, et al: Impaired restitution of blood volume after large hemorrhage. *J Trauma* 21:598, 1981.
36. Friedman SG, Pearce FJ, Drucker WR: The role of blood glucose in defense of plasma volume during hemorrhage. *J Trauma* 22(1):86, 1982.
37. Stone JP, Schutzer SF, McCoy S: Contribution of glucose to the hyperosmolality of prolonged hypovolemia. *Am Surg* 43(1):1, 1977.
38. Jarhult J: Osmotic fluid transfer from tissue to blood during hemorrhagic hypotension. *Acta Physiol Scand* 89:213, 1973.
39. Shires GT, Cunningham JN Jr, Baker CRF, et al: Alterations in cellular membrane function during hemorrhagic shock in primates. *Ann Surg* 176:288, 1972.
40. Depalma RG, Holden WD, Robinson AV: Fluid therapy in experimental hemorrhagic shock: Ultrastructural effects in liver and muscle. *Ann Surg* 175(4):539, 1972.
41. Demaria EJ, Lilly MP, Gann DS: Potential hormonal responses in a model of traumatic injury. *J Surg Res* 43:45, 1987.
42. Gann DS, Amaral JF: Endocrine and metabolic responses to injury, in Schartz SI (ed): *Principles of Surgery.* New York, McGraw-Hill, 1989.
43. Lucas CE: Resuscitation of the injured patient: The three phases of treatment. *Surg Clin North Am* 57(1):49, 1977.
44. Peitzman AB: Shock, in Simmons RL, Steed DL (eds): *Basic Science Review for Surgeons.* Philadelphia, Saunders, 1992.
45. Bell DR, Watson PD, Renkin EM: Exclusion of macromolecules in the interstitium of tissue from the hind paw. *Fed Proc* 37:314, 1978.
46. Mathews MB: *Connective Tissue: Macromolecular Structure and Evolution.* Berlin, Springer, 1975.
47. Comper WD, Laurent TC: Physiologic function of connective tissue polysaccharides. *Physiol Rev* 58:255, 1978.
48. Varga L: Studies on hyaluronic acid prepared from the vitreous body. *J Biol Chem* 217:651, 1955.
49. Granger HJ: Physiological properties of the extracellular matrix, in Hargens AR (ed): *Tissue Fluid Pressure and Composition.* Baltimore, Williams & Wilkins, 1982.
50. Anderson JC: Glycoproteins of the connective tissue matrix. *Int Rev Connective Tissue Res* 7:251, 1976.
51. Arnott S, Winter WT: Details of glycosaminoglycan conformations and intermolecular interactions. *Fed Proc* 36:78, 1977.
52. Weiderheilm CA, Black LL: Osmotic interaction of plasma proteins with interstitial macromolecules. *Am J Physiol* 231:638, 1976.
53. Laurent TC: Physiochemical properties of interstitial tissue. *Pfleugers Arch* 336:S21, 1972.
54. Laurent TC: The interaction between polysaccharides and other macromolecules: IX. The exclusion of molecules hyaluronic gels and solutions. *Biochem J* 93:106, 1964.
55. Laurent TC, Ogston AG: The interaction between polysaccharides and other macromolecules: IV. The osmotic pressure of mixtures of serum albumin and hyaluronic acid. *Biochem J* 89:249, 1963.
56. Granger HJ: Role of the interstitial matrix and lymphatic pump in regulation of transcapillary fluid balance. *Microvasc Res* 18:209, 1979.
57. Granger HJ, Shepard AP: Dynamics and control of the microcirculation, in Brown JHU (ed): *Advances in Biomedical Engineering,* vol 7. New York, Academic Press, 1979.

58. Unpublished data, interstitial fluid laboratories, 1981.

59. Lucas CE, Benishek DJ, Ledgerwood AM: Reduced oncotic pressure after shock. *Arch Surg* 117:675, 1982.

60. Denis R, Smith RW, Grabow D, et al: Relocation of nonalbumin proteins after albumin resuscitation. *J Surg Res* 43(5):413, 1987.

61. Saxe JM, Guan ZX, Grabow D, et al: The myth of hyperglycemia-induced plasma volume expansion during shock. *Surg Forum* 39:73, 1988.

62. Lowry SF, Fong Y: Cytokines and the cellular response to injury and infection, in Wilmore DW, Brennan MF, Harken AH, et al (eds): *Care of the Surgical Patient.* New York, Scientific American Press, 1989.

63. Lucas CE, Ledgerwood AM: The fluid problem in the critically ill. *Surg Clin North Am* 63(2):439, 1983.

64. Harrigan C, Lucas CE, Ledgerwood AM, Mammem EF: Primary hemostasis after massive transfusion for injury. *Am Surg* 48(8):393, 1982.

65. Martin DJ, Lucas CE, Ledgerwood AM, et al: Fresh frozen plasma supplement to massive red blood cell transfusion. *Ann Surg* 202(4):505, 1985.

66. Dawson CW, Lucas CE, Ledgerwood AM: Altered interstitial fluid space dynamics and post-resuscitation hypertension. *Arch Surg* 116:657, 1981.

67. Lucas CE, Ledgerwood AM, Higgins RF: Impaired salt and water excretion after albumin resuscitation for hypovolemic shock. *Surgery* 86:544, 1979.

68. Lucas CE, Ledgerwood AM: Cardiovascular and renal response to hemorrhagic and septic shock, in Clowes GH (ed): *Trauma, Sepsis, and Shock: The Physiological Basis of Therapy.* New York, Marcel Dekker, 1988.

69. Clift DR, Lucas CE, Ledgerwood AM, et al: The effect of albumin resuscitation for shock on immunoglobulin activity. *J Surg Res* 32:449, 1982.

70. Lucas CE, Ledgerwood AM, Rachwal WJ, et al: Colloid oncotic pressure and body water dynamics in septic and injured patients. *J Trauma* 31(7):927, 1991.

71. Bock JC, Barker BC, Clinton AG, et al: Post-traumatic changes in and effect of colloid oncotic pressure on the distribution of body water. *Ann Surg* 208:139, 1989.

72. Ladegaard-Pedersen AJ, Engell HC: A comparison between the changes in the distribution volumes of inulin and (^{51}Cr)EDTA after major surgery. *Scand J Clin Lab Invest* 35:103, 1975.

73. Lucas CE, Denis R, Ledgerwood AM, et al: The effects of hespan on serum and lymphatic albumin, globulin, and coagulant protein. *Ann Surg* 207:416, 1988.

74. Lucas CE, Ledgerwood AM, Shief MR, Bradley VE: The renal factor in the post traumatic "fluid overload" syndrome. *J Trauma* 17:667, 1977.

75. Starling EH: On the absorption of fluids from the connective tissue spaces. *J Physiol* 19:312, 1896.

76. Lucas CE, Ledgerwood AM, Higgins RF, et al: Impaired pulmonary function after albumin resuscitation from shock. *J Trauma* 20:446, 1980.

77. Faillace DF, Ledgerwood AM, Lucas CE, et al: Immunoglobulin changes after varied resuscitation regimes. *J Trauma* 22:1, 1982.

78. Lucas CE, Ledgerwood AM, Mammem EF: Altered coagulation protein content after albumin resuscitation. *Ann Surg* 196:198, 1982.

79. Unpublished data, interstitial fluid laboratories, 1988.

80. Elliot LA, Ledgerwood AM, Lucas CE, et al: The role of Fluosol-Da 20% in pre-hospital resuscitation. *Crit Care Med* 17:166, 1989.

81. Moncada S, Vane JR: Arachidonic acid metabolites and the interactions between platelets and blood vessel walls. *N Engl J Med* 300:1142, 1979.

82. Wilson JW: Treatment or prevention of pulmonary cellular damage with pharmacologic doses of corticoid steroid. *Surg Gynecol Obstet* 134:675, 1972.

83. Lucas CE, Ledgerwood AM: Pulmonary response of massive steroid in seriously injured patients. *Ann Surg* 194:256, 1981.

84. Glen TM, Lefer AM: Anti-toxic action of methylprednisolone in hemorrhagic shock. *Eur J Pharmacol* 13:230, 1971.

85. Howland DS, Scheizer O, Graziano CC, Goldiner PL: The cardiovascular effects of low levels of ionized calcium during massive transfusions. *Surg Gynecol Obstet* 145:581, 1977.

86. White BC, Winegar CD, Wilson RF, Krause GS: Calcium channel blockers in cerebral resuscitation. *J Trauma* 23:788, 1983.

87. Porter DL, Ledgerwood AM, Lucas CE, Harrigan C: Effect of calcium infusion on heart function. *Am Surg* 49:304, 1983.

88. Lucas CE, Sennish JC, Ledgerwood AM, Harrigan C: Parathyroid response to hypocalcemia after treatment of hemorrhagic shock. *Surgery* 96:711, 1984.

89. Shatney CH, Shirakawa Y, Smith RA: Thyroidectomy improves survival in canine hemorrhagic shock. *Surg Forum* 35:10, 1984.

90. Gallick HL, Lucas CE, Ledgerwood AM, et al: Detrimental effect of recent thyroidectomy on hemorrhagic shock and resuscitation. *Circ Shock* 21:11, 1987.

91. Sugiura A, Smith RA, Shatney CH: Thyrotropin-releasing hormone increase survival in canine hemorrhagic shock. *J Surg Res* 40:63, 1986.

6

TECHNIQUES OF RESUSCITATION

Robert F. Wilson

HISTORY

One of the earliest authenticated resuscitations in the medical literature is the "miraculous deliverance of Anne Green" who was executed by hanging on December 14, 1650.[1,2] Until the middle of the sixteenth century, anatomic dissections of the human body were conducted in Oxford, as in most European universities, according to ritual that had not been altered for centuries.[3] The dissection of the cadaver was performed by an assistant, while the professor sat on a raised throne above the dissection table and read aloud from the works of either Galen or Mondino.

In 1549, however, the statutes of the University of Oxford were revised after the visitation of King Edward VI, and from that time on, Oxford medical students were required to view two anatomic dissections and then to perform two dissections. Obtaining the human cadavers for these dissections was a difficulty that was solved in 1636 by a section of the great Charter of Charles I to the University of Oxford. This part of the charter permitted the anatomy reader to demand, for the purpose of anatomic dissection, the body of any person executed within 21 miles of Oxford.

Anne Green was executed in the customary way by being turned off a ladder to hang by the neck (Fig. 6–1). She hanged for half an hour, during which time some of her friends pulled "with all their weight upon her legs, sometimes lifting her up, and then pulling her down again with a sudden jerk, thereby the sooner to despatch her out of her pain." When everyone thought she was dead, the body was taken down and put in a coffin and carried to the private house of Dr. William Petty, the reader in anatomy.

When the coffin was opened, Anne Green was observed to take a breath, and a rattle was heard in her throat. William Petty and Thomas Willis abandoned all thoughts of a dissection and proceeded to try to revive their patient. They held her up in the coffin and then, by wrenching her teeth apart, poured hot cordial

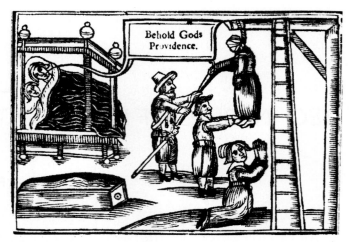

FIG. 6–1. The execution and resuscitation of Anne Green. (*From Hughes JT: The miraculous deliverance of Anne Green: An Oxford case of resuscitation in the seventeenth century. Br Med J 285:1792, 1982, with permission.*)

into her mouth, which caused her to cough. They then rubbed and chafed her fingers, hands, arms, and feet, and, after a quarter of an hour of this, put more cordial into her mouth. Then after tickling her throat with a feather, she opened her eyes momentarily. At this stage the doctors opened a vein and bled her off 5 ounces of blood. They then continued administering the cordial and rubbing her arms and legs. Compressing bandages were applied to her arms and legs. Heating plasters were put to her chest, and another was inserted as an enema "to give heat and warmth to her bowels." They then placed her in a warm bed with another woman to lie with her (see Fig. 6–1) to keep her warm.

After 12 hours, she began to speak, and 24 hours after her revival, she was answering questions freely. At 2 days her memory was normal, apart from the period of the execution and the resuscitation. At 4 days she was eating solid food, and 1 month after the event she was fully recovered except for the period of amnesia. William Petty and Thomas Willis achieved considerable fame from their conduct of the case. Although Petty left the practice of medicine shortly thereafter, Willis went on to become an Oxford professor and then a wealthy London physician.

THE ORIGINS OF INTRAVENOUS THERAPY

The first record available on someone understanding the need for fluid in injured patients is apparently from Ambroise Paré (1510–1590), who urged the use of clysters (administration of fluid into the rectum) to prevent "noxious vapors from mounting to the brain."[4,5]

According to Garrison,[6] intravenous injection of drugs and transfusion of blood had their scientific origins in the seventeenth century. Sir Christopher

Wren (1632–1723), assisted by Boyle and Wilkins, first injected opium and *Crocus metallorum* into the veins of dogs in 1656. This experiment was repeated by Carlo Fracassato in 1658. Johann Daniel Major (1662), Caspar Scotus (1664), and Elsholtz (*Clysmata nova,* 1665) made the first successful intravenous injections in humans. Major published his efforts in *Chirurgia infusoria* at Kiel in 1667. Major believed that intravenous injection could lead to thinning of blood that was excessively viscous and thus could be of assistance in certain illnesses.[6,7]

Priority in blood transfusions has been claimed for Francesco Folli (1654), but the first authenticated records are those of Richard Lower (1665–1667) and Coga (1667). Transfusion is mentioned on November 14, 1666, in Pepys' diary.

The first clear description of intravenous fluid therapy was in response to an epidemic of cholera which reached England by way of India (1827) and then Russia (1829). The tremendous loss of fluid in cholera and the resulting clinical picture were generally recognized by the physicians of that period. Hermann[7,8] attempted to treat this in 1830 by injecting water into the veins of cholera patients. According to Howard-Jones,[7,9] Jaehnichen, a physician in the same institute as Hermann, injected 6 ounces of water into the vein of a cholera patient who showed initial improvement but died 2 hours later. Howard Jones does, however, credit Jaehnichen and Hermann "for grasping the fundamental principle that governs cholera therapy today, i.e., rehydration by intravenous infusion."

In the midst of the severe cholera epidemic of 1831–1832, Dr. William Brook O'Shaughnessy, a 22-year-old recent Edinburgh graduate, wondered whether "the habit of practical chemistry which I have occasionally pursued might lead to the application of chemistry to its cure."[10,11] Within a few days of seeing some cholera patients firsthand and analyzing their blood, he published his results in *The Lancet* on December 29, 1831, as follows:

> The blood drawn in the worst cases . . . has lost a large proportion of its water. . . . Of the free alkali contained in healthy serum, not a particle is present. . . . Urea exists in those cases where suppression of urine has been a marked symptom. . . . All the salts deficient in the blood, especially the carbonate of soda, are present in large quantities [in the diarrhea fluid].[11]

Pursuing this theme logically to its "therapeutic conclusions," O'Shaughnessy[12] wrote:

> . . . the indications of cure . . . are two in number—*viz.* 1st to restore the blood to its natural specific gravity; 2nd to restore its deficient saline matters. . . . The first of these can only be effected by absorption, by imbibition, or by the injection of aqueous fluid into the veins. The same remarks, with sufficiently obvious modifications, apply to the second. . . . When absorption is entirely suspended . . . in those desperate cases . . . the author recommends the injection into the veins of tepid water holding a solution of the normal salts of the blood.

Thomas Latta (1832) then "resolved to throw the fluid immediately into the circulation."[13] According to Masson,[14] the solution used by Latta was about a half-normal concentration of muriate of soda ($NaCl$) and subcarbonate of soda ($NaHCO_3$); however, in later cases, the concentrations of both salts were increased by about a third. The solutions were strained through leather and warmed before injection. A large syringe directed the fluid through a tube previously inserted into the basilic vein. Latta's first subject was an aged woman who had "reached the last moments of her earthly existence." As he stated:

> Having no precedent to direct me, I proceeded with caution. . . . Cautiously—anxiously, I watched the effects; ounce after ounce was injected but no visible change was produced. Still persevering, I thought she began to breathe less laboriously, soon the sharpened features, and sunken eye, and fallen jaw, pale and cold, bearing the manifest impress of death's signet, began to glow with returning animation; the pulse, which had long ceased, returned to the wrist; at first small and quick, by degrees it became more and more distinct, fuller, slower and firmer, and in the short space of half an hour, when six pints had been injected, she expressed in a firm voice that she was free from all uneasiness, actually became jocular, and fancied all she needed was a little sleep; her extremities were warm, and every feature bore the aspect of comfort and health.[13]

The patient then experienced a relapse, and she was given more fluids. In the space of 12 hours this patient received 10,000 ml of fluid. Of the first 15 patients treated, all of whom were moribund, 5 survived.[8]

Latta had great insight into the usefulness of fluid resuscitation, and in summarizing his experiences, he concluded that the failure of saline therapy in the patients who died was due to one of three causes: (1) the quantity injected was too small, (2) the time of injection was too late, or (3) the effect was rendered abortive by the disease.[15,16]

DIAGNOSIS OF SHOCK

To be able to adequately describe resuscitation, one must also be able to describe what shock is and how to monitor the process before and during treatment. The clinical diagnosis of shock is usually made on the basis of (1) evidence of poor tissue perfusion, (2) a low or greatly decreased systolic blood pressure, and/or (3) development of a metabolic (lactic) acidosis (Fig. 6–2).

CLINICAL EVIDENCE OF POOR TISSUE PERFUSION

Clinical evidence of hypovolemic shock, most cardiogenic shock, and late septic shock includes a cold, clammy skin which may be pale, cyanotic, or blotchy in color. The pulse rate is usually rapid, and the pulse feels thready. Mentation is usually impaired, and the patient often seems anxious, restless, and/or confused and obtunded.

In early (warm) septic shock, the pulse rate tends to be rapid, but it feels more full.[17,18] The skin tends to be warm and dry, and it is more apt to be pink. Patients in neurogenic shock resemble patients with early septic shock, but they tend to have a slower, frequently normal, pulse rate in spite of hypotension.

BLOOD PRESSURE

A systolic blood pressure of less than 80 mmHg is usually considered evidence of septic or traumatic shock in patients with the appropriate clinical background,

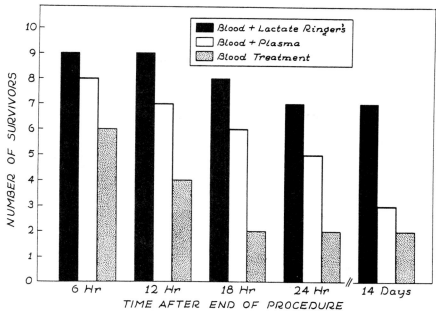

FIG. 6–2. Survival after acute hemorrhagic shock. Black bars: blood + Ringer's lactate. White bars: blood + plasma. Gray bars: blood. (*From Shires GT, Canizaro PC, Lowry SE, et al: In Schwartz SI: Principles of Surgery, 4th ed. New York, McGraw-Hill, 1984, p 115–164. Reproduced with permission.*)

while a systolic pressure less than 90 mmHg is generally used as a criterion for cardiogenic shock. In previously hypertensive patients, a relatively rapid fall in systolic blood pressure exceeding 30 to 40 mmHg is also considered to be evidence of shock. However, a low blood pressure by itself is poor evidence for shock, since other signs of impaired perfusion also should be present.

METABOLIC ACIDOSIS

As a patient develops shock, there is usually a strong tendency to hyperventilate and develop an acute respiratory alkalosis. However, once shock is established, there is usually an increasing metabolic (lactic) acidosis with a progressive fall in arterial bicarbonate levels. Even though the patients tend to hyperventilate even more as the bicarbonate levels fall, the compensation is not complete, and the arterial pH falls.

Electrolyte studies tend to indicate that the metabolic acidosis of poor tissue perfusion is usually of the increased anion gap type. Direct measurement of lactate may show increased lactate levels before the arterial bicarbonate and pH fall below normal; however, the increased lactate levels usually make up only a fraction of the increased anion gap.[19,20]

Basal oxygen consumption ($\dot{V}_{O_2}$) in adults is usually about 120 to 160 ml/min/m². In patients who are not hypothyroid, hypothermic, or hypometabolic for other reasons, a $\dot{V}_{O_2}$ less than 100 ml/min/m² is generally inadequate for the cell to metabolize properly and will eventually be associated with a rise in lactate levels and a metabolic acidosis.[20] If the $\dot{V}_{O_2}$ stays less than 100 ml/min/m² for more than 30 to 60 min, the patients almost invariably die.

MONITORING

Appropriate monitoring is important to identify patients who are beginning to go into shock and to properly evaluate the effects of therapy. This should include clinical, ventilatory, oxygenation, and hemodynamic monitoring. The sooner hypovolemia, hypotension, or hypoxemia is recognized and treated aggressively, the better the outcome.

CLINICAL MONITORING

MENTATION

It is important to keep a close watch on central nervous system (CNS) function in patients who may have poor tissue perfusion. Patients who are awake, alert, and comfortable probably have a satisfactory perfusion of the brain and other vital organs, regardless of the blood pressure and cardiac output. Restless, anxious, confused, or uncooperative patients should be considered to have CNS hypoxemia or ischemia until proven otherwise. A cloudy sensorium may be a particularly helpful early sign of sepsis; however, at times it may be difficult to differentiate between cerebral ischemia-hypoxia, sepsis, and early delirium tremens.

SKIN

A cool, clammy skin implies poor skin perfusion and sympathetic nervous system hyperactivity. This coolness and clamminess tend to be worse in the distal extremities, and the abdomen and chest may stay relatively warm and dry. The tips of digits, and sometimes the tip of the nose and ears, may even be cyanotic. A cold, clammy skin is usually associated with a systemic vascular resistance that is higher than normal.

The skin will usually not look cyanotic unless there is at least 5.0 g/dl of reduced hemoglobin at the capillary level. In a patient with a hemoglobin of less than 10.0 g/dl, the capillary oxygen saturation would have to be less than 50 percent for the patient to appear cyanotic. Since the venous oxyhemoglobin saturation is seldom less than 40 to 50 percent, the arterial oxyhemoglobin saturation would have to be less than 50 to 60 percent for the patient to look cyanotic. However, if the hemoglobin is 15.0 g/dl, the arterial oxyhemoglobin saturation only has to fall below 74 to 84 percent for the patient to appear cyanotic.

LUNGS

Tachypnea and obvious hyperventilation are usually seen with stress, hypoxemia, metabolic acidosis, or shock. A persistent rapid respiratory rate exceeding

30 to 40 breaths per minute and/or use of accessory muscles of ventilation often indicates impending respiratory failure. Diffuse rales, poor breath sounds, and neck vein distension may indicate the presence of heart failure.

HEART

Tachycardia is very nonspecific and is typical of all types of stress. The presence of a gallop may indicate cardiac failure. Failure to develop tachycardia after trauma or in shock doubly jeopardizes the patient; the physician may remain less concerned about the patient's hemodynamic status, and the lack of an appropriate tachycardia also will tend to keep cardiac output less than it should be. This is especially important in older individuals who tend to have a relatively low fixed stroke volume.

An enlarged heart by percussion may be due to cardiac enlargement or a pericardial fluid collection. Murmurs often reflect valvular or septal abnormalities.

BLOOD PRESSURE

The systemic arterial blood pressure can be considered to have three parts: the diastolic pressure, which correlates primarily with the amount of arteriolar vasoconstriction present; the pulse pressure, which is related both to stroke volume and to the rigidity of the aorta and its major branches; and the systolic pressure, which is determined by a combination of these factors.

Systolic and Diastolic Pressures. Diastolic pressure often rises initially with hemorrhage, pain, or stress because of sympathoadrenal stimulation, particularly if there is excess pain. However, since vasoconstriction can only increase to a certain maximum, continued blood loss will eventually result in a fall in diastolic pressure.

In previously normal patients, the systolic pressure is often maintained relatively well until a blood volume deficit of at least 25 percent has developed. In the average 70-kg man with a normal blood volume of 5000 ml, a rapid blood loss of 500 to 1000 ml may cause some decrease in the pulse pressure, but the systolic pressure often does not fall significantly until more than 1500 ml (30 percent of the normal blood volume) has been lost; this is usually associated with a blood volume deficit of at least 20 to 25 percent. An acute blood loss of 30 to 40 percent of the blood volume (2100 to 2800 ml in a 70-kg man) will usually cause the systolic blood pressure to fall below 80 mmHg. With a blood volume deficit exceeding 40 percent, the blood pressure is often not obtainable by the standard cuff technique.

Pulse Pressure. Pulse pressure is usually the most important pressure to monitor in patients who are in shock or may be going into shock because it often provides some indication of whether the stroke volume is increasing or decreasing. Although cardiac output and stroke volume tend to decrease with advancing age, pulse pressure tends to rise in the elderly because of increasing stiffness of the aorta and its larger branches.[21]

There is a great deal of difference in systolic and diastolic pressures among individuals, and consequently, the correlation between stroke volume and pulse pressure in large groups of patients is poor. However, in an individual patient, the percentage change in pulse pressure often correlates quite well with the percentage change in stroke volume. For example, if a patient's blood pressure changes from 120/80 to 110/90 mmHg, the pulse pressure has fallen by 50 percent from 40 to 20 mmHg, and it is likely that the stroke volume also has decreased by about 50 percent.

Sphygmomanometer (Cuff) Pressures. The usual method for obtaining the systolic and diastolic blood pressure with a sphygmomanometer relies on the amount of blood going past the area constricted by the partially inflated cuff and the ability of the listener to hear Korotkoff's sounds. The amount of blood going past the constricted area determines the amount of turbulence and amplitude of the vibrations produced. If the patient has a low cardiac output or is very vasoconstricted, Korotkoff's sounds may not be heard in spite of a relatively normal blood pressure. Although an "unobtainable" cuff blood pressure is usually associated with a systolic blood pressure of less than 50 mmHg, occasional patients with systolic pressures over 200 mmHg also will have unobtainable cuff pressures.

Doppler Blood Pressures. If there is any difficulty obtaining a blood pressure by the cuff technique, a Doppler device may be used. The Doppler signal can generally be heard clearly even at very low levels of systolic pressure. Doppler measurements of blood pressure at the radial artery usually correlate fairly well with intraarterial pressures, even in patients with hypotension.[22] A number of devices are now available to measure blood pressure by this technique automatically every 1 to 5 min.

Pulsus Paradoxus. During spontaneous inspiration, venous return to the right atrium is increased, but venous return to the left atrium is decreased. As a consequence, stroke volume tends to fall during inspiration, producing a 3- to 10-mmHg decrease in systolic pressure. If the patient is hypovolemic, has bronchospasm, or has a pericardial tamponade, the fall in systolic blood pressure during spontaneous inspiration will often exceed 15 mmHg, and this is considered abnormal.[23]

Respirophasic Variations. Exaggerated respirophasic variations in systolic blood pressure during mechanical ventilation may be an early indication of hypovolemia.[24,25] The difference between the highest and lowest systolic pressures usually exceeds 10 mmHg if the patient is hypovolemic, has a pericardial tamponade, or has severe bronchospasm. In hypovolemic patients, the magnitude of the difference usually correlates with the severity of the volume deficit.[24] In animals, respirophasic variations correlate better with hypovolemia than central venous pressure.[25] Respirophasic changes also have been observed on pulse oximetry recordings from hypovolemic patients, but the accuracy of this variation as an indicator of hypovolemia remains to be determined.

PRELOAD

If a patient has an inadequate blood pressure and tissue perfusion despite what appears to be adequate fluid loading, one can gain some impression of the patient's fluid status by examining the patient and performing certain maneuvers. If the patient is on a ventilator, certain other maneuvers can be performed.

Breathing Spontaneously. *Hand veins.* The veins of a hand will normally, except in some overweight individuals, distend to some degree after the arm hangs straight down over the side of the bed for a few minutes. If the veins do not distend, it suggests that the patient is hypovolemic. If the hand veins do distend, one can get some idea of the peripheral venous pressure (PVP) by slowly raising the hand and arm to the level of the heart (midaxillary line if the patient is lying flat or slightly lower if the patient has an increased anteroposterior diameter to his or her chest).

If the hand veins disappear at this level or at less than 5 to 10 cm above the presumed level of the heart, the patient is probably still hypovolemic. If the hand veins are distended after the hand is more than 20 to 30 cm above the heart, the patient may be overloaded with fluid.

It must be remembered that the central venous pressure (CVP) will be lower than the PVP. Thus, although a low PVP means that the CVP is also low, a high PVP may be present with either a high or a low CVP.

Neck veins. If the patient is lying flat and no neck veins are visible at all, even after turning the head slightly to one side, the patient is probably hypovolemic. If the neck veins are visible for several centimeters above the clavicle while the patient is sitting up at a 30- to 45-degree angle and breathing spontaneously, the patient is usually overloaded with fluid.

Rales. Obviously, if there are diffuse crackly rales in the lung without retained secretions or a pulmonary infection and they do not clear with a cough, the patient is apt to be overloaded with fluid. On the other hand, lungs can be clear to auscultation with relatively high cardiac filling pressures, particularly in patients with chronically high left atrial pressures due to mitral stenosis.

Response to leg raising. If the legs are raised without causing pain or discomfort and the blood pressure rises more than 10 to 20 mmHg, the patient is probably hypovolemic. Even if there is no rise in blood pressure with leg raising, but there is a fall in blood pressure when the patient sits up, the patient has orthostatic hypotension and is probably hypovolemic. If sitting up makes the blood pressure improve, the patient is probably overloaded with fluid.

On a Ventilator. If the patient is on a ventilator and adding 1 to 2 cmH$_2$O of positive end-expiratory pressure (PEEP) up to a total of 5 to 10 cmH$_2$O causes a drop in blood pressure, the patient is probably hypovolemic. On the other hand, if the patient's hemodynamics improve with increased PEEP, the patient is probably overloaded with fluid.

MONITORING OF VENTILATION AND OXYGENATION

BLOOD GASES

Invasive Techniques of Analysis. *Arterial puncture or catheters.* Blood for analysis of pH, P_{CO_2}, and P_{O_2} can be obtained from systemic arteries by intermittent percutaneous needle aspiration or withdrawal from an indwelling catheter. Mixed venous blood can be obtained from indwelling pulmonary artery catheters.

Intravascular probes. A further development in the area of blood gas tension analysis is the intravascular probe. Although intravascular oxygen sensors have been available for some time, their usefulness has been limited by the loss of sensitivity of the electrode as protein deposits accumulate on the membrane. Recently, intravascular probes using fiberoptic light channels and specific fluorescent compounds to continuously measure pH, arterial P_{O_2}, and arterial P_{CO_2} have been developed.[26] One of the newer probes is so small that it can pass through a 20-gauge catheter and still leave enough room for pressure measurements and blood sampling. Clinical experience with these intravascular fiberoptic "blood gas machines" is limited; however, these catheters should be widely accepted as the technology is perfected.

Arterial P_{CO_2}. With adequate alveolar ventilation, the arterial P_{CO_2} (Pa_{CO_2}) will be closely related to the arterial pH (pHa). The respiratory compensation for metabolic acidosis, as a rough rule, in millimeters of mercury should be equal to half the change in pH units (i.e., the last two digits of the pHa). Thus, if the pHa is 7.40, the arterial P_{CO_2} should be 40 mmHg or less. If the pHa falls to 7.30 because of a metabolic acidosis, the arterial P_{CO_2} should fall to 35 mmHg or less. If the pHa is 7.20, the arterial P_{CO_2} should be 30 mmHg or less. If the arterial P_{CO_2} is higher than these expected values, it usually indicates an inadequate ventilatory effort.

If cardiac output is normal, the mixed venous P_{CO_2} (Pv_{CO_2}) is an average of 6 to 7 mmHg higher than the arterial P_{CO_2}.[27] If the $Pa_{CO_2} - Pv_{CO_2}$ difference is greater than 10 to 15 mmHg, the cardiac output (pulmonary blood flow) is probably significantly reduced below normal. For example, it is not unusual in patients receiving CPR for a cardiac arrest to respond to IV $NaHCO_3$ with little or no change in the arterial P_{CO_2} but to have an abrupt rise in the mixed venous P_{CO_2}. Thus, in patients with a very low cardiac output, one should measure both arterial and mixed venous blood gases prior to giving bicarbonate.

Arterial P_{O_2}. *On room air.* When evaluating the arterial P_{O_2} on room air, it is important to know the arterial P_{CO_2}. If the arterial P_{CO_2} is 40 mmHg, the alveolar P_{O_2} (PA_{O_2}) is about 105 mmHg, and the arterial P_{O_2} will be about 90 to 100 mmHg. The arterial P_{O_2} (Pa_{O_2}) will normally fall about 2 to 3 mmHg per decade after 20 years of age.

If a patient is on room air at sea level, the alveolar P_{O_2} (PA_{O_2}) plus the alveolar P_{CO_2} (PA_{CO_2}) add up to about 145 mmHg, and normally the arterial P_{CO_2} and alveolar P_{CO_2} are equal. Thus, if the patient is hyperventilating and has an arterial P_{CO_2} of 25 mmHg, the alveolar P_{O_2} should be about 120 mmHg. Consequently, patients who have a respiratory alkalosis can have a normal arterial P_{O_2} but abnormally functioning lungs with a significantly increased alveolar-arterial P_{O_2} difference [$P(A-a)_{O_2}$]. Thus, in patients with a low arterial P_{CO_2}, one should use the $P(A-a)_{O_2}$ rather than the arterial P_{O_2} to monitor pulmonary function. This is also true of patients who have a severe metabolic alkalosis. In such patients, the arterial P_{CO_2} will be elevated in an effort to compensate for the metabolic alkalosis, even if the lungs are normal.

As a general rule, a $P(A\text{-}a)_{O_2}$ of 5 to 20 mmHg on room air is normal and a $P(A\text{-}a)_{O_2}$ of 40 to 55 mmHg on room air is considered evidence of a moderate impairment in oxygenation.

On oxygen. If the patient is receiving oxygen, one can estimate the $F_{I_{O_2}}$ being inhaled by assuming that nasal O_2 raises the $F_{I_{O_2}}$ by about 0.04 for each 1.0 liter/min given. Thus nasal O_2 given at 4 liters/min provides an $F_{I_{O_2}}$ of about 0.37.

If the percentage of inhaled oxygen is known, one can estimate the alveolar P_{O_2} as 6 times the percentage of inspired O_2. Thus a patient on 40% oxygen would be expected to have an alveolar P_{O_2} of about 240 mmHg. If the arterial P_{O_2} is less than a third of the alveolar P_{O_2} in a patient with sepsis or trauma, the patient should probably receive ventilator support.

The arterial $P_{O_2}/F_{I_{O_2}}$ ratio is one way to look at the effect that an increased $F_{I_{O_2}}$ has on the arterial P_{O_2}. For example, if the arterial P_{O_2} is 80 mmHg on 40% oxygen, the arterial $P_{O_2}/F_{I_{O_2}}$ ratio is $80/0.4 = 200$, and if the arterial P_{O_2} is 90 mmHg on 60% O_2, the arterial $P_{O_2}/F_{I_{O_2}}$ ratio is 150.

As a general rule, a normal arterial $P_{O_2}/F_{I_{O_2}}$ ratio is about 600, and this ratio is equivalent to a pulmonary shunt (Q_{sp}/Q_t) of about 5 percent. The percentage shunts (Q_{sp}/Q_t) usually present at various arterial $P_{O_2}/F_{I_{O_2}}$ ratios are as follows:

$F_{I_{O_2}}$	Pa_{O_2}	$Pa_{O_2}/F_{I_{O_2}}$ Ratio	Estimated Shunt (%)
0.50	300	600	5
0.50	250	500	10
0.50	150	300	15
0.50	100	200	20
0.50	75	150	30
0.50	50	100	40

Although arterial blood gases in themselves are usually adequate to get some impression of the pulmonary function present, simultaneous analysis of mixed venous gases also permits calculation of the physiologic shunting in the lung (Q_{sp}/Q_t) utilizing the following modified Berggen formula (assuming an $F_{I_{O_2}}$ of 0.30 or more):

$$Pc_{O_2} = \text{approximately } 6 \times \text{percentage } O_2 \text{ inhaled}$$

i.e., on 40% O_2, $Pc_{O_2} = 6 \times 40 = 240$ mmHg

$$\frac{Q_{sp}}{Q_t} = \frac{Cc_{O_2} - Ca_{CO_2}}{Cc_{O_2} - Cv_{O_2}}$$

$$Cc_{O_2} = (Hb)(1.34) + (Pc_{O_2})(0.003)$$

$$Ca_{O_2} = (Hb)(1.34)\frac{(Sa_{O_2})}{100} + (Pv_{O_2})(0.003)$$

$$Cv_{O_2} = (Hb)(1.34)\frac{(Sv_{O_2})}{100} + (Pv_{O_2})(0.003)$$

where Cc_{O_2} = pulmonary capillary oxygen content, Pc_{O_2} = pulmonary capillary

P_{O_2}, Hb = hemoglobin, S_aO_2 = arterial oxygen saturation, $C_{\bar{v}}O_2$ = mixed venous oxygen content.

In general, the Q_{sp}/Q_t is a more accurate and sensitive index of pulmonary function than the arterial P_{O_2}, $P(A\text{-}a)_{O_2}$, or the arterial P_{O_2}/FI_{O_2} ratio. Normally the Q_{sp}/Q_t is 3 to 5 percent. If the Q_{sp}/Q_t rises above 15 to 20 percent acutely, the patient generally will benefit from ventilatory assistance. If the Q_{sp}/Q_t rises acutely above 20 to 25 percent, the patient may benefit from positive end-expiratory pressure (PEEP).

Noninvasive Techniques. Several noninvasive transcutaneous techniques for measuring O_2 and CO_2 have been studied by a number of investigators. Pulse oximetry monitors oxygen saturation, whereas other techniques of transcutaneous monitoring measure P_{O_2} and P_{CO_2} directly.

Pulse oximetry. The use of pulse oximetry for monitoring oxygen saturation and pulse amplitude can often provide early warning of pulmonary or cardiovascular deterioration before it is clinically apparent.[27] This technique employs a microprocessor that continuously measures pulse rate and oxyhemoglobin saturation. The photosensor is not heated and does not require calibration. Oxyhemoglobin (HbO_2) is red, and reduced hemoglobin (Hb) is blue, each of which has a different absorption of light at a given wavelength. Because the ratio of transmittance of each of the two wavelengths (660 nm, red; 940 nm, infrared) varies according to the percentage of oxygen saturation at each pulse, there is a predictable correlation between noninvasive Sa_{O_2} and arterial oxygen saturation over a wide range of Sa_{O_2} values. Pulse oximetry has many advantages which makes it ideal for use in the intensive care unit.[28]

There are several situations in which pulse oximetry changes do not adequately reflect changes in lung function or arterial P_{O_2}. These include impaired local perfusion, abnormal hemoglobins, and very high levels of arterial P_{O_2}.[28] Carboxyhemoglobin and fetal hemoglobin falsely raise oximeter saturation readings, while methemoglobin lowers them.

Pulse oximetry helps to reduce the number of arterial blood gas determinations performed and can provide rapid feedback on the effects of therapeutic interventions. Despite its limitations, it is increasingly becoming the standard of care in neonatal, pediatric, and adult intensive care units.

Transcutaneous monitoring. Electrochemical sensors have been developed to noninvasively detect the partial pressures of O_2 and CO_2 at the skin surface. Using the current technology, oxygen molecules which diffuse from "arterialized" capillaries to the skin surface are consumed at the surface electrode in an electrochemical reaction that alters current flow between a cathode and anode proportional to the oxygen tension present.[28]

Transcutaneous oxygen and carbon dioxide tensions (Ptc_{O_2} and Ptc_{CO_2}) are important variables for the early warning of disturbed pulmonary function or systemic circulation as well as for the evaluation of local tissue perfusion. Comparative studies indicate that Ptc_{O_2} and Ptc_{CO_2} are more sensitive indicators of circulatory changes than conventional monitoring variables such as arterial pressure, heart rate, CVP, ECG, and urine output.[29] If tissue perfusion is severely reduced, Ptc_{O_2} and Ptc_{CO_2} values deviate from their relationship with arterial partial pressures and become flow-dependent.[30]

In adults, the Ptc_{O_2} is nearly always substantially lower than the arterial P_{O_2}, partially because the thicker skin layer acts as a barrier to oxygen diffusion. Heating of the skin tends to raise Ptc_{O_2} levels and make them more closely approximate the arterial P_{O_2}. It does this through three major effects: (1) vasodilation of the cutaneous blood vessels, (2) right shift of the oxyhemoglobin dissociation curve, and (3) altered lipid structure of the stratum corneum, allowing more rapid diffusion of oxygen.[31]

The transcutaneous carbon dioxide electrode is separated from skin by a thin hydrophobic membrane that is permeable to carbon dioxide. Carbon dioxide molecules diffuse through the membrane and form carbonic acid (H_2CO_3), which alters the pH across a conventional pH-sensitive glass electrode.

Carbon dioxide diffuses fairly rapidly through the skin. Heating the skin causes (1) faster diffusion of carbon dioxide to the skin surface, (2) decreased solubility of carbon dioxide, and (3) increased local metabolism and carbon dioxide production.[29] These three heating effects can cause transcutaneous P_{CO_2} readings to be 1.2 to 2 times greater than the arterial values.

In critically ill adults, the Ptc_{O_2} responds rapidly to changes in arterial P_{O_2} and cardiac output. Its 95 percent response time is less than 2 minutes, even in patients with low-flow circulatory shock.[28] In a study of high-risk surgical patients monitored perioperatively with Ptc_{O_2} sensors and pulmonary artery catheters, a decrease in Ptc_{O_2} was one of the earliest warning signs of impending circulatory deterioration.[32]

Although transcutaneous monitoring is a noninvasive technique and can provide constant real-time monitoring, it has a number of disadvantages. For example, if the electrode site is not changed every 2 to 6 h, there is a risk of burns from the heated electrode. There also may be skin irritation from the adhesive ring.

Transconjunctival measurements. Measurement of conjunctival oxygen tension (Pcj_{O_2}) also allows noninvasive monitoring of arterial P_{O_2}, and this also can help provide early warning of inadequate tissue perfusion.[33] A Pcj_{O_2}/Pa_{O_2} ratio of 0.57 or less may be a good sign that hypovolemia is present. Other causes of a low conjunctival-arterial P_{O_2} ratio include impaired local perfusion or impaired ventilation or oxygenation. To a certain extent, conjunctival P_{O_2} also may reflect O_2 delivery to the brain, since the ophthalmic artery is the first branch of the internal carotid artery.[34]

Capnography. Capnography is a technique for measuring the P_{CO_2} in expired gases. If cardiac output is relatively normal and there is no increased dead space in the lungs, the end-tidal P_{CO_2} in the expired gases should closely approximate the alveolar P_{CO_2}.[28,35,36] This is a useful and accurate means of assessing ventilatory adequacy, respiratory gas exchange, carbon dioxide production, and cardiovascular status (particularly cardiac output). Although the end-tidal P_{CO_2} (Pet_{CO_2}) usually underestimates the arterial P_{CO_2} by about 1 to 2 mmHg, the difference is constant for a given patient provided the dead space/tidal volume (V_d/V_t) ratio and airway resistance are not changing.

Mainstream and sidestream infrared capnometers are available commercially. A mainstream capnometer connects directly to the endotracheal tube, thus providing real-time, breath-by-breath analysis. The major disadvantage of this system is its size and bulk and the fact that it cannot be used in nonintubated patients. Sidestream capnometers aspirate gas at the sample site. The principal advantage of this system is that it reduces mechanical factors related to gas sampling that can affect the results and which can require much expert attention and time.[35,36]

Because carbon dioxide production is directly dependent on metabolic rate, there are a large number of conditions that can lower end-tidal P_{CO_2}. However, sudden decreases in end-tidal P_{CO_2} suggest a mechanical problem in the airway, hypoventilation, or increased dead space. A gradual decrease in end-tidal P_{CO_2} is usually due to changes in the lung itself. Increases are generally due to hypermetabolic states.[37]

If a simultaneous arterial P_{CO_2} is available, one can estimate the alveolar-arterial P_{CO_2} difference [$P(A-a)_{CO_2}$]. Normally, this is zero, and if it suddenly increases, one should suspect a pulmonary embolus or drastic reduction in cardiac output producing increased dead space in the lungs.

The most frequent use of end-tidal P_{CO_2} is to evaluate the adequacy of ventilation; however, if cardiac output is severely reduced, the difference between the end-tidal P_{CO_2} and the arterial P_{CO_2} will reflect the amount of reduction in effective blood flow to the lung.

Inadvertent esophageal intubation, tracheal extubations, and endotracheal tube obstruction usually can be detected rapidly by a sudden decrease in capnographic P_{CO_2} levels. Capnography can reduce the number of arterial blood gas determinations needed, and it can be very useful in weaning patients from mechanical ventilatory support. All in all, capnographs are relatively inexpensive, and they are reliable in a wide variety of clinical settings.

Mass spectrometry. A mass spectrometer is an expensive and very complex machine that allows measurement of all clinically relevant respiratory gases (carbon dioxide, oxygen, and nitrogen) and anesthetic gases on a breath-by-breath basis. Analysis of inspired and expired respiratory gases by mass spectrometry is rapid and accurate to within 0.1 percent of the measured value.[38]

A mass spectrometer can be used to continuously monitor several patients at a time. Data analyzed by the mass spectrometer are generally delayed by at least 9 to 22 s, and as the number of monitored beds increases, so does the time between the machine obtaining a gas sample for analysis and displaying the results.[39] Much of this delay occurs because of the time it takes for the aspirated sample to reach the mass spectrometer. In a system with more than 10 monitoring stations, sample determinations may be delayed by more than 2 min.

A mass spectrometer can evaluate carbon dioxide partial pressures and thereby determine which samples are inspired and expired gas. Sudden changes may indicate mechanical problems in the ventilatory system or airway. Slower changes usually indicate progressive changes in cardiopulmonary function.

One of the main disadvantages of mass spectrophotometers are their high cost (at least $35,000). If used to monitor many patients, sample data are provided too infrequently to prevent serious injury to individual patients. Unless sampling from each patient can occur at least once a minute, alarms for low oxygen levels or low ventilator pressures or flow should be included.[28]

Arterial and Venous Oxygen Content. *Arteriovenous oxygen differences.* Trends in cardiac output may be indicated by changes in arteriovenous oxygen differences or pulmonary artery (mixed venous) oxygen saturation. If the $C(a\text{-}v)_{O_2}$ is greater than 6.0 vol % or if the Sv_{O_2} is less than 60 percent, tissue perfusion is probably impaired. A fall in arteriovenous O_2 differences may be an early sign of sepsis, while a rise in arteriovenous differences often indicates a reduction in blood volume and/or cardiac output.

Oxygen delivery. Oxygen delivery (D_{O_2}) is the amount of oxygen delivered to the entire body per minute and is equal to the cardiac output multiplied by the arterial oxygen content. Arterial oxygen content (Ca_{O_2}) can be calculated by the following formula:

$$Ca_{O_2} = (Hb)(1.34)(\% \text{ saturation}/100) + (Pa_{O_2})(0.0031)$$

Thus a patient with a hemoglobin level of 15.0 g/dl, an arterial oxygen saturation (Sa_{O_2}) of 98 percent, and Pa_{O_2} of 100 mmHg would have a Ca_{O_2} of 20.0 ml/dl, which is equivalent to 200 ml/liter of blood. Therefore, if the cardiac output is 5.0 liters/min, the patient would have a D_{O_2} of 1000 ml/min. It should be noted that the oxygen dissolved in the plasma, i.e., the Pa_{O_2}, only contributes a small percentage (1.5 percent in this example) to the Ca_{O_2} and can for practical purposes be ignored in calculating D_{O_2}.

Because of wide variations in patient size, physicians are increasingly describing D_{O_2} in terms of an oxygen delivery index ($D_{O_2}I$). This is obtained by dividing the D_{O_2} by the body surface area (BSA) in square meters (m²) or by multiplying the Ca_{O_2} by the cardiac index (CI) rather than the cardiac output (CO). Thus, if the patient in the preceding example had a body surface area of 1.73 m², the CI would be 5.0 divided by 1.73 = 2.89 liters/min/m² and the $D_{O_2}I$ would be 578 ml/min/m².

Oxygen consumption. Oxygen consumption ($\dot{V}_{O_2}$) can be measured directly with a metabolic cart or it can be calculated by multiplying the cardiac output by the arteriovenous oxygen content. Thus $\dot{V}_{O_2} = CO(Ca_{O_2} - Cv_{O_2})$. If a patient has a CO of 5 liters/min, a Ca_{O_2} of 20.0 ml/dl, and a Cv_{O_2} of 15.0 ml/dl, $\dot{V}_{O_2} = 5.0(20.0 - 15.0)(10) = 250$ ml/min.

Note that the factor 10 is included in the calculation to convert oxygen content from milliliters per deciliter to milliliters per liter. Normal $\dot{V}_{O_2}$ under basal conditions in adult males is said to be about 250 to 300 ml/min. If the body surface area is 1.73 m², one can calculate the oxygen consumption index as

$$\begin{aligned}
\dot{V}_{O_2}I &= CI(Ca_{O_2} - Cv_{O_2}) \\
&= (5.0/1.73)(20 - 15)(10) \\
&= (2.89)(5)(10) \\
&= 144.5 \text{ ml/min/m}^2
\end{aligned}$$

The $\dot{V}_{O_2}$ under basal conditions is normally 110 to 160 ml/min/m².

Optimizing D_{O_2} and $\dot{V}_{O_2}$. In critically ill or injured patients, D_{O_2} and $\dot{V}_{O_2}$ should be increased to higher than normal levels.[40] After resuscitation from shock, the $\dot{V}_{O_2}$ will usually have to be at least 25 to 50 percent above normal for 24 to 48 h to repay the O_2 debt that developed while the tissues were inadequately perfused. The oxygen debt is due not only to the anaerobic metabolism that occurred while blood flow was inadequate but also to the hypermetabolism caused by increased release of catecholamines, glucagon, and corticosteroids.

In many shock studies, returning the left atrial pressure (LAP) to normal has returned the blood pressure to control values, but under such circumstances, splanchnic blood flow may remain lower than control for several hours. However, if one increases O_2 delivery (D_{O_2}) to values up to 50 percent greater than normal or until O_2 consumption ($\dot{V}_{O_2}$) no longer rises with an increased D_{O_2}, resuscitation of the splanchnic tissues will usually also be complete.

Many years ago we noted that patients with a $\dot{V}_{O_2}$ persistently less than 100 ml/min/m^2 almost invariably died, while patients who kept their $\dot{V}_{O_2}$ above 160 ml/min/m^2 tended to have an improved outcome.[21,41] Other investigators also have noted improved survival with high oxygen delivery and oxygen consumptions.[42,43]

Bland et al.[43] noted that postoperative patients who died generally had a decreased oxygen delivery despite maintenance of normal arterial blood gases and hemoglobin values of 10.0 g or higher. Shoemaker et al.[44] concluded that tissue oxygen debt reflected by an insufficient oxygen consumption appears to be a major determinant of organ failure and outcome.[6] Shoemaker et al.[45] studied 223 consecutive critically ill postoperative patients and found that one-half to two-thirds of the postoperative deaths were secondary to physiologic problems that could have been identified or prevented with the use of hemodynamic monitoring. Shoemaker et al.[40] also have shown in a randomized, prospective trial that optimizing D_{O_2} and $\dot{V}_{O_2}$ can significantly reduce mortality rates, organ failure, and ICU stay over protocols that only restore D_{O_2} and $\dot{V}_{O_2}$ to normal values.

MONITORING VENTILATOR PERFORMANCE

Factors that can cause the delivered gas volume in patients on a ventilator to be less than desired include poor compliance, high flow rates, undetected circuit leaks, and high temperature of the water in the humidifier. Consequently, it is important to monitor the delivered tidal volume (V_t) by inserting a spirometer in the circuit.

Other parameters requiring frequent monitoring are respiratory rate, ventilatory pressures (both peak airway and PEEP), $F_{I_{O_2}}$, minute ventilation, and the heat level of the humidifier. The patient and the ventilatory equipment should be monitored at least every 2 h, and preferably much more frequently. This includes auscultation of the chest for bilateral air entry and the presence and location of rales and rhonchi. The pressure in the balloon cuff on the endotracheal or tracheostomy tube should be checked at least once or twice per shift, and the balloon should be inflated just enough to allow a small air leak during peak inspiration.

Peak inflation pressure (PIP) should be monitored closely. A rapid increase in PIP may be the result of a mucous plug, pneumothorax, or the endotracheal tube kinking or slipping into the right mainstem bronchus. A slow increase in airway pressure may be an early indication of pulmonary edema or other interstitial disease. A rapid decrease in pressure usually indicates a ventilator or circuit disconnection or an endotracheal cuff leak. A very slow decrease in airway pressure may indicate improvement in lung compliance, a decrease in airway resistance, or a slow air leak.

In patients with a high minute ventilation and rapid respiratory rate, a phenomenon known as *auto-PEEP* may develop because the gas in the lungs does not have enough time to escape from the alveoli and terminal bronchi during the expiration phase of ventilation.[46] As the volume of gas in the lungs increases with auto-PEEP, there will be a progressive increase in inflation pressures, dead space, and P_{CO_2}. One should suspect the presence of auto-PEEP if an increased minute ventilation causes the arterial P_{CO_2} to rise. A quick way to determine if auto-PEEP is present is to stop the ventilator at the end of expiration and note the pressure in the system. If no auto-PEEP is present, the pressure in the tracheobronchial tree will fall to whatever level of PEEP is being used.

An inspiratory hold of 0.5 s will allow one to calculate the dynamic and static compliance of the lungs and chest wall. If the patient is being ventilated with 1.0 liter of gas with each breath, if PIP is 55 cmH_2O PEEP, and if 5.0 cmH_2O PEEP is used, then

$$\text{Dynamic compliance} = \frac{\text{tidal volume}}{\text{PIP} - \text{PEEP}} = \frac{1000 \text{ cc}}{55 - 5} = 20 \text{ cc/cmH}_2\text{O}$$

If the pressure in the ventilatory system is 45 cmH_2O during the inspiratory hold (PIH),

$$\text{Static compliance} = \frac{\text{tidal volume}}{\text{PIH} - \text{PEEP}} = \frac{1000 \text{ cc}}{45 - 5} = 25 \text{ cc/cmH}_2\text{O}$$

The normal dynamic compliance is about 60 to 70 cc/cmH_2O, and the normal static compliance is about 100 cc/cmH_2O.

HEMODYNAMIC MONITORING

The word *hemodynamic* comes from the Greek words *haima,* meaning "blood," and *dynamica,* meaning "power," and it is defined as the study of the movement of blood in the body and the forces involved in its circulation. Although a wide array of calculations can be made from the changes in pressure and flow, they should be used to complement, not replace, clinical judgment.

Wherever possible, the numbers generated by monitoring should be graphed. Rapid scanning of columns of numbers does not facilitate appreciation of subtle trends. However, graphic recordings of vital signs, particularly the pulse pressure, can be extremely helpful.

ECG MONITORING

Continuous monitoring of heart rate and rhythm is essential in critically ill or injured patients. The heart rate may correlate to some degree with the amount of hypovolemia present. Thus, if a high pulse rate is falling during treatment, this is usually a sign that the blood volume is returning to normal; however, if the pulse rate is relatively low despite severe hypovolemia and a very low cardiac output, this usually indicates an intrinsic cardiac problem.

Arrhythmias are frequent in critically ill or injured patients. Tachyarrhythmias may serve as a warning of impending complications, such as congestive heart failure or sepsis,[47] or they may represent the first sign of hypovolemia or pulmonary embolism. However, as recently emphasized by Little,[48] in the presence of tissue trauma, the pulse rate response to hypovolemia tends to be somewhat blunted.

INTRAARTERIAL BLOOD PRESSURE

If there is any difficulty obtaining a consistent and clear cuff blood pressure, and if the patient's condition is not improving with therapy, an intraarterial catheter should be inserted. In treating patients with shock, it is extremely important to be able to follow changes in blood pressure accurately. Although arterial lines are indicated primarily for continuous monitoring of blood pressure, they also are often used to facilitate frequent arterial blood sampling.

The systolic pressure obtained via a radial artery line is often at least 10 to 20 mmHg higher than central aortic or cuff blood pressure. This discrepancy occurs because of the peripheral buildup of pressure waves proximal to small arterioles. Thus as the arterial pressure pulse wave passes to the periphery (1) the ascending limb of the pressure wave becomes steeper, (2) the systolic pressure becomes higher, and (3) the diastolic pressure becomes lower. Nevertheless, mean blood pressure determinations via a radial artery catheter usually reflect mean central aortic pressures quite well. However, if there is excessive proximal vasoconstriction, the mean radial artery pressure may be significantly lower than the mean central aortic pressure.

The radial artery is generally the preferred site for insertion of an intraarterial catheter because of its accessibility. Complications of ischemia to the fingers or thumb are quite rare, particularly if (1) an Allen's test done with a Doppler flowmeter reveals that the ulnar artery and palmar arch are patent, (2) the intraarterial catheter is small (20 gauge) and is inserted percutaneously, and (3) the catheter is removed within 48 to 72 h.

Thrombosis of the radial artery occurs in 30 to 40 percent of patients with an indwelling percutaneous catheter, but these vessels frequently recanalize.[49] Nevertheless, transient vascular insufficiency with necrosis of the tip of the thumb and/or index finger occasionally occurs. Factors that increase the risk of this problem include hypotension and use of the intraarterial catheter for more than 6 days. Thromboembolic complications are also more likely with an 18-gauge catheter than with a 20-gauge catheter.

Catheter-related sepsis (CRS) is demonstrated by (1) positive blood cultures from another site,· (2) cultures from the catheter tip or intracutaneous portion yielding at least 10 to 15 colonies of the same organism, and (3) no other apparent source of infection. The incidence of CRS with radial artery catheters is about 4 percent.[50] Sepsis is more likely to occur with cutdowns and if the catheter is left in place for more than 4 days. The pressure transducer or flushing solutions also can become infected if they are left in place for more than 48 h.

URINE OUTPUT AND CONTENT

The kidney has been referred to as the "window of the viscera" because renal perfusion, as reflected by the urine output, can be a rather accurate gauge of vital organ blood flow. Indeed, renal blood flow and urine output often fall long before other vital organ perfusion is significantly reduced.

Correlation with Cardiac Output. With any decrease in cardiac output or blood pressure, there is usually a prompt renal artery and arteriolar vasoconstriction resulting in a rapid reduction in renal blood flow (RBF). In addition, with a decrease in RBF, blood tends to be diverted toward the less numerous glomeruli in the juxtamedullary portion of the renal cortex. This results in a further decrease in glomerular filtration. Since the juxtamedullary glomeruli have long loops of Henle, there is increased absorption of water and sodium from the glomerular filtrate. As a result, urine sodium concentrations will tend to fall and urine osmolality will tend to rise as hypovolemia develops. These changes in urine composition tend to occur before there is any significant change in the urine output.

Decreased perfusion pressure in the renal arterioles stimulates the juxtaglomerular apparatus to secrete renin. Renin enzymatically converts angiotensinogen in the blood to angiotensin I. This in turn is converted by angiotensin-converting enzyme (ACE) in the lung into angiotensin II. This very potent octapeptide can cause severe vasoconstriction, and it also stimulates increased aldosterone release from the adrenal cortex. Aldosterone is a powerful mineralocorticoid hormone that causes the kidney to retain sodium, bicarbonate, and water. The four most important stimuli to renin secretion are sympathetic stimulation, hypotension, decreased sodium in distal tubule fluid, and hyperkalemia.

The other important hormone that causes renal retention of water is antidiuretic hormone (ADH) from the posterior pituitary gland. The four main stimuli to the release of ADH in order of their potency are nausea, abdominal pain, hypovolemia, and hyperosmolality. It is important to note that a patient who is hypovolemic and has hypotonic plasma will tend to retain water and his or her plasma will become even more hypotonic.

As a result of all these changes, the urine output often falls before other signs of impaired tissue perfusion become apparent. On the other hand, if the urine output is adequate without diuretics, it suggests that vital organ perfusion is also adequate. However, in patients with sepsis or severe trauma, urine flow may be normal despite a renal blood flow as low as 25 percent of normal.[51]

Urine Flow in Sepsis. Monitoring urine output is extremely helpful in detecting fluid deficits. Although severe sepsis often causes a reduction in urine output, early sepsis may be associated with an "inappropriate" polyuria.[51] Polyuria is termed *inappropriate* if urine output is greater than normal despite an absolute or relative hypovolemia. The polyuria may be particularly deceptive because many aspects of the clinical picture in severe sepsis suggest that the patient is overloaded with fluid. These patients tend to be edematous, have been given large quantities of fluids, often have rales over much of their lungs, and often have a chest x-ray that shows evidence of increasing congestion or even early pulmonary edema. Under such circumstances, the polyuria may appear to be appropriate. However, if the intravenous fluid intake is restricted without close observation of the patient, the blood pressure and urine output may fall abruptly and oliguric renal failure may develop.

Urine Sodium. One way to detect an "inappropriate" polyuria is to check the urine sodium concentrations in spot or random samples. If the polyuria is "appropriate," the urine sodium level will tend to exceed 40 to 60 mEq/liter. If the polyuria is "inappropriate," the urine sodium concentration will tend to fall to less than 10 to 20 mEq/liter as the patient becomes more hypovolemic. If the urine sodium concentration falls to less than 10 to 20 mEq/liter, the kidneys are usually functioning quite well but are probably not being perfused adequately.

Urine Osmolality. A urine osmolality greater than 450 to 500 mosmol/kg or a urine-to-serum osmolality ratio greater than 1.5 is usually a reliable index of dehydration and/or reduced renal perfusion. Although the reduced renal blood flow under such circumstances may occasionally be caused by renal artery stenosis or cardiac failure, in most instances it is due to hypovolemia.

Standard Renal Function Tests. Urine output, blood urea nitrogen (BUN), and serum creatinine are generally used as the standard clinical renal function tests; however, they may not reflect significant degrees of dysfunction in critically ill patients, especially if large quantities of fluid are given and the patient has a high urine output. Of the patients we have monitored in the ICU with a good urine output (at least 1.0 ml/kg/h) and normal BUN and serum creatinine levels, 40 percent have had a creatinine clearance of less than 40 ml/min.[52]

Septic patients often have a greatly reduced creatinine excretion, which may be less than 600 mg/d (versus 1500 mg/d in normal patients). As a consequence, the correlation between serum creatinine and creatinine clearance can be very poor, and urine creatinine should be determined at the same time as the serum creatinine to calculate creatinine clearance. Standard formulas attempting to calculate creatinine clearance without measuring urine values are extremely inaccurate in critically ill or injured patients.

CENTRAL VENOUS PRESSURE

Preload is the end-diastolic stretch of a muscle fiber. The intrinsic ability of the heart to adjust its output in response to changing amounts of inflowing blood was expounded by Starling in his Linacre lecture, which was published in 1918.[53] He and his associates noted that increases in diastolic volume (fiber stretch) determine the magnitude of each succeeding cardiac contraction. They further concluded that "the mechanical energy set free on passage from the resting to the contracted state depends on the available chemical active surfaces on the length of the myocardial muscle fiber." Thus the greater the end-diastolic stretch of a muscle fiber, the harder it will contract.

In the 1950s and 1960s, the central venous pressure (CVP) began to be used increasingly to monitor the filling of the heart. Although the CVP is determined by blood volume, vascular tone, and the heart's pumping action, vascular tone and cardiac contractility tend to remain relatively constant, at least for short periods of time, and consequently, changes in the CVP during a fluid challenge can provide important information on the preload of the heart.

The normal CVP is considered to be about 0 to 5 mmHg, and a CVP exceeding 15 mmHg is generally considered to be high and may be evidence of fluid overload. However, other factors that affect the CVP level besides the blood volume include right-sided heart contractility, the amount of systemic arterial and venous constriction, and the resistance to blood flow in the lungs. Therefore, when monitoring the CVP, the response to a fluid challenge (usually 3 ml/kg of a balanced electrolyte solution over 10 min) is much more important than the actual CVP level.[54] Nevertheless, some physicians still say that if the CVP is above 15 mmHg, fluid administration should be stopped because the patient is probably overloaded.

In most instances, the outputs of the right and left ventricles are quite similar. Consequently, changes in the filling pressures in the right side of the heart normally correlate fairly well with changes in filling pressures of the left side of the heart. However, in a number of instances, the CVP and pulmonary artery wedge pressure (PAWP) may be quite disparate. For example, myocardial infarction may transiently produce an isolated acute left ventricular failure that can cause a low CVP and high PAWP.[55,56] Such patients may develop acute pulmonary edema despite a CVP that is initially less than 5.0 cmH$_2$O. It is important to note that this is more likely to occur if hypotensive patients with a very low CVP are given large quantities of fluid rapidly without considering the possibility of isolated left ventricular failure.

The CVP in critically ill patients is extremely variable and frequently correlates poorly with fluid needs. I have seen a number of patients, particularly those with severe sepsis or respiratory failure, who have had a CVP above 20 cmH$_2$O but had a relatively low PAWP and responded to a fluid challenge with an increased cardiac output and improved tissue perfusion with little or no change in the CVP.[57] In such instances, the high CVP is probably due to an increased pulmonary vascular resistance. Consequently, one should not rely on absolute CVP levels to determine fluid needs, particularly in patients with adult respiratory distress syndrome (ARDS) or pulmonary hypertension.

The use of high tidal volumes and large amounts of PEEP may increase the PAWP and CVP. This must be taken into account if the patient cannot be taken off the ventilator while the CVP or PAWP is being measured. As a general rule, if more than 10 cmH$_2$O of PEEP is used, a third of the PEEP pressure should be subtracted from the CVP or PAWP to obtain a "corrected" or "true" value.

The CVP and PAWP also may be deceptively high if the patient is receiving large doses of vasopressor drugs. The arterial vasoconstriction caused by vasopressors increases the resistance against which the heart must pump, thereby tending to reduce cardiac output. Increased venous constriction also reduces vascular capacity, thereby increasing venous return to the heart. Both these factors will tend to increase diastolic volumes and pressures, even if the patient is hypovolemic.

As mentioned previously, the response of the CVP or PAWP to a fluid challenge can provide much more important information than isolated readings. If a fluid challenge of 3 ml/kg of a balanced electrolyte solution is given over 10 min and it improves the blood pressure, cardiac output, stroke volume, and/or left ventricular stroke work index (LVSWI) with little or no rise in CVP or PAWP, further fluid can generally be given safely and with benefit. On the other hand, if the fluid challenge causes no rise in blood pressure or cardiac output and the CVP and PAWP rise abruptly by more than 5.0 cmH$_2$O and/or remain more than 2.0 mmHg above the baseline value after another 10 min, further fluid challenges are probably hazardous. Additional fluid should probably not be given until the CVP and PAWP fall back to within 2.0 mmHg of the baseline value.

Initially, CVP was measured with a water manometer. Although this technique is relatively easy to perform and the apparatus is inexpensive, it usually takes several minutes for each reading to be performed, and the results may vary by 3 to 5 cmH$_2$O between individuals taking such readings. Furthermore, Mann et al.[58] demonstrated that manometrically determined CVP measurements tend to average 4 to 6 cmH$_2$O higher than levels obtained with a transducer. Consequently, CVP is now generally measured electronically and continuously.

It is also important to note that the CVP is a pressure measurement and hence does not directly indicate preload, which is determined by the end-diastolic volume. If the heart is poorly compliant, such as with a myocardial infarction or hypertrophy, the filling pressure may be high despite a low filling (end-diastolic) volume. The reverse also may be true at times. In other words, the CVP and PAWP may be low, but the right ventricular end-diastolic volume may be high.[59,60]

PULMONARY ARTERY PRESSURES

Pulmonary Artery Wedge Pressure (PAWP). There are many circumstances, such as sepsis, chronic obstructive pulmonary disease (COPD), and ARDS, which can increase pulmonary vascular resistance so that the CVP will not adequately reflect left-sided heart filling pressures. Consequently, floatation pulmonary artery catheters to measure PAWP have been used increasingly to monitor the preload and function of the left side of the heart.

In patients with a normal pulmonary vascular bed, mitral valve, and left ventricular function, the PAWP, mean left arterial pressure, and left ventricular end-diastolic pressure will be approximately equal. In addition, for the PAWP to reflect left atrial pressure (P_{LA}) accurately, the vessels between the tip of the pulmonary artery catheter and the left atrium must be filled with blood at all times.

If the catheter tip is located in the least dependent portion of the lung (West's zone I) where alveolar pressure (P_A) is greater than pulmonary artery (P_a) and pulmonary venous (P_v) pressure, the peak pressure tracing will record alveolar pressure (P_A) rather than P_{LA}.[61] In West's zone II, where $P_a > P_A > P_v$, the pressure tracing will reflect P_a during systole and P_A during diastole. It is only in the most dependent portion of the lung (West's zone III) that $P_a > P_v > P_A$, and in this zone a PAWP tracing with the balloon occluded will reflect P_v and P_{LA} rather than P_A throughout the ventilatory cycle.[62] In addition to having the pulmonary artery catheter tip in zone III, the mitral valve must be normal for the PAWP to adequately reflect left ventricular end-diastolic pressure.

Falsely high PAWP. In about 5 to 15 percent of our patients with pulmonary artery catheter monitoring, the recorded PAWP is higher than the pulmonary artery diastolic pressure (PADP).[57] The PAWP is normally at least 1 to 2 mmHg lower than the PADP, except transiently in severe mitral insufficiency. A recorded PAWP that is continuously higher than the PADP is obviously erroneous, unless blood is flowing backwards from the left atrium to the right atrium. The PAWP will appear to be higher than the PADP if the catheter tip is in West's zone II and, therefore, reflects alveolar pressure from the ventilator rather than the pulmonary venous pressure. This can occur if the catheter was malpositioned or if the catheter was positioned correctly initially but the size of zone III was reduced by increasing PEEP and/or allowing hypovolemia to develop.

Another factor that can make the PAWP seem higher than the PADP at times is the use of digital readouts. Because digital readouts often average the highest readings for systolic pressures and the lowest readings for diastolic pressures over a 3- to 5-s span, wide variation in pressures can cause deceptive mean digital readings. Pressures taken off individual waveforms are usually much more accurate than digital readouts, particularly if there are wide swings in ventilatory and pulmonary artery pressures.

Clinical uses. PAWP and cardiac output can be particularly helpful in monitoring (1) patients with suspected cardiopulmonary disorders, (2) hypotensive patients with clinically unclear volume status, (3) during afterload reduction in patients with impaired myocardial function, (4) during treatment of shock in patients with acute myocardial infarction, sepsis, or ARDS, and (5) to differentiate between cardiac and noncardiac causes of diffuse pulmonary infiltrates.

Maintenance of optimal ventricular filling intraoperatively and postoperatively may be of help in reducing postoperative complications. The optimal PAWP on a Starling curve is determined by progressively raising the PAWP to that level at which the cardiac output reaches a maximum without an abrupt rise in the PAWP. In high-risk surgical patients, maintenance of the PAWP within 4 mmHg of the optimal value during surgery and postoperatively may greatly reduce complication rates.[63]

PADP-PAWP gradients. The PADP-PAWP gradient is normally only 1 to 2 mmHg. If the PADP is more than 5 mmHg higher than the PAWP, the patient usually has an increased pulmonary vascular resistance (PVR). As lung water increases or the patient becomes more hypoxic, the PADP-PAWP gradient tends to increase. As a general rule, the greater the PADP-PAWP gradient, the higher is the mortality rate, particularly in patients with ARDS. In one series, the patients with a PADP-PAWP gradient less than 5 mmHg had a mortality rate of 30 percent, but if the PADP-PAWP gradient was greater than 5 mmHg, the mortality rate was 83 percent.[64]

Clinical correlations. Although there has been some concern that the PAWP is overused, such monitoring can be extremely helpful in critically ill patients, particularly those with severe pulmonary problems and those not responding favorably to standard fluid therapy.

At least three major studies have compared the accuracy of clinical estimates of pulmonary artery pressure (PAP), PAWP, and cardiac output with the values obtained from a pulmonary artery catheter.[65–67] Clinical assessments of PAWP (in terms of whether they were low, normal, or high) were only 47 ± 20 percent correct, and the estimates of cardiac output (in terms of whether they were low, normal, or high) were only 48 ± 5 percent correct.[67] Additionally, in two of the studies, the information obtained after pulmonary artery catheterization prompted major changes in therapy in 48 and 58 percent of the patients, respectively.[65,66]

In 1980, DelGuerico and Cohn[68] conducted a study in 148 consecutive elderly patients who had been cleared for surgery by standard clinical assessment. However, only 13.5 percent of these patients had normal hemodynamic, respiratory, and oxygen transport functions when measured invasively. When the patients with inadequate cardiopulmonary function had surgery without correction of these variables, morbidity and mortality rates were very high.

Some investigators have had an interest in determining effective pulmonary capillary pressure (P_c) using the pressure profile after pulmonary artery occlusion.[49] As the pulmonary artery is occluded by a balloon, the distal pressure falls rapidly and then more slowly to the PAWP level. The junction of fast and slow pressure decline represents the P_c, which is probably the primary factor determining the rate of formation of extravascular fluid in the lungs. In most instances, the P_c is equal to the PAWP plus about 40 percent of the PADP-PAWP difference. Thus a patient with a PAP of 50/20 mmHg and a PAWP of 10 mmHg would probably have a P_c of about 14 mmHg.

Even when the PAWP is measured accurately, variances in left ventricular compliance may result in a poor correlation between the PAWP and left ventricular end-diastolic volume as measured by radionuclide angiography. In such circumstances, the responses of the blood pressure, stroke volume (SV), and PAWP to fluid challenges are far more informative than absolute PAWP levels.

Complications. Pulmonary artery lines can be associated with numerous complications related to both the catheter insertion and its presence in the pulmonary artery. Complications associated with catheter insertion include pneumothorax (uncommon with internal jugular vein insertion), air embolism, and arrhythmias.[69] Because of the rare (3 percent) but grave consequences of pulmonary artery catheter insertion causing a right bundle branch block (RBBB) in patients with preexisting left bundle branch block (LBBB), standby external and transvenous pacemaker equipment should be readily available during pulmonary artery catheterization if the patient already has a LBBB.[70]

Complications related to the continued presence of a pulmonary artery catheter include infections, thromboembolism, and rupture of the pulmonary artery. The incidence of catheter-related sepsis is about 2 percent, but this is increased if the patient is bacteremic or if the catheter is left in place for more than 3 days.[71]

The most serious of all complications related to pulmonary artery catheters is rupture of the pulmonary artery resulting in massive pulmonary hemorrhage. Such ruptures are usually caused by using more than the minimal amount of air to obtain a wedge waveform. The massive bleeding that is apt to result may be preceded by small amounts of hemoptysis, and it is more likely to occur in elderly patients with pulmonary hypertension.[72]

Nevertheless, errors in management due to inadequate understanding of the physiologic data obtained are common. Other problems using the data include reliance on displayed digital pressures and use of *absolute numbers* rather than *trends* or *changes*.

Mixed Venous Oxygen Saturation (Sv_{O_2}). The potential value of continuous monitoring of mixed venous (pulmonary artery) oxygen saturation (Sv_{O_2}) has been recognized for many years. For the catheter to function optimally, the catheter tip should be in the proximal portion of one of the pulmonary arteries. This can be determined by positioning the catheter so that a good PAWP tracing is obtained with inflation of the catheter balloon to 75 to 95 percent of its total capacity. Pulmonary artery blood gases also should be checked against the continuous Sv_{O_2} catheter at least once every 24 h. If there is more than a 4 percent difference in saturation, the system should be recalibrated.[73]

Mixed venous oxygen saturation (Sv_{O_2}) reflects the balance between oxygen supply and overall tissue oxygen demand. Normally, the Sv_{O_2} is about 70 to 75 percent. If $\dot{V}_{O_2}$ is relatively constant, reductions in Sv_{O_2} values should reflect decreases in cardiac output or arterial O_2 content.

This can be seen from the Fick equation, which is

$$\dot{Q} \text{ (liters/min)} = \frac{\dot{V}_{O_2} \text{ (ml/min)}}{[Ca_{O_2} - Cv_{O_2} \text{ (ml/100 ml)}] \ (10)}$$

$$= \frac{\dot{V}_{O_2}}{(Sa_{O_2} - Sv_{O_2}) \ (1.34) \ (Hb) \ (10)}$$

The relationship between cardiac output ($\dot{Q}$) and Sv_{O_2} does not hold true in situations when $\dot{V}_{O_2}$ is changing rapidly (shivering, agitation, sepsis, etc.). If $\dot{V}_{O_2}$ remains relatively constant, there is a good correlation between changes in the Sv_{O_2} and changes in the cardiac output. Furthermore, if the Sv_{O_2} and the patient's clinical condition appear to be stable, the number of blood gas determinations and cardiac output measurements can generally be reduced.

An Sv_{O_2} fall of more than 5 percent may be an early warning either of a reduced cardiac output or decreased oxygenation of blood.[74] A decrease in Sv_{O_2} of greater than 10 percent, particularly to values less than 60 percent, usually indicates inadequate oxygen delivery to tissues. An Sv_{O_2} less than 50 percent is often associated with hypotension and increasing lactic acidosis.

If the cause of a low or falling Sv_{O_2} is not clear, cardiac output, arterial blood gases, and hemoglobin should be measured to determine the cause. Thus an Sv_{O_2} change can be quite sensitive, but it is not specific. Continuous Sv_{O_2} monitoring also can be helpful in evaluating the efficacy of various therapeutic interventions, especially those designed to correct an oxygen supply/demand imbalance.[59] Sv_{O_2} monitoring may be particularly helpful in patients with poor left ventricular function, severe acute respiratory failure, or multisystem failure.

Although use of the Sv_{O_2} catheter can be cost-effective by reducing the number of arterial and venous blood gas and cardiac output determinations, it has a number of limitations. Routine use is not justified in all patients selected for pulmonary artery catheter monitoring, and the catheter is more expensive than a conventional pulmonary artery catheter.

Right Ventricular End-Diastolic Volume. Although measurements of ventricular volumes more accurately reflect preload, until relatively recently, this has only been possible clinically with echocardiography or radionuclide angiography. Recently, a modification of the flow-directed pulmonary artery catheter has been developed that allows rapid and frequent measurements of right ventricular end-systolic volume (RVESV) and right ventricular end-diastolic volume (RVEDV).

RVESV and right ventricular ejection fraction (RVEF) can be determined with a modified pulmonary artery catheter equipped with a fast-response thermistor and with electrodes for an intracardiac ECG. Cardiac output (CO) and RVEF are measured by the thermodilution technique. The injection of the thermal indicator is started at end inspiration in ventilated patients, as suggested by Daper et al.,[75] to minimize variability of CO and RVEF measurements. Several investigators have validated the right ventricular volumes obtained with this technique by using concurrent radionuclide angiocardiography, two-dimensional echocardiography, and contrast ventriculography.[75-77]

Several studies have suggested that right ventricular volumes provide a better index of the patient's volume status than PAWP determinations. Martyn et al.[78] have shown that cardiac output correlated best with RVEDV ($r = 0.75$) and only weakly with PAWP ($r = 0.32$) in acutely burned patients. In a study of 41 critically ill patients who were fluid challenged, Reuse et al.[79] showed that changes in stroke volume index (SVI) correlated with right ventricular end-diastolic volume index (RVEDVI), CVP, and PAWP. However, when RVEDVI exceeded 140 ml/m², no further increases in SVI or cardiac index (CI) occurred with volume loading. Earlier work by Calvin et al.[80] also demonstrated that PAWP did not provide a reliable assessment of left ventricular preload or accurate prediction of the response to volume expansion.

In a recent study by Diebel et al.,[59] regression analysis of 131 hemodynamic studies in 29 critically ill patients demonstrated that CI correlated better with RVEDVI ($r = 0.61$) than did PAWP ($r = 0.42$). Comparisons of PAWP and RVEDVI also showed that misleading information concerning filling volumes was provided by the PAWP at some time in 15 (52 percent) of these patients.

In 15 patients given 22 fluid challenges, those with a high PAWP (≥ 18 mmHg) actually "responded" favorably with a rise in CI more frequently than patients with a low PAWP (< 12 mmHg). However, the patients with a high PAWP who responded favorably had a RVEDVI of less than 138 ml/m². All 8 patients with a RVEDVI of less than 90 ml/m² responded with a rise in CI, and all 7 patients with a RVEDVI of 139 ml/m² or more failed to respond regardless of their PAWP level. Thus RVEDVI more accurately predicted preload-recruitable increases in cardiac output than did the PAWP.

CARDIAC OUTPUT

Indicator (Dye) Dilution Technique. Until the thermodilution technique with pulmonary artery catheters was developed, cardiac output (CO) was usually measured by a dye dilution technique described by Hamilton et al.[81] in 1932. With this technique, a measured amount of dye (usually indocyanine green) is injected rapidly via a CVP catheter, and arterial blood, which is removed by a constant-withdrawal syringe, is assayed by a photodensitometer. The concentrations of dye in the arterial blood each second are used to construct a curve from which the CO can be calculated quite accurately.

Thermodilution. Cardiac output is now usually measured clinically by a thermal indicator dilution technique using iced saline rather than dye and a pulmonary artery catheter that contains a calibrated thermocouple 10 to 25 cm upstream from the site of injection. For greatest accuracy, there should be less than a 5 percent difference between serial determinations of CO, and at least three values should be averaged. Mean values obtained with a carefully performed thermodilution technique correlate relatively well with the Fick and dye dilution techniques as long as the volume and temperature of the injectate are precisely known and the CO is not very high or very low. However, the differences between thermodilution and dye dilution studies often exceed 15 to 25 percent if the cardiac output is high or low or if circulation times are abnormal.

Fick Technique. If oxygen consumption is determined by indirect calorimetry and the arterio-venous oxygen difference [$C(a\text{-}v)_{O_2}$] is calculated from arterial and mixed venous gases, the cardiac output ($\dot{Q}$) can be calculated using the principle postulated by Adolf Eugene Fick, a German physiologist (1829–1901). For example, if the oxygen consumption ($\dot{V}_{O_2}$) is 250 ml/min, if the arterial oxygen content (Ca_{O_2}) is 13.0 ml/dl, and if the mixed venous oxygen content (Cv_{O_2}) is 8.0 ml/dl, the $C(a\text{-}v)_{O_2}$ is 5 ml/dl, or 50 ml/liter. Therefore, $\dot{Q} = 250/50 = 5$ liters/min.

Sv_{O_2} and Pulse Oximetry. An interesting spinoff of monitoring Sv_{O_2} is the possibility of measuring CO almost continuously using a modified Fick principle. With steady-state hemoglobin concentrations and hemoglobin oxygen affinity, hemoglobin oxygen saturation and blood oxygen content correlate very closely. Therefore, pulse oximetry and Sv_{O_2} measurement can be used to determine arterio-venous oxygen content differences continuously. If this value is coupled with continuous assessment of oxygen consumption from measurements of inspired and expired gases, substitution of the known values into the Fick equation allows continuous computer determination of the cardiac output.

Noninvasive Techniques. The main advantage of noninvasive cardiac monitoring is its safety and lack of discomfort to the patient.[82] Because of the risk of pulmonary artery rupture, catheter sepsis, arrhythmias, and death and the relatively minor benefits achieved by some physicians with this monitoring, Robin[82] has proposed that the practice of pulmonary artery catheterization be halted.

The two most frequently used noninvasive techniques for measuring cardiac output include Doppler studies and thoracic bioimpedance. These techniques also have the advantage that they can be used to monitor CO continuously. Therefore, even if the values determined by these techniques are not very accurate, they can still be used to monitor relative changes in overall tissue blood flow.

Doppler studies. Continuous-wave Doppler ultrasound can be used to measure CO by placing a Doppler transducer in the suprasternal notch, aiming it toward the ascending aorta, and measuring aortic blood flow velocity. The aortic diameter, determined from a nomogram, is used with the measured aortic systolic blood flow velocity to calculate stroke volume (SV). This is multiplied by the heart rate to calculate the Doppler cardiac output. Clinical studies have shown that the correlation coefficient (*r*) between Doppler and thermodilution CO values is 0.85 to 0.97.[83]

Thoracic bioimpedance. Thoracic bioimpedance devices measure CO by placing two opposing pairs of surface ECG electrodes on the neck and two opposing pairs of surface ECG electrodes on the lower chest at the level of the xiphoid process in the midcoronal plane.[82] The outer pairs of electrodes transmit a 70-kHz, 2.5-mA current into the thoracic tissue, and the current is then measured with the inner pairs of electrodes. The resistance to the injected current depends on the fluid and electrolyte characteristics of the thoracic volume and will vary with the SV. Pulsatile changes in thoracic electrical resistance (bioimpedance) are timed to ventricular electrical depolarization and mechanical systole and then are used to calculate the SV. Clinical studies have shown that the correlation coefficient between thoracic bioimpedance and thermodilution CO values is 0.83 to 0.90.[82]

Thoracic electrical bioimpedance (TEB) is currently the only noninvasive method for on-line determination of CO continuously with little technical effort. Most critics of TEB admit that even if there is a weak correlation with absolute CO values, this technique accurately reflects trends.

PULMONARY AND SYSTEMIC VASCULAR RESISTANCE

With mean pulmonary artery pressure (mPAP), PAWP, and CO data available from a pulmonary artery catheter, one can calculate pulmonary vascular resistance (PVR) by the following formula:

$$PVR = \frac{mPAP - PAWP}{CO} \times 80$$

Normal values are 80 to 160 dyn·s·cm^{-5}.

If the mean arterial BP (mBP), CVP, and CO are available, one can calculate the systemic vascular resistance (SVR) by the following formula:

$$SVR = \frac{mBP - CVP}{CO} \times 80$$

Normal values are 800 to 1500 dyn·s·cm^{-5}. If the SVR and PVR are very high, one may wish to use vasodilators to reduce them to normal levels.

ACID-BASE CHANGES

The characteristic acid-base abnormality in established shock is a lactic (metabolic) acidosis. However, early shock is often characterized by hyperventilation producing a respiratory alkalosis. Terminally, the patient may have a combined metabolic and respiratory acidosis.

Respiratory Alkalosis. *Stimuli to ventilation.* An increasing respiratory alkalosis is an important sign that a patient's condition is deteriorating, and it should stimulate a search for hypoxemia, sepsis, hypovolemia, or pulmonary emboli. Sepsis and shock can be very powerful stimuli to ventilation. Therefore, arterial blood gas analyses in septic patients just beginning to go into shock generally reveal a low arterial P_{CO_2} (25 to 35 mmHg), a relatively normal bicarbonate level, and an elevated pH. This initial respiratory alkalosis is generally not a compensatory mechanism, but rather a nonspecific response to stress. If the effects of the trauma, shock, or sepsis are not rapidly corrected, however, and oxygen consumption falls below critical levels, metabolic acidosis develops, causing a further increase in the hyperventilation. If the arterial P_{CO_2} is driven below 20 mmHg, this severe hypocapnia may in itself cause some hemodynamic impairment, especially of blood flow to the brain.

Tachypnea is often a valuable sign that an otherwise stable patient may be deteriorating. Noticeable breathing is not normal, yet it may initially be interpreted as "good" ventilation. If breathing is clearly noticeable, the patient usually has a minute ventilation that is 1.5 to 2.0 times normal, and the work of respiration is probably 2 to 3 times normal.

Work of breathing. The work of breathing compared with normal can be estimated by multiplying the respiratory rate by the effort with each breath and dividing by 10. The effort with each breath is 1.0 with normal quiet breathing, 2.0 with noticeable breathing, and 3.0 to 4.0 if there is obviously increased effort with each breath. Thus a patient breathing 40 times a minute and working hard with each breath is working 12 to 16 times harder than normal. As a general rule, a patient cannot maintain a work of breathing greater than 6 times normal for more than a few hours, at which time a respiratory arrest may suddenly occur. On the other hand, if a patient with shock or sepsis is not hyperventilating to some degree, one should suspect that the patient may be developing ventilatory failure.

Arteriovenous CO$_2$ differences. It is important to emphasize that during severe shock there may be large differences between the arterial and central or mixed venous P_{CO_2}. Normally, the arteriovenous CO_2 difference is only 6 to 7 mmHg. In severe shock, the difference may exceed 20 to 30 mmHg.[84] During cardiopulmonary resuscitation, the arteriovenous P_{CO_2} difference tends to be even higher. If the venous P_{CO_2} is high, giving bicarbonate will produce a more severe intracellular acidosis. The administered bicarbonate will further increase P_{CO_2} levels, and the CO_2 moves into cells easily while bicarbonate does not. In addition, with very low blood flow to the lungs, the end-tidal P_{CO_2} will be very low and is often much lower than the arterial P_{CO_2}.

Metabolic Alkalosis. Metabolic alkalosis may be found in many critically ill and injured patients prior to their going into severe shock. Some of the more frequently recognized causes of metabolic alkalosis in the ICU include administration of large amounts of antacids to reduce gastric acidity, hypokalemia due to excessive diuresis, the use of corticosteroids, and metabolism of citrate (from blood transfusions) or lactate (from Ringer's lactate). If there is also a respiratory alkalosis because of CNS or hepatic disease or sepsis, the resulting severe combined alkalosis may be fatal.[85]

Metabolic Acidosis. Metabolic (lactic) acidosis often indicates a fairly advanced state of hypoperfusion or impaired cell metabolism. Normal oxygen consumption ($\dot{V}_{O_2}$) at rest is about 110 to 160 ml/min/m². As shock progresses, impaired cellular metabolism associated with a reduction in $\dot{V}_{O_2}$ to below 100 ml/min/m² eventually results in the development of metabolic (lactic) acidosis. This acidosis first develops intracellularly and then at the capillary and venous levels. A metabolic acidosis in arterial blood occurs later. Indeed, alterations in cell membrane potential and intracellular pH may occur long before changes are apparent in the arterial blood gas samples. Nevertheless, blood lactate determinations can be very helpful as an indicator of the progress of the resuscitation and the patient's prognosis.[19] It also has been shown that patients with elevated lactate levels are more apt to have a rise in their $\dot{V}_{O_2}$ when D_{O_2} is increased than patients with normal lactate levels.

In the early phases of metabolic acidosis, the acid-base abnormality can usually be corrected by improving tissue perfusion. Later, however, sodium bicarbonate may be necessary, particularly if the arterial pH falls below 7.10. If cell metabolism continues to deteriorate, the amount of bicarbonate needed for correction increases almost geometrically.

Combined Metabolic and Respiratory Acidosis. Ordinarily, the lungs excrete carbon dioxide readily. However, in the terminal stages of prolonged shock, pulmonary blood flow and/or the number of functional pulmonary capillaries can be so critically reduced that it may be impossible for the patient to eliminate carbon dioxide properly despite a minute ventilation that is 2 to 3 times normal. If a combined metabolic and respiratory acidosis is allowed to develop, the chances for ultimate survival are extremely poor.[86] A rise in the venous P_{CO_2} with an increasing arteriovenous P_{CO_2} usually indicates a severe reduction in perfusion of functional pulmonary tissue.

BLOOD VOLUME

Blood volume determinations as guides to the rate or amount of fluid administration are seldom used except during research studies, and they can be very deceptive. Blood volume normally varies widely from patient to patient. One standard deviation for blood volume in normal individuals averages about 10 percent.[54] Furthermore, the actual blood volume is not nearly as important as its dynamic relationship with vascular capacity.

Vascular capacity can change rapidly with vasoconstriction or vasodilation. For example, vasoconstriction can reduce vascular capacity by up to 25 percent, and vasodilation can increase vascular capacity by 50 percent or more. Blood volume determinations with radioiodinated serum albumin (RISA) are particularly deceptive because the normal RISA disappearance rate of 6.0 to 8.0 percent per hour may rise to more than 30 to 35 percent per hour in patients with shock or severe sepsis. A method using serial sampling every 10 min can provide more accurate results than "one-shot" techniques by allowing one to plot a logarithmic disappearance curve and thereby determine the concentration of the marker at time zero.

TREATMENT

CORRECTION OF THE PRIMARY PROCESS

Although it is sometimes necessary to treat patients who are in shock without knowing the initial or primary cause of the problem, a strong effort should be made to establish an accurate etiologic diagnosis as soon as possible. Left uncorrected for more than a few hours, problems such as intraabdominal abscesses, necrotic bowel, a torn spleen, or a ruptured ectopic pregnancy can carry an extremely high mortality rate, regardless of how well the cardiovascular, respiratory, and metabolic changes are managed.

ACTUAL RESUSCITATION

AIRWAY MANAGEMENT

Upper Airway. The most frequent cause of upper airway obstruction after trauma, particularly in unconscious victims, is prolapse of the tongue into the oropharynx. Teeth, dental plates, vomitus, or blood also may be present in the upper airway. If the patient is unconscious, a finger may be inserted into the mouth and oral pharynx to remove any foreign bodies. A metal tonsil sucker is ideal for removing blood or thick secretions from the mouth and pharynx.

Since the genioglossus connects the tongue and the mandible, moving the mandible forward will pull the tongue anteriorly up and away from the posterior pharynx and open the airway. Three maneuvers to pull or push the mandible forward include the chin lift, jaw lift, and jaw thrust. The chin lift involves grasping the chin between the thumb and index finger and lifting it forward. The jaw lift is accomplished by placing the thumb inside the mouth and grasping the lower incisors and anterior mandible and lifting them forward. The jaw thrust involves placing the thumbs of both hands behind the angle of the mandible and the fingers along the sides of the jaw to push it forward.

A soft nasopharyngeal tube placed through a nostril down into the hypopharynx also may be helpful in providing an upper airway, particularly if the mouth cannot be opened properly. It also may help one to aspirate secretions from the hypopharynx.

Lower Airway. *Esophageal obturator airway (EOA).* If a patient has inadequate ventilation prior to reaching the hospital, and if an endotracheal tube cannot be inserted, an EOA may be used; however, insertion of this tube must be done very carefully because it can cause injury to the esophagus. The EOA consists of a face mask and an attached tube that is hollow and has multiple holes in the portion that lies in the mouth and pharynx. The tube is inserted via the mouth into the esophagus below the level of the carina of the trachea. When the balloon at its tip is inflated, the distal esophagus is occluded. If air is then blown into the tube of the attached face mask, it enters the mouth and pharynx and then must enter the larynx and lungs because the esophagus is occluded.

Esophagogastric tube airway (EGTA). The EGTA is a newer modification of the EOA that allows a nasogastric tube to be passed through its center to empty the stomach. If the EOA or EGTA is to be removed in an unconscious patient, an endotracheal tube should be inserted prior to its removal to prevent aspiration as the EOA is removed.

Endotracheal intubation. Endotracheal intubation is preferable to mask ventilation in severely traumatized patients because it (1) allows control of ventilation, (2) helps protect against aspiration of gastric or oral contents, and (3) provides a means for removal of tracheal secretions. Although endotracheal intubation can be lifesaving, if it is done incorrectly or if excessive ventilatory pressures are used, it can cause a cardiac arrest (Table 6–1).

Orotracheal intubation. As a general rule, one should make at least one or two attempts to insert an orotracheal tube in patients who are not ventilating adequately, even if injury to the cervical spine has not been ruled out. However, if an orotracheal tube is to be inserted in someone with even a vague possibility of cervical spine injury, someone else must stabilize the head in the midline, and the intubation must be done carefully with little or no motion of the patient's neck.

TABLE 6–1. Causes of Cardiac Arrest During or Just After Endotracheal Intubation

1. Severe hypoxemia during prolonged attempts at intubation, especially if no preintubation attempted with a bag and mask
2. Intubation of the esophagus
3. A properly inserted endotracheal tube moving into the right main stem bronchus
4. Excessive ventilatory pressure by hand bagging raising intrathoracic pressure and reducing further an already marginal venous return
5. Development of a tension pneumothorax
6. Systemic air embolism, especially if a penetrating lung wound and hemoptysis are present
7. Vasovagal responses—rare unless patient already had inappropriate bradycardia
8. Sudden severe respiratory alkalosis dropping ionized calcium or potassium levels too rapidly

Nasotracheal intubation. With a possible cervical spine injury, insertion of a nasotracheal tube is considered safer than orotracheal intubation by some physicians because less neck movement is required. However, a nasotracheal tube is narrower and is usually at least 5 cm longer than an orotracheal tube. Consequently, it may be much more difficult to aspirate pulmonary secretions through it. Insertion also can cause severe nasal hemorrhage at times.

Since the nasal mucosa is very sensitive, the nostril to be used should be anesthetized with cetacaine spray. If time is available, packing the nose with gauze soaked in 4% cocaine will provide even better anesthesia and will help shrink the turbinates. The tube is then passed blindly into the trachea by following the characteristic sounds made when the end of the tube is directly over the glottis and the patient is exhaling. Pulling the tongue forward may help line up the tip of the tube with the glottis.

Cricothyroidotomy. If the patient has an inadequate upper airway, is in acute respiratory distress, and an endotracheal tube cannot be inserted, a cricothyroidotomy (coniotomy) should be performed promptly. After identifying the cricothyroid membrane, which is just above the cricoid cartilage and about 1 to 2 cm below the thyroid prominence, it is incised transversely with a knife for 1.5 to 2.0 cm, and then a 6- to 7-mm tracheostomy or endotracheal tube is inserted.

There are several types of rapid insertion cricothyroidotomy sets now available. After a needle is inserted through the cricothyroid membrane, a soft wire is passed into the larynx and trachea, and then successive dilators are passed over the wire until a proper-sized cricothyroid cannula can be inserted.

In smaller patients, particularly children under the age of 10 to 12 years, even the smaller cricothyroidotomy tubes may be too big for the space, and it may be preferable to ventilate the patient through a large (8-gauge) cricothyroid needle attached to intermittent wall oxygen.

Tracheostomy. In general, a tracheostomy should not be performed to provide an emergency airway; however, if there is laryngeal injury, no other technique may be suitable for ventilating the patient.

If the upper trachea can be identified with a needle and syringe, a rapid tracheostomy insertion kit may be used to progressively dilate the needle hole over a wire.

BREATHING

Ventilatory Assistance. Ventilatory assistance is extremely important in resuscitating critically ill or injured patients, particularly if they are in shock, comatose, elderly, or have a large lung contusion, multiple rib fractures, multiple large-bone fractures, or preexisting pulmonary disease. If ventilation is still not clearly adequate after endotracheal intubation and bagging, one must rapidly examine the patient for a hemopneumothorax or distended abdomen.

Need for Increased Minute Ventilation. Patients with severe sepsis or shock typically have a minute ventilation that is more than double normal. In such patients, a "normal" minute ventilation of 6 liters is usually inadequate. If the patient has severe sepsis or shock and is not hyperventilating, one must suspect a significant ventilatory problem and provide early mechanical assistance.

Blood gases also may indicate a need for ventilatory assistance. Ventilatory assistance is generally required if (1) the arterial P_{O_2} is low and does not improve substantially with an $F_{I_{O_2}}$ of 0.50 or (2) the arterial P_{CO_2} is inappropriately high relative to the pH.

The arterial P_{CO_2} in early to moderate shock is usually 25 to 35 mmHg. If the arterial P_{CO_2} is greater than 45 mmHg and the pH is less than 7.35, the patient should be intubated and ventilation mechanically assisted. If the pH is less than 7.20 and the arterial P_{CO_2} is greater than 30 mmHg, a ventilator is probably also required; however, in patients who have severe COPD with CO_2 retention, the P_{CO_2} should not be reduced by more than 5 mmHg/h.

Problems Causing Reduced Effective Ventilation. If a tension pneumothorax is present, a large needle can be inserted into the pleural cavity through the second intercostal space in the midclavicular line to temporarily decompress the pneumothorax while a chest tube is being inserted. If a sucking chest wound is present, the sucking wound should be sealed with a sterile dressing, and a chest tube should be inserted promptly high in the midaxillary line.

If the patient is in severe acute respiratory distress and there is clinical evidence of a hemopneumothorax, it is important to insert a chest tube rapidly without waiting for a chest x-ray. Whenever a chest tube is inserted without an x-ray showing a hemopneumothorax space, the tube must be inserted high in the axilla (fourth or fifth intercostal space), and a finger should be inserted into the pleural cavity prior to inserting the chest tube. This is done to be sure that the lung is not stuck to the chest wall by adhesions and to prevent diaphragmatic or other visceral injury if the diaphragm is very high or ruptured. Once a properly functioning chest tube is in place, it should be connected to 20- to 30-cmH$_2$O suction.

Occasionally, hypotension and/or respiratory distress may be due to severe gastric dilatation, which can limit diaphragmatic motion or result in vomiting and aspiration. Consequently, a gastric tube should be inserted in virtually all trauma patients who have shock or pulmonary failure, particularly if the patient has had head or abdominal injury.

OXYGEN

Oxygenation in the lungs in critically ill or injured patients is often impaired, and if cardiac output is decreased, tissue oxygenation may be inadequate. Consequently, even if ventilation appears to be adequate, virtually all patients in shock will benefit from the administration of 100% oxygen. If wall oxygen is used, it is given at 12 liters/min, preferably by mask with a partial rebreathing bag.

All patients in shock should be given extra oxygen during the initial resuscitation to maintain an arterial P_{O_2} of at least 80 mmHg (oxyhemoglobin saturation of 95 percent). At this stage, providing sufficient oxygen to the tissues is the primary concern; oxygen toxicity is a very secondary consideration. If the patient does not respond promptly to resuscitative efforts and there is evidence of bleeding, the patient should be taken promptly to the operating room. If there is no evidence of bleeding but the blood pressure and tissue perfusion are not improving as they should with the fluid resuscitation, a pulmonary artery catheter should be inserted to monitor filling pressures and cardiac output and to obtain parameters for calculating oxygen delivery and oxygen consumption.

In critically ill or injured patients with severe hemodynamic or pulmonary failure, oxygen delivery (D_{O_2}) should be increased until oxygen consumption ($\dot{V}_{O_2}$) is either significantly above normal or no longer rises with further increases in D_{O_2}.[40,41] If the $\dot{V}_{O_2}$ does not rise with further increases in D_{O_2}, the $\dot{V}_{O_2}$ is said to no longer be flow-dependent.

CONTROLLING BLOOD LOSS

Blood loss should be controlled promptly in critically ill or injured patients. Even the best resuscitation cannot make up for continuing loss of erythrocytes and all the other components in blood. For example, if the patient has a leaking abdominal aortic aneurysm, two IVs are started, a type and crossmatch is obtained, and the aorta is controlled surgically in the operating room as soon as possible with little or no preoperative resuscitation.

With external blood loss, digital control at the bleeding site(s) is usually adequate. In some instances, a tourniquet may be required; however, if a tourniquet is not properly applied, it can cause severe tissue damage and may actually increase the blood loss. Proper splinting also tends to reduce blood loss from fracture sites. External fixation of pelvic fractures may also help reduce blood loss.

PNEUMATIC ANTISHOCK GARMENT

Application of military antishock trousers (MAST), which is a type of pneumatic antishock garment (PASG), has been recommended for the temporary treatment of traumatic hypovolemic shock and to try to control internal hemorrhage into the pelvis and lower extremities.[87] This concept of external counterpressure to combat hypovolemia was first employed by Crile[88] in 1903 and reintroduced by Gardner and Dohn[89] in 1956. Since then, MAST has been used extensively as an effective therapeutic modality in the treatment of shock.[89,90] It also has been a mainstay in prehospital treatment of shock at the accident scene and during prolonged transportation to medical centers.[91]

Despite its widespread use, experimental and clinical data have indicated that MAST may not be universally applicable for hypotensive injury because of the variable clinical responses and lack of a significant effect on the trauma score or mortality.[92,93] Experimental studies have further demonstrated that external counterpressure consistently increases systemic arterial pressure by increasing systemic vascular resistance.[94] However, the response in cardiac output and tissue perfusion is quite variable.[95,96]

Acute left-sided heart failure is considered a contraindication to the use of PASG, and diaphragmatic injury and pregnancy are contraindications to inflating the abdominal compartment.

A number of complications, including the development of lactic acidosis and decreased survival, have been noted in phlebotomized canines treated by MAST.[95,97] Other untoward effects of this treatment modality, including an increased incidence of atelectasis, pneumonia, and ventilatory failure, also have been observed.[98] Finally, lower extremity complications, such as compartment syndrome, arterial thrombosis and embolism, crush syndrome, and increased bleeding from vascular injuries and amputations, have all been shown to be associated with MAST treatment.[99-101]

CORRECTING HYPOVOLEMIA

Blood Volume Deficits. The goal in the obviously hypovolemic patients with severe hypotension and no apparent continued severe bleeding is to infuse 2000 to 3000 ml of fluid within 10 to 15 min or until the patient is out of shock. If it is thought that the patient may still be bleeding, as with a leaking abdominal aortic aneurysm, aggressive fluid resuscitation probably should not be instituted until the bleeding site is controlled. At least 95 percent of shock in trauma victims is due to hypovolemia, and if shock is allowed to persist for more than 30 min, particularly in someone who is bleeding massively, the mortality rate often exceeds 50 percent.

It is important to differentiate the amount of *blood lost* from the *blood volume deficit*. If a patient lost 2000 ml of blood over a period of 1 h, 500 to 1000 ml of extravascular fluid might move from the interstitial space into the vascular space to partially correct the hypovolemia; thus the actual blood volume deficit at the end of 1 h might only be 1000 to 1500 ml (Table 6–2).

The severity of acute blood loss may be divided into four classes (Table 6–3). In a previously normal 70-kg man, a class I blood loss is up to 750 ml (or 15 percent) of the expected blood volume (BV). A class II hemorrhage is 750 to 1500 ml (15 to 30 percent of BV). A class III hemorrhage is 1500 to 2000 ml (30 to 40 percent of BV), and class IV is any greater loss. Class I and II hemorrhages usually can be treated with crystalloid resuscitation alone, while class III and IV hemorrhages generally also require blood transfusions.

A 70-kg man normally has a blood volume of about 5000 ml. His blood pressure usually does not fall below 80 mmHg until there is a blood volume deficit of at least 25 percent. An acute blood volume deficit of 50 percent usually is

TABLE 6–2. Time-Related Restoration After Single Acute Hemorrhage, Untreated

	Restoration Time
Blood volume	24–48 h
Plasma volume	24–48 h
Plasma protein concentration	
Maximal dilution	2 h
Normal concentration restored	79–96 h
Total circulating plasma protein restored	48–72 h
Red blood cell mass	20–25 days

Source: From Cope O, Litwin SB: Contribution of the lymphatic system to the replenishment of the plasma volume following a hemorrhage. *Ann Surg* 156:655, 1962, with permission.

TABLE 6–3. Grading of Shock

Degree of Shock	Blood Pressure (Approx.)	Pulse Quality	Skin				Thirst	Mental State
			Temperature	Color	Circulation (Response to Pressure Blanching)			
None	Normal	Normal	Normal	Normal	Normal		Normal	Clear and distressed
Slight	To 20% decrease	Normal	Cool	Pale	Definite slowing		Normal	Clear and distressed
Moderate	Decreased 20–40%	Definite decrease in volume	Cool	Pale	Definite slowing		Definite	Clear and some apathy unless stimulated
Severe	Decreased 40% to nonrecordable	Weak to imperceptible	Cold	Ashen to cyanotic (mottling)	Very sluggish		Severe	Apathetic to comatose; little distress except thirst

Source: From Beecher HK, Simeone FA, Burnett CH, et al: The internal state of the severely wounded man on entry to the most forward hospital. *Surgery* 22:672, 1947, with permission.

promptly fatal. Thus a previously normal 70-kg patient who is in shock probably has a blood volume of between 2500 to 3750 ml. Consequently, rapid administration of 2000 to 3000 ml of a balanced electrolyte solution should get him out of shock unless he is bleeding rapidly. If the blood pressure does not respond to this rapid infusion, prompt surgical control of the bleeding is indicated.

IV Lines. Two or three large IV catheters should be inserted promptly in hypovolemic hypotensive patients. Peripheral veins should be used for starting these IVs whenever possible. Subclavian or internal jugular lines can be inserted rapidly by most physicians working in busy emergency departments, but insertion of these central lines can cause complications, such as pneumothorax.

Central lines are usually not as large as those which can be inserted peripherally, particularly if a cutdown is used, and this can reduce the rate at which resuscitation can be provided. If a subclavian vein catheter is inserted, it should be placed on the side of the chest that has been injured so that if the catheter insertion causes a pneumothorax, it will not collapse the uninjured lung.

Although there is a tendency in some centers to insert subclavian vein catheters in all trauma patients who are in shock, they are often not needed. Indications for central venous catheters in trauma resuscitation should probably be restricted whenever possible to (1) venous access when no other site is available, (2) CVP measurements, (3) insertion of a pulmonary artery catheter, or (4) pacemaker insertion.

Trendelenburg Position. If adequate IV sites cannot be found rapidly, sometimes the central veins can be distended by placing the patient in the Trendelenburg (head-down) position. Head-down positioning of hypovolemic patients has been practiced since World War I in an attempt to improve central blood volume and cardiac output.[102,103] However, using radionuclide scanning techniques, Bivins et al.[104] demonstrated only a 1.8 percent increase in central blood volume in awake normovolemic volunteers in a 15-degree Trendelenburg position. Sibbald et al.[105] and others[103] found no beneficial hemodynamic effect of this position in either normotensive or hypotensive patients. In anesthetized patients with coronary artery disease, a 20-degree Trendelenburg position caused a slight (10 percent) increase in systemic blood pressure, cardiac index, and filling pressures; right ventricular dilatation and decreased right ventricular ejection fraction also were noted.[106]

Thus the Trendelenburg position appears to offer little, if any, beneficial hemodynamic effect during the treatment of shock. In addition, in normal individuals, this position has been shown to decrease cerebral blood flow, probably by increasing the jugular venous pressure and thereby impeding venous drainage.[107] In patients with increased intracranial pressure (ICP), the Trendelenburg position tends also to increase the ICP and may reduce the cerebral perfusion pressure. The head-down position also may cause respiratory embarrassment because of cephalad displacement of intraabdominal contents against the diaphragm. The hemodynamic effects of passive leg raising are similar to those of the Trendelenburg position, but it has less tendency to elevate the diaphragm and retard ventilation and to impede venous return from the head.[106]

If no peripheral or central veins can be found in children less than 3 years of age, insertion of an 18-gauge spinal needle into the proximal tibia or distal femur may allow flow rates averaging 1.7 ml/min.[108,109]

Fluid Administration. Fluid should continue to be administered rapidly until the resuscitation is adequate, as reflected by (1) a systolic blood pressure of at least 100 to 110 mmHg, (2) the patient is alert (assuming no head injuries), (3) the skin is warm and dry, (4) the urine output is at least 0.5 to 1.0 ml/h, (5) the tachycardia is beginning to abate, preferably to rates less than 110 to 120 beats per minute, and (6) the core body temperature is at least 35°C.

If the patient's neck veins begin to distend but the patient is still in shock, the patient may have cardiac failure and/or fluid overload. However, before fluid administration is stopped and diuretics are started, one must rule out (1) pericardial tamponade, (2) tension pneumothorax, (3) mediastinal hematoma, (4) air embolism, and (5) Valsalva maneuvers by the patient.

The cause of neck vein distension with persistent shock must be found and corrected as rapidly as possible. In addition, inotropes, such as dopamine or dobutamine, may be required.

Rapid Fluid Administration Sets. A rapid solution administration set (RSAS) utilizing a 40-μm screen blood transfusion filter, a heat exchanger, and a no. 8.5 French IV catheter has been developed and is capable of infusing 37°C fluid at up to 1600 ml/min. Use of such equipment may be lifesaving with certain types of trauma or surgery by preventing hypothermia and correcting hypovolemia rapidly.

TYPES OF FLUIDS USED IN RESUSCITATION

Crystalloids. *Physiology and pharmacokinetics.* Resuscitation from shock is usually begun with a balanced electrolyte (crystalloid) solution. The terms *crystalloid* and *colloid* were coined by Thomas Graham in 1861 and refer, respectively, to solute particles that will or will not pass through semipermeable membranes and are smaller or larger than an arbitrarily determined particle weight, usually taken as 10,000 Da.

Isotonic fluids such as Ringer's lactate and normal saline distribute evenly throughout the extracellular space. In normal, healthy adults, equilibration of such fluids throughout the extracellular space occurs within 20 to 30 min of IV infusion, and after 1 h, only about a third of the volume infused remains in the intravascular space. Glucose-in-water, in contrast, tends to equilibrate with the total body water so that only about one-fifteenth (60 to 70 ml out of a liter) will remain in the vascular space. Although crystalloids can usually restore blood pressure fairly rapidly, in critically ill or injured patients, only 10 to 20 percent of these solutions will remain in the circulation after 1 to 2 h.[110]

Normal (0.9%) saline and Ringer's lactate are the most frequently used crystalloids, and they can generally be given interchangeably. Three problems that can occur with Ringer's lactate are related to its calcium concentration of 3 mEq/liter, its lactate concentration of 28 mEq/liter, and its potassium concentration of 4 mEq/liter. The calcium may cause clots if it comes into contact with bank blood. The lactate present in Ringer's lactate solution does not usually increase the lactic acidemia associated with shock, unless the patient has severe liver dysfunction. Furthermore, the use of Ringer's lactate does not usually alter the reliability of blood lactate measurements,[111] except perhaps in patients with hepatic failure. In patients who are oliguric and have high serum potassium levels, one should probably not give Ringer's lactate.

The theoretical concern that large volumes of normal saline can produce a "dilution acidosis" or hyperchloremic acidosis is seldom a problem clinically. The excess circulating chloride ions are normally excreted by the kidney quite readily. However, if the patient has severe persistent shock and very poor renal function, the extra chloride could be a problem.

Indications. Crystalloid solutions are indicated for plasma volume expansion in the initial resuscitation of almost all shock patients. They are inexpensive, readily available, easily stored, reaction-free, and can readily correct most extracellular volume deficits. Crystalloids also decrease blood viscosity and can thereby improve capillary blood flow. Shires et al.[111a] have found that resuscitation with a combination of blood and crystalloid provides better survival from hemorrhagic shock than blood alone or blood plus plasma.

Side effects. Nonsanguinous fluids dilate the remaining red cells and protein, thereby reducing the oxygen-carrying capacity, buffering ability, and colloid osmotic pressure of the blood. In severe trauma, sepsis, or shock, where capillary permeability may be increased, these solutions may leave the intravascular space so rapidly that only transient blood volume expansion is provided. For the same reason, severe edema may develop in tissues, including the brain and lung, particularly if they are injured.

Recommendations for use. Acute blood loss of up to 30 percent of the blood volume may be adequately replaced with crystalloid if given rapidly in quantities equal to three to four times the blood lost.[112,113] Nevertheless, in the most critically ill or injured patients, hemoglobin levels should be kept above 10.0 g/dl and albumin levels should probably be kept above 2.0 g/dl. Consequently, after the initial 3000 to 4000 ml of crystalloids is given to a critically injured patient, consideration should be given to administering blood and some colloid as needed to maintain reasonable hemoglobin and colloid levels.

Studies by Shires et al.[111a] suggest that even in advanced shock, lactate metabolism by the liver may be adequate. Nevertheless, in patients with advanced cirrhosis, I prefer to use normal saline with an ampule of sodium bicarbonate added to each liter of fluid.

Colloids. Clinically, the term *colloid* refers to solutions containing substances of high molecular weight (usually at least 10,000 Da) which cannot readily diffuse through normal capillary membranes. These agents are used primarily to expand intravascular volume and to try to raise colloid osmotic pressure (COP) or oncotic pressure back to normal.[114]

The colloids used most frequently now include albumin, dextran, hydroxyethyl starch, pentastarch, and fresh frozen plasma. Other colloids sometimes used, particularly in other countries, include plasma protein fraction and gelatin.

Albumin. Human serum albumin can be very effective in rapidly restoring blood volume in intravascular volume depletion, particularly if plasma protein levels are extremely low. However, its clinical indications are controversial, and it costs much more than other plasma expanders. In fact, it costs at least 30 times as much as the crystalloids required to produce an equivalent blood volume expansion.[114]

The average molecular weight of endogenous albumin is 65,000. Normally, 12 to 14 g is made by the liver daily. It is the major oncotically active plasma protein, accounting for about 80 percent of the plasma colloid oncotic pressure.[114]

An adult has 4 to 5 g of albumin per kilogram of body weight in the extracellular space, but only about 30 to 40 percent of this is present in the intravascular compartment. Normal serum albumin levels are about 3.5 to 5.0 g/dl. The plasma level varies with the rate of hepatic synthesis and metabolic breakdown and the flux of albumin between the interstitial and intravascular spaces.[116] Much of the endogenous albumin in the interstitial space is tissue-bound and unavailable to the circulation. Unbound or "free" interstitial space albumin returns to the intravascular compartment via lymphatic drainage. The half-life of albumin in the body is approximately 20 to 22 days.[115] In severe injury or stress, hepatic albumin synthesis falls acutely, and the liver production of acute phase reactants (such as fibrinogen and C-reactive protein) increases markedly.

Administered albumin rapidly distributes itself throughout the extracellular space. The plasma half-life of exogenous albumin is usually about 12 to 16 h. However, in severe shock or sepsis, the hourly disappearance rate of exogenous albumin increases from 7 to 8 percent per hour to over 30 percent per hour.[54]

Albumin is clinically available as a 5% or 25% solution in isotonic saline. It is prepared by fractionating blood from healthy donors and heating it to 60°C for 10 h. This apparently inactivates the hepatitis and human immunodeficiency (HIV) viruses. The 5% solution contains 50 g albumin per liter in normal saline, and it exerts an oncotic pressure of approximately 20 mmHg. Thus 1 g of intravascular albumin can bind about 18 ml of water by its oncotic activity.[116] However, the effects of 5% albumin on plasma volume expansion are not entirely predictable. Reports of plasma volume expansion due to infusion of 500 ml of 5% albumin range anywhere from 250 up to 750 ml.[116] These reported differences may be caused by variability of the volume deficits, initial colloid oncotic pressure, vascular permeability, and the adequacy of the volume resuscitation itself.

The 25% albumin solution contains 12.5 g of albumin in 50 ml of a buffered solution containing approximately 130 to 160 mEq/liter of sodium. The oncotic pressure of 25% albumin is approximately 100 mmHg. When 100 ml of a 25% albumin solution (25 g albumin) is infused, intravascular volume increases by about 300 to 600 ml (average of 450 ml) over 30 to 60 min.[116]

Albumin is generally used in critically ill patients with extremely low protein levels for its oncotic properties. Because the 25% albumin solution is quite expensive to prepare, the 5% solution of human serum albumin is what is used generally in the resuscitation of hypovolemic shock.[114] The more concentrated 25% solution is usually reserved for patients in whom the interstitial space is expanded but the plasma volume and albumin concentration are severely decreased. Postoperative patients, as well as burn patients, after their initial resuscitation, may benefit from infusion of 25% albumin. This colloid can expand their total plasma volume by transcapillary movement of fluid from the interstitial to the intravascular space.

In addition to its plasma volume-expanding effects, albumin may have other unique properties that make it clinically useful. These include binding and inactivation of toxic products, including proteolytic enzymes, maintenance of normal microvascular permeability to protein, and scavenging of free radicals.[117]

Although albumin generally is a very safe plasma expander, many studies have documented a number of adverse effects.[118]

Trauma patients with hypovolemia who are resuscitated with albumin have been described as having increased requirements for both total and blood resuscitation volumes and an increased tendency to heart and pulmonary failure.[119] In sepsis, the increased pulmonary capillary permeability may allow increased albumin to enter and remain in the interstitial fluid space raising the COP there, thereby contributing to the formation of increased extravascular lung water. However, the pulmonary capillary pressure is much more important than the COP.[120] It is also clear that the overall volume of fluid used[121] and the presence or absence of sepsis[122] affect pulmonary function to a far greater extent than does the type of resuscitation fluid.

Trauma patients resuscitated with large amounts of albumin may have low hourly urine volumes, suggesting that, at least in some patients, the use of albumin may prolong the renal insult by transiently maintaining the intravascular volume at the expense of the depleted interstitial fluid volume.[119] Another study[123] showed that seriously injured patients receiving supplemental albumin therapy had an effective expansion of plasma volume and renal blood flow, but paradoxically, there was a drop in glomerular filtration rate. This may have been caused by increased oncotic pressure within the glomerulus and peritubular vessels, causing a decrease in excretion of sodium and water during the early phase of extravascular fluid sequestration.

Each gram of albumin binds about 1.0 mg calcium and may temporarily lower ionized calcium levels, producing a negative inotropic effect on the myocardium.[124] In one series of trauma patients, resuscitation with large amounts of albumin maintained normal serum albumin levels and high total calcium levels but significantly depressed the levels of ionized calcium.[124] Thus the albumin, by binding ionized calcium, appeared to depress myocardial function.

Albumin occasionally causes mild allergic reactions. The incidence of short-lived urticaria, fever, chills, and nausea ranges between 0.5 and 1.5 percent.[114] However, changes in blood pressure, heart rate, and respirations are very uncommon.

Patients in hypovolemic shock who have been resuscitated with albumin have been shown to have decreased levels of immunoglobulins and a reduced immune response to tetanus toxoid compared with similar patients resuscitated with crystalloid solutions.[125,126] The reduced levels of immunoglobulins may be due to nonspecific binding to the albumin, with a subsequent passive loss as albumin-immunoglobulin complexes extravasate out of the intravascular space.

Lucas et al.[123] have shown that use of large quantities of albumin can reduce plasma concentrations of various coagulation proteins. The mechanism for this is not clear.

Hepatic albumin production may be regulated by the albumin concentration within the interstitial space of the liver.[127] Exogenously administered albumin may elevate this level, leading to suppression of subsequent endogenous production of albumin.

In 1975, a National Institutes of Health task force examined the appropriate use of albumin in the light of its increasing cost and apparent indiscriminate use.[128] It was agreed that for major volume resuscitation (replacement of greater than 30 percent of the blood volume), colloids such as albumin can be used as part of the resuscitation regimen. If the patient is edematous, 25% albumin can be used to help mobilize the patient's own interstitial fluid into the vascular space. A COP of 20 mmHg or more, a serum albumin of 2.5 g/dl or more, or a total serum protein of 5.0 g/dl or more indicates an adequate plasma oncotic activity for most clinical situations.

Albumin can be provided as normal serum albumin (NSA), 5% and 25%, and purified protein fraction (PPF). The protein content of NSA preparations is 96 percent albumin, and the sodium content of all albumin preparations is 145 ± 15 mEq/liter. PPF preparations contain only 83 percent albumin, with the remainder being alpha and beta globulins. Use of PPF is occasionally associated with development of some hypotension, which is thought to be secondary to kinins or prekallikrein activator activity present in the solution.[129]

Dextran. Dextran is a glucose polymer with primarily 1,6-glucosidic linkages. In its native form, dextran is a branched polysaccharide of about 200,000 glucose units.[114] Partial hydrolysis produces polysaccharides of smaller size, which are available commercially as preparations having average molecular weights of 40,000 (Rheomacrodex, Dextran 40, D-40) or 70,000 (Dextran 70, D-70).

Dextran molecules quickly equilibrate with the entire extracellular space. Particles of less than 15,000 molecular weight are rapidly filtered by the kidney, and 50 to 75 percent of these are lost in the urine in 15 to 30 min; however, while in the circulation, they exert osmotic activity.

Up to 60 to 70 percent of D-40 and 30 to 40 percent of D-70 are cleared from the plasma into the urine or interstitial fluid space within 12 h. After 24 h, the particles remaining in the circulation have an average molecular weight of more than 80,000. These particles are gradually taken up by the reticuloendothelial system and enzymatically degraded to glucose at a rate of 70 to 90 mg/kg per day and metabolized to carbon dioxide and water. Some of the larger dextran molecules also may be excreted through the gut.

Dextran infusion increases the intravascular volume by an amount equal to or greater than the volume infused; a 500-ml bolus of D-40 may produce an intravascular volume expansion of 750 ml at 1 h and 1050 ml at 2 h.[130] This volume expansion may persist for up to 8 h in hypovolemic patients; however, the osmotic diuresis limits the duration of the volume expansion. Urine flow also may increase because dextran resuscitation is associated with increased renal plasma flow and a fall in plasma antidiuretic hormone levels.[131]

Dextran tends to improve blood flow in the microvasculature by coating endothelial and blood cell surfaces, decreasing viscosity, and preventing red blood cell sludging in the microcirculation. It also reduces platelet adherence and degranulation,[130] and it may decrease platelet factor 3.[132] These changes decrease the activation of the clotting cascade mechanism and limit thrombus formation.[133] Dextran is also reported to copolymerize with fibrin monomers, resulting in a less stable clot that is more susceptible to endogenous lysis.[130] All these changes increase the likelihood of oozing from raw surfaces.

The incidence of anaphylactoid reactions to dextran prior to 1977 was between 0.34 and 5.3 percent.[134] Since that time, however, improved testing methods for the presence of antigens, as well as manufacturing of dextrans with more linear molecules and fewer antigenic properties, have drastically reduced the number of severe allergic reactions.

Allergic reactions usually occur within $\frac{1}{2}$ h after the infusion is begun and may include rash, urticaria, nausea, bronchospasm, shock, and death. Dextran is a potent antigen that has cross-reactivity with several bacterial polysaccharide antigens. Gut flora can make endogenous dextran from dextrose, and patients with *Streptococcus* pneumonia or *Salmonella* infections are more prone to dextran reactions. Consequently, a small portion of the patient population has never received dextran but has circulating precipitins to the dextran molecule.

If the blood bank is not informed of the recent administration of dextran to a patient who requires blood transfusions, it may fail to obtain a proper type and crossmatch. Dextran can interfere with typing and crossmatching of blood. This problem is handled best by drawing blood prior to the dextran infusion and/or notifying blood bank personnel that the patient is receiving dextran so that they can wash the dextran off the red blood cells prior to their tests.

If dextran is given to patients with large open wounds, excessive oozing and blood loss may occur. In addition to a dilutional effect on the various coagulation factors, dextran inhibits erythrocyte aggregation in vivo. It also adheres to vessel walls and cellular elements of the blood, decreases platelet adhesiveness, and precipitates fibrinogen, factor VIII, fibrin monomers, and probably, von Willebrand factor. This can result in prolonged bleeding times and increased incisional bleeding.[135] Such oozing can be a particular problem in patients with large open wounds. However, at doses less than 20 ml/kg per day (1.5 g/kg per day), clinical bleeding is usually not encountered.[136]

Because dextran particles with molecular weights less than 50,000 are rapidly filtered through the glomerulus, a highly viscous urine may result, and if unrecognized hypovolemia is allowed to persist, acute renal failure can develop rapidly.[137] The risk of renal dysfunction is particularly great if the lower-molecular-weight dextrans are used in patients who have a persistent decrease in renal blood flow or glomerular filtration rate. The mechanism for the renal failure appears to be tubular obstruction due to concentration and precipitation of dextran in the tubules. Therefore, patients receiving dextran should be kept well-hydrated by aggressive concomitant administration of crystalloid solutions.[138]

An osmotic diuresis can occur almost immediately with dextran because the smaller molecules are filtered by the glomeruli and not absorbed. The effect is greater with D-40 than with D-70. In the face of this obligate osmotic diuresis, urine volume cannot serve as a guide to the adequacy of intravascular volume repletion.

Because the larger dextran molecules are cleared by the reticuloendothelial system, there is some concern that the larger molecules will adversely affect immune function.[139] Although dextran may temporarily impair reticuloendothelial system function and immune competence in experimental animals, there have been no reports of this in patients.

Blood glucose levels can be falsely elevated in patients receiving dextran if the glucose measurement is done by an analysis using acid, which converts dextran to dextrose. Dextran also may cause false elevations of total protein and serum bilirubin levels.[139] Other adverse effects that may occur with administration of dextran include depression of plasma levels of several important plasma proteins, such as fibrinogen, haptoglobin, C3, C4, and the immunoglobulins.[140]

Dextran 40 (Rheomacrodex) (low-molecular-weight dextran) is commercially available as a 10% solution in normal saline or 5% dextrose in water. Dextran 70 (Macrodex) is commercially available as a 6% solution in normal saline, 5% dextrose in water, or 10% invert sugar in water.

For restoration of blood volume in shock, approximately 1000 ml of 10% D-40 (for a 70-kg man) may be given acutely in conjunction with crystalloid, packed red blood cells, and plasma as necessary. To avoid excessive bleeding, the total dosage should be less than 15 ml/kg per day of D-40 or 20 ml/kg per day of D-70.[141]

Gelatin. Gelatin is prepared by hydrolysis of bovine collagen. The solutions prepared for clinical use have a rather wide range of molecular weights but average under 100,000.[114] Although no gelatin solutions are available for use in the United States now, there are two types of commercially prepared gelatin solutions for intravenous infusion in the United Kingdom. Urea-linked gelatin (Haemaccel) has a 10-fold higher content of calcium (6.26 mmol/liter) and potassium (5.1 mmol/liter) than succinylated gelatin (Gelofusine), in which the concentration of both elements is less than 0.4 mmol/liter. Because of its higher calcium content, Haemaccel can cause clotting in the warming coils if it is infused with bank blood.

Although it was originally claimed that the new-generation gelatins were nonantigenic, all types have been associated with occasional allergic reactions. Haemaccel has been associated with over twice the incidence of anaphylactoid reactions (0.14 percent) as the Gelofusine. Histamine release and complement activation also may occur with both types. Gelatins also may cause prolonged depression of plasma fibronectin levels in postoperative patients.[142] Although there is a dose-dependent dilution of clotting factors, the newer gelatins neither impair hemostasis nor interfere with blood typing and crossmatch reactions.

Hydroxyethyl starch (hetastarch) (HES). Hydroxyethyl starch (hetastarch) (HES) is a synthetic starch molecule derived from a waxy starch composed almost entirely of amylopectin.[114] Its production involves introduction of hydroxyethyl ether groups into the glucose units of the starch to retard degradation by serum amylase.

Plasma volume expansion after infusion of hetastarch is approximately 100 to 170 percent of the infused volume of HES. This is equal to or slightly greater than the volume expansion produced by D-70 or 5% albumin, and it has a slightly longer plasma retention time, which has been reported to be between 12 and 48 h.[143] The increase in colloid pressure is similar to that seen with albumin.

Hydroxyethyl starch subunits that are less than 50,000 Da are rapidly filtered and excreted by the kidney. Larger subunits persist in the circulation until they are hydrolyzed intravascularly or sequestered extravascularly by reticuloendothelial cells.[144]

After intravenous infusion, there is an almost immediate appearance of smaller HES particles in the urine. In normal volunteers, an average of 46 percent of an administered dose is excreted in the urine by 2 days and 64 percent by 8 days.[145] However, the reported half-life of hetastarch varies from 2 to 65 days, depending on the time and duration of sampling. This variability in half-life is due to the heterogeneous molecular weight of the particles found in the commercially available product, as well as to the complexity of distribution and degradation within the body. The rate of disappearance of the larger particles of HES from the plasma depends on their absorption by tissues, gradual return to the circulation, uptake by the reticuloendothelial system (RES), and subsequent degradation by the RES to smaller particles which are then cleared into urine and bile.

As with dextran, the uptake of hetastarch molecules by the cells of the RES has caused concern that the immune function of the patient could be compromised. However, clinically significant RES dysfunction has not been demonstrated.[146]

One of the main concerns with hetastarch is its effects on blood coagulation. The exact mechanism of the hemostatic defect is not clear. Although hetastarch precipitates factors I and VIII, fibrin monomer, and von Willebrand factor from plasma, the amount of precipitation appears to vary widely between patients.[136] Platelet coating with hetastarch and dilutional changes in the serum also have been implicated. All these effects can cause a number of coagulation and bleeding changes, including (1) transient reduction in fibrinogen levels and platelet count, largely because of hemodilution, (2) minor prolongation of prothrombin, partial thromboplastin, and bleeding times, (3) shortening of thrombin-, reptilase-, and urokinase-activated clot lysis times, and (4) a reduction in factor VIII complex concentration to a greater degree than accounted for by hemodilution.[147,148] There is also evidence that hetastarch results in impaired fibrin clot formation and decreased clot tensile strength. These findings, suggestive of enhanced fibrinolysis and a direct interaction with factor VIII, may result in varying degrees of subclinical coagulopathy. If the daily dose of HES exceeds the recommended maximum (>20 ml/kg) and is administered repeatedly, clinically significant coagulopathies have been reported. However, other studies have failed to demonstrate clinically significant bleeding or increased requirements for blood transfusion.[147]

Hetastarch is not immunogenic and does not induce histamine release. Consequently, the incidence of anaphylactic reactions to hetastarch is very low (0.0004 to 0.006 percent), and the incidence of severe reactions, including shock or cardiopulmonary arrest, is even lower. However, a number of miscellaneous adverse effects including chills, itching, mild temperature elevations, submaxillary and parotid gland enlargement, and erythema multiforme have been reported.[115]

Serum amylase levels may rise to values about twice normal, reaching a maximum at about 20 h and persisting for 3 to 5 days following hetastarch administration. This occurs because plasma amylase forms complexes with hetastarch molecules, creating large macroamylase particles that are excreted in the urine at a much slower rate than the usual amylase molecule.[149] There is no alteration of pancreatic function.

Because the larger molecules of hetastarch are cleared to a large degree by macrophages and other members of the reticuloendothelial system (RES), a theoretical concern over its potential depression of the immune system has been raised.[115] However, no evidence has been found clinically to confirm this.

Hetastarch may be used whenever colloid is required to restore plasma volume. At doses of 1500 ml/d or less, bleeding complications are rare.[150] Nevertheless, hetastarch should be used with extreme caution in the presence of a known bleeding problem. Adequate monitoring for early detection of volume overload is important. However, the immediate osmotic diuresis associated with its use protects somewhat from this phenomenon.

Hetastarch costs about one-fourth as much as an equivalent amount of 5% albumin. Although hetastarch costs more than dextran, it has fewer side effects.

Hetastarch is available as a 6% solution in 0.9% sodium chloride. Its pH is 5.5, and its osmolarity is 310 mosmol/liter. Although the total dosage should not exceed 20 ml/kg per day, this volume may be administered over 1 h or less if the clinical situation demands very rapid volume resuscitation.

Pentastarch. Pentastarch is a low-molecular-weight form of hydroxyethyl starch.[114] It is more rapidly and completely degraded by circulating amylase than is hetastarch, and therefore, it is more rapidly and effectively eliminated directly in the urine. Larger particles are phagocytized by the RES. The volume expansion produced by pentastarch is about 1.5 times the administered volume; however, this effect usually lasts less than 12 h.[151]

Preoperative infusion of 500 ml of 10% pentastarch during a 30-min period can produce a plasma volume increase of about 700 ml. In contrast to hetastarch, the degree of plasma volume expansion is typically greater (although variable results have been reported), but the duration of volume expansion is shorter. Thus the potential advantages of pentastarch include a greater degree of plasma volume expansion per volume infused, faster onset of action, and more rapid elimination from the blood than hetastarch.

When administered to normal persons undergoing leukapheresis, pentastarch is associated with lengthening of the activated partial thromboplastin time, reduction in fibrinogen and factor VIII levels, and shortening of the thrombin time; however, urokinase-activated clot lysis time and bleeding time are usually unchanged. Furthermore, the effects on factor VIII levels, urokinase-activated clot lysis time, and bleeding times are of a lesser magnitude (despite a greater degree of hemodilution) than those previously reported from hetastarch. Therefore, the effects of pentastarch on coagulation appear to be proportional to its degree of hemodilution only. The lesser presumed interaction with factor VIII may be related to its smaller average molecular size.

Although clinical data are lacking, it is likely that the incidence of anaphylactoid reactions occurring with pentastarch is similar to that of hetastarch.

Comparable groups given pentastarch or albumin have revealed no differences in respiratory, oncotic, or coagulation measurements, no untoward reactions attributable to the colloids, and no differences in total chest tube drainage or blood product usage.

Pentastarch has been used very successfully as an adjunct to leukapheresis, but it also may be a useful colloid in fluid resuscitation. Given its favorable elimination profile and lack of clinically significant effects on coagulation, it appears that pentastarch may be safer than hetastarch. If commercially available at a lower cost than albumin, pentastarch would appear to be a reasonable first choice for postoperative plasma volume expansion.

Pentastarch is available for use as a 10% solution in normal saline. Doses of pentastarch up to 2000 ml appear to be well tolerated, and its volume-expanding capability is similar to or greater than that of 5% albumin.

Fresh frozen plasma. Fresh frozen plasma is prepared from whole blood by separating and freezing the plasma within 6 h of phlebotomy. The typical unit has a volume of 200 to 300 ml. When frozen, the labile clotting factors (V and VIII) deteriorate to a minimal extent.[152]

Fresh frozen plasma can correct deficiencies in clotting factors (not platelets) and antithrombin, but it can transmit bloodborne diseases, especially hepatitis. Therefore, it is used primarily in individuals with multiple coagulation factor problems.[153] Fresh frozen plasma should not be used solely to provide volume expansion.

Although there is a possibility of fluid overload when using fresh frozen plasma, its main risk is that of transmission of various serious infections. Fresh frozen plasma has a risk of hepatitis and AIDS transmission equal to that of whole blood.[152] Allergic reactions and noncardiogenic pulmonary edema also may occur, but they are unusual.

The dose of fresh frozen plasma depends on the clinical situation and the degree of clotting abnormality noted clinically or by measurement of prothrombin time, partial thromboplastin time, or specific factor assay. Fresh frozen plasma takes 20 to 40 min to thaw and must be given through a filter. If used within 2 h of thawing, it contains normal levels of coagulation factors. However, longer delays decrease the coagulation factor activity, especially for factor VII.[152] Compatibility testing is not required, but it should be ABO-compatible whenever possible.

Liquid plasma. Liquid plasma is a blood component obtained by separating plasma from whole blood any time up to 5 days after the expiration date of a unit of blood. It contains all the stable coagulation factors, but it has reduced levels of factors V and VIII. The main indication for liquid plasma is treatment of patients with deficiencies of coagulation factors other than V or VIII. The contraindications and precautions, dosage, and administration are the same as those for fresh frozen plasma.

Plasma protein fraction. Plasma protein fraction (PPF) is a 5% solution of stabilized human plasma proteins in normal saline.[115] It is a mixture of plasma proteins, of which at least 83 percent is albumin, no more than 17 percent is alpha and beta globulins, and no more than 1 percent is gamma globulin. There are no clotting factors in PPF. PPF is prepared from large pools of normal human plasma by fractionation, involving a series of controlled precipitations with cold ethanol. Viral hepatitis and HIV are probably not a hazard because this product is heated to 60°C for 10 h.

The pharmacologic properties of PPF are very similar to those of its primary constituent, albumin, but the presence of the globulins seems to induce a larger number of side effects, such as hypersensitivity reactions and hypotension. Originally, bradykinin was thought to be the offending substance causing the hypotension which was occasionally seen during rapid infusions of PPF; however, it now appears that the primary vasodilators are Hageman-factor fragments present in the solution.[154]

Crystalloids versus Colloids. Successful resuscitation is primarily dependent on the rapidity and adequacy of fluid repletion, not on the composition of the resuscitation fluid. Controversies over the selection of the type of fluid for resuscitation center mainly on issues relating to philosophy, side effects, and economics.

Proponents of colloids usually argue that (1) since the key problem in shock is a loss of circulating blood volume, replacement with colloid is more appropriate and more rapidly effective, (2) crystalloids reduce the colloid osmotic pressure, thus favoring the development of pulmonary edema,[155] and (3) crystalloids, because of their prompt equilibration with extracellular fluid (ECF), must be infused in amounts exceeding estimated blood losses by at least three to four times. Patients who are older, who have more significant hemodynamic instability, or who require both volume and an increase in plasma colloid osmotic pressure may do better with a colloid resuscitation.[114] In critically ill patients, 1000 ml of a balanced crystalloid solution increases plasma volume by only 194 ml, whereas 500 ml of 5% albumin produces an increase of about 700 ml.[155]

Proponents of crystalloid solutions, on the other hand, argue that (1) since the main problem in shock is shrinkage of the entire ECF, replacement with crystalloid is more appropriate, (2) fluid overload causing congestive heart failure and/or pulmonary edema is less likely to occur with crystalloids because of their rapid equilibration with ECF, (3) crystalloids do not cause anaphylactoid reactions, (4) colloids, except possibly for FFP,[156,157] have adverse effects on coagulation either by dilution of the factors or by actually interfering with their production or function, (5) administered colloids may cross the pulmonary capillary membrane in patients with increased microvascular permeability pulling water along with them, (6) all commercially available colloid solutions are capable of supporting bacterial growth and transmitting infection, and (7) fluid resuscitation with colloids is 10 to 100 times more expensive than equivalent blood volume expansion with crystalloid infusions.

Appropriate use of either crystalloids or colloids with comprehensive monitoring should lead to successful resuscitation in most patients. Careful judgment is often required to provide the rate of fluid administration needed for optimal tissue perfusion without producing fluid overload.

Hypertonic Saline Solutions. Hypertonic saline (7.5% NaCl) may be useful in resuscitation from shock because of the small volume required to produce significant hemodynamic improvements. Velasco et al.[158] demonstrated that a single bolus of hypertonic saline (HTS), given in a volume equal to 10 percent of the shed blood, produced permanent recovery from hemorrhagic shock in anesthetized dogs. Other investigators have shown similar beneficial results with HTS in dogs with endotoxic shock[159] and in swine with hemorrhagic shock.[160]

Hypertonic saline appears to be more effective in resuscitation from shock than other solutions of equal osmolarity.[161] Several mechanisms may contribute to the hemodynamic response seen with HTS resuscitation from hemorrhagic shock. Hyperosmotic solutions increase plasma osmolarity, which increases blood volume.[162] In addition, HTS has been demonstrated to transiently increase myocardial contractility and catecholamine levels.[163] Permanent survival after HTS resuscitation from severe hemorrhagic shock in dogs has been reported to involve a pulmonary reflex resulting in selective vasoconstriction.[164] Lung denervation or arterial injection has been shown to prevent permanent resuscitation from hemorrhagic shock with a single injection of HTS.[165] Angiotensin II antagonism also has been shown to block the selective venoconstriction and prevent the long-term hemodynamic improvements.[166] Finally, increased osmolarity may result in release of vasopressin, which produces vasoconstriction.[167]

Hypertonic saline solutions (HSS) (1200 to 2500 mosmol/liter) have been shown to effectively resuscitate patients with less volume,[168] less edema formation,[169] and better tissue perfusion than normal (0.9%) saline solutions (NSS).[170,171] By decreasing the amount of interstitial fluid that might accumulate in the heart, gastrointestinal tract, skin, and brain, HSS is less apt to cause the reduced organ function, impaired healing, and increased risk of infection seen in some patients after an otherwise successful resuscitation with isotonic solutions. There is no risk of transmission of infectious agents with HSS, and the cost is approximately 1 percent of that for colloid agents producing a similar ECF expansion.[172]

In addition to pulling intracellular fluid into the extracellular space,[173] hypertonic saline is also reported to (1) exert direct inotropic actions on the myocardium,[174] (2) cause vasodilation,[175] (3) decrease intracranial pressure,[175] and (4) enhance vagally mediated reflex venoconstriction.[174] Interestingly, these effects seem to be most prominent if the HSS is given intravascularly to animals that have intact innervation to their lungs.

In a study that used several different hypertonic solutions to treat sheep with moderate hemorrhagic shock, 2400 mosmol NaCl with 6% Dextran 70 (colloid osmotic pressure = 70 mmHg) produced a higher and more sustained rise in blood pressure and cardiac output than several other hypertonic solutions. In patients with head trauma and shock, it may be advantageous to keep intracranial pressure (ICP) as low as possible. In a recent study in dogs, HSS (2500 mosmol/liter) raised the ICP 45 percent less than Ringer's lactate (RL) for an equivalent resuscitation.[176]

Preliminary data also suggest that HSS attenuates the ACTH, cortisol, and aldosterone responses to trauma.[177] There also was suppression of the angiotensin II response, and this might increase perfusion to the intestines, heart, and kidney.

Although HSS apparently has many benefits, it should not be used in every patient. Most patients, in fact, do very well with isotonic crystalloid resuscitation. In addition, some studies on HTS resuscitation from hemorrhagic and septic shock in dogs[178,179] and humans[180] have reported only transient improvements in cardiac output (CO) and mean arterial pressure (MAP). Nevertheless, HSS may be more effective than isotonic crystalloids in reducing third-space losses in selected patients with hypotension and large volume requirements. It also may be very helpful when peripheral or central edema would be detrimental.

Autologous Transfusion (Autotransfusion). Autotransfusion involves the collection of shed blood from a body cavity with acute reinfusion into that patient's circulation. The first reported use of autotransfusion was in 1886 when Duncan reinfused blood which he collected during an amputation of the crushed legs of a victim of a railway accident.[176]

Autotransfusion offers many advantages. Blood can be available for administration without waiting for a type and crossmatch. Of greater importance to many individuals, however, has been the concern over transmission of disease with bank blood. With autotransfusion, the risk of transmitted disease such as hepatitis, AIDS, malaria, and syphilis is eliminated. Furthermore, no hemolytic, febrile, or allergic reactions have been reported during autotransfusion.

Autotransfusion practices and devices fall into three main categories. Direct reinfusion of pleural blood was popularized by Symbas et al.,[181] who pointed out that blood drained from the pleural space is usually already defibrinated and requires little or no anticoagulant. The only real problem is that relatively few patients have enough bleeding into the chest to justify setting up for an autotransfusion. Most chest tube placements in trauma result in the collection of less than 500 ml of blood.

The second category is suction collection,[182] such as with a Sorenson apparatus, to recover blood lost during an operation. A collection trap is placed in the suction line, and blood collected there is reinfused using a transfusion filter to catch and remove whatever aggregates, fat particles, and debris also may have been collected. The apparatus is simple and easy to set up, and the overall cost is about half as much as bank blood. It is ideal for bleeding inside the chest. In the abdomen, it can be used for bleeding from solid organ or vascular injuries. Most surgeons feel that intestinal injury is a contraindication to autotransfusing intraabdominal blood; however, some surgeons feel that even if intestinal contents are present, they can be removed by washing the red cells thoroughly, and antibiotics will take care of any residual bacteria.[183]

Blood collected during operations may or may not be washed, but it must be filtered prior to reinfusion. Although the washing takes some time, it is advantageous because it removes fibrin, cellular debris, free hemoglobin, potassium, and various procoagulants and anticoagulants.

The third category of autotransfusion devices is the blood concentrator, which uses a special console that is capable of rapidly washing the aspirated blood and concentrating it to a hematocrit of about 45 percent. However, there is usually only one washing, and this may not clear bacteria reliably. Also, it takes 15 to 30 min to set up the blood concentrator, and the setup pack costs $200. In one study,[184] the device was set up for 85 trauma patients, but only 22 actually received blood from it, and only 28 percent of the total blood received was from the autotransfusor. The major reasons for patients not receiving autotransfused blood were inadequate collection (60 percent), colon contamination (21 percent), and death before reinfusion (19 percent). Whether a hospital should spend $40,000 for a blood concentrator and intensively train its personnel for the relatively small number of patients who would benefit from autotransfusion is an important question. However, this type of autotransfusor would be appropriate for major trauma centers or for hospitals with busy cardiac or vascular programs.

Several disadvantages of autotransfusion have been described. Air embolism used to be a disastrous complication; however, most reports of air embolism occurred with early autotransfusion systems that are no longer in use. The administration of large volumes of autotransfused blood also may result in an increased bleeding tendency or coagulopathy.

AMOUNT OF FLUID GIVEN

The amount of fluid to be given to a critically ill or injured patient is determined by multiple factors, including the patient's blood pressure, heart rate, urinary output, and skin perfusion. One also must continuously listen and watch for rales or distended neck veins that might indicate fluid overload.

The response of the central venous pressure (CVP) to a fluid load can be very helpful in estimating further fluid requirements. However, if the amount of fluid given seems excessive, or if the patient has severe sepsis, respiratory failure, or an acute myocardial infarction, a pulmonary artery catheter should be inserted to help monitor cardiovascular function.

Central Venous Pressure (CVP). Fluid can usually be given until the CVP rises from a normal of 0 to 5 mmHg to about 10 to 15 mmHg. However, since there are many factors affecting the CVP, it is best to note the response to a fluid challenge.

In patients without obvious cardiac problems, a fluid challenge of 200 ml (3 ml/kg) of isotonic crystalloid can be given over a period of 10 min, while the CVP is monitored constantly. If the CVP rises by more than 5.0 mmHg, the fluids should be stopped until the CVP returns to within 2.0 mmHg of baseline.

Pulmonary Artery Wedge Pressure (PAWP). If the patient's volume status is still in question despite CVP monitoring, pulmonary artery wedge pressure (PAWP) monitoring should be used, particularly in patients with severe sepsis or other causes of myocardial or pulmonary dysfunction. With a pulmonary artery catheter in place in a patient with persistent shock, fluid and blood can usually be given until the PAWP is at least 15 mmHg. However, the response of the PAWP to a fluid challenge is more indicative of the fluid status of the patient than is the absolute PAWP level.

Fluid challenges may be performed in a wide variety of ways. A technique frequently used is to administer a balanced electrolyte solution in a dose of 3 ml/kg (200 ml for a 70-kg man) over 10 min to patients thought to have a normal heart and over 20 to 30 min if there is evidence of compromised cardiac function. If the patient's blood pressure or cardiac output improves and the PAWP does not rise rapidly, further fluid can generally be given. However, if the blood pressure or cardiac output does not improve and the PAWP rises more than 5.0 mmHg, further fluid should not be given until the PAWP is within 2 to 3 mmHg of the baseline value before the last fluid challenge. If the cardiac output is still low, such patients should be given inotropic agents and/or vasodilators.

If the oxygen saturation in mixed venous blood (Sv_{O_2}) in the pulmonary arteries is being measured, fluid and/or inotropes should be given until the Sv_{O_2} is at least 60 percent or until it rises no further with therapy.

End-Diastolic Volume. If a patient has severe sepsis with ARDS or if the patient has a low PAWP and does not seem to be responding properly to fluid administration, one should consider inserting a special pulmonary artery catheter that can be used to determine right ventricular end-diastolic volume index. As a general rule, if the index is less than 90 ml/m², fluid can be given with the expectation that the cardiac output and stroke volume will probably increase.[59,60] However, if the index is 140 ml/m² or more, tissue perfusion is not likely to improve with further fluid administration. If the index is 90 to 139 ml/m², one should give a fluid challenge and watch the response of the index and cardiac output. If the index increases only slightly but cardiac output increases, further fluids can usually be given with benefit until the index begins to approach 140 ml/m².

Cardiac Output. Since shock is usually defined in terms of inadequate tissue perfusion, one should attempt to increase cardiac output (CO) in critically ill or injured patients to normal or higher levels. In fact, in such individuals, a CO that is 25 to 50 percent greater than normal appears to be needed to adequately perfuse vital organs, especially the intestine and liver. Although measurement of CO is difficult in the emergency department, it should be measured in the intensive care unit and in high-risk patients in the operating room.

In general, fluid should be given rapidly to shock patients as long as CO is rising and there is little or no increase in filling pressure. At the point at which further fluid causes no increase in CO but causes the filling pressure to rise rapidly, additional fluid challenges should be withheld, and further attempts at raising CO should rely on inotropic agents and/or vasodilators.

Oxygen Delivery and Oxygen Consumption. It is becoming increasingly apparent that in addition to optimizing CO, one also should increase oxygen delivery (D_{O_2}) until oxygen consumption ($\dot{V}_{O_2}$) is no longer flow-dependent.[40]

The normal oxygen delivery index ($D_{O_2}I$) in healthy young adults is about 600 to 700 ml/min/m². For example, the $D_{O_2}I$ with a hemoglobin of 15.0 g/dl, a cardiac index (CI) of 3.5 liter/min/m², and a 95 percent arterial oxyhemoglobin saturation would be

$$D_{O_2}I = (CI)(Hb)(1.34) \frac{(\% \text{ Saturation})}{100} \quad (10)$$
$$= (3.5)(15)(1.34)(0.95)(10)$$
$$= 668 \text{ ml/min/m}^2$$

In a similar manner, a CI of 4.5 liter/min/m², a hemoglobin of 12.0 g/dl, and an Sa_{O_2} of 95 percent will provide a $D_{O_2}I$ of 687 ml/min/m².

Shoemaker et al.[40] have shown that using pulmonary artery catheter monitoring to raise the CI to 4.5 liter/min/m² and oxygen delivery to >600 ml/min/m² will significantly reduce morbidity and mortality in high-risk postoperative patients. In their landmark paper of 1988, they divided 90 postoperative patients who were at high risk for developing sepsis and organ failure into three groups.[40] Group I (30 patients) was monitored with only a CVP catheter. Group II (30 patients) was monitored with a PAWP catheter, but CI, D_{O_2}, and $\dot{V}_{O_2}$ were only restored to normal levels. Group III (30 patients) was monitored with a PAWP catheter, and the CI, D_{O_2}, and $\dot{V}_{O_2}$ were optimized to >4.5 liter/min/m², >600 ml/min/m², and >170 ml/min/m², respectively. The postoperative mortality rates in groups I, II, and III were 23, 33, and 4 percent, respectively. The days on a ventilator were 4.6 ± 1.4, 9.4 ± 3.4, and 2.3 ± 0.5 days, respectively.

To provide these optimal values, one should raise the CI as high as possible with fluid loading. If the patient has already had as much fluid loading as he or she can tolerate, one should consider giving inotropic agents and/or vasodilators to increase the CO further. However, if the CI is driven much above 5.0 liter/min/m², there may be difficulty off-loading the oxygen in the tissues because of the rapidity with which the blood will be passing through the capillaries.

Although there is a great deal of controversy concerning the ideal hemoglobin or hematocrit level for critically ill or injured patients, my own studies suggest that a hematocrit of 35 to 40 percent or higher is optimal, especially in patients with severe sepsis. As a general rule, each unit of packed red cells given to normovolemic or slightly hypervolemic septic patients with hematocrits of 30 percent or higher increases arterial oxygen content 8 to 10 percent but increases oxygen delivery by only 5 to 8 percent because of a slight drop in CO, probably due to the increased viscosity of the blood at the higher hematocrit. As a general rule, patients with lower $\dot{V}_{O_2}$ and higher lactate levels are more apt to have an increase in their $\dot{V}_{O_2}$ if the $\dot{D}_{O_2}$ is increased by raising the hemoglobin or the cardiac output.[20,41,185]

Although I am usually satisfied with an arterial P_{O_2} of about 70 mmHg, which is normally equivalent to an oxyhemoglobin saturation of 92 to 93 percent, in my critically ill patients who are severely septic and/or have a relatively low D_{O_2} or $\dot{V}_{O_2}$, I may increase the arterial P_{O_2} to 80 to 100 mmHg (equivalent to an oxyhemoglobin saturation of 95 to 98 percent).

INOTROPIC AGENTS

In patients in whom the CO, D_{O_2}, or $\dot{V}_{O_2}$ is not optimal despite fluid loading, I attempt to increase the CO with inotropic agents.

Digoxin. Digoxin is used only rarely in the management of hypotensive patients because of (1) the difficulty and time delay in obtaining optimal tissue levels, (2) frequent prolonged side effects, and (3) relatively minor inotropic effects. However, digoxin can be very helpful in patients with a dilated, failing heart, especially if atrial fibrillation is present.

The amount of digoxin needed in shock patients can vary greatly. Although the ECG response is generally not a good criterion for regulating digoxin dosage, it may be the only rapid means to obtain some reasonable idea if an adequate amount of drug has been given. Patients who are elderly or in shock may be adequately digitalized or may even develop digitalis toxicity with half the usual dosage.

Dopamine. Dopamine in doses of 0.5 to 3.0 μg/kg per minute affects dopaminergic receptors primarily, thereby dilating renal and splanchnic vessels and increasing renal blood flow, urine output, and urine sodium excretion. At doses of 2.0 to 5.0 μg/kg per minute, beta receptors are also stimulated, resulting in an increased CO.

Most physicians consider dopamine the inotropic agent of choice in patients with hypotension and a low CO. In doses of 5 to 15 μg/kg per minute, dopamine acts primarily as a positive inotrope. At doses exceeding 20 to 30 μg/kg per minute, it tends to cause increasing vasoconstriction. However, in some septic patients, the vasoconstrictor effect of dopamine may not be apparent, even at doses exceeding 50 μg/kg per minute. Thus, in choosing between dopamine and another catecholamine, the decision is less dependent on the pharmacologic characteristic of the agents than it is on the clinical and hemodynamic circumstances of the patient.

In vasodilated septic patients with hypotension and oliguria, dopamine is probably the inotrope of choice. In patients who are vasoconstricted and have a normal blood pressure but a low CO, dobutamine is preferred.

The most frequent problem limiting the use of dopamine is tachycardia. Occasionally, it may be difficult to wean a patient from small doses of dopamine because he or she has become catecholamine-depleted, and the exogenous dopamine acts as a precursor for norepinephrine and epinephrine. Dopamine also inhibits thyroid-stimulating hormone (TSH) and prolactin release, and this blunts the response to thyroxine-releasing hormone.[186]

Dobutamine. Dobutamine is generally the inotrope of choice in patients with a low CO and a normal or increased blood pressure. In doses of 5 to 20 μg/kg per minute, it has a positive inotropic effect and is a vasodilator. It is particularly helpful in patients with acute myocardial infarction shock, characterized by a low CO, normal blood pressure, and high systemic vascular resistance.[187] As a rule, dobutamine causes less of an increase in heart rate, pulmonary artery pressure, and PAWP than dopamine and also may be a good agent for treating shock due to massive pulmonary embolism. Frequently, combinations of dopamine (5 to 10 μg/kg/min) and dobutamine (5 to 15 μg/kg/min) are used to improve myocardial function and raise CO in patients who are elderly or may have impaired cardiac contractility.[188]

Amrinone. Amrinone (Inocor) can be a potent inotropic agent with vasodilator properties. Its mode of action is not completely understood, but it probably causes an inhibition of phosphodiesterase, the substance that breaks down cyclic adenosine monophosphate (cAMP). Consequently, by increasing cAMP levels, amrinone can potentiate the actions of various adrenergic agents.[186]

Since amrinone is not inhibited by beta-adrenergic blocking agents, it can be very helpful in patients receiving beta blockers. Amrinone also can be a good vasodilator, especially in the lungs, and because of this property, it is being used increasingly in intensive care unit patients with pulmonary hypertension, especially after cardiac surgery.

One problem with amrinone is that of having to use a loading dose (0.75 mg/kg) and then a maintenance dose (5 to 10 μg/kg/min). It also has a long half-life (3.6 to 5.8 h), which can be a problem if undesirable side effects develop.[189]

Epinephrine. Epinephrine in doses of 1 to 5 μg/min can be used to improve the blood pressure and CO if they remain low despite fluid loading and rather large doses of dopamine and/or dobutamine. However, dopamine tends to produce a somewhat more uniform response, and it is less likely to cause tachyarrhythmias.

Isoproterenol. In patients who are in shock and have a slow pulse rate and a low CO, isoproterenol in doses of 1 to 2 μg/min may dramatically improve CO. However, since isoproterenol has a strong chronotropic effect on the heart and is a vasodilator, it is of little or no benefit in the usual shock patient who has hypotension and tachycardia. Indeed, if the heart rate exceeds 120 beats per minute, isoproterenol can increase myocardial O_2 consumption ($M\dot{V}_{O_2}$) much more than it increases coronary blood flow and thereby cause severe myocardial ischemia and/or dangerous tachyarrhythmias. For these reasons, isoproterenol should generally not be given to patients with an acute myocardial infarction or a pulmonary embolus.

Glucagon. Glucagon can be an effective inotropic and chronotropic agent in patients with heart failure or cardiogenic shock. In about 20 to 30 percent of patients in whom relatively large doses (4-mg bolus and then 10 mg/h by constant IV infusion) are used, it has produced some hemodynamic improvement, although often only temporarily. Glucagon may be particularly helpful in the treatment of shock in patients taking beta blockers because its effectiveness is based on an entirely different mechanism of action.[190] However, it can cause nausea and severe hyperglycemia.

Glucagon should be reconstituted hourly, because it rapidly loses its potency at room temperature. This agent acts at least partially by stimulating adenyl cyclase activity and thereby increasing cAMP production in the myocardium. Consequently, its effectiveness may be increased by the simultaneous administration of aminophylline, which inhibits phosphodiesterase, the enzyme that converts cAMP into an inactive form. The cardiovascular actions of glucagon are calcium-dependent and require adequate plasma ionized calcium levels.[191]

Calcium. Shock, sepsis, and rapid massive blood transfusions can cause ionized calcium levels to fall to very low levels.[192–194] Administration of calcium to patients with shock or sepsis and very low ionized calcium levels may dramatically improve myocardial function, CO, and blood pressure. However, if tissue perfusion and cell function are not restored to normal, much of the calcium that was administered will move into myocardial and vascular smooth muscle cells, and after 30 to 45 min, hemodynamic function and tissue perfusion may be worse than before the calcium was given.[195] Furthermore, if cell metabolism is still impaired, the additional calcium entering the cytoplasm will move into the mitochondria, where it will further interfere with ATP production.

As a consequence, calcium should probably only be given to patients in persistent shock or heart failure if they are receiving massive blood transfusions rapidly (more than 1 unit every 5 min) or if the patient has been on beta-adrenergic blockers or calcium channel blockers.

In hypotensive and bradycardiac individuals taking beta blockers and/or calcium blockers, IV calcium chloride may produce an immediate and dramatic beneficial hemodynamic response. Hypocalcemia in patients receiving rapid blood transfusions may sometimes be picked up early by noting prolongation of the QT interval.

Glucose-Insulin-Potassium (GIK). An occasional patient who is unresponsive to inotropes and vasoconstrictors will respond, at least transiently, to "polarizing" solutions containing increased quantities of glucose, insulin, and potassium. The usual GIK solution is a liter of 10% to 20% glucose containing 20 to 40 units of insulin and 40 to 80 mEq of KCl. This solution is usually given at 150 to 250 ml/h, but care should be taken not to overload the patient with fluid. Experimental studies suggest that GIK solutions may improve myocardial blood flow and metabolism.[196] They also have been shown to reduce the incidence of arrhythmias in acute anterior myocardial infarctions.

CARDIAC PACING

Cardiac pacing for heart block or severe bradycardia in patients with a fixed low stroke volume can be extremely helpful, particularly if atropine or isoproterenol have not been effective. Overdrive pacing also may improve CO in some patients with tachyarrhythmias.

Cardiac pacing also may be of benefit in some patients with right ventricular infarctions. The syndrome of right-sided heart failure, low CO, and hypotension following right ventricular infarction is seen in 3 to 8 percent of all acute myocardial infarctions.[197] Some of these patients will have the Beck I triad (hypotension, distended neck veins, and muffled heart tones) and will be suspected of having pericardial tamponade.[198] Heart block and bradyarrhythmias are common in these patients, and atrioventricular sequential pacing may significantly increase CO and blood pressure.

VASODILATORS

In patients who show evidence of excessive vasoconstriction and poor tissue perfusion despite all other therapy but have a blood pressure that is normal or high, a vasodilator may greatly improve tissue perfusion. However, vasodilators must be used with great care because they can cause a sudden drop in blood pressure, especially if the patient is hypovolemic.

Vasodilators may increase vascular capacity by 2 to 3 liters, making hypovolemic patients have an even greater discrepancy between vascular capacity and intravascular volume. This can cause sudden, severe hypotension. Even if the patient has a normal blood volume, vasodilators will often cause the blood pressure to fall by at least 5 to 10 mmHg. If the patient is already hypotensive, the further decrease in blood pressure can jeopardize coronary and cerebral blood flow. This is particularly dangerous if these vessels have a 70 to 80 percent occlusion that makes flow through them pressure-dependent. Consequently, to use a vasodilator effectively and safely, one should have catheters in place to constantly monitor systemic arterial pressure and PAWP. One also should be prepared to give fluid rapidly if the blood pressure falls significantly as the vasodilator is started.

Nitroprusside in doses of 0.3 to 3.0 μg/kg per minute acts on both arteries and veins and therefore tends to reduce afterload more than preload, thereby increasing CO in patients with a normal or increased blood volume.[199] Nitroglycerin in similar doses primarily reduces preload but also dilates coronary arteries. In addition to causing occasional sudden, severe drops in blood pressure, especially if the patient is not adequately fluid loaded, nitroglycerin can cause a reduction in the arterial P_{O_2} by inhibiting pulmonary vasoconstriction in poorly ventilated areas of the lungs.[200] Large doses (>3 to 5 μg/kg/min) of nitroprusside given for more than 36 to 48 h may cause blood levels of thiocyanate to rise to toxic levels. This toxicity may be manifested by confusion, hyperreflexia, and convulsions.[199]

Other agents that can decrease total peripheral vascular resistance include dobutamine, isoproterenol, prostacyclin, ATP-MgCl$_2$, narcotics, sedatives, and glucose-insulin-potassium solutions.

ACID-BASE THERAPY

Most acid-base problems in shock will improve spontaneously if adequate ventilation and tissue perfusion are provided. However, if severe metabolic acidosis with a pH less than 7.10 persists despite optimal fluid loading and inotropic drugs and the patient is hypotensive or has a low CO, enough bicarbonate should be given to raise the arterial pH to 7.20.[201] However, if bicarbonate is given, it is important to provide a greater than normal alveolar ventilation and to monitor the arterial and mixed venous P_{CO_2}. If the arterial P_{CO_2} rises above 40 to 45 mmHg and/or the venous P_{CO_2} rises above 50 to 55 mmHg, the bicarbonate administration may actually cause increasing cellular acidosis and thereby increase mortality rates.[202]

If hyperventilation is used to raise the arterial pH, one should not reduce the P_{CO_2} below 25 mmHg because of the possible adverse effects that severe hypocarbia can have on the cerebral circulation. Since cerebral blood flow falls about 2 to 4 percent for each 1.0 mmHg drop in the arterial P_{CO_2}, an arterial P_{CO_2} below 15 to 20 mmHg can cause cerebral ischemia. One also must be careful not to produce an overshoot alkalosis because it can markedly reduce the P_{O_2}, O$_2$ availability, and ionized calcium and magnesium levels. Each 0.10 pH rise reduces the oxygen availability to tissues about 10 percent. It reduces sodium potassium levels by an average of 0.5 mEq/liter and reduces ionized calcium and magnesium levels about 4 to 8 percent.

When determining how much bicarbonate to give, the total bicarbonate deficit can generally be calculated by considering the bicarbonate space in humans to be equal to 30 percent of the body weight if the base deficit (BD) is mild (5 to 10 mEq/liter), and 50 percent of the body weight if the BD is severe (>15 mEq/liter). Thus a BD of 10 mEq/liter in a 70-kg man can generally be corrected with about 210 mEq bicarbonate, but only if oxygen demand and supply are balanced. As a general rule, it takes at least 100 to 125 mEq bicarbonate to raise the pH from 7.10 to 7.20 in an average-sized adult male.

ADRENOCORTICAL-LIKE STEROIDS

Physiologic Doses. Subclinical adrenal cortical insufficiency may be present in up to 5 to 15 percent of critically ill patients. *Adrenal insufficiency* refers to adrenal cortical secretion that is below normal and low plasma cortisol levels, and *adrenal inadequacy* refers to less secretion than is needed for the degree of stress that is present. Thus many critically ill patients have increased adrenal cortical activity, but it may not be adequate for the degrees of stress present. Consequently, patients with shock that is unresponsive to fluid loading and inotropic agents should probably be given at least 200 mg hydrocortisone by rapid IV injection. If the patient responds, 50 to 100 mg hydrocortisone can then be given every 6 to 12 h as needed. After 24 to 48 h of such treatment, the steroids can usually be tapered off quite safely over the next 3 to 4 days.

IV ACTH (cosyntropin) can be used to determine if adrenal insufficiency is present. If 250 μg cosyntropin is given IV, plasma cortisol levels should double or rise by at least 7 μg/dl or adrenal insufficiency is probably present and should be treated.[203]

Pharmacologic Doses. Experimentally, adrenocortical-like steroids in massive doses equivalent to 150 mg hydrocortisone per kilogram of body weight have been thought to be helpful in shock by (1) preventing uncoupling of mitochondrial electron transport and oxidative phosphorylation,[204] (2) reducing lysosomal fragility and capillary membrane permeability,[205] (3) improving cardiovascular function,[206] and (4) reducing excessive activation of complement and formation of prostaglandins and leukotrienes.[207] More recently, steroids also have been shown to block transcription and mobilization of tumor necrosis factor messenger RNA in macrophages. Thus, if given early enough, massive steroids can prevent excessive activation of the various proteolytic cascades seen as a response to endotoxin in many experimental animals.[208] Hinshaw et al.[209] have shown that baboons can achieve a 100 percent survival in spite of a lethal infusion of endotoxin or bacteria by administration of appropriate antibiotics plus early massive steroids.

In the largest prospective, randomized, double-blind study performed at a single institution with pharmacologic doses of corticosteroids in patients with septic shock, Schumer et al.[210] found that patients treated with a placebo had a mortality rate of 43 percent, while those treated very early with steroids, usually less than 2 h from the onset of shock, had a mortality rate of only 14 percent.

Sprung et al.[211] also performed a double-blind, prospective, randomized study on 59 medical patients with septic shock. The patients were given either dexamethasone (DXM) (6 mg/kg), methylprednisolone sodium succinate (MPSS) (30 mg/kg), or a placebo every 4 h as needed. These patients were treated an average of 17 ± 5 h after the onset of shock. Of those treated within 4 h of the onset of the shock, reversal of the shock occurred in 73 percent (8 of 11) of those given steroids as compared with 20 percent (1 of 5) of controls. This difference was statistically significant ($p < 0.05$).

The two large multi-institutional, prospective, double-blind studies on the use of massive steroids in sepsis suggest that there is little or no place for massive steroids in the treatment of sepsis or septic shock.[212,213] Although a favorable response in patients with gram-negative sepsis was found in one of the studies and was almost significant, the result with gram-positive organisms was poor. Other steroid problems included an increased tendency to ARDS and increased mortality rates in patients with elevated serum creatinine levels. However, very early and more sustained administration of large doses of adrenocorticosteroids may still be helpful.

INCREASING AFTERLOAD

Vasopressors. Vasopressors should be considered potentially lethal drugs. They should probably only be given to correct a very low blood pressure in normo-volemic, neurogenic shock or temporarily when there appears to be no other rapidly effective method for restoring an adequate coronary or cerebral blood flow in patients with severe vascular disease. They should generally be administered only after an adequate trial with ventilation, oxygen, fluids, acid-base correction, and inotropic agents. Dopamine, particularly if doses greater than 20 to 30 μg/kg per minute are used, can raise the blood pressure quite adequately in about 80 to 90 percent of patients who require drugs to correct their hypotension. Thus only a small number of patients with shock require relatively pure vasoconstrictors, such as neosynephrine or norepinephrine.

Agents such as phenylephrine and methoxamine that have only a peripheral vasoconstrictor effect also can raise blood pressure, but at the same time they tend to cause a decrease in CO and tissue perfusion. Norepinephrine and metaraminol, which are predominantly vasoconstrictors but also have some cardiac effect, generally cause less of a drop in CO than the pure vasopressors. With norepinephrine, doses less than 1 to 2 μg/min cause relatively less vasoconstriction and more of a positive inotropic effect than larger doses.

My current favorite vasopressor in appropriate patients is dopamine in large doses (20 to 60 μg/kg/min). If this is ineffective, I may use four ampules (16 mg) of norepinephrine plus two ampules (10 mg) of phentolamine in 500 ml of D_5W. Phentolamine (Regitine) in this dosage can prevent the excessive vasoconstriction that is usually caused by norepinephrine, but it does not significantly reduce the blood pressure rise. Furthermore, if the norepinephrine should extravasate into tissues around the IV catheter, the phentolamine prevents the local necrosis that would otherwise tend to occur. In instances when the patient already seems excessively vasoconstricted, the concentration of phentolamine may be increased to two ampules for each ampule of norepinephrine. Low doses (1 to 2 μg/min) of norepinephrine combined with moderate doses (5 to 15 μg/kg/min) of dopamine also may be of value in septic shock.

In patients with significant coronary artery disease, raising the mean blood pressure to 80 mmHg may increase coronary blood flow more than it increases myocardial oxygen demand ($M\dot{V}_{O_2}$), and CO also may rise. However, raising the blood pressure to even higher levels is apt to increase $M\dot{V}_{O_2}$ more than myocardial oxygen delivery (MD_{O_2}), and this may cause increasing myocardial ischemia. Furthermore, there is no clinical evidence that vasopressors such as dopamine or norepinephrine increase survival of patients with cardiogenic shock.

Newer Agents. *Naloxone.* ACTH and beta-endorphins are derived from a common precursor (preopiocortin) and are secreted in equimolar amounts in response to stress at the hypothalamic level. The beta-endorphins appear to relieve pain and inhibit central autonomic sites that regulate the release of pressor substrates from the adrenal medulla in large doses. In large amounts, they may even cause shock. Consequently, it was thought that antagonists of the endorphins might be useful for the treatment of hypotension. The first report of such action by naloxone, a beta-endorphin antagonist, was by Holaday and Faden[214] in

1978, who noted that naloxone blocked the hypotension caused by endotoxin administration in rats. Naloxone was particularly beneficial if large doses were given before systemic deterioration was present. However, it had minimal, if any, hemodynamic effect in normal animals.

The majority of studies on naloxone have related its overall beneficial effects to a central (CNS) mechanism of action. However, experiments in rats with adrenalectomy or with selective adrenal demedullation (with adrenal cortical function remaining intact) show not only enhanced sensitivity to endotoxin but also lack of the normal pressor response to naloxone during the endotoxic shock.[215]

Relatively few studies have evaluated the effects of naloxone on hypotension in humans. Although it can usually increase the blood pressure in hypotensive individuals, it has not improved survival rates in humans.[216]

Thyrotropin-releasing hormone (TRH). TRH has been found to improve cardiovascular function and survival in experimental hemorrhagic[217] and endotoxic shock.[218] These effects appear to be independent of its pituitary-thyroid regulatory function.

TRH, like naloxone, appears to function largely through central CNS effector sites and is dependent on an intact sympathetic-adrenal complex.[219] In contrast to naloxone, TRH does not bind to opiate receptors or alter the analgesic properties of various opiate drugs. However, it does antagonize many of the other biologic effects of endorphins that seem to cause hypotension. TRH may be of particular benefit if an antiendorphin is to be used in settings where adequate pain control is also important.

MECHANICAL CARDIOVASCULAR SUPPORT

Intraaortic Balloon Pumping (IABP). Intraaortic balloon pumping (IABP) can be of great value in treating acute myocardial infarction shock and severe postoperative myocardial dysfunction that is refractory to all other therapy.[220] However, the longer one waits to try IABP in a patient in cardiogenic shock, the more the myocardium becomes damaged and the less likely the IABP is to be helpful.

The IABP catheter is generally inserted through the common femoral artery and passed up into the proximal aorta. A 27- to 35-cc balloon is positioned in the descending thoracic aorta, just distal to the left subclavian artery. The balloon is rapidly deflated in the descending aorta as the aortic valve is opening, and this causes the systolic pressure, time in systole, and heart size to decrease. The resulting decrease in systolic tension-time index can greatly reduce myocardial oxygen consumption ($M\dot{V}_{O_2}$). The balloon is then inflated at the beginning of diastole. This causes diastolic aortic pressure to increase, thereby improving myocardial blood flow.

Extracorporeal Membrane Oxygenation (ECMO). In patients who have had cardiogenic shock that is refractory to all measures, including IABP, one may try to support the circulation with arteriovenous extracorporeal membrane oxygenation (ECMO).[221] Reedy et al.[222] reported their experience with 38 patients supported with ECMO. They found that ECMO is useful for 12 to 24 h and is best applied to (1) patients < 60 years of age, (2) patients with acute events (such as a failed PTCA amenable to surgical correction), and (3) candidates for cardiac transplantation who can be switched to more sophisticated support devices within 12 to 24 h. There also has been renewed interest in the use of ECMO to help adults with severe acute respiratory failure.[223]

NONSTEROIDAL ANTI-INFLAMMATORY DRUGS (NSAID)

During shock and sepsis there is a greatly increased conversion of membrane phospholipids to arachidonic acid.[215] Increased quantities and/or abnormal relationships between these arachidonic acid metabolites may be responsible for many of the changes seen in both experimental endotoxin and clinical septic shock.

A number of prostaglandin inhibitors, including aspirin,[224] indomethacin,[225] and ibuprofen,[226] have been beneficial in experimental shock, especially when used as pretreatment. However, benefit in proper clinical trials has not been demonstrated.

ANTIENDOTOXIN THERAPY

E. coli Antisera and Vaccines. Certain cell wall components of gram-negative bacteria contribute to the development of severe sepsis and septic shock. The outermost layer of the cell wall of gram-negative bacteria is a polysaccharide referred to as O, or *somatic, antigen.* This chain of repeating oligosaccharide units is unique for each serotype of gram-negative organism, and it is responsible for the smooth appearance of the colonies when grown on culture medium. The colonies of mutant organisms that lack the O antigen and show only core polysaccharide or the second layer of endotoxin on their surface appear rough on culture. The core polysaccharide layer is attached via 2-keto-3-deoxyoctulosonate (KDO) to a third layer composed of a lipid moiety called *lipid A.*

The KDO–lipid A segment appears to be immunologically identical in almost all aerobic gram-negative bacteria studied. Together, the three component layers—O antigen, R core antigen, and lipid A—make up *endotoxin,* which is also called *lipopolysaccharide* (LPS). Although the term *endotoxin* was originally chosen because it was felt that this toxic bacterial component was an integral part of the bacterial cell wall, it has since been noted that endotoxin can exist in a free state, can be released by bacteria growing in culture, and can retain its biologic activity after extraction from bacteria.

Studies indicate that antibodies to core lipopolysaccharides (R core antigen plus lipid A) can be cross-protective. In a study reported by Ziegler et al.,[227] antiserum containing polyclonal antibodies to core lipopolysaccharide was randomly given to 103 of 212 patients with gram-negative infections. The mortality rate of the control group was 39 percent compared with 22 percent in the antiserum group. Its effect in patients in shock was even greater, with mortality rates of 77 percent in the controls and 44 percent in the antiserum group.

In another prospective, randomized study, Lachman et al.[228] used freeze-dried human plasma which was rich in antilipopolysaccharide (anti-LPS) IgG to treat septic shock in patients. The mortality was 47 percent (9 of 19) in conventionally treated patients and 7 percent (1 of 14) with anti-LPS. Anti-LPS also caused a mean arterial blood pressure rise from 45 ± 8 to 69 ± 9 mmHg within 75 min of administration.

Interestingly, another study showed markedly different results.[229] In a randomized, double-blind trial of human antilipopolysaccharide (anti-LPS) specific globulin versus placebo in the treatment of severe septic shock, the hospital mortality rate was 53 percent (9 of 17) in the treated group and 59 percent (10 of 17) in the control group. Measurement of serum endotoxin and anti-LPS levels at the time of admission to the study and 24 h later revealed no significant difference between controls and treatment patients.

Monoclonal Antibodies. Difficulty in preparation, lack of homogeneity, and risks associated with administration of antiserum led to the concept of developing immunotherapy based on monoclonal antibody (mAb) technology. Dunn et al.[230] experimentally produced monoclonal antibodies directed against certain common antigens on core lipopolysaccharide (LPS). They found that anti-J5 mAb significantly protected mice from various bacterial challenges, including organisms that were stereotypically distinct from *E. coli* J5. Antonacci et al.[231] found that monoclonal antibodies were effective in significantly decreasing mortality rates in mice given an LD_{60-70} dose of gram-negative bacteria. Thus an increasing number of studies suggest that monoclonal and polyclonal antibodies to endotoxin can significantly improve survival rates in severe sepsis and/or septic shock.

In a phase I trial, Fisher et al.[232] evaluated the safety, pharmacokinetics, and immunogenicity of the human monoclonal antibody HA-1A for 14 to 21 days in septic patients. This human monoclonal antibody had cross-reacted with endotoxins from a large number of unrelated species of gram-negative bacteria. Thirty-four patients received either 25, 100, or 250 mg of HA-1A as a single intravenous infusion over 15 min. There were no reports of adverse or allergic reactions thought to be related to HA-1A infusion, and there was no evidence of an antibody response to HA-1A during the study period.

Ziegler et al.[233] evaluated the efficacy and safety of HA-1A in gram-negative bacteremia and sepsis in a large prospective, placebo-controlled, double-blind study. In this study, there were 543 patients with suspected gram-negative sepsis. Of these, 200 patients were diagnosed as having gram-negative bacteremia and sepsis. These 200 patients received either a 100-mg single dose of HA-1A or a placebo and were evaluated for a 28-day study period. Mortality with gram-negative bacteremia was significantly reduced from 49 percent in patients on the placebo to 30 percent in those on HA-1A. In addition, mortality with gram-negative bacteremia and shock was significantly reduced from 57 percent in patients on placebo to 33 percent in those on HA-1A.

A murine (E5) antiendotoxin monoclonal antibody also has been studied. Greenman et al.[234] in a double-blind, randomized, multicenter trial of E5 in 486 patients with suspected gram-negative sepsis, gave either 2 mg/kg of E5 antibody or a placebo over 1 h, followed by a second infusion 24 h later. Among patients not in refractory shock at study entry, E5 significantly improved survival and resolution of organ failure.

REFERENCES

1. Hughes JT: The miraculous deliverance of Anne Green: An Oxford case of resuscitation in the seventeenth century. *Br Med J* 285:1792, 1982.
2. *Newes from the Dead or A True and Exact Narration of the Miraculous Deliverance of Anne Green.* Written by a Scholler in Oxford. Printed by Leonard Lichfield for Tho Robinson, 1651.
3. Sinclair HM, Robb-Smith AHT: *A Short History of Anatomical Teaching in Oxford.* Oxford, Oxford University Press, 1950.
4. Scholten D: Electrolytes and plasma volume regulation in hypovolemic shock. *Am J Emerg Med* 2:82, 1984.
5. Paré A: *Oeuvres completes D'ambroise Paré.* Paris, JB Bailiniers, 1840.
6. Garrison FH: *The History of Medicine,* 4th ed. Philadelphia, Saunders, 1929, p 273.
7. Bartecchi CE: Intravenous therapy: From humble beginnings through 150 years. *South Med J* 75:61, 1982.
8. Hermann R: Über die veraenderungen, die die sekretionen des menschlichen organismus durch die cholera erleiden. *Poggendorffs Ann* 22:161, 1831.
9. Howard-Jones N: Cholera therapy in the nineteenth century. *J Hist Med* 27:373, 1972.
10. Cosnett JE: The origin of intravenous fluid therapy. *Lancet* 1:768, 1989.
11. O'Shaughnessy WB: Proposal of a new method of treating the blue epidemic cholera by the injection of highly oxygenated salts into the venous system. *Lancet* 1:366, 1831–1832.
12. O'Shaughnessy WB: Experiments on the blood in cholera. *Lancet* 1:490, 1831–1832.
13. Latta T: Malignant cholera. *Lancet* 2:274, 1831–1832.
14. Masson AHB: Latta: Pioneer in saline infusion. *Br J Anaesthesiol* 43:681, 1832.
15. Latta T: Injections into the veins in cholera. *Lond Med Gaz* 379, 1832.
16. Latta T: Reply to some objectives offered to the practice of venous injections in cholera. *Lancet* 2:428, 1831–1832.
17. Wilson RF, Jablonski DV, Thal AP: The usage of dibenzyline in clinical shock. *Surgery* 56:172, 1962.
18. Wilson RF, Thal AP: Hemodynamic measurements in septic shock. *Arch Surg* 91:121, 1965.
19. Groenveld ABJ, Kester ADM, Nauta JJPM, et al: Relation of arterial blood lactate to oxygen delivery and hemodynamic varices in human shock states. *Circ Shock* 22:35, 1987.
20. Wilson RF, Christensen C, Al M, et al: Oxygen consumption in critically ill surgical patients. *Ann Surg* 176:801, 1972.
21. Ross J Jr: Dynamics of the peripheral circulation, in West JB (ed): *Best and Taylors Physiological Basis of Medical Practice,* 11th ed. Baltimore, Williams & Wilkins, 1985, pp 142–143.
22. Kaye W: Invasive monitoring techniques: Arterial cannulation, bedside pulmonary artery catheterization and arterial puncture. *Heart Lung* 12:395, 1983.
23. Coyle JP, Teplick RS, Long MC, et al: Respiratory variations in systemic arterial pressure as an indicator of volume status. *Anesthesiology* 59:A53, 1983.
24. Perel A, Pizov R, Cotev S: Systolic blood pressure variation is a sensitive indicator of hypovolemia in ventilated dogs subjected to graded hemorrhage. *Anesthesiology* 67:498, 1987.
25. Hurst JW, Schlant RC: Examination of the arteries, in Hurst JW, Louge RB (eds): *The Heart.* New York, McGraw-Hill, 1966, pp 75–77.
26. Shapiro BA, Cane RD, Chomka CM, et al: Preliminary evaluation of an intraarterial blood gas system in dogs and humans. *Crit Care Med* 17:455, 1989.
27. Taylor MB, Whiteman JG: The current status of pulse oximetry. *Anesthesia* 41:943, 1989.
28. Stasic AF: Continuous evaluation of oxygenation and ventilation, in Civetta JM, Taylor RW, Kirby RR (eds): *Critical Care.* Philadelphia, Lippincott, 1988, p 317.
29. Nolan LS, Shoemaker WC: Transcutaneous O_2 and CO_2 monitoring of high risk surgical patients during the perioperative. *Crit Care Med* 10:762, 1982.

30. Temper KK, Waxman K, Shoemaker WC: Effects of hypoxia and shock and transcutaneous PO$_2$ values in dogs. *Crit Care Med* 7:526, 1979.

31. Ritchalia SVS, Booth S: Factors influencing transcutaneous oxygen tension. *Intensive Care World* 2:126, 1985.

32. Shoemaker WC, Vidyasagar D: Physiological and clinical significance of P$_{tc}$O$_2$ and P$_{tc}$CO$_2$ measurements. *Crit Care Med* 9:689, 1981.

33. Kram HB, Shoemaker WC: Transcutaneous, conjunctival, and organ PO$_2$ and PCO$_2$ monitoring during carotid endarterectomy. *Arch Surg* 121:914, 1986.

34. Kram HB, Shoemaker WC, Bratanow N, et al: Noninvasive conjunctival oxygen during carotid endarterectomy. *Arch Surg* 121:914, 1986.

35. Smalhout B, Kalenda Z: *An Atlas of Capnography,* 2d ed, vol 1. The Netherlands, Zerckebosch-Zeist, 1981, p 20.

36. Schena J, Thompson J, Crone RK: Mechanical influences on the capnagram. *Crit Care Med* 12:672, 1984.

37. Triner L, Sherman J: Potential value of expiratory carbon dioxide measurement in patients considered to be susceptible to malignant hyperthermia. *Anesthesiology* 55:482, 1981.

38. Linko K, Paloheimo M, Tammisto T: Capnography for detection of accidental oesophageal intubation. *Acta Anaesthesiol Scand* 27:199, 1983.

39. Ozanne GM, Young WG, Mazzel WG, et al: Multipatient anesthetic mass spectometry: Rapid analysis of gas of long catheters. *Anesthesiology* 55:62, 1981.

40. Shoemaker WC, Appel PL, Kram HB, et al: Prospective trial of supranormal values of survivors as therapeutic goals in high risk surgical patients. *Chest* 94:1176, 1988.

41. Wilson RF, Gibson DB: The use of arterio-central venous oxygen differences to calculate cardiac output and oxygen consumption in critically ill surgical patients. *Surgery* 84:362, 1978.

42. Tuchschmidt J, Fried J, Swinney R, et al: Early hemodynamic correlates of survival in patients with septic shock. *Crit Care Med* 17:719, 1989.

43. Bland RD, Shoemaker WC, Abrahamm E, et al: Hemodynamic and oxygen transport patterns in surviving and nonsurviving postoperative patients. *Crit Care Med* 13:85, 1985.

44. Shoemaker WC, Appel PL, Kram HB: Tissue oxygen debt as a determinant of lethal and nonlethal postoperative organ failure. *Crit Care Med* 16:117, 1988.

45. Shoemaker WC, Appeal P, Bland R: Use of physiologic monitoring to predict outcome and to assist in clinical decision in critically ill postoperative patients. *Am J Surg* 146:43, 1983.

46. Blalock A: *Principles of Surgical Care, Shock, and Other Problems.* St. Louis, Mosby, 1940.

47. Kirkpatrick JR, Wilson RF: The significance of cardiac arrhythmias in the septic patient. *Mich Med* 74:645, 1975.

48. Little RA: 1988 Fitts Lecture: Heart rate changes after hemorrhage and injury: A reappraisal. *J Trauma* 29:903, 1989.

49. Cope DK, Allison RC, Parmentier JC, et al: Using pulmonary arterial pressure profile after occlusion. *Crit Care Med* 14:16, 1986.

50. Goldenheim PD, Kazemi H: Cardiopulmonary monitoring of critically ill patients. *N Engl J Med* 311:717, 1984.

51. Lucas CE: The renal response to acute injury and sepsis. *Surg Clin North Am* 56:953, 1976.

52. Wilson RF, Soullier G, Antonenko D: Creatinine clearance in critically ill surgical patients. *Arch Surg* 114:461, 1979.

53. Starling EH: *The Linacre Lecture on the Law of the Heart.* London, Longmore, Green, 1918.

54. Wilson RF, Sarver E, Birks R: Central venous pressure and blood volume determinations in clinical shock. *Surg Gynecol Obstet* 132:631, 1971.

55. Wilson RF, Quadros E, Chiscano A: Some observations on 58 patients with cardiac shock. *Anesth Analg* 46:764, 1967.

56. Wilson RF, Sarver EJ, Rizzo J: Hemodynamic changes, treatment and prognosis in clinical shock. *Arch Surg* 102:21, 1971.

57. Wilson RF, Beckman B, Tyburski JG, Scholten D: Pulmonary artery diastolic and wedge pressure relationships in critically ill and injured patients. *Arch Surg* 123:933, 1988.

58. Mann RL, Carlon GC, Turnbull AD: Comparison of electronic and manometric central venous pressures. *Crit Care Med* 9:98, 1981.

59. Diebel LN, Wilson RF, Tagett MG, Kline RA: End-diastolic volume: A better indicator of preload in the critically ill. *Arch Surg* 127:817, 1992.

60. Reuse C, Vincent CL, Pinsky MR: Measurement of right ventricular volume during fluid challenge. *Chest* 98:1450, 1990.

61. West JB, Dollery CT, Naimark A: Distribution of blood flow in isolated lung. Relation to vascular and alveolar pressure. *J Appl Physiol* 19:713, 1964.

62. Gengiz M, Crapo RO, Gardner RM: The effect of ventilation on the accuracy of pulmonary artery and wedge pressure measurements. *Crit Care Med* 11:502, 1983.

63. Yang SC, Puri VK: Role of preoperative hemodynamic monitoring in intraoperative fluid management. *Am Surg* 52:536, 1986.

64. Sibbald WJ, Holliday RL, Lobb TR: Pulmonary hypertension in sepsis. *Chest* 73:583, 1978.

65. Conners AF Jr, McCaffree DR, Gray BA: Evaluation of right-heart catheterization in the critically ill patient without acute myocardial infarction. *N Engl J Med* 380:263, 1983.

66. Eisenberg PR, Jaffe AS, Schuster DP: Clinical evaluation compared to pulmonary artery catheterization in the hemodynamic assessment of critically ill patients. *Crit Care Med* 12:549, 1984.

67. Fein AM, Goldberg SK, Walhenstein MD, et al: Is pulmonary artery catheterization necessary for the diagnosis of pulmonary edema? *Am Rev Respir Dis* 129:1006, 1984.

68. Del Guercio LRM, Cohn JD: Monitoring operating risk in the elderly. *JAMA* 243:1350, 1980.

69. Patel C, Laboy V, Venus B, et al: Acute complications of pulmonary artery catheter insertion in critically ill patients. *Crit Care Med* 14:195, 1986.

70. Sprung CL, Elser B, Schein RMH, et al: Risk of right bundle-branch block and complete heart block during pulmonary artery catheterization. *Crit Care Med* 17:1, 1989.

71. Pinilla JC, Ross DF, Martin T, et al: Study of the incidence of intravascular catheter infection and associated septicemia in critically ill patients. *Crit Care Med* 11:21, 1983.

72. Barash PG, Nardi D, Hammond G, et al: Catheter-induced pulmonary artery perforation, mechanisms, management and modification. *J Thorac Cardiovasc Surg* 82:5, 1981.

73. Nelson LD: Application of venous saturation monitoring, in Civetta JM, Taylor RW, Kirby RR (eds): *Critical Care*. Philadelphia, Lippincott, 1988, p 327.

74. Watson CB: The PA catheter as an early warning system. *Anesthesiol Rev* 10:34, 1983.

75. Daper A, Parquier J, Preiser J, et al: Timing of cardiac output measurements during mechanical ventilation. *Acute Care* 12:113, 1986.

76. Kay HR, Afshari M, Barash P, et al: Measurement of ejection fraction by thermal dilution techniques. *J Surg Res* 34:337, 1983.

77. Urban P, Scheidegger D, Gabathuler J, et al: Thermodilution determination of right ventricular volume and ejection fraction: A comparison with biplane angiography. *Crit Care Med* 15:652, 1987.

78. Martyn JA, Snider MT, Farago LF, et al: Thermodilution right ventricular volume: A novel and better predictor of volume replacement in acute thermal injury. *J Trauma* 21:619, 1981.

79. Reuse C, Vincent JL, Pinsky MR: Measurement of right ventricular volume during fluid challenge. *Chest* 98:1450, 1981.

80. Calvin JE, Driedger AA, Sibbald WJ: The hemodynamic effect of rapid fluid infusion in critically ill patients. *Surgery* 90:61, 1981.

81. Hamilton WF, Moore JW, Kinsman JM, et al: Studies on the circulation: IV. Further anal-

ysis of injection methods, and of changes in hemodynamics under physiological and pathological conditions. *Am J Physiol* 99:534, 1932.

82. Robin ED: Death by pulmonary artery flow-directed catheter. *Chest* 92:727, 1987.

83. Wong DH, Onishi R, Tremper KK, et al: Thoracic bioimpedance and Doppler cardiac output measurement: Learning curve and interobservor reproducibility. *Crit Care Med* 17:1174, 1989.

84. Sutton RN, Wilson RF, Walt AJ: Differences in acid-base levels and oxygen saturation between central venous and arterial blood. *Lancet* 2:748, 1967.

85. Wilson RF, Gibson DB, Percinel AK, et al: Severe alkalosis in critically ill patients. *Arch Surg* 105:197, 1972.

86. Wilson RF, Krome R: Factors affecting prognosis in clinical shock. *Ann Surg* 169:93, 1969.

87. Flint LM Jr, Brown A, Richardson Polk HC: Definitive control of bleeding from severe pelvic fractures. *Ann Surg* 189:709, 1979.

88. Crile GW: *Blood Pressure in Surgery.* Philadelphia, Lippincott, 1903, pp 289–291.

89. Gardner WJ, Dohn DF: The antigravity suit (G suit) in surgery. *JAMA* 126:274, 1956.

90. McSwain NE Jr: Pneumatic trousers and the management of shock. *J Trauma* 17:719, 1977.

91. Hoffman J: External counterpressure and the MAST suit: Current and future roles. *Ann Emerg Med* 9:419, 1980.

92. Mackensie RC, Christensen JM, Lewis FR: The prehospital use of external counterpressure: Does MAST make a difference? *J Trauma* 24:882, 1984.

93. Mattox KL, Bikell WH, Pepe PE, et al: Prospective, randomized evaluation of antishock MAST in post-traumatic hypotension. *J Trauma* 26:779, 1986.

94. Gaffney F, Thal E, Taylor W, et al: Hemodynamic effects of medical antishock trousers (MAST garment). *J Trauma* 21:931, 1981.

95. Wagensteen SL, deHoll JD, Ludewig RM, Magdden JJ Jr: The detrimental effect of the G-suit in hemorrhagic shock. *Ann Surg* 170:187, 1969.

96. McSwain NE: Pneumatic anti-shock garment: State of the art 1988. *Ann Emerg Med* 17:506, 1988.

97. Ransom KJ, McSwain NF: Metabolic acidosis with pneumatic trousers in hypovolemic dogs. *JACEP* 8:184, 1979.

98. McCabe JB, Seidel DR, Jagger JA: Antishock trouser inflation and pulmonary vital capacity. *Ann Emerg Med* 12:290, 1983.

99. Maull KI, Capehart JE, Cardea JA, Haynes BW: Limb loss following military antishock trousers (MAST) application. *J Trauma* 21:60, 1981.

100. Godbout B, Burchard KW, Stolmen GJ, Gann DS: Crush syndrome with death following pneumatic antishock garment application. *J Trauma* 24:1052, 1984.

101. Templeman D, Lange R, Harms B: Lower extremity compartment syndrome associated with use of pneumatic antishock garments. *J Trauma* 27:79, 1987.

102. Lucas CE, Ledgerwood AM: Hemodynamic management of the injured, in Capan LM, Miller SM, Turndorf H (eds): *Trauma: Anesthesia and Intensive Care.* Philadelphia, Lippincott, 1991, pp 83–113.

103. Taylor J, Weil MH: Failure of the Trendelenburg position to improve circulation during clinical shock. *Surg Gynecol Obstet* 124:1005, 1967.

104. Bivins HG, Knopp R, dos Santos POL: Blood volume distribution in the Trendelenburg position. *Ann Emerg Med* 14:641, 1985.

105. Sibbald WJ, Paterson MAM, Holliday RL, et al: The Trendelenburg position: Hemodynamic effects in hypotensive and normotensive patients. *Crit Care Med* 7:218, 1979.

106. Reich DL, Konstadt SN, Raissi S, et al: Trendelenburg position and passive leg raising do not significantly improve cardiopulmonary performance in the anesthetized patient with coronary artery disease. *Crit Care Med* 17:313, 1989.

107. Shenkin HA, Sheuerman EB, Spitz EB, et al: Effect of change of posture upon cerebral circulation of man. *J Appl Physiol* 2:317, 1949.

108. Harte FA, Chalmers PC, Walsh RF, et al: Intraosseous fluid administration: A parenteral alteration in pediatric resuscitation. *Anesth Analg* 66:687, 1987.

109. Rosetti VA, Thompson BM, Miller J, et al: Intraosseous infusion: An alternative route for pediatric intravascular access. *Ann Emerg Med* 14:885, 1985.

110. Carey JS, Scharschmidt BF, Culliford AT: Hemodynamic effectiveness of colloid and electrolyte solutions for replacement of simulated operative blood loss. *Surg Gynecol Obstet* 131:679, 1970.

111. Lowery BD, Cloutier CT, Carey LC: Electrolyte solutions in resuscitation in human hemorrhagic shock. *Surg Gynecol Obstet* 133:273, 1971.

111a. Shires GT, Canizaro PC: Fluid, electrolyte, and nutritional management of the surgical patient, in Schwartz SI: *Principles of Surgery*, 4th ed. New York, McGraw-Hill, 1984.

112. Davidson I, Eriksson B: Statistical evaluations of plasma substitutes based on 10 variables. *Crit Care Med* 10:653, 1982.

113. Virgilio RW, Rice CL, Smith DE: Crystalloid vs colloid resuscitation: Is one better? A randomized clinical study. *Surgery* 85:129, 1979.

114. Rainey TG, English JF: Pharmacology of colloids and the crystalloids, in Chernow B (ed): *The Pharmacologic Approach to the Critically Ill Patient*. Baltimore, Williams & Wilkins, 1983, p 219.

115. Rothschild MA, Oratz M, Schreiber SS: Albumin synthesis. *N Engl J Med* 286:748, 1972.

116. Hauser CJ, Shoemaker WC, Turpin I: Oxygen transport responses to colloids and crystalloids in critically ill surgical patients. *Surg Gynecol Obstet* 150:811, 1980.

117. Emerson TE: Unique features of albumin: A brief review. *Crit Care Med* 17:690, 1989.

118. Nearman HS, Herman ML: Toxic effects of colloids in the intensive care unit. *Crit Care Clin* 7:713, 1991.

119. Ledgerwood AM, Lucas CE: Postresuscitation hypertension, etiology, morbidity and treatment. *Arch Surg* 108:531, 1974.

120. Lewis RT: Albumin: Role and discriminative use in surgery. *Can J Surg* 23:322, 1980.

121. Poole GV, Meredity JW, Pernell T, et al: Comparison of colloids and crystalloids in resuscitation from hemorrhagic shock. *Surg Gynecol Obstet* 154:577, 1982.

122. Esrig BC, Fulton RL: Sepsis, resuscitated hemorrhagic shock and "shock lung": An experimental correlation. *Ann Surg* 182:218, 1975.

123. Lucas CE, Ledgerwood AM, Mammen EF: Altered coagulation protein content after albumin resuscitation. *Ann Surg* 196:198, 1982.

124. Kovalik SG, Ledgerwood AM, Lucas CE: The cardiac effect of altered calcium homeostasis after albumin resuscitation. *J Trauma* 21:275, 1981.

125. Faillace D, Ledgerwood AM, Lucas CE, Kithier K: Effects of different resuscitation regimens on immunoglobulins. *Surg Forum* 30:18, 1979.

126. Clift DR, Ledgerwood AM, Lucas CE, et al: The effect of albumin resuscitation for shock on the immune response to tetanus toxoid. *J Surg Res* 32:449, 1982.

127. Rothschild MA, Oratz M, Schreiber SS: Albumin metabolism. *Gastroenterology* 64:324, 1973.

128. Tullis JL: Albumin: I. Background and use. *JAMA* 237:355, 1977.

129. Alving BM, Hojima Y, Pisano JJ: Hypotension associated with prekallikrein activator (Hageman-factor fragments) in plasma protein fraction. *N Engl J Med* 299:66, 1978.

130. Aberg M, Hedner V, Bergentz S: Effect of dextran on factor VIII and platelet function. *Ann Surg* 189:243, 1979.

131. Shoemaker WC: Comparison of the relative effectiveness of whole blood transfusions and various types of fluid therapy in resuscitation. *Crit Care Med* 4:71, 1976.

132. Sashahara AA, Sharma Gurk, Parisi AF: New developments in the detections and prevention of venous thromboembolism. *Am J Cardiol* 43:1214, 1979.

133. Lewis JH, Szetol LF, Beyer WL: Severe hemodilution with hydroxyethyl starch and dextrans. *Arch Surg* 93:941, 1966.

134. Ring J, Messmer K: Incidence and severity of anaphylactoid reactions to colloid volume substitutes. *Lancet* 1:466, 1977.

135. Thompson WL: Rational use of albumin and plasma substitutes. *Johns Hopkins Med J* 136:220, 1975.

136. Alexander B, Odake K, Lawlor J, et al: Coagulation, hemostasis and plasma expanders: A quarter-century enigma. *Fed Proc* 34:1429, 1975.

137. Feest TG: Low molecular weight dextran: A continuing cause of acute renal failure. *Br Med J* 2:1300, 1976.

138. Bergentz SE, Falkheden T, Olson S: Diuresis and urinary viscosity in dehydrated patients: Influence of dextran-40,000 with and without mannitol. *Ann Surg* 161:562, 1965.

139. Lamke JH, Liljedahl SO: Plasma volume expansion after infusion of 5%, 20%, and 25% albumin solutions in patients. *Resuscitation* 5:85, 1976.

140. Skrede S, Ro JS, Mjolnerod O: Effects of dextrans on the plasma protein changes during the postoperative period. *Clin Chim Acta* 48:143, 1973.

141. Abramowicz M (ed): *Med Lett Drug Ther* 10(1):3, 1968.

142. Perttila J, Salo M, Peltola O: Effects of different plasma substitutes on plasma fibronectin concentrations in patients undergoing abdominal surgery. *Acta Anaesthesiol Scand* 34:304, 1990.

143. Lazgrove S, Waxman K, Shippy C: Hemodynamic blood volume and oxygen transport responses to albumin and hydroxyethyl starch infusions in critically ill postoperative patients. *Crit Care Med* 8:302, 1980.

144. Yacobi A, Stoll RG, Sum CY, et al: Pharmacokinetics of hydroxyethyl starch in normal subjects. *J Clin Pharmacol* 22:206, 1982.

145. Yacobi A, Stoll RG, Sum CY: Pharmacokinetics of hydroxyethyl starch in normal subjects. *J Clin Pharmacol* 22:206, 1982.

146. Lenz G, Hempel V, Jurger H, Worle H: Effect of hydroxyethyl starch, oxypolygelatin and human albumin on the phagocytic function of the reticuloendothelial system in healthy subjects. *Anaesthetist* 35:423, 1986.

147. Strauss RG, Stump DC, Henriksen RA, et al: Effects of hydroxyethyl starch on fibrinogen, fibrin clot formation, and fribrinolysis. *Transfusion* 25:230, 1985.

148. Stump DC, Strauss RG, Heinriksen RA, et al: Effects of hydroxyethyl starch on blood coagulation, particularly factor VIII. *Transfusion* 25:349, 1985.

149. Kohler H, Kirch W, Horstmann HJ: Hydroxyethyl starch induced macroamylasemia. *Int J Clin Pharmacol* 15:428, 1977.

150. Shatney CH, Deapiha K, Militello PR, et al: Efficacy of hetastarch in the resuscitation of patients with multisystem trauma and shock. *Arch Surg* 118:804, 1983.

151. London MJ, Ho JS, Triedman JK, et al: A randomized clinical trial of 10% pentastarch (low molecular weight hydroxyethyl starch) versus 5% albumin for plasma volume expansion after cardiac operations. *Thorac Cardiovasc Surg* 97:785, 1989.

152. Pisciotto PT, Synder EL: Use and administration of blood and components, in Chernow B (ed): *Critically Ill Patients.* Baltimore, Williams & Wilkins, 1988, p 254.

153. Office of Medical Applications of Research, National Institutes of Health: Fresh frozen plasma: Indications and risks. *JAMA* 253:551, 1985.

154. Oh MS, Carroll HT, Goldstein DA: Hyperchloremic acidosis during the recovery phase of diabetic ketosis. *Ann Intern Med* 89:925, 1978.

155. Rackow EC, Falk JL, Fein IA, et al: Fluid resuscitation in circulatory shock. *Crit Care Med* 11:839, 1983.

156. Lucas CE, Martin DJ, Ledgerwood AM, et al: Effect of fresh-frozen plasma resuscitation on cardiopulmonary function and serum protein flux. *Arch Surg* 121:559, 1986.

157. Martin DJ, Lucas CE, Ledgerwood AM, et al: Fresh frozen plasma supplement massive red blood cell transfusion. *Ann Surg* 202:505, 1985.

158. Velasco IT, Pontieri V, Silva MR, et al: Hyperosmotic NaCl and severe hemorrhagic shock. *Am J Physiol* 239:H664, 1980.

159. Mullins RJ, Hudgens RW: Hypertonic saline resuscitates dogs in endotoxin shock. *J Surg Res* 43:37, 1987.

160. Traverso LW, Bellamy RF, Hollenbaugh SJ, et al: Hypertonic sodium chloride solutions: Effect on hemodynamics and survival after hemorrhage in swine. *J Trauma* 27:32, 1987.

161. Silva MR, Velasco IT, Nogueira RI, et al: Hyperosmotic sodium salts reverse severe hemorrhagic shock: Other solutes do not. *Am J Physiol* 253:H751, 1987.

162. Mazzoni MC, Borgstrom P, Arforse KE, et al: Dynamic fluid redistribution in hyperosmotic resuscitation of hypovolemic hemorrhage. *Am J Physiol* 255:H629, 1988.

163. Liang CS, Hood WB: Mechanism of cardiac output response to hypertonic sodium chloride infusion in dogs. *Am J Physiol* 235:H18, 1978.

164. Silva MR, Negraes GA, Soares AM, et al: Hypertonic resuscitation from severe hemorrhagic shock: Patterns of regional circulation. *Circ Shock* 19:165, 1986.

165. Younes RN, Aun F, Tomida RM, et al: The role of lung innervation in the hemodynamic response to hypertonic sodium chloride solutions in hemorrhagic shock. *Surgery* 98:900, 1985.

166. Velasco IT, Baena RC, Rocha e Silva M, et al: Central angiotensinergic system and hypertonic resuscitation from severe hemorrhage. *Am J Physiol* 259:H1752, 1990.

167. Wallace AW, Tunin CM, Shoukas AA: Effects of vasopressin on pulmonary and systemic vascular mechanics. *Am J Physiol* 257:H1228, 1989.

168. Holcroft JW, Vassar MJ, Turner JE, et al: 3% NaCl and 7.5% NaCl/dextran 70 in the resuscitation of severely injured patients. *Ann Surg* 206:279, 1987.

169. Bowser BH, Caldwell FT: The effects of resuscitation with hypertonic vs hypotonic vs colloid on wound and urine fluid and electrolyte losses in severely burned children. *J Trauma* 23:916, 1983.

170. Monafo WW, Halverson JD, Schectman K: The role of concentrated sodium solutions in the resuscitation of patients with severe burns. *Surgery* 95:129, 1984.

171. Shackford SR, Fortlage DA, Peters RM, et al: Serum osmolar and electrolyte changes associated with large infusions of hypertonic sodium lactate for intravenous volume expansion of patients undergoing aortic reconstruction. *Surg Gynecol Obstet* 164:127, 1987.

172. Moss GS, Gould SA: Plasma expanders: An update. *Am J Surg* 155:425, 1988.

173. Kramer GC, Perron PR, Lindsey C, et al: Small-volume resuscitation with hypertonic saline-dextran solution. *Surgery* 100:239, 1986.

174. Wildenthal K, Mierzwiak DS, Mitchell JH: Acute effects of increased serum osmolality on left ventricular performance. *Am J Physiol* 216:898, 1969.

175. Nerlick M, Gunther R, Demling RH: Resuscitation from hemorrhagic shock with hypertonic saline or lactated Ringer's: Effect on the pulmonary and systemic microcirculations. *Circ Shock* 10:179, 1983.

176. Gervin AS: Transfusion, autotransfusion, and blood substitutes, in Mattox KL, Moore EE, Feliciano DV (eds): *Trauma*. Norwalk, Conn, Appleton & Lange, 1988, p 159.

177. Cross JS, Gruber DP, Burchard KW, et al: Hypertonic saline fluid therapy following surgery: A prospective study. *J Trauma* 29(6):817, 1989.

178. Prough DS, Johnson JC, Stump DA, et al: Effects of hypertonic saline versus lactated Ringer's solution on cerebral oxygen transport during resuscitation from hemorrhagic shock. *J Neurosurg* 64:627, 1986.

179. Johnston WE, Alford PT, Prough DS, et al: Cardiopulmonary effects of hypertonic saline in canine oleic acid-induced pulmonary edema. *Crit Care Med* 13:814, 1985.

180. Armistead CS, Vincent JL, Preiser JC, et al: Hypertonic saline solution-hetastarch for fluid resuscitation in experimental septic shock. *Anesth Analg* 69:714, 1989.

181. Symbas PN, Levin JM, Ferrier FL, et al: A study of autotransfusion from hemothorax. *South Med J* 62:671, 1969.

182. Popovsky MA, Devine PA, Taswell HF: Intraoperative autologous transfusion. *Mayo Clin Proc* 60:125, 1985.

183. Glover JL, Smith R, Yaw PB, et al: Autotransfusion of blood contaminated by intestinal contents. *J Am Coll Emerg Physicians* 7:142, 1978.

184. Jurkovich GJ, Moore EE, Medina G: Autotransfusion in trauma: A pragmatic analysis. *Am J Surg* 148:782, 1984.

185. Wilson RF: Special problems in the diagnosis and treatment of surgical sepsis. *Surg Clin North Am* 65:965, 1985.

186. Zaritsky AL, Chernow B: Catecholamines and other inotropes, in Chernow B (ed): *The Pharmacological Approach to the Critically Ill Patient,* 2d ed. Baltimore, Williams & Wilkins, 1988, pp 584–602.

187. Fowler MB, Alderman EL, Oesterle SN, et al: Dobutamine and dopamine after cardiac surgery: Greater augmentation of myocardial blood flow with dobutamine. *Circulation* 70(suppl):103, 1984.

188. Richard C, Ricome JL, Rimailho A, et al: Combined hemodynamic effects of dopamine and dobutamine in cardiogenic shock. *Circulation* 67:620, 1983.

189. Edelson J, Stroshane R, Benziger DP, et al: Pharmacokinetics of the bipyridines amrione and milrinone. *Circulation* 73(suppl):145, 1986.

190. Peterson CD, Leeder JS, Sterner S: Glucagon therapy for beta-blocker overdose. *Drug Intel Clin Pharmacol* 18:394, 1984.

191. Zaloga GP, Malcom DS, Holaday JW, et al: Glucagon, in Chernow B (ed): *The Pharmacological Approach to the Critically Ill Patient,* 2d ed. Baltimore, Williams & Wilkins, 1988, pp 659–670.

192. Sibbald WJ, Sardesai V, Wilson RF: Hypocalcemia and nephrogenous cyclic AMP production in critically ill or injured. *J Trauma* 17:677, 1977.

193. Wilson RF, Soullier G, Antonenko D: Ionized calcium levels in critically ill surgical patients. *Am Surg* 45:485, 1979.

194. Wilson RF, Dulchavsky SA, Soullier G, Beckman B: Problems with 20 or more blood transfusions in 24 hours. *Am Surg* 53:410, 1987.

195. White BC, Winegar CD, Wilson RF, Trombler JH: The possible role of calcium blockers in cerebral resuscitation: A review of the literature and synthesis for future studies. *Crit Care Med* 11:202, 1983.

196. Bronsveld W, VanLambalgen AA, Vandenbos GC, et al: Effects of glucose-insulin-potassium (GIK) on myocardial blood flow and metabolism in canine endotoxic shock. *Circ Shock* 12:325, 1984.

197. Dell'Italia LJ: Right ventricular infarction. *J Intensive Care Med* 1:246, 1986.

198. Lorell B, Leinbach RC, Pohost GM, et al: Right ventricular infarction: Clinical diagnosis and differentiation from cardiac tamponade and pericardial constriction. *Am J Cardiol* 43:465, 1979.

199. Parillo JE: Vasodilator therapy, in Chernow B (ed): *The Pharmacological Approach to the Critically Ill Patient,* 2d ed. Baltimore, Williams & Wilkins, 1988, pp 346–364.

200. Pierpont G, Hale KA, Franciosa JA, et al: Effects of vasodilators on pulmonary hemodynamics in gas exchange in left ventricular failure. *Am Heart J* 99:208, 1980.

201. Narins RG, Cohen JJ: Bicarbonate therapy for organic acidosis: The care for its continued use. *Ann Intern Med* 106:615, 1987.

202. Wilson RF, Binkley LE, Sabo FM, et al: Electrolyte and acid-base changes with massive blood transfusions. *Am Surg* 58:535, 1992.

203. Sibbald WJ, Short A, Cohen MP, Wilson RF: Variations in adrenocortical responsiveness during severe bacterial infections: Unrecognized adrenocortical insufficiency in bacterial infections. *Ann Surg* 186:29, 1977.

204. DePalma RG, Glickman MH, Hartman P, et al: Prevention of endotoxin induced changes in oxidative phosphorylation in hepatic mitochondria. *Surgery* 82:68, 1977.

205. Sibbald WJ, Anderson RR, Reid B, et al: Alveolar capillary permeability in human septic ARDS: Effect of high dose corticosteroid therapy. *Chest* 79:133, 1981.

206. Altura BM, Altura BT: Peripheral vascular actions of glucocorticoids and their relationship to protection in circulatory shock. *J Pharmacol Exp Ther* 190:300, 1976.

207. Jacob HS: Complement induced vascular leukostasis. *Arch Pathol Lab Med* 104:617, 1980.

208. Beutler B, Krochin N, Milsark IW, et al: Control of cachectin (tumor necrosis factor) synthesis: Mechanisms of endotoxin resistance. *Science* 232:977, 1986.

209. Hinshaw LB, Beller-Todd BK, Archer LT: Current management of the septic shock patient: Experimental basis for treatment. *Circ Shock* 9:543, 1982.

210. Schumer W: Steroids in the treatment of clinical septic shock. *Ann Surg* 184:333, 1976.

211. Sprung CL, Caralis PV, Marcial EH, et al: The effects of high dose corticosteroids in patients with septic shock. *N Engl J Med* 311:1137, 1984.

212. Bone RC, Fisher CJ Jr, Clemmer TP, et al: A controlled trial of high-dose methyprednisolone in the treatment of severe sepsis and septic shock. *N Engl J Med* 317:653, 1987.

213. The Veterans Administration Systemic Sepsis Cooperative Study Group: Effect of high-dose glucocorticoid therapy on mortality in patients with clinical signs of systemic sepsis. *N Engl J Med* 317:659, 1987.

214. Holaday JW, Faden AI: Naloxone reversal of endotoxin hypotension suggests role of endorphins in shock. *Nature* 275:450, 1978.

215. Schein RMH, Long WM, Sprung CL: Controversies in the management of septic shock: Corticosteroid, naloxone and non-steroidal anti-inflammatory agents, in Sibbald WJ, Sprung CL (eds): *Perspectives on Sepsis and Septic Shock: New Horizons.* Fullerton, Calif, Society of Critical Care Medicine, 1986.

216. DeMaria A, Craven DE, Hefferman JJ, et al: Naloxone vs placebo in treatment of septic shock. *Lancet* 1:1363, 1985.

217. Gurll NJ, Holaday JW, Reynolds DG, et al: Thyrotropin-releasing hormone: Effects in monkeys and dogs subjected to experimental circulatory shock. *Crit Care Med* 15(6):574, 1987.

218. Holaday JW, Ruvio BA, Faden AI: Thyrotropin-releasing hormone improves blood pressure and survival in endotoxic shock. *Eur J Pharmacol* 74:101, 1981.

219. McIntosh TK, Faden AI: Thyrotropin-releasing hormone (TRH) and circulatory shock. *Circ Shock* 18:241, 1986.

220. Mueller HS: Management of acute myocardial infarction, in Shoemaker WC, Ayere S, Grenvik A, et al (eds): *Textbook of Critical Care,* 2d ed. Philadelphia, Saunders, 1989, pp 341–353.

221. Zwischenberger JB, Bartlett R: Extracorporeal circulation for respiratory or cardiac failure, in Civetta JM, Taylor RW, Kirby RR (eds): *Critical Care.* Philadelphia, Lippincott, 1988, pp 1629–1637.

222. Reedy JE, Swartz MT, Raithel SC, et al: Mechanical cardiopulmonary support for refractory cardiogenic shock. *Heart Lung* 19:514, 1990.

223. Gattinoni L, Presenti A, Mascheroni D, et al: Low-frequency positive pressure ventilation with extracorporeal CO_2 removal in severe acute respiratory failure. *JAMA* 256:881, 1986.

224. Halushka PV, Wise WC, Cook JA: Studies on the beneficial effects of aspirin in endotoxin shock (Aspiron Symposium). *Am J Med* 77:91, 1983.

225. Tempel GE, Cook JA, Wise WC, et al: The improvement in endotoxin induced redistribution of organ blood flow by inhibition of thromboxane in prostaglandin synthesis. *Adv Shock Res* 7:209, 1982.

226. Bone RC, Jacobs ER: Research on ibuprofen for sepsis and respiratory failure: Symposium on Motrin (ibuprofen), past, present and future. *Am J Med* 77:114, 1983.

227. Ziegler EJ, McCutchan A, Fierer J, et al: Treatment of gram-negative bacteremia and shock with human antiserum to a mutant *Escherichia coli. N Engl J Med* 307:1225, 1982.

228. Lachman E, Pitsoe SB, Gaffin SL: Anti-lipopolysaccharide immunotherapy in management of septic shock of obstetric and gynecological origin. *Lancet* 1:981, 1984.

229. Aitchison JM, Arbuckle DD: Anti-endotoxin in the treatment of severe surgical septic shock: Results of a randomized double-blind trial. *S Afr Med J* 68:787, 1985.

230. Dunn DL, Mach PA, Cerra FB: Monoclonal antibodies protect against lethal effect of gram-negative bacterial sepsis. *Surg Forum* 34:142, 1983.

231. Antonacci AC, Chio J, Calcano SE, et al: Development of monoclonal antibodies against virulent gram-negative bacteria: Efficacy in a septic mouse model. *Surg Forum* 35:116, 1984.

232. Fisher CJ Jr, Zimmerman J, Khazaeli MB, et al: Initial evaluation of human monoclonal anti-lipid A antibody (HA-1A) in patients with sepsis syndrome. *Crit Care Med* 18:1311, 1990.

233. Ziegler EJ, Fischer CJ Jr, Sprung CL, et al: Treatment of gram-negative bacteremia and septic shock with HA-1A human monoclonal antibody against endotoxin. *N Engl J Med* 324:429, 1991.

234. Greenman RL, Schein RM, Martin MA, et al: A controlled clinical trial of E5 murine monoclonal IgM antibody to endotoxin in the treatment of gram-negative sepsis. *JAMA* 266:1097, 1991.

6A

RESUSCITATIVE THORACOTOMY

Robert F. Wilson

INDICATIONS

The use of emergency room thoracotomy should be determined by at least three considerations: the type of injury, emergency department and hospital resources, and the local surgical experience.[1,2]

TYPE OF INJURY

Since 1966, most trauma surgeons have agreed that with the proper personnel and facilities, an emergency department resuscitative thoracotomy should be performed on patients who have a cardiac arrest due to a penetrating wound of the chest or extremities just prior to or soon after arrival in the emergency department.[3,4]

In general, the highest salvage rates with emergency room thoracotomy are found in patients who have a cardiac arrest just before or soon after arrival in the emergency department due to a stab wound of the heart with pericardial tamponade.[1,4–11] Trauma patients in the emergency department who are otherwise salvageable but are in severe shock either from bleeding or pericardial tamponade and are not likely to reach the operating room alive also should have an emergency resuscitative thoracotomy.

An emergency department resuscitative thoracotomy should probably not be performed on trauma patients who have no vital signs at the scene or for more than 5 min before arriving in the emergency department. Patients with cardiac arrest from blunt trauma prior to emergency department arrival seldom, if ever, benefit from a resuscitative thoracotomy. In one series of 177 patients with no signs of life (absent pulses, no pupil reactivity, and no breathing) at the scene reported by Moore et al.,[12] only 1 survived with intact neurologic function following an emergency department resuscitative thoracotomy. This patient had multiple stab wounds, but the only significant injury was a transected brachial artery, which was rapidly controlled by direct pressure in the field. Of 136 patients arriving in the emergency department with no signs of life but with vital signs at the scene, only 3 were salvaged, and all 3 had sustained penetrating wounds.

If blunt trauma to the chest or abdomen is the cause of cardiac arrest in a patient of any age, the chance of salvage by emergency department thoracotomy is less than 5 percent.[1,9,10] Of 175 patients seen at San Francisco General Hospital who underwent an emergency department thoracotomy, there was only 1 survivor (1.7 percent) among the 63 who had blunt trauma.[7] This patient was agonal upon admission and arrested in the emergency room. Of 150 patients with blunt trauma arriving in the emergency department with no vital signs, Moore et al.[12] reported no survivors with neurologic recovery. The poor prognosis of patients arriving without vital signs following blunt trauma has been corroborated by other surgeons, including Bodai et al.[8] However, this does not imply that emergency department thoracotomy should never be employed in blunt trauma, because salvage of such patients is occasionally described.[7,11]

EMERGENCY DEPARTMENT AND HOSPITAL RESOURCES

Not all hospitals are set up to perform emergency department thoracotomies. Proper planning and resources are needed if one is to perform emergency thoracotomies outside the operating room.[1] Optimal results can be achieved with an emergency thoracotomy in an emergency department where (1) properly trained individuals are immediately available to perform the procedure, (2) proper lighting and instrument trays are available at all times, and (3) a full-scale operating room is held open for use without delay to provide definitive care.

SURGICAL EXPERIENCE

Properly trained individuals with experience in performing emergency department thoracotomies should be present before one decides to open the chest of a patient with a traumatic cardiac arrest.[1] The individual opening the chest should not only be able to make the incision but also should be able to immediately clamp or repair almost any structure in the chest as needed.

Although the initial incision may be made by a properly trained emergency physician, considerable thoracic trauma experience may be necessary to ensure proper management once the chest is open. Furthermore, emergency department thoracotomies should not continue to be performed at an institution unless they are done with acceptable rates of patient salvage.

POTENTIAL BENEFITS

The objectives of an emergency department resuscitative thoracotomy after trauma, in addition to optimizing cardiac output by performing open cardiac massage,[1,12] are (1) to release cardiac tamponade, (2) to control intrathoracic bleeding, (3) to treat or prevent air embolism, and (4) to redistribute the available blood flow to vital organs (brain and heart) by cross-clamping the descending aorta.

RELIEF OF PERICARDIAL TAMPONADE

CLINICAL DIAGNOSIS

Early recognition and prompt relief of pericardial tamponade is essential to improve survival in patients with cardiac wounds.[12] Pericardial tamponade is said to be characterized by the Beck I triad, which includes hypotension, distended neck veins, and muffled heart tones. However, if the patient is hypovolemic, distended neck veins may not appear until the patient has been given IV fluids. Even then, however, presence or absence of the Beck I triad is frequently inaccurate.[4] Kussmaul signs also may be present with pericardial tamponade; these include pulsus paradoxus and increased neck vein distension during inspiration.

PHASES OF PERICARDIAL TAMPONADE

The hemodynamic and cardiac perfusion abnormalities seen with rising intrapericardial pressures can be divided into four phases according to the adequacy of the compensatory mechanisms.[12–14] In the first phase, the increased pericardial pressure restricts ventricular diastolic filling and reduces subendocardial blood flow. The resultant reduction in cardiac output, however, is adequately compensated by an increased heart rate, systemic vascular resistance, and central venous pressure.

In the second phase of pericardial tamponade, the rising intrapericardial pressure further reduces coronary perfusion, and the resultant subendocardial ischemia begins to compromise ventricular ejection.[15] Although systemic blood pressure may be maintained relatively well during the second phase, signs of impaired tissue perfusion, such as anxiety, diaphoresis, and pallor, become increasingly apparent.

During the third phase, the intrapericardial pressure approaches ventricular filling pressure, and the stroke volume may fall to less than 20 to 25 ml per beat with a corresponding severe reduction in systemic blood pressure. In the fourth and final phase, intrapericardial pressures exceed atrial and ventricular diastolic pressures, and profound coronary hypoperfusion results in an unobtainable blood pressure that will be followed rapidly by a cardiac arrest if uncorrected.

The quickest, safest way to raise the blood pressure in a patient with pericardial tamponade, prior to pericardiocentesis or thoracotomy, is to give IV fluids. If the bleeding into the pericardium has stopped, volume loading may raise diastolic filling pressures enough to restore a reasonable blood pressure. However, bleeding into the pericardial cavity may recur, and if it does, an immediate thoracotomy is usually the only possible way to save the patient.

If a reasonable systemic blood pressure is obtained after aggressive fluid loading, the patient should be brought immediately to the operating room for emergency thoracotomy. If the patient remains in severe shock despite the aggressive fluid resuscitation and is likely to have a cardiac arrest before he or she reaches

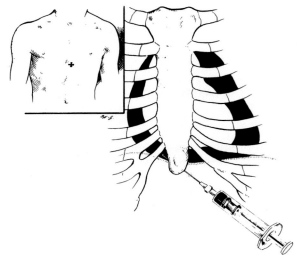

FIG. 6A–1. The paraxiphoid technique for pericardiocentesis is usually performed with the needle directed toward the left shoulder or left scapula tip. However, if one
aims toward the tip of the right scapula, the needle tends
to go parallel to the lateral border of the right heart and
is less apt to penetrate the coronary artery or myocardium. (*From Wilson RF: Injury to the heart and great vessels,
in Henning RJ, Grenvik A (eds): Critical Care Cardiology. New
York, Churchill Livingston, 1989, p 415. Reprinted with permission.*)

the operating room, an emergency department thoracotomy or pericardiocentesis should be performed promptly.

With persistent shock and a suspected pericardial tamponade, some surgeons
favor performing an immediate pericardiocentesis (Fig. 6A–1). However, there
are many false-positive and false-negative results with pericardiocentesis, and
most surgeons prefer rushing the patient to the operating room for a thoracotomy. Furthermore, a negative pericardiocentesis does not rule out tamponade,
and an emergency anterolateral thoracotomy can be performed almost as
quickly.

In stable patients with a possible pericardial tamponade, some surgeons, such
as Arom et al.,[16] prefer an initial subxiphoid incision under local anesthesia for
diagnosis. Using such an incision, the diaphragmatic portion of the pericardium
can be opened directly, and pericardial tamponade can be ruled in or out with
certainty. However, most surgeons believe that these patients are better served
by an emergency thoracotomy. If it is unlikely that the patient will survive
movement to the operating room, emergency department thoracotomy should
be performed.

CONTROL OF INTRATHORACIC HEMORRHAGE

Life-threatening intrathoracic hemorrhage requiring a thoracotomy occurs in
about 5 percent of patients admitted to a hospital following penetrating trauma

to the chest,[17,18] and most frequently this is due to bleeding from a severe injury of the lung.[19] A hemithorax can rapidly fill with a third to a half of the total blood volume before obvious physical signs of a hemothorax appear.[12]

In patients with severe continuing hypotension, the injured lung should be clamped at the hilum as soon as the chest is entered rather than making an attempt to repair the injured area of lung.[19] If a major systemic vessel is involved, the bleeding should be controlled digitally at first or with proximal and distal clamping. If the aorta is involved, side clamping, digital pressure, or a rapid running suture can be used to control the bleeding until an adequate heart beat is obtained.

PREVENTION AND/OR TREATMENT OF SYSTEMIC AIR EMBOLISM

A sudden change in central nervous system (CNS) or cardiovascular function after endotracheal intubation and positive-pressure ventilation is begun should be considered due to systemic air embolism until proven otherwise. Major air embolism following thoracic trauma is probably much more common than generally recognized.[19–21] The typical scenario of air embolism is the patient who sustains a penetrating chest wound and then develops an arrhythmia, severe shock, cardiac arrest, or sudden severe CNS changes immediately following endotracheal intubation and positive-pressure ventilation. Many of these patients also have hemoptysis.[19] The incidence of systemic air embolism, theoretically at least, is increased if pulmonary venous pressures are low and the airway pressures are high due to aggressive hyperventilation. A similar process also may occur in patients with blunt pulmonary lacerations.[12]

Massive hemoptysis or a suspected air embolism should be an indication for an emergency thoracotomy. Immediate thoracotomy with pulmonary hilar cross-clamping is essential to prevent further air embolism and bleeding into the undamaged lung.[12,19] The patient's head should be lowered immediately to reduce the risk of air embolism to the brain. Air should be aspirated from the left side of the heart and ascending aorta with a needle and syringe as soon and as completely as possible. Cardiopulmonary bypass may be very helpful for clearing the coronary arteries of air and for supporting systemic perfusion until adequate coronary perfusion and myocardial function can be obtained. Hyperbaric oxygenation may be helpful for reducing the CNS signs and symptoms due to cerebral air embolism.

THORACIC AORTIC CROSS-CLAMPING

If the cardiac output is kept constant, temporary occlusion of the descending thoracic aorta not only can increase blood flow to the heart and brain by two- to threefold but also can reduce subdiaphragmatic blood loss.[22–27] Canine studies by Dunn et al.[28] demonstrated that left ventricular stroke work index and myocardial contractility increased in response to thoracic aortic occlusion during hypovolemic shock. Although the improvement in myocardial function in this study occurred without an increase in pulmonary capillary wedge pressure or a significant change in systemic vascular resistance, I have found that both these parameters usually rise abruptly in my patients after thoracic aortic clamping.

Dunn et al.[28] felt that an improved coronary perfusion due to an increase in the aortic diastolic pressure accounted for the enhanced cardiac contractility following aortic cross-clamping. This experimental observation suggests that temporary aortic occlusion may be valuable in patients with continued shock during or following repair of cardiac wounds or other exsanguinating injuries.[12,28]

Although thoracic aortic cross-clamping can be very helpful, it should be considered a potentially dangerous temporary maneuver designed to keep the patient alive while life-threatening problems are rapidly corrected. Thoracic aortic cross-clamping may be particularly deleterious in normovolemic patients because of the significantly increased myocardial oxygen demands caused by the elevated systemic vascular resistance.[29] Blood flow to the abdominal viscera, spinal cord, and kidneys may be reduced to 10 percent of normal following thoracic aortic occlusion, and femoral systolic blood pressure falls to about 10 to 20 mmHg. Consequently, aortic occlusion can induce a high degree of anaerobic metabolism in tissues below the clamp, resulting in lactic acidemia, generalized vasodilatation, and release of numerous inflammatory mediators, such as thromboxane and other prostanoids.[30] The hypotension following aortic declamping may be largely related to these substances getting back to the heart and systemic circulation.

Vasomotor tone below the aortic clamp is partially reestablished over time by increased levels of epinephrine and angiotensin. However, some ischemic damage to abdominal vital organs is thought to be inevitable if the thoracic aortic clamping is prolonged beyond 30 min.[31] Although thoracic aortic occlusion has been tolerated for as long as 75 min without spinal sequelae,[32] clinical experience with elective thoracic aortic procedures indicates that 30 min is generally the safe limit for reversible normothermic ischemia.[12] Intermittent declamping to allow periodic systemic perfusion has not been studied adequately and, theoretically, could actually cause more harm than continued clamping by increasing the production of toxic oxygen metabolites.[12]

Resuscitative thoracotomy and descending thoracic aortic occlusion prior to laparotomy to control exsanguinating abdominal hemorrhage have been applied routinely in many trauma centers with improved survival.[22–25] Recently, use of intraaortic balloon occlusion to control traumatic abdominal hemorrhage has been resurrected as a concept to avoid the thoracic incision.

TECHNIQUES

THORACIC INCISION

A left anterolateral thoracotomy incision is the preferred approach for performing open cardiac massage and for treating left-sided penetrating chest wounds if the patient is in severe shock.[12,33] It should extend from about 2 cm lateral to the sternum (to avoid cutting the internal mammary vessels that run about 0.5 to 1.0 cm from lateral border of the sternum) out laterally to the axilla (Fig. 6A–2). If needed, the incision can be extended across into the right side of the chest to obtain exposure of both pleural spaces as well as virtually all the anterior mediastinal structures. An initial right thoracotomy is used in severely hypoten-

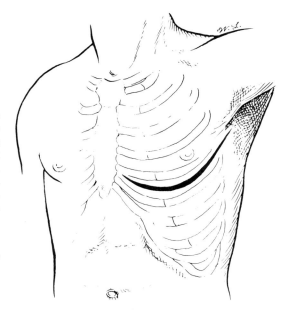

FIG. 6A–2. Emergency thoracotomy to treat a stab wound of the heart or to perform open cardiac massage is usually done through an anterolateral thoracotomy approach. The incision extends along the fifth intercostal space with the skin incision placed in the inframammary crease. It extends from just lateral to the sternum to the midaxillary line. (*From Wilson RF: Injury to the heart and great vessels, in Henning RJ, Grenvik A (eds): Critical Care Cardiology. New York, Churchill Livingston, 1989, p 418. Reprinted with permission.*)

sive patients with penetrating injuries to the right side of the chest to control massive blood loss from that side. Of course, if an associated cardiac wound is encountered, transsternal extension into the left side of the chest can be done as needed for repairing the heart and/or clamping the descending thoracic aorta.

Emergency median sternotomy can be used for treating anterior wounds in relatively stable patients. However, it takes special equipment (sternal saw or Lebschke knife), takes longer to perform, and does not provide good exposure to posterior wounds in the heart, lungs, or mediastinum.

In women, the incision is made through the inframammary crease, and the breast is then retracted superiorly to gain better access to the fourth or fifth intercostal space. The intercostal muscles are divided initially with a knife and then with heavy scissors. The intercostal incision should avoid the inferior margin of the upper rib in the interspace to reduce the chances of damaging the intercostal neurovascular bundle.

A standard (Finichetto) rib spreader is inserted into the incision with the handle directed inferiorly toward the axilla. Resistance in opening the chest incision with the rib spreader can be reduced by cutting the intercostal muscles back further laterally and posteriorly and by cutting the costal cartilages medially. If the incision extends too far medially, or if the sternum is transected for additional exposure, the internal mammary vessels must be clamped and ligated.

Extension of the incision into the other hemithorax can be accomplished quickly with a Lebsche knife or rib shears. A bilateral anterolateral thoracotomy can provide wide exposure of both pleural cavities. If better exposure of the superior mediastinum is needed, the superior sternum can be split in the midline. This incision can then be extended into the right or left neck or supraclavicular fossa as needed for control of more distal injuries to arch vessels.

PERICARDIOTOMY

The pericardial sac is opened to provide optimal internal cardiac massage, to relieve any suspected tamponade, and to control any heart wounds. It is not always obvious that a tamponade is present because, not infrequently, the blood will pool posteriorly in the pericardial cavity.

At times, the pericardium may be so tight that it is difficult to grasp and cut with scissors, and one may have to carefully make a small nick in the pericardium with a knife to get the incision started. The pericardial incision is extended vertically 1 to 2 cm anterior to the phrenic nerve up along the ascending aorta to the top of the pericardium and then down to the diaphragm. If a bilateral anterior thoracotomy incision is used, the pericardium may be opened vertically in the midline. Blood clots should be evacuated rapidly from the pericardium. If some cardiac activity is present, it is not unusual for the heart to stop beating just as the pericardial tamponade is relieved.

Further attempts at resuscitation should cease if, at the time of thoracotomy, there is (1) no cardiac activity, (2) the heart is completely empty, and (3) the patient has had no signs of life for over 5 min. Moore et al.[12] noted that of 139 patients with no cardiac activity when the heart was exposed at emergency thoracotomy, only one eventually survived to leave the hospital. This patient had sustained a ventricular laceration with pericardial tamponade and resultant cardiac arrest, and this was remedied quickly in the emergency department.

If there were any recent signs of life in a patient with a penetrating wound of the lung or heart, one can try to rapidly resuscitate the patient by (1) controlling or repairing any major bleeding injuries, (2) rapid fluid infusions, (3) clamping of the descending thoracic aorta, and (4) open cardiac massage for 5 to 10 min. Epinephrine, as an IV push of 0.5 mg (5 ml of a 1:10,000 solution) repeated every 1 to 2 min, may produce enough vasoconstriction to get a reasonable proximal aortic blood pressure. Intracardiac injection of 3 to 4 ml of 1:10,000 epinephrine also may help convert asystole to ventricular fibrillation.

CARDIORRHAPHY

Bleeding sites from the heart can usually be controlled immediately with digital pressure. Sometimes a partial occluding vascular clamp can be used to control bleeding from an atrium or a great vessel. In some instances, bleeding from a ventricle can best be controlled by inserting a Foley catheter through the wound into the cardiac chamber, blowing up the Foley balloon, and then pulling the inflated balloon up against the inside of the cardiac wound.

If the heart is beating adequately and the bleeding can be controlled digitally, efforts at cardiorrhaphy should be delayed, if possible, until the initial resuscitative measures have been completed. In the nonbeating heart, the suturing should generally be done rapidly prior to defibrillation.

Ventricular wounds are generally closed with 2-0 nonabsorbable horizontal mattress sutures. If available, buttresses of Teflon pledgets on the sutures reduce the chances of the sutures pulling through the myocardium when they are tied. Low-pressure venous and atrial lacerations can be repaired with simple running 3-0 nonabsorbable sutures. Posterior cardiac wounds may be particularly treacherous to expose and repair. When the heart is lifted up to expose posterior wounds, severe bleeding can ensue, and the wound may enlarge.

Definitive closure of ventricular wounds or wounds that are difficult to expose is best accomplished in the operating room with optimal lighting and equipment. Cardiopulmonary bypass should be considered if there is a large cardiac injury or if severe bleeding and/or ventricular fibrillation occur every time the heart is moved to try to expose an injury. If cardiopulmonary bypass is not available rapidly enough, one can temporarily occlude the superior and inferior vena cava to facilitate repair.

If there is a suspicion that coronary or systemic air embolism has occurred, further air embolism usually can be prevented by placing a vascular clamp across the pulmonary hilum proximal to the injured lung. An attempt should then be made to evacuate air from the left atrium, the left ventricle (after raising the apex), and the proximal aorta with a syringe and needle. If the heart is in asystole or ventricular fibrillation, clamping the ascending aorta just proximal to the innominate artery and alternatively squeezing the heart and ascending aorta may help rid the coronary arteries of any air they may contain. However, total cardiopulmonary bypass is preferable for clearing air from the coronary arteries.

INTERNAL CARDIAC MASSAGE

If no effective cardiac activity is present but it seems worthwhile to continue aggressive attempts at resuscitation, internal cardiac massage should be instituted promptly. If the sternum is intact, I prefer to hold the sternum with a thumb and squeeze the heart up against the sternum with the palm of the hand and other fingers. If the sternum has been transected, two-handed massage should be performed.

Moore et al.[12] specifically describe using a hinged clapping motion with the wrists apposed to squeeze the heart. The ventricular compression should proceed from the apex of the heart toward its base. Massaging the heart while it is held with the fingers and thumb of one hand increases the risk of myocardial perforation by the tip of the thumb or one of the fingers.

THORACIC AORTIC OCCLUSION

If the heart is completely empty and/or internal electrical defibrillation does not rapidly produce spontaneous cardiac activity, the descending thoracic aorta should be occluded to maximize coronary and cerebral perfusion. Markison and Trunkey[1] feel that manual occlusion of the descending aorta is simpler and safer than using a clamp.

If the descending aorta is to be clamped, it should be done under direct vision rather than by palpation alone (Fig. 6A–3). Visualizing the lower thoracic aorta usually requires a rather large anterolateral thoracotomy incision and retraction of the lung anteriorly by two hands of an assistant standing on the right side of the patient.

Under direct vision, the thoracic aorta can usually be separated from the esophagus anteriorly by blunt dissection. The prevertebral fascia, which is much stronger, is then incised posterior to the aorta. Some surgeons feel that the aorta

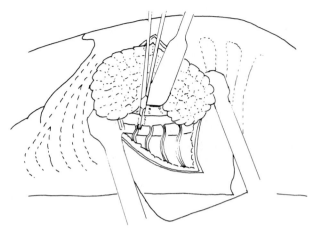

FIG. 6A–3. If the descending thoracic aorta is to be cross-clamped, it is best done under direct vision. To accomplish this, the anterior thoracotomy must be large and the incision opened as widely as possible. The left lung is pulled up anteriorly as far as possible by an assistant standing at the right side of the table. The pleura and fascia anterior to the aorta is thin, but the tissue between the aorta and the vertebral column is often rather tough and must be incised for the surgeon to get around the aorta properly. A straight clamp is often easier to put around the aorta than a curved clamp and is less likely to rupture the intercostal vessels. (*From Wilson RF: Surgical indications in trauma, in Webb WR, Besson A (eds): Thoracic Surgery: Surgical Management of Chest Injuries. St. Louis, Mosby–Year Book, 1991, p 201. Reprinted with permission.*)

should not be completely encircled because this increases the likelihood of avulsing intercostal branches off the aorta.[1] However, the occlusion is less apt to be complete and the aortic clamp is more likely to slip off if the aorta is not completely dissected. When properly exposed and freed up from the surrounding tissue, the thoracic aorta can usually be readily occluded with a large curved Satinsky or straight DeBakey vascular clamp.

The blood pressure response to aortic clamping should be monitored very closely. If the systolic blood pressure in the proximal aorta after proximal clamping is allowed to exceed 160 to 180 mmHg, the strain on the left ventricle can cause acute left ventricular distension with resultant acute failure and pulmonary edema. If there is coincident head or eye trauma, the hypertension may cause increased bleeding into those injured tissues.

The proximal aorta pressure after aortic clamping also provides some prognostic information on the patient. Moore et al.[12] have had no survivors among 180 patients in whom the systolic blood pressure proximal to an aortic clamp remained less than 70 mmHg despite full resuscitative efforts. In the studies of Wiencek and Wilson,[22,23] the critical systolic blood pressure was 90 mmHg. None of their patients left the operating room alive unless the proximal systolic blood pressure exceeded 90 mmHg within 5 min of the aortic clamping.

OPTIMIZING OXYGEN DELIVERY AND CONSUMPTION

The traditional approach to salvage of cardiac muscle and reduction of peri-infarction mortality has been directed toward optimization of the myocardial oxygen supply/demand.[12,34] This may be accomplished at least partially by early coronary reperfusion and vasodilation combined with beta blockade (if blood pressure and cardiac output are reasonable) and left ventricular afterload reduction; however, improved myocardial reperfusion has not been uniformly associated with preservation of regional wall motion.[35] Continuing abnormalities in cardiac metabolism include (1) conversion from free fatty acid–based to glucose-based metabolism for myocardial energy production, (2) loss of tricarboxylic acid cycle intermediates, and (3) depletion of energy-production enzymes depending on sulfhydryl groups.[36,37] Following CPR, there is also the problem of production of toxic oxygen metabolites because of ischemia-reperfusion injury in the lungs, intestine, liver, and heart.[38,39]

The combination of direct myocardial injury, ischemia, circulating cardiac depressants, and pulmonary hypertension can have an adverse impact on cardiac work. In addition, the aortic clamping causes washout of metabolic products and inflammatory mediators from the previously ischemic areas below the diaphragm back into the central circulation. The oxygen debt in tissues distal to the aortic cross-clamp and resultant ischemic damage increase exponentially when the occlusion time exceeds 30 min. Correcting this oxygen debt in a timely fashion may be extremely difficult, especially in patients with multisystem trauma.[12] Consequently, the aortic clamp should be removed as soon as possible.

Evidence is emerging that controlled reperfusion directed toward restoration of intermediary metabolism, use of toxic radical scavengers, and reduced activation of neutrophils by various drugs can help reduce the amount of tissue damage associated with ischemia-reperfusion injury.[38]

MECHANICAL CARDIAC SUPPORT

INTRAAORTIC BALLOON PUMPING

My experience with the intraaortic balloon pump (IABP) for severe cardiac failure or persistent shock after chest trauma has been very disappointing. The degree of cardiovascular failure developing by the time I have inserted the IABP has been too severe to get much benefit from this modality.

CARDIOPULMONARY BYPASS (CPB)

TOTAL BYPASS

Although the concept of cardiopulmonary support by extracorporeal circulation of oxygenated blood was proposed in 1813 by LeGallios, the first successful use of cardiopulmonary bypass for open cardiac surgery was not reported until 1954 by John Gibbon.[40] Extracorporeal circulation was first utilized for the treatment of cardiac arrest by Fell et al.[41] in 1968. These clinicians described a patient who presented with ventricular fibrillation and profound hypothermia. He was refractory to open cardiac massage and internal defibrillation. Following rewarming with the aid of cardiopulmonary bypass, the patient was successfully defibrillated and discharged alive from the hospital.

PARTIAL BYPASS

Partial cardiopulmonary bypass (PCPB) was used in conjunction with closed chest CPR in 1972 by Towne et al.[42] Utilizing femoral vein–femoral artery vascular access, a patient with ventricular fibrillation unresponsive to conventional CPR was successfully resuscitated by PCPB and discharged alive from the hospital. I have also found femoral vein–femoral artery partial cardiopulmonary bypass to be helpful in the management of severe hypothermia.[43]

In 1976, Mattox et al.[5] reported on 39 moribund patients (6 with cardiac arrest) who were treated with a portable PCPB system. Three of these 6 patients with cardiac arrest were successfully resuscitated, and 1 was discharged alive from the hospital. When used for management of cardiac arrest, vascular access via a femoral artery and femoral vein was usually accomplished within 5 min without interrupting external massage.[44] More recent reports have been controversial on the value of CPB for treating cardiac arrest.[45,46] It appears that such mechanical support should be limited to cardiac arrest in patients without advanced organic heart disease, and it should be instituted prior to the development of irreversible cerebral ischemia.

Experimental studies indicate that CPB may be able to sustain systemic, myocardial, and cerebral blood flow at levels that can prevent irreversible injury, even after prolonged periods of cardiac arrest. CPB also may extend the time for successful resuscitation beyond those which have been documented experimentally with open or closed chest cardiac massage.[47,48] Thus CPB has the potential for increasing both initial cardiac resuscitability and short-term survival.

The technique of CPB is attractive because it is much less invasive than open cardiac massage, and it can be used with a preprimed battery-powered pump-oxygenator system that is mobile and of small size. However, partial CPB will probably only be effective if used for a brief time as a "jump-start for resuscitation."[47]

The advent of centrifugal pumps (BioMedicus pump and Sarns centrifugal pump) which allow partial cardiac bypass with little or no systemic anticoagulation offers another potential mechanism for increasing salvage of moribund patients.[12,48,49] Indeed, this device has revamped the approach of many surgeons to the treatment of a torn descending thoracic aorta, especially in patients with an associated myocardial contusion.[50] Adjunctive use of extracorporeal membrane oxygenation (ECMO) also may play a role in supporting patients with early multiple organ failure.[12]

DIRECT MECHANICAL VENTRICULAR COMPRESSION

Direct mechanical ventricular actuation (DMVA) or compression is achieved with a biventricular circulatory support device that can be rapidly applied to the exterior of the heart. DMVA is described by Anstadt et al.[51] as an improved method of internal cardiac massage. The heart is placed inside a contoured cup that is pneumatically driven to intermittently compress the ventricular myocardium. The drive system regulates cycle rate, systolic duration, force, and rate of force delivery, and it also supplies a continuous vacuum to maintain the cup's attachment to the ventricles. This vacuum creates a constant seal between the ventricular myocardium and the actuating diaphragm of the cup. During the actuation (compression), the ventricular myocardium is "pushed" into systolic and "pulled" into diastolic configurations that appear to be remarkably effective compared with other modalities for supporting ventricular function.[6,52,53]

DMVA was initially described in 1968 by Anstadt et al.[54] Subsequent laboratory and clinical investigations over the next 6 years demonstrated a number of potential applications,[55,56] including improved salvage of ischemic myocardium.[57]

The feasibility of using DMVA for emergent cardiovascular stabilization in patients suffering a witnessed but refractory cardiac arrest was evaluated in a recent study by Anstadt et al.[51] Application of the DMVA took less than 2 min from the time of skin incision and resulted in immediate hemodynamic improvement. During DMVA, the systolic and diastolic blood pressures produced averaged 78 ± 4 and 41 ± 4 mmHg, respectively, with a mean cardiac output of 3.1 ± 0.2 liters/min during a mean of 228 ± 84 min of circulatory support (range of 25 min to 18 h). In selected patients, the device was temporarily removed for 2 to 3 min and open chest cardiac massage (OCCM) was performed at similar compression rates. DMVA was able to maintain arterial pressures and cardiac outputs that were 65 and 190 percent greater than with OCCM.

Although there was an average of 1.5 h of closed chest massage before the DMVA was applied, four patients were successfully defibrillated. However, two had inadequate cardiac function and died within 1 h, and the other two were successfully resuscitated but later died from cardiac failure and respiratory insufficiency.[51] No complications resulted from the device.

CLINICAL RESULTS

The results of emergency department thoracotomy vary considerably from hospital to hospital due to the heterogeneity of the patient populations studied. It is critical to distinguish between patients with "no vital signs" and those with "no signs of life."[12] *No vital signs* usually describes a patient who is alive but has no obtainable cuff blood pressure or palpable pulse. *No signs of life* describes a patient who is "dead" and has no vital signs, no movements or reflexes (even to pain), no pupil reactivity, and no respiratory efforts.

The best results with thoracotomy are found in patients who have severe shock in the emergency department from a knife wound of the heart causing pericardial tamponade. In-hospital survival approaches 50 percent in patients arriving with profound shock from a penetrating cardiac wound and 20 percent for all emergency department thoracotomies performed for penetrating wounds.[12] In Houston, a 59 percent survival rate was achieved in patients with cardiac wounds arriving without an obtainable blood pressure.[58] However, patient outcome is dismal when an emergency department thoracotomy is done either in patients with a cardiac arrest from blunt trauma or in patients arriving without any signs of life for more than 5 min regardless of the injury mechanism.

COMPLICATIONS

Technical complications of emergency department thoracotomy may involve every intrathoracic structure and have included lacerations of the heart, coronary arteries, aorta, phrenic nerves, esophagus, and lungs, as well as avulsion of intercostal arteries off the aorta.[12] Adhesions from a previous thoracotomy make emergency department thoracotomy extremely difficult and represent a relative contraindication to the procedure. However, in such cases, a midsternotomy for heart lesions may still be possible.

In individuals who survive an emergency department thoracotomy, the more frequent postoperative morbidities include recurrent intrathoracic bleeding, pneumonia, empyema, chest wall infections, and postpericardiotomy syndrome.[12]

A rather unique syndrome of postresuscitation pulmonary edema occasionally occurs after open cardiac massage with aortic cross-clamping; however, its mechanism is not well understood.[31] It is still not clear whether this represents hydrostatic (high pulmonary capillary pressure) and/or permeability (normal pulmonary capillary pressure) pulmonary edema.

WHEN TO STOP ATTEMPTS AT CARDIAC RESUSCITATION

The only definite contraindication to beginning cardiac resuscitation is terminal disease in which the patient's suffering would be prolonged. If cardiac resuscitation is begun, it should not be continued if there are unreconstructable injuries, uncontrollable bleeding, or apparent brain death, as demonstrated by fixed, dilated pupils and absence of all reflexes for more than 20 to 30 min at normothermia and without drugs. Even without these injuries or signs, if adequate myocardial function cannot be restored after 30 to 60 min of effective cardiac massage, it is extremely unlikely that further attempts will be successful. If the descending thoracic aortic is clamped and open cardiac massage plus fluids and epinephrine will not raise proximal aortic systolic pressure to at least 90 mmHg within 5 to 10 min, survival is essentially impossible.

REFERENCES

1. Markison RE, Trunkey DD: Establishment of care priorities, in Capan LM, Miller SM, Turndorf H (eds): *Trauma: Anesthesia and Intensive Care.* Philadelphia, Lippincott, 1991, pp 29–42.
2. Moore EE, Moore JB, Galloway AC, Eiseman B: Postinjury thoracotomy in the emergency department. *Surgery* 86:590, 1979.

3. Beall AC, Diethrich EB, Crawford HW, et al: Surgical management of penetrating cardiac injuries. *Am J Surg* 112:686, 1966.

4. Wilson RF, Bassett JS: Penetrating wounds of the pericardium or its contents. *JAMA* 195: 513, 1966.

5. Mattox KL, Beall AC Jr: Resuscitation of the moribund patient using portable cardiopulmonary bypass. *Ann Thorac Surg* 22:435, 1976.

6. Hall CW, Liotta D, Henly WS, et al: Development of artificial internal circulatory pumps. *Am J Surg* 108:685, 1964.

7. Baker CC, Thomas AN, Trunkey DD: The role of emergency room thoracotomy in trauma. *J Trauma* 20:848, 1980.

8. Bodai BI, Smith JP, Blaisdell FW: The role of emergency thoracotomy in blunt trauma. *J Trauma* 22:487, 1982.

9. Cogbill TH, Moore EE, Millikan JA, et al: Rationale for selective application of emergency department thoracotomy in trauma. *J Trauma* 23:453, 1983.

10. Baxter BT, Moore EE, Moore JB, et al: Emergency department thoracotomy following injury: Critical determinants for patient salvage. *World J Surg* 12:671, 1988.

11. Carveth S, Reese HE, Buchman RJ, Gangahar DM: The place for open chest cardiac compression, in Donegan JH (ed): *Cardiopulmonary Resuscitation.* Springfield, Ill, Charles C Thomas, 1982, p 180.

12. Moore JB, Moore EE, Harken AH: Emergency department thoracotomy, in Moore EE, Mattox KL, Feliciano DV (eds): *Trauma,* 2d ed. Norwalk, Conn, Appleton & Lange, 1991, pp 181–193.

13. Breaux ED, Dupont JB, Albert HM, et al: Cardiac tamponade following penetrating mediastinal injuries: Improved survival with early pericardiocentesis. *J Trauma* 19:461, 1979.

14. Shoemaker WC, Carey JS, Rao ST, et al: Hemodynamic alterations in acute cardiac tamponade after penetrating injuries to the heart. *Surgery* 67:754, 1970.

15. Wechsler AS, Auerback BJ, Graham TC, et al: Distribution of intramyocardial blood flow during pericardial tamponade. *J Thorac Cardiovasc Surg* 68:847, 1974.

16. Arom KV, Richardson JD, Webb G, et al: Subxiphoid pericardial window in patients with suspected traumatic pericardial tamponade. *Ann Thorac Surg* 23:545, 1977.

17. Wilson RF, Sarver E, Birks R: Central venous pressure and blood volume determinations in clinical shock. *Surg Gynecol Obstet* 132:631, 1971.

18. Washington B, Wilson RF, Steiger Z: Emergency thoracotomy: A four-year review. *Ann Thorac Surg* 40:188, 1985.

19. Weincek RG, Wilson RF: Central lung injuries: A need for early vascular control. *J Trauma* 28:1418, 1988.

20. Thomas AN, Stephens BG: Air embolism: A cause of morbidity and death after penetrating chest trauma. *J Trauma* 14:663, 1974.

21. King MW, Aitchism JM, Nel JP: Fatal air embolism following penetrating lung trauma: An autopsy study. *J Trauma* 24:753, 1984.

22. Wiencek RG, Wilson RF: Injuries to the abdominal vascular system: How much does aggressive resuscitation and prelaparotomy thoracotomy really help? *Surgery* 102:731, 1987.

23. Wiencek RG, Wilson RF: Inferior vena cava injuries: The challenge continues. *Am Surg* 54:423, 1988.

24. Millikan JS, Moore EE: Outcome of resuscitative thoracotomy and descending aortic occlusion performed in the operating room. *J Trauma* 24:387, 1984.

25. Ledgerwood AM, Kazmers M, Lucas CE: The role of thoracic aortic occlusion for massive hemoperitoneum. *J Trauma* 16:610, 1976.

26. Symbas PN, Pfuender LM, Drucker MH, et al: Cross-clamping of the descending aorta: Hemodynamic and neurohumoral effects. *J Thorac Cardiovasc Surg* 85:300, 1983.

27. Michel J, Bardon A, Tedqui A, et al: Effect of descending thoracic aortic clamping and unclamping on phasic coronary blood flow. *J Surg Res* 36:17, 1984.

28. Dunn EL, Moore EE, Moore JB: Hemodynamic effects of aortic occlusion during hemorrhagic shock. *Ann Emerg Med* 11:238, 1982.

29. Peng CF, Kane JJ, Jones EM, et al: The adverse effects of systemic hypertension following myocardial reperfusion. *J Surg Res* 34:59, 1983.

30. Huval WV, Leluck S, Allen PD, et al: Determinants of cardiovascular stability during abdominal aneurysmectomy. *Ann Surg* 199:216, 1983.

31. Oyama M, McNamara JJ, Sueniro GT, et al: The effects of thoracic aortic cross-clamping on visceral organ blood flow. *Ann Surg* 197:459, 1983.

32. Katz NM, Blackstone EH, Kirklin JW, et al: Incremental risk factors for spinal cord injury following operation for acute traumatic aortic transection. *J Thorac Cardiovasc Surg* 81:669, 1981.

33. Wilson RF, Thoms N, Arbulu A, Steiger Z: Cardiopulmonary resuscitation, in Walt AJ, Wilson RF (eds): *The Management of Trauma: Practice and Pitfalls.* Philadelphia, Lea & Fibiger, 1975, pp 149–162.

34. Braumwald E: The aggressive treatment of acute myocardial infarction. *Circulation* 71:1087, 1985.

35. Lazar HL, Piehn JF, Shick EM, et al: Effects of coronary revascularization on regional wall motion. *J Thorac Cardiovasc Surg* 98:498, 1989.

36. Schwaiger M, Schelbert HR, Ellison D: Sustained regional abnormalities in the cardiac metabolism after transient ischemia in the chronic dog model. *J Am Coll Cardiol* 6:336, 1985.

37. Beyersdorf F, Acar C, Buckberg GD, et al: Studies in prolonged acute regional ischemia. *J Thorac Cardiovasc Surg* 98:567, 1989.

38. Brown JM, Grosso MA, Whitman GH, et al: The coincidence of myocardial reperfusion injury and H_2O_2 production in the isolated rat heart. *Surgery* 105:496, 1989.

39. Kharazmi A, Andersen LW, Back L, et al: Endotoxemia and enhanced generation of cardiac radicals by neutrophils from patients undergoing cardiopulmonary bypass. *J Thorac Cardiovasc Surg* 98:381, 1989.

40. Gibbon JH Jr: Application of a mechanical heart and lung apparatus to cardiac surgery. *Minn Med* 37:171, 1954.

41. Fell RH, Gunning AJ, Bardhan KD, et al: Severe hypothermia as a result of barbiturate overdose complicated by cardiac arrest. *Lancet* 1:392, 1968.

42. Towne WD, Geiss WP, Vanes HO, et al: Intractable ventricular fibrillation associated with profound accidental hypothermia: Successful treatment with partial cardiopulmonary bypass. *N Engl J Med* 287:1135, 1972.

43. Splittgerber FH, Talbert JG, Sweezer WP, Wilson RF: Partial cardiopulmonary bypass for core rewarming in profound accidental hypothermia. *Am Surg* 52:407, 1986.

44. Phillips SJ, Ballentine B, Slonine D, et al: Percutaneous initiation of cardiopulmonary bypass. *Ann Thorac Surg* 36:223, 1983.

45. Hartz R, LoCicero J, Sanders J, et al: Portable bypass does not improve survival in cardiac arrest patients (abstract). *J Am Coll Cardiol* 13:121A, 1989.

46. Overlie PA, Reichman RT, Smith SC, et al: Emergency use of portable cardiopulmonary bypass in patients with cardiac arrest (abstract). *J Am Coll Cardiol* 13:160A, 1989.

47. Weil MH, Gazmuri RJ, Rackow EC: The clinical rational of cardiac resuscitation. *Dis Mon* 36:431, 1990.

48. Hess PJ, Howe HR, Bobiesek F: Traumatic tears of the thoracic aorta: Improved results using the BioMedicus pump. *Ann Thorac Surg* 48:6, 1989.

49. Walls JT, Curtis JJ, Boley T: Sarns centrifugal pump for repair of thoracic injury. *J Trauma* 29:1283, 1989.

50. McCroskey BM, Moore EE, Moore FA, et al: Torn descending thoracic aorta: Evolution of a technical approach. *Am J Surg* 162:473, 1991.
51. Anstadt MP, Bartlett RL, Malone JP, et al: Direct mechanical ventricular actuation for cardiac arrest in humans. *Chest* 100:86, 1991.
52. Bencini A, Parola LP: The pneumomassage of the heart. *Surgery* 39:375, 1956.
53. Wolcott MW, Wherry CG: A mechanical heart massager: A preliminary report. *Surgery* 48:903, 1960.
54. Anstadt GL, Blakemore WS, Baue AE: A new instrument for prolonged mechanical massage (abstract). *Circulation* 32(suppl 2):II-43, 1965.
55. Skinner DB: Experimental and clinical evaluations of mechanical ventricular assistance. *Am J Cardiol* 27:146, 1971.
56. Brown GH, Hamlin R, Anstadt MP, et al: The effect of direct mechanical ventricular assistance on myocardial hemodynamics during ventricular fibrillation. *Crit Care Med* 17:1175, 1989.
57. Anstadt MP, Malone JP, Brown GR, et al: Direct mechanical ventricular assistance promotes salvage of ischemic myocardium. *Trans Am Soc Artif Internal Organs* 33:720, 1987.
58. Mattox KL, Beall AC, Jordon GI, et al: Cardiorrhaphy in the emergency center. *J Thorac Cardiovasc Surg* 68:886, 1974.

7

PHARMACOLOGY OF RESUSCITATION

Stephen A. Vitkun

The use of resuscitative drugs is part of the entire picture of emergency care. The practitioner must always secure the airway, ensure breathing, and then evaluate the circulation and consider how to optimize it. It is in this area that drugs will be most helpful. When evaluating a patient with injuries, one must consider all causes of cardiac arrest (including surgical causes) that are not primary considerations when faced with a cardiac arrest secondary to medical causes. These surgical conditions include, but are not limited to, pericardial tamponade, tension pneumothorax, brainstem herniation, and massive hemorrhage (laceration/rupture of internal organs or major blood vessel injury) resulting in severe hypovolemic shock. They must be treated quickly and appropriately, since no combination of pharmacologic agents will be effective without other concurrent therapies. Therefore, the primary resuscitative effort in the trauma patient will most likely focus on fluid, blood, or plasma infusions and control of bleeding or treatment of a life-threatening surgical condition. Pharmacologic agents will be an adjuvant therapy in this effort. The use of resuscitative drugs will be helpful to suppress ventricular arrhythmias, providing a rhythm that will maintain adequate blood pressure, maintain coronary and cerebral perfusion, correct acidosis, and improve hemodynamics.

Almost by definition, a chapter on resuscitative drugs is broad and must consider a variety of agents, irrespective of their specific pharmacologic classification. Therefore, within any given pharmacologic class of drugs, some but not necessarily all agents are discussed. Furthermore, this discussion will consider primarily the use of these drugs in the emergent treatment of cardiac arrhythmias and cardiac arrest. The discussion considers the drugs' effects on the cardiovascular system, with less regard to their effects on other organ systems or long-term effects. Table 7–1 lists the agents to be discussed in this chapter and their pharmacologic classification.

This chapter is divided into two main sections. The first section will discuss general principles, the pharmacology of specific agents used during resuscitation, their indications, dosages, and routes of administration. In addition, other

TABLE 7–1. Drugs Used in Resuscitation and Their Pharmacological Classification

Drug	Pharmacological Classification
Epinephrine	Catecholamine (natural)
Norepinephrine	Catecholamine (natural)
Dopamine	Catecholamine (natural)
Dobutamine	Catecholamine (synthetic)
Isoproterenol	Catecholamine (synthetic)
Lidocaine	Antiarrhythmic (class Ib), local anesthetic
Bretylium	Antiarrhythmic (class III)
Procainamide	Antiarrhythmic (class Ia), local anesthetic
Atropine	Parasympatholytic
Nitroglycerin	Nitrate (vasodilator)
Sodium nitroprusside	Nitrate (vasodilator)
Amrinone	Noncatecholamine nonglycoside bipyridine
Propranolol	Beta-adrenergic antagonist (class II antiarrhythmic)
Metoprolol	Beta-adrenergic antagonist
Verapamil	Calcium channel blocker (class IV antiarrhythmic)
Diltiazem	Calcium channel blocker
Adenosine	Purine nucleotide
Calcium chloride	Electrolyte
Sodium bicarbonate	Electrolyte
Magnesium sulfate	Electrolyte
Furosemide	Loop diuretic
Naloxone	Opiate antagonist
Flumazenil	Benzodiazepine receptor antagonist

agents such as narcotic and benzodiazepine antagonists are reviewed. Although they are not used in resuscitation per se, they may be useful agents in the initial resuscitation of a patient in shock. Drug dosages and routes of administration in the pediatric patient are presented. The second section consists of algorithms for treatment of various cardiac arrhythmias, cardiac arrest, and hypotension. The algorithms also show the indications for defibrillation and cardioversion; however, detailed discussion of these therapies is beyond the scope of this chapter.

GENERAL PRINCIPLES

The general pharmacologic and physiologic principles of resuscitation, irrespective of the cause of the condition, include correction of hypoxemia, reestablishment of spontaneous cardiac rhythm, and optimization of the circulation. Cardiac arrhythmias must be suspected and treated should they occur. Acid-base balance must be ascertained and corrected if necessary. Ideally, all medications should be administered intravenously (IV) through a cannula that allows injection directly into the central circulation. Usually, this is a central venous catheter. However, such a catheter is not always available and may be relatively time consuming to place, particularly in a situation of cardiac arrest, where chest compressions will need to be stopped. Other options include a long femoral venous catheter or a brachial catheter in adults. If medication is given through a peripheral venous catheter, injection of drugs should be followed by a bolus of 50 ml normal saline to enhance the delivery to the central circulation.[32] In infants, because of the difficulties in obtaining venous access, any venous access is acceptable.[33] Furthermore, in pediatric patients, intraosseous injection may be used as an access site for the administration of fluids and drugs.[34,35]

If intravenous access is not available, epinephrine and atropine may be given by endotracheal instillation. The endotracheal dose to produce comparable hemodynamic effects is not established; however, some studies suggest that as much as 10 times the usual IV dose is needed. In clinical practice, the higher-range IV dose is usually used.[32,36,37]

Although we may not even think of oxygen as a drug, it is an essential component of cardiac resuscitation. During mouth-to-mouth breathing, the oxygen concentration is about 16 to 17 percent, which can produce a maximum partial pressure of oxygen of about 80 mmHg. Normally, the partial pressure of oxygen is approximately 100 mmHg on room air, and in addition, there are many other factors during resuscitation which may impair oxygen delivery and uptake.[38] Supplemental oxygen should be given to all patients with chest pain, possible hypoxemia, or cardiopulmonary arrest. As with any drug, there are precautions to consider before administering oxygen. Pure oxygen is toxic to the lungs, but this is not a consideration during the relatively brief period of resuscitation. Particular care should be used when giving supplemental oxygen to a patient with chronic pulmonary disease who may have a hypoxemic respiratory drive. Ultimately, if clinically indicated, oxygen should never be withheld.[1]

PHARMACOLOGY OF SPECIFIC AGENTS

CATECHOLAMINES AND POSITIVE INOTROPES

Sympathomimetic agents may be divided into naturally occurring catecholamines (epinephrine, norepinephrine, dopamine), synthetic catecholamines (dobutamine, isoproterenol), noncatecholamines (ephedrine, phenylephrine, amphetamine, and others), and other inotropes (amrinone, milrinone). All these agents produce varying degrees of vasoconstriction, vasodilation of skeletal muscle, bronchodilation, and cardiac stimulation (increased force of contraction and increased heart rate). Other uses of these agents include treatment of bronchospasm, life-threatening allergic reactions, and addition to local anesthetic solutions to slow the systemic absorption of the anesthetic agent.

All catecholamines are derivatives of beta-phenylethylamine (Fig. 7–1A). Addition of hydroxyl groups on the number 3 and 4 carbon atoms of the benzene ring defines a catecholamine (Fig. 7–1B). Dopamine is an endogenous cate-cholamine, from which epinephrine and norepinephrine are derived (Fig. 7–2). In addition, synthetic catecholamines, such as isoproterenol and dobutamine, are derived from substitutions to the terminal amine of norepinephrine (Fig. 7–3). The synthetic noncatecholamines lack hydroxyl groups on the number 3 and 4 carbon atoms of the benzene ring. Hydroxylation of the number 3 and 5 carbon atoms of the ring increases beta-2 agonist activity. Amrinone has a bi-pyridine structure. Milrinone is the methylcarbonitrile derivative of amrinone.

Sympathomimetic agents directly or indirectly activate alpha-adrenergic (al-pha-1 or alpha-2), beta-adrenergic (beta-1 or beta-2), or dopaminergic (DA-1 or DA-2) receptors. This is thought to increase the production of cyclic adeno-sine monophosphate (cyclic AMP) by stimulation of adenylate cyclase.[2] Adren-ergic receptors may be broken down into subtypes, and stimulation of various subtypes produces different effects as shown in Table 7–2. Ahlquist[6] evaluated the physiologic effects of sympathomimetic agents on different tissues and noted two sequences of agent potency, suggesting two types of adrenergic receptors. The first sequence in descending order was epinephrine > norepinephrine > isoproterenol, while the second was isoproterenol > epinephrine > norepi-nephrine. The effects as described by the first sequence are termed *alpha effects,* while the second sequences effects are called *beta effects.* In many instances, these effects oppose each other. While alpha effects cause vasoconstriction, beta stim-ulation causes vasodilation. The beta receptors are divided into two separate subtypes called *beta-1* and *beta-2.*[5] Stimulation of beta-1 receptors increases the force of myocardial contraction, while beta-2 stimulation results in relaxation of vascular and bronchial smooth muscle. The alpha receptors also have two dis-tinct subtypes.[7] Alpha-1 receptors are located postsynaptically and cause exci-tation, while alpha-2 receptors are located presynaptically and are inhibitory in nature. This system has subsequently been modified because further studies have demonstrated that alpha-2 receptors may exist both pre- and postsynapti-cally.[3]

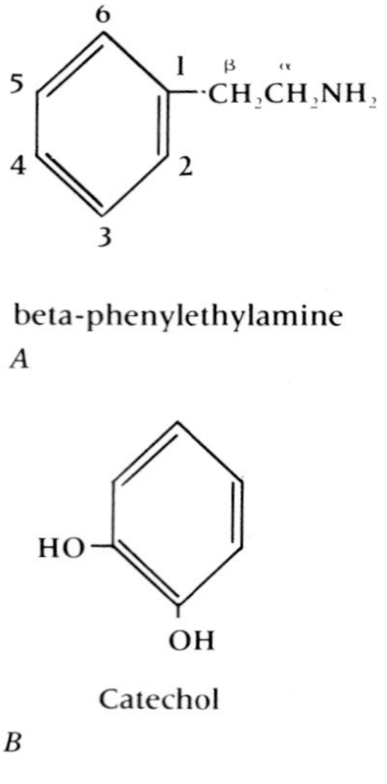

beta-phenylethylamine

A

Catechol

B

FIG. 7–1. Beta-phenylethylamine (*A*) represents the basic compound from which catecholamines are de-rived. Hydroxyl substitution on the number 3 and 4 carbons of the benzene structure defines a catechol-amine (*B*).

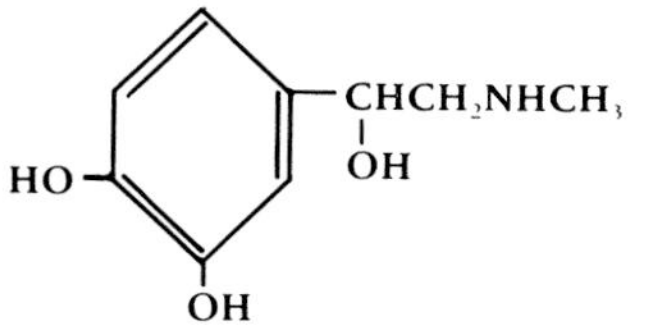

Epinephrine

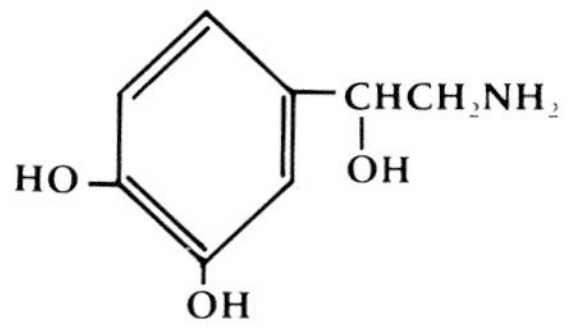

Norepinephrine

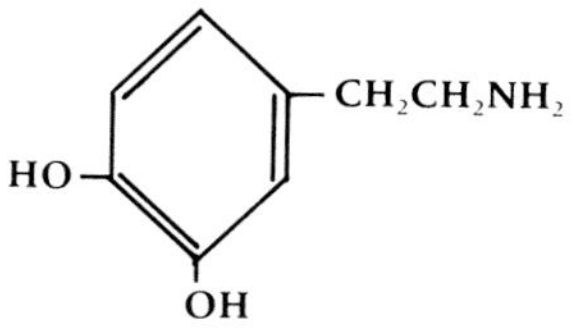

Dopamine

FIG. 7–2. The catecholamines. All have —OH substitutions on the number 3 and 4 ring positions.

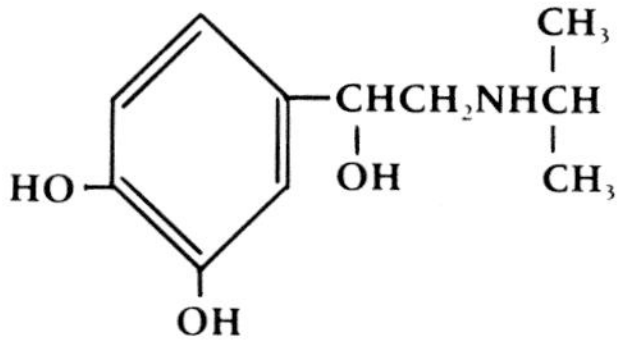

Isoproterenol

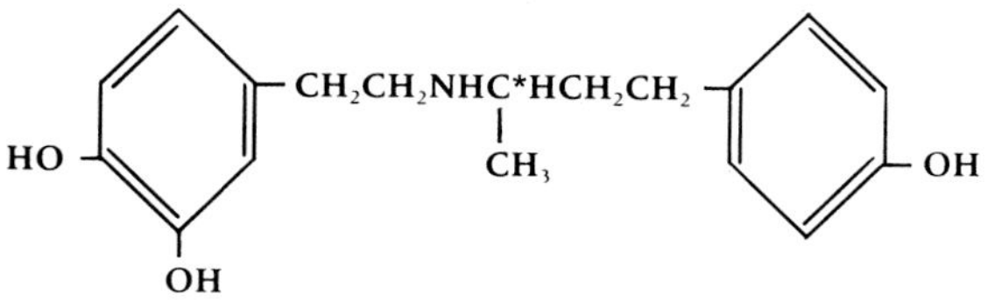

Dobutamine

FIG. 7–3. The synthetic catecholamines. Dobutamine possesses a chiral center (*).

TABLE 7–2. Cardiopulmonary Effects of Specific Adrenergic/Dopaminergic Receptor Stimulation

Alpha-1 (Postsynaptic) Receptors	Alpha-2 (Presynaptic)
Vasoconstriction	Inhibition of norepinephrine release
Increased peripheral resistance	
Increased blood pressure	
Beta-1 (Postsynaptic)	**Beta-2 (Postsynaptic)**
Tachycardia	Vasodilation
Increased myocardial contractility	Decrease of peripheral resistance
	Bronchodilation
Dopamine-1 (Postsynaptic)	**Dopamine-2 (Presynaptic)**
Vasodilation	Inhibition of norepinephrine release

Source: Adapted from Stoelting RK: *Pharmacology and Physiology in Anesthetic Practice,* Philadelphia, Lippincott, 1991; and Harvey RA, Champe PC: *Pharmacology,* Philadelphia, Lippincott, 1992, with permission.

EPINEPHRINE (ADRENALIN)

Epinephrine, 1-β-(3,4-dihydroxyphenyl)-α-methylaminoethanol, has been a significant part of the therapy for cardiac arrest during most of the twentieth century. The first use of epinephrine during cardiac arrest was described in 1906. Epinephrine is normally released from the adrenal medulla. It regulates cardiac contractility, heart rate, vascular and bronchial smooth muscle tone, and various metabolic processes. It is the most potent alpha agonist (stimulating both alpha-1 and alpha-2 receptors with similar potency) in addition to activating beta-1 and beta-2 receptors.[3] Epinephrine is one of the most potent vasopressor drugs known. It increases blood pressure in a dose-dependent fashion, causing a relatively greater rise in systolic blood pressure compared with diastolic blood pressure, thereby causing an increase in the pulse pressure. This primary beneficial effect of epinephrine is due to peripheral vasoconstriction. In addition, the alpha effects make ventricular fibrillation more susceptible to electrical countershock.[9,22–24]

The increase in blood pressure produced by epinephrine is due to three factors: direct myocardial stimulation causing an increase in the force of the ventricular contraction (increased inotropy) and increasing heart rate (increased chronotropy), both effects being mediated through beta-1 receptors, and, perhaps most important, vasoconstriction. Vasoconstriction occurs in many different vascular beds through effects on the smaller arterioles and precapillary sphincters. Veins and large arteries also respond to epinephrine.

Epinephrine also has a variety of metabolic effects, including increasing blood glucose, free fatty acid, and lactate concentrations. Insulin secretion is inhibited through alpha-2 effects. The uptake of glucose by peripheral tissues is decreased.[4]

Epinephrine may not be administered orally. It is broken down rapidly by the gastrointestinal mucosa and liver. It is absorbed slowly when given subcutaneously because of local vasoconstriction. Circulating epinephrine is metabolized primarily in the liver by catechol-O-methyl transferase (COMT) and monoamine oxidase (MAO).[4]

The toxicity of epinephrine, as well as other catecholamines, causes myocardial damage (the microscopic appearance of which has been called *contraction band necrosis*[12,13]) and vascular injury.[13,14] Epinephrine also has been shown to cause an increase in pulmonary shunting during spontaneous circulation.[15] During cardiopulmonary resuscitation, epinephrine administration can cause a decrease in end-tidal carbon dioxide, a decrease in arterial oxygen, and an increase in arterial carbon dioxide levels.[16-18] These effects should not be significant, except in patients with marginal blood gases. This may represent an advantage of pure alpha agonists. Ultimately, concerns about toxicity are secondary when epinephrine is being administered during cardiac arrest. Epinephrine may induce or exacerbate ventricular ectopy, especially in patients receiving digoxin preparations.

Administration of epinephrine to a conscious person can produce anxiety reactions, fear, a sense of impending doom, tenseness, tremor, dizziness, and palpitations. These effects are usually transient.

Many animal studies have demonstrated the efficacy of epinephrine during experimental cardiac arrest. Animal studies have demonstrated that the alpha effects are more important than the beta effects during resuscitation. There are no controlled human trials to demonstrate the efficacy of epinephrine compared with placebo, since these studies would be ethically difficult to perform. Use of a pure alpha agonist (methoxamine) was much more effective compared with isoproterenol (a pure beta agonist) during cardiac arrest; also, some patients were resuscitated successfully with methoxamine after failure of epinephrine.[8-11] In fact, the beta-mediated increases in myocardial oxygen consumption may be clinically detrimental during cardiac arrest.[3] When administered at lower doses during spontaneous circulation, epinephrine causes a decrease in blood pressure through stimulation of beta receptors; however, at the higher doses used during cardiac arrest, its alpha effects predominate.[19,20] Despite the theoretical advantages of alpha-agonist agents, there have not been any clear demonstrations that they offer significant improvement over epinephrine, particularly when epinephrine has been demonstrated to increase cerebral blood flow compared with pure alpha agonists.[21]

Specific indications for epinephrine during resuscitation include asystole, ventricular fibrillation (especially to convert "fine" ventricular fibrillation to "course" ventricular fibrillation, which is more amenable to electrical countershock), and circulatory shock. The optimal dose of epinephrine to augment diastolic blood pressure is unknown. The recommended dose of epinephrine is 7.5 to 15 µg/kg (0.5 to 1.0 mg in a 70-kg patient) given intravenously. The dose should be repeated every 5 min.[1] Tachyphylaxis may develop in response to synthetic noncatecholamines; however, repeated doses of epinephrine will produce similar cardiovascular effects.[2]

Epinephrine is a potent renal artery vasoconstrictor, which limits its usefulness in patients with shock. Epinephrine infusions as low as 0.035 µg/kg/min have been shown to cause a 10 percent decrease in renal plasma flow. The net effect is to reduce renal blood flow and ultimately urine output. However, despite these problems, epinephrine may increase urine output by increasing cardiac output and renal blood flow.[43,44]

If IV access has not been established, 1 mg of epinephrine diluted with 10 ml sterile water or normal saline may be instilled directly into the tracheobronchial tree via the endotracheal tube. The plasma concentration and hemodynamic effects of intratracheal epinephrine are about 10 percent of an equivalent IV dose.[42] In children, the dilution is not necessary. Intracardiac epinephrine may be administered in those rare circumstances when it cannot be given either intravenously or intratracheally.

Continuous infusion of epinephrine is useful to maintain the arterial pressure and/or the heart rate. The initial infusion rate is 2 µg/min, and it is then titrated to effect (to a maximum of 20 µg/min). At the lower infusion rate (2 µg/min), the primary effect is stimulation of beta-2 receptors in the peripheral vasculature. At higher doses (4 µg/min), stimulation of beta-1 receptors occurs. Larger doses (10 to 20 µg/min IV) stimulate both alpha and beta receptors.[2] Rapid infusion may precipitate hypertension and/or ventricular ectopy.[1]

NOREPINEPHRINE (LEVARTENENOL)

Norepinephrine, 1-β-[3,4-dihydroxyphenyl]-α-aminoethanol, is also a naturally occurring catecholamine. It differs chemically from epinephrine by the lack of a methyl group on the terminal amine (see Fig. 7–2). Norepinephrine is released from postganglionic adrenergic nerves. It normally constitutes about 10 to 20 percent of the catecholamines released from the adrenal medulla, although it may account for a much higher percentage of catecholamines released from a pheochromocytoma.[4]

Norepinephrine differs from epinephrine mainly in the ratio of its effectiveness in stimulating alpha-2 and beta-2 receptors. Both agents are equipotent in stimulating beta-1 cardiac receptors. Norepinephrine is a potent alpha agonist, with little beta-2 effects. Intravenous infusion causes an increase in systolic and diastolic blood pressure. Cardiac output is unchanged, and total peripheral resistance is increased. It is important to realize that the blood pressure increases observed with norepinephrine are predominantly due to increases in systemic vascular resistance, which may also diminish cardiac output. This, in turn, increases myocardial oxygen demand and may cause cardiac ischemia to develop. Therefore, norepinephrine should be used as the last resort in patients with coronary artery disease. Furthermore, it is a potent renal and splanchnic vasoconstrictor, which limits its clinical usefulness.[40] In dogs, low-dose dopamine used with norepinephrine decreases the vasoconstrictive effect in the renal vasculature, suggesting that the combination may provide the desired increase in coronary perfusion pressure as well as maintain adequate renal function.[45] Heart rate may decrease due to reflex vagal stimulation. Metabolic effects are similar to those produced by epinephrine. Like epinephrine, norepinephrine will not work if given orally, since it is metabolized in a similar fashion to epinephrine.

Norepinephrine is usually administered by infusion to treat refractory hypotension, which may occur during a state of septic shock.[41] It is usually administered by central intravenous infusion from 2 to 16 µg/min. It is contraindicated in the presence of hypotension resulting from hypovolemia, except as a temporary means of maintaining blood pressure until appropriate volume replacement is achieved. Peripheral infusion of norepinephrine, as well as epinephrine, should be avoided because of the potential for necrosis and sloughing at the injection site due to extravasation of the drug. Norepinephrine (16 mg in

200 ml iced saline) also may be used in gastric lavage solutions to treat acute gastrointestinal bleeding.[46] The hemodynamic effects of epinephrine and norepinephrine are compared in Table 7–3.

Norepinephrine is metabolized by the same enzymes that methylate and oxidatively deaminate epinephrine. The side effects and toxicity of norepinephrine are similar to those described for epinephrine.

DOPAMINE

Dopamine, 3,4-dihydroxyphenylethylamine, is a naturally occurring catecholamine (see Fig. 7–2). It is a metabolic precursor to norepinephrine and epinephrine, in addition to its role as a neurotransmitter. Chemically, it differs from norepinephrine by the absence of a beta-hydroxyl group. Like the other catecholamines, it is not effective when given orally.

Dopamine acts at dopamine-1 receptors located postsynaptically and mediates vasodilation of renal, mesenteric, coronary, and cerebral blood vessels.[39] Dopamine-2 receptors are located presynaptically and inhibit the release of norepinephrine. The cardiovascular effects of dopamine are dose-related. It stimulates dopaminergic, beta-2-adrenergic, and alpha-adrenergic receptors.[25] At lower concentrations (0.5 to 2 μg/kg/min), dopamine interacts with dopaminergic receptors in the renal, mesenteric, and coronary beds. This interaction causes vasodilation and increases in glomerular filtration rate and renal blood flow. It is a very important agent in the management of cardiogenic and hypovolemic shock, particularly when decreased cardiac output compromises renal function.

TABLE 7–3. Comparision of Hemodynamic Effects of Epinephrine and Norepinephrine

Hemodynamic Effects	Epinephrine	Norepinephrine
Cardiac		
Heart rate	+	−
Stroke volume	+ +	+ +
Cardiac output	+ + +	0, −
Arrhythmias	+ + + +	+ + + +
Coronary blood flow	+ +	+ +
Blood pressure		
Systolic (arterial)	+ + +	+ + +
Diastolic	+ ,0, −	+ +
Mean	+	+ +
Pulmonary artery (mean)	+ +	+ +
Peripheral circulation		
Total peripheral resistance	−	+ +
Cerebral blood flow	+	0, −
Renal blood flow	−	−
Metabolic effects		
Oxygen consumption	+ +	0, +

Note: + = increase; − = decrease; 0 = no change.

Source: Adapted from *Goodman and Gilman's Pharmacological Basis of Therapeutics*, 8th ed. New York, Pergamon Press, 1990, p. 194, with permission.

At higher concentrations (2 to 10 μg/kg/min), dopamine has positive inotropic effects, mediated through beta-1-adrenergic receptors as well as alpha effects through release of norepinephrine from nerve terminals. When infused at 10 to 20 μg/kg/min, the alpha effects predominate over the beta effects. Infusions in excess of 20 μg/kg/min have predominately alpha-adrenergic effects. Studies in dogs pretreated with reserpine to deplete endogenous norepinephrine stores suggests that as much as 50 percent of dopamine's hemodynamic action may be due to release of norepinephrine.[47] Infusion of dopamine increases norepinephrine plasma concentrations in a dose-dependent fashion.[28] When used at the higher concentrations (above 10 μg/kg/min), dopamine has its predominant effects on alpha-1-adrenergic receptors, leading to vasoconstriction. With infusions above 20 μg/kg/min, it has hemodynamic effects similar to those of norepinephrine.

Dopamine is useful in the treatment of shock (hypotensive states), particularly when associated with oliguria and low or normal peripheral vascular resistance (in the absence of hypovolemia). It is also beneficial in treating cardiogenic and septic shock. It is the only catecholamine that can increase renal blood flow and glomerular filtration rate in addition to improving myocardial contractility. Dopamine should be used in lower doses (as little as 1/10 the normal dose) in patients who take MAO inhibitors or tricyclic antidepressants, since these agents will potentiate its effects. Additionally, the initial infusion of bretylium tosylate may have synergistic effects with dopamine. The mechanism of this action is unknown.[26]

Dopamine undergoes rapid metabolism, requiring that it be used as a continuous IV infusion. The infusion rate may vary between 1 and 20 μg/kg/min; however, the infusion may be increased as high as 20 to 50 μg/kg/min, as dictated by the clinical situation. It is diluted to a concentration of 0.4 to 1.6 mg/ml and infused at an initial rate of 2 to 5 μg/kg/min. The infusion rate may be increased until blood pressure, urine output, and other parameters of organ perfusion improve.

DOBUTAMINE

Dobutamine is a synthetic catecholamine. It is structurally similar to dopamine but possesses a large aromatic substituent on the amino group (see Fig. 7–3). Dobutamine is the only catecholamine to possess an asymmetric center yielding two enantiomeric forms that are present in the racemic mixture which is used clinically. It stimulates beta- and alpha-adrenergic receptors, with somewhat greater selectivity for beta-1 than for beta-2 receptors. The (−)-isomer is an alpha-adrenergic agonist, while the (+)-isomer is a competitive alpha-adrenergic antagonist. The (+)-isomer is also a more potent beta-adrenergic agonist.[28] It does not appear to act through dopaminergic receptors or through release of norepinephrine.[27,28]

Dobutamine has relatively more inotropic than chronotropic effects on the heart when compared with isoproterenol. In animal studies, dobutamine infusion at 2.5 to 15 μg/kg/min increases cardiac contractility and cardiac output, while total peripheral resistance is not affected.[29] In clinical concentrations, dobutamine is less likely to cause tachycardia than either isoproterenol or dopamine. However, at higher doses, increases in heart rate do occur. Renal blood flow is usually increased, but in contrast to dopamine, it is probably related to the increased cardiac output rather than to effects on dopaminergic receptors.[30] The overall hemodynamic effect of dobutamine is similar to that of a combination of dopamine with a vasodilator such as nitroprusside.[31] Dobutamine generally lowers the central venous and pulmonary wedge pressures and has little effect on pulmonary vascular resistance.[50] Dobutamine lacks a selective renal vascular effect but may enhance urine output secondary to improvements in cardiac output and renal perfusion.[51] Unlike dopamine, dobutamine's effects do not depend on the body's stores of norepinephrine.[28]

Some studies suggest that the combined administration of dopamine and dobutamine may have advantages over the administration of either agent alone in the treatment of cardiogenic shock.[49] When given alone, dopamine at 15 μg/kg/min increases mean arterial pressure, but also increases pulmonary capillary wedge pressure and reduces alveolar P_{O_2}. Infusion of dobutamine alone at 15 μg/kg/min did not increase mean arterial pressure but improved stroke volume. When given in combination at 7.5 μg/kg/min each, dopamine and dobutamine had beneficial effects on mean arterial pressure, cardiac index, and stroke volume without increasing the pulmonary capillary wedge pressure.

Dobutamine is indicated in situations where increases in contractility with little effect on peripheral vascular resistance are needed. This situation usually occurs in a normotensive patient with congestive heart failure. Dobutamine, combined with volume loading, is very effective in the treatment of hemodynamically significant right ventricular infarction.[53] Dobutamine increases stroke volume and cardiac output while reducing the filling pressures.[51] When lower doses are used, there may be minor changes in heart rate, and dobutamine improves the balance between myocardial oxygen supply and demand in patients with heart failure secondary to coronary artery disease.[27] In the setting of hypotensive cardiogenic shock, dopamine may be more effective because of its greater effect on peripheral vascular resistance; furthermore, owing to a lack of vasoconstrictive effects, dobutamine may be disadvantageous in patients with septic shock and hypotension.

The usual initial infusion rates of dobutamine in adults or children are 2 to 5 μg/kg/min. Maximal benefits usually occur with infusions of 10 to 15 μg/kg/min, and the usual dose range is from 2.5 to 20 μg/kg/min. Infusion rates should be guided by measurement of hemodynamic parameters, and the smallest clinically effective dose should be used. Dobutamine has a plasma half-life of about 2.4 min, being cleared by catechol-*O*-methyl transferase and distribution from the central compartment. Similar to other catecholamines, dobutamine should be administered directly into the central circulation. Dysrhythmias are the most frequently observed side effect. Other side effects include tachycardia, headaches, anxiety, and extremes of blood pressure.[27] Dobutamine also can worsen myocardial ischemia at higher doses.

ISOPROTERENOL (ISUPREL)

Isoproterenol hydrochloride (see Fig. 7–3) is a synthetic *N*-alkylated amine with almost pure beta-adrenergic receptor activity. As a beta agonist, it is from 2 to

10 times more potent than epinephrine and over 100 times more potent than norepinephrine. Its effects include increasing heart rate, cardiac contractility, and conduction velocity through stimulation of beta-1 receptors, while beta-2 stimulation causes a relaxation of vascular smooth muscle. Ultimately, isoproterenol increases cardiac output, providing the circulating volume is adequate; otherwise, vasodilation may impair venous return and cardiac output may fall. Much of the improvement in cardiac output is related to increases in heart rate rather than stroke volume, particularly in pediatric patients.[54,55] Enhanced contractility, which increases myocardial oxygen demand, and increases in heart rate, which shorten the diastolic filling time and impair myocardial oxygen supply, may result in myocardial ischemia.[56]

Although isoproterenol is an inotrope, the tendency to produce tachycardia and myocardial ischemia has limited its clinical use. It is used to treat hemodynamically significant bradycardia (which is refractory to treatment with atropine) usually associated with heart block. It is generally used temporally until a more definitive treatment such as a pacemaker is instituted. It is also potentially useful in the treatment of refractory torsades de pointes,[52] a specific type of ventricular tachycardia demonstrating a gradual alteration in the amplitude and direction of electrical activity. In addition, isoproterenol has been used in the treatment of status asthmaticus and pulmonary artery hypertension.[57,58] It also appears to be useful in treating pulmonary hypertension and is a bronchodilator. However, more selective beta-2 agonists have replaced it as a bronchodilating agent.

Intravenous infusions usually range from 1 to 5 μg/min and are adjusted to produce the desired hemodynamic effect. Doses in excess of 10 μg/min are rarely necessary. Heart rate and blood pressure must be monitored closely. The major side effects of isoproterenol are tachycardia and tachydysrhythmias. Angina and myocardial infarction also may occur, while palpitations, headaches, and flushing of the skin are less common.[56]

AMRINONE

Amrinone (5-amino[3,4'-bipyridine]-6(1H)-one) is a phosphodiesterase inhibitor with the chemical structure shown in Fig. 7–4. The structure of amrinone is unique (a bipyridine); unlike any of the other inotropic agents it is not a catecholamine. Milrinone is the methyl carbonitrile derivative of amrinone, which has recently been approved for intravenous use. Amrinone has positive inotropic and chronotropic properties as well as being a vasodilator. Amrinone does not stimulate alpha- or beta-adrenergic receptors, and its effects are not antagonized by adrenergic blocking agents or norepinephrine depletion.[62] It does not inhibit cell membrane sodium-potassium ATPase like the cardiac glycosides, nor does it release either histamine or prostaglandins.[60,61]

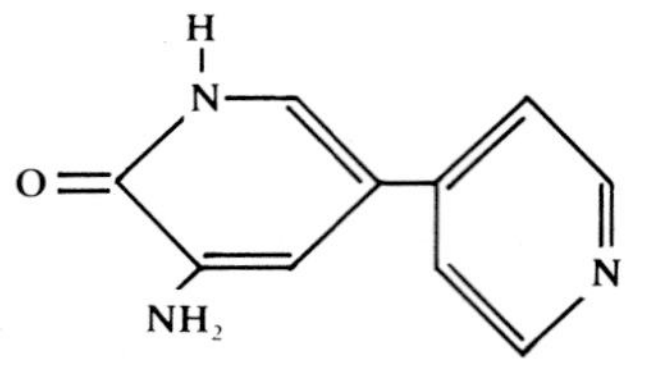

FIG. 7–4. Amrinone.

Amrinone-induced inhibition of the phosphodiesterase enzyme, similar to methylxanthines, leads to increased intracellular concentrations of cyclic AMP. This enhances myocardial contractility by increasing delivery of calcium to the myocardial contractile apparatus.[59] Although amrinone's effects are similar to those of digoxin, they may be used together without causing digitalis toxicity, suggesting that the mechanism of action of these agents is different.

Although it has been used successfully in patients with congestive heart failure, it may induce or worsen myocardial ischemia. It is a useful agent in the treatment of severe congestive heart failure which is refractory to treatment with diuretics, vasodilators, and the usual inotropic agents. It has dose-dependent positive inotropic and vasodilator effects resulting in an increase in cardiac output (increased contractility and stroke volume) and lowering of left ventricular end-diastolic pressure.[63,64] An increase in heart rate may also occur. Pulmonary vascular pressures usually decrease and peripheral vasodilation will reduce afterload, enhancing contractility without an increase in myocardial oxygen consumption.[65] Despite decreases in the systemic vascular resistance, the blood pressure is unchanged with lower doses of amrinone because the increase in stroke volume can compensate for the fall in peripheral vascular resistance.[69,70]

Amrinone may be given intravenously in a single loading dose of 0.5 to 1.5 mg/kg over 3 to 5 min. Following an initial injection, a continuous infusion of 2 to 10 μg/kg/min produces positive inotropic effects. The recommended maximum dose is 10 mg/kg. A side effect of amrinone is hypotension due to vasodilation. The therapeutic index of amrinone is approximately 100:1 compared to 1.2:1 for the cardiac glycosides. The mean half-life of amrinone is approximately 3.6 h with slower elimination in patients with congestive heart failure (5 to 8 h).[66,67] The principal route of excretion is through the kidney, yielding unchanged drug in the urine.[68]

Milrinone produces hemodynamic effects similar to dobutamine in patients with congestive heart failure. It has positive inotropic and vasodilating effects, but its mechanism of action appears to be different than that of dobutamine. Milrinone probably produces greater decreases in arterial impedance, which increases cardiac index, and it does so without increasing myocardial oxygen consumption as is seen with dobutamine.[191] In studies comparing intravenous milrinone with dobutamine and nitroprusside, milrinone produced greater improvement in pulmonary capillary wedge pressure, with lower myocardial oxygen consumption than dobutamine, and in addition it produced comparable hemodynamic improvement to nitroprusside with less associated hypotension.[192]

Milrinone is indicated in the treatment of congestive heart failure. The recommended loading dose of milrinone is 50 μg/kg IV over 10 min with continuous IV infusions of 0.375 μg/kg/min to 0.75 μg/kg/min. The infusion is titrated to hemodynamic effects. Dose reductions may be necesssary in patients with renal impairment.

ANTIARRHYTHMIC AGENTS

The antiarrhythmic drugs are divided into four major classes based on their major effects on the electrophysiologic properties of isolated normal cells.[71] Agents

TABLE 7–4. Classification of Antiarrhythmic Agents

	Major Effect	Effects on Electrocardiogram	Principal Clearance	Elimination Half-Time	Therapeutic Plasma Conc.	Indication(s)*
Class I	Sodium channel blockade					
Class Ia: Procainamide		Moderate decrease in conduction Moderate increase in repolarization	Renal/hepatic	2.5–5 h	4–10 µg/ml	A.fib. (+), PSVT (++), PVC (++), VT (++)
Class Ib: Lidocaine		Mild increase in conduction Little effect on repolarization	Hepatic	1.4–1.8 h	1–5 µg/ml	PVC (++), VT (++)
Class Ic: Flecainide (not discussed)		Marked decrease in conduction Little effect on repolarization				
Class II: Propranolol/ Metoprolol	Beta-adrenergic antagonist	Reduce catecholamine effects	Hepatic	2–4 h	10–30 ng/ml	A.fib. (+), PSVT (++), PVC (+) < VT (+)
Class III: Bretylium	Variable/mixed actions	Prolongs action potential duration	Renal	8–12 h	75–100 ng/ml	PVC (+), VT (++)
Class IV: Verapamil	Calcium channel blockade	Slows conduction in AV node	Hepatic	4.5–12 h	100–300 ng/ml	A.fib. (=), PSVT (++)

Note: A.fib. = conversion of atrial fibrillation; PSVT = paroxysmal supraventricular tachycardia; PVC = premature ventricular contractions; VT = ventricular tachycardia; (+) = effective; (++) = very effective.

Source: Adapted from Chernow B: *The Pharmacologic Approach to the Critically Ill Patient,* 2d ed. Baltimore, Williams & Wilkins, 1988; and Stoelting, RK: *Pharmacology and Physiology in Anesthetic Practice,* 2d ed. Philadelphia, Lippincott, 1991, with permission.

in class I are local anesthetics. They have their predominant effect on sodium conductance. They cause a depression of sodium conductance during phase 0 of the action potential. They slow conduction velocity and decrease excitability. Most class I agents also suppress automaticity and affect potassium repolarization. Class I agents have been subdivided, based on the variation in their effects on conduction and repolarization, as shown in Table 7–4. Class I agents include quinidine, procainamide, lidocaine, and flecainide, among others. Drugs in class II are beta-adrenergic blocking agents. They include propranolol and metoprolol. The principal effects of class II agents are depression of the phase 4 depolarization in the sinus node, slowing of conduction through the AV node, and antagonizing catecholamine-induced changes. Class III agents produce a prolongation of the duration of the action potential. The mechanism of action of drugs in class III are generally poorly understood. Drugs in class III include bretylium and amiodarone. Agents in class IV depress the activity of the calcium-dependent slow channels (calcium channel blockers).[71] Agents in this category include verapamil and diltiazem.

The antiarrhythmic agents are a heterogeneous group. Not all are used in the management of medical or surgical resuscitation. This section will consider only those drugs with specific indications in the management of resuscitation. These agents include lidocaine, procainamide, propranolol, metoprolol, bretylium, verapamil, and possibly, diltiazem.

LIDOCAINE

Lidocaine (Fig. 7–5) is the drug of choice for the immediate management of many ventricular arrhythmias, including ventricular tachycardia, ventricular fibrillation, and premature ventricular contractions (PVCs). It reduces the incidence of primary ventricular fibrillation in patients with acute myocardial infarction.[76–78] However, prophylactic use in acute myocardial infarction is controversial because conflicting data exist.[84,85] Although lidocaine is a class Ib drug, having different electrophysiologic properties from procainamide, which is designated a class Ia drug, it decreases automaticity by reducing the rate of the phase 4 diastolic depolarization.[72] Its effects on sodium channels are more prominent in partially depolarized fibers. In depolarized fibers or those damaged by ischemia, the action potential is prolonged and conduction is slowed.[74,75] The threshold for induction of ventricular fibrillation is reduced during acute myocardial ischemia, and lidocaine has been shown to increase the fibrillation threshold.[73] Usually, lidocaine does not affect blood pressure or myocardial contractility.[72]

Lidocaine is well absorbed orally; however, extensive first-pass metabolism in the liver makes oral administration unreliable. The drug, when given intrave-

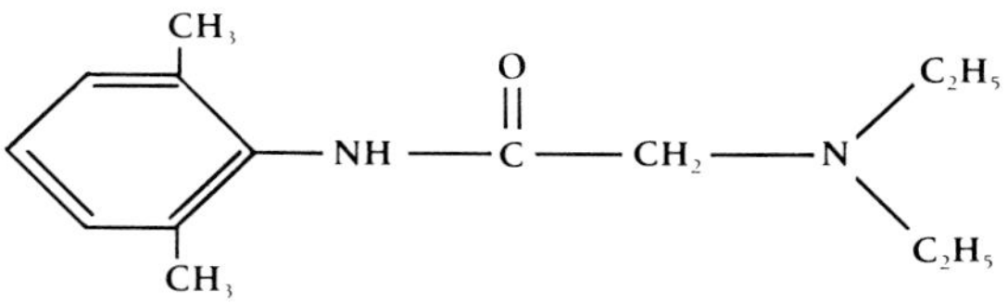

FIG. 7–5. Lidocaine.

nously, is distributed into the central compartment. In the blood, about 50 percent of lidocaine is bound to plasma albumin. The desired serum concentration of lidocaine is between 1 and 5 µg/ml. Toxicity occurs at higher levels. Toxicity is manifested by alterations of central nervous system function and circulatory depression. Dysarthria is usually the first sign of toxicity, and it is followed by paresthesias, muscle twitching, disorientation, and agitation.[82] At higher drug concentrations, seizures can occur.[72] Signs of circulatory depression include hypotension and slowing of the conduction of electrical impulses in the heart, resulting in bradycardia, a prolonged PR interval, and widened QRS complexes.

Lidocaine is eliminated by hepatic metabolism; therefore, the dose of lidocaine should be decreased (as much as 50 percent) in patients with impaired hepatic blood flow (congestive heart failure, acute myocardial infarction, or shock).[79,80] The dose of lidocaine also should be decreased in patients over 70 years of age because of decreased metabolism.[83] Less than 10 percent of lidocaine is excreted unchanged in the urine; therefore, little adjustment of the infusion rate is required in renal failure. The elimination half-life is about 1.5 to 2.5 h.

The loading dose of lidocaine is 1 mg/kg IV, followed by 0.5 mg/kg IV every 2 to 10 min, up to a total dose of 3 mg/kg.[81] IV infusions of lidocaine can range from 2 to 4 mg/min.

PROCAINAMIDE

Procainamide is a cinchona alkaloid. Cinchona alkaloids were used as far back as the 1700s to treat malaria. Even at that time, it was observed that patients would occasionally be cured of arrhythmias when treated for malaria. Today, procainamide (Fig. 7–6) is classified as a group Ia antiarrhythmic agent and is used to suppress PVCs and paroxysmal ventricular tachycardia. It also may be effective in situations where lidocaine is not effective in suppressing the arrhythmia.[86]

Physiologically, the effect of procainamide is to decrease the slope of phase 4 depolarization and shift the voltage threshold toward zero. This results from a blockade of the fast sodium channels and causes a small increase in the duration of the action potential and the effective refractory period. Reentry arrhythmias are eliminated as a result of the increase in the effective refractory period. On the electrocardiogram (ECG), drugs in class Ia can produce small increases in heart rate and PR and QRS intervals.

Procainamide is administered intravenously at a rate of 20 mg/min until either the arrhythmia responds, hypotension develops, the QRS complex is widened by 50 percent of its original width, or a dose of 1 g has been administered.[86] Continuous infusions of procainamide range between 1 and 4 mg/min. Blood pressure and ECG monitoring is essential during procainamide administration.

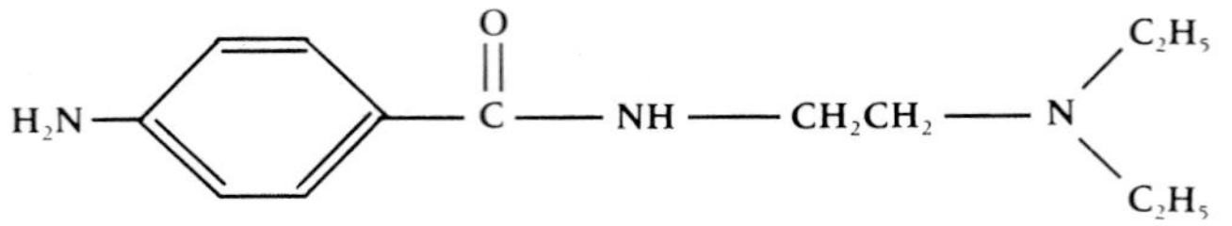

FIG. 7–6. Procainamide.

The dosage should be reduced in patients with left ventricular dysfunction or renal failure. Procainamide is eliminated by hepatic metabolism and renal excretion. In the liver, acetylation to N-acetyl procainamide (NAPA) occurs. The rate of acetylation is genetically determined (levels of the N-acetyltransferase enzyme), and the half-life varies from 2.5 to 5 h between slow and fast acetylators. The NAPA metabolite contributes to the antidysrhythmic effects; however, in renal failure, NAPA levels may become excessively high. Between 40 and 60 percent is excreted unchanged in the urine by the kidneys. Therapeutic blood levels range from 4 to 10 μg/ml.[87]

Rapid IV administration of procainamide may cause hypotension because it is a ganglionic blocker with potent vasodilating properties, in addition to having some negative inotropic properties.[86–88] High plasma levels may cause a slowing of conduction through the AV node. Ventricular fibrillation or asystole may occur if procainamide is given in the presence of heart block. A systemic lupus erythematosus–like syndrome[89] presenting as arthralgias and hepatomegaly may occur with chronic (but not acute) procainamide administration. Lupus-like symptoms subside after the drug has been discontinued. Gastrointestinal side effects (nausea and vomiting) may limit therapy. Procainamide is also associated with fever, leukopenia, and agranulocytosis.

BRETYLIUM TOSYLATE

Bretylium tosylate is a benzyl quarternary ammonium compound (Fig. 7–7). It is a class III antiarrhythmic agent (see Table 7–4), having both adrenergic and direct myocardial effects. The mechanism of its antiarrhythmic action is not well understood. Bretylium is effective in the treatment of ventricular tachycardia and ventricular fibrillation. Its electrophysiologic effects are due to interactions with sympathetic nerve terminals.

Initially, bretylium causes release of norepinephrine from presynaptic nerve endings. These effects last for approximately 20 min and may cause hypertension, tachycardia, and increases in cardiac output.[90–92] Subsequently, accumulation of bretylium at the nerve endings inhibits norepinephrine release and blocks reuptake of catecholamines. This may potentiate the effects of exogenous catecholamines.[98] These second-phase effects begin after 20 min and peak at 45 to 60 min[93] but may last as long as 6 h. During this period of time, significant hypotension may develop,[94] particularly with changes in position.

Initial administration of bretylium increases the sinus rate, AV conduction, and ventricular automaticity, probably due to catecholamine release. Bretylium and lidocaine have similar effects on the fibrillation threshold.[95,96] However, lidocaine may increase the defibrillation threshold, while this is not the case with

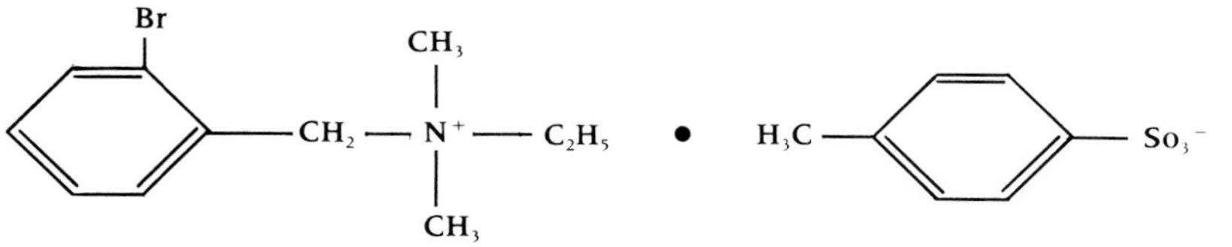

FIG. 7–7. Bretylium tosylate.

bretylium.[95,97] The effects of bretylium on ventricular fibrillation may occur within a few minutes, buts its effects may take as long as 20 min to develop in the treatment of ventricular tachycardia.

Bretylium has an apparent volume of distribution of 3 to 5 liters/kg and is not bound to plasma proteins, but it is highly bound in tissues, making the plasma level an unreliable indicator of antiarrhythmic activity. It is not metabolized, being excreted unchanged by the kidneys. The dosage should be reduced in patients with reduced renal function. It has an elimination half-life of 8 to 13 h.[99,100]

Bretylium is useful in the treatment of ventricular fibrillation and ventricular tachycardia which is refractory to other agents/therapy (lidocaine, procainamide, electrical cardioversion).[101,102] However, bretylium has not been shown to be superior to lidocaine in treating either ventricular tachycardia or ventricular fibrillation, and since it has a greater potential to cause adverse hemodynamic side effects,[103] it is not recommended as a first-choice treatment. It should be considered when lidocaine and electrical therapy fail to treat ventricular tachycardia or ventricular fibrillation or when lidocaine and procainamide fail to treat ventricular tachycardia.

To treat ventricular fibrillation, a loading dose of 5 mg/kg bretylium is given intravenously. Intramuscular therapy is possible, requiring no dose adjustment if the peripheral circulation is intact. The dose may be increased to 10 mg/kg and repeated to a maximum of 30 mg/kg.[98] For persistent ventricular tachycardia, a continuous intravenous infusion of 2 mg/min may be used.[104]

VERAPAMIL AND DILTIAZEM

Verapamil hydrochloride is a papaverine derivative (Fig. 7–8) chemically designated benzeneacetonitrile, α-[3-[[2-(e,4-dimethoxyphenyl)ethyl]methylamino]-propyl]-3,4-dimethoxy-α-(1-methylethyl) hydrochloride.[105,106] It is a class IV antiarrhythmic agent (see Table 7–4) producing its effects through blockade of the inward passage of calcium ions through the slow channel (calcium) in cardiac cell membranes. Verapamil also blocks calcium channels in vascular smooth muscle.[107] Verapamil slows the rate of spontaneous phase 4 depolarization in the sinoatrial and AV nodes. It is effective for the treatment of reentrant supraventricular tachycardia. Intravenous verapamil is beneficial for terminating narrow-complex paroxysmal supraventricular tachycardia (PSVT); however, adenoside is the drug of choice for treating narrow-complex PSVT.[52] It also can slow the ventricular response during atrial fibrillation or atrial flutter.[108–110] In

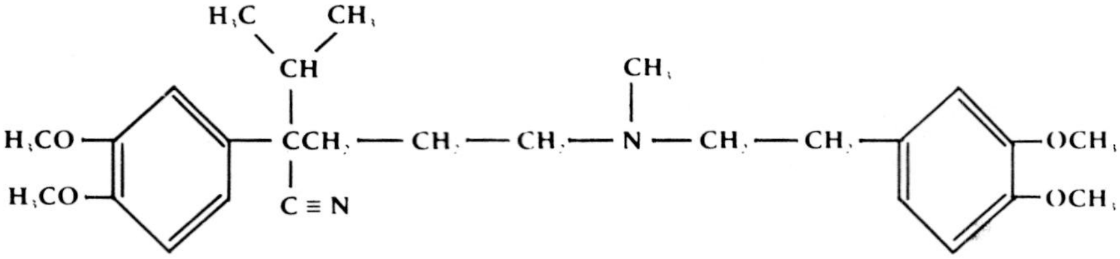

FIG. 7–8. Verapamil.

emergency situations, verapamil is used to treat paroxysmal supraventricular tachycardia not requiring cardioversion.[107,108,111–113] It possesses negative inotropic effects in addition to causing relaxation of vascular smooth muscle. Most patients will experience a decrease in blood pressure after receiving intravenous verapamil; this is principally due to peripheral vasodilation. This decrease in afterload may be beneficial during myocardial ischemia.[113]

Verapamil has minimal effects on the bypass pathways in patients with Wolff-Parkinson-White (WPW) syndrome.[116] It should be avoided in patients with WPW syndrome who have atrial fibrillation or atrial flutter because the ventricular response during atrial fibrillation may be increased in response to verapamil and ventricular fibrillation may occur.[117–122] There is no predictable effect on ventricular arrhythmias, and since it may cause hypotension or predispose to ventricular fibrillation, verapamil should not be given in this situation. In principle, it should be avoided when there is a wide-complex tachycardia of undetermined origin.[123,124] Verapamil may be used in patients who are taking digitalis preparations unless there is AV node dysfunction; however, it should not be used in patients receiving beta-blocking agents. The electrophysiologic and hemodynamic effects of this combination are synergistic and may result in cardiac arrest.[105,125]

Verapamil is administered intravenously or orally. A single IV loading dose of 0.075 to 0.15 mg/kg (5 to 10 mg total) is administered over 1 min. A repeat intravenous dose of 0.15 mg/kg may be administered 30 min later if needed. After IV administration, verapamil has a volume of distribution of 4 liters/kg when the steady state is achieved. Ninety percent of verapamil is bound to plasma proteins. It is metabolized by the liver to norverapamil, which has some antiarrhythmic activity, but much less than verapamil. The elimination half-life is from 3 to 6 h.[114,115]

Diltiazem, another calcium channel blocking agent, has been used in the emergent treatment of supraventricular arrhythmias. However, the experience with intravenous diltiazem is less extensive. Given in a dose of 0.25 mg/kg IV, followed by a second dose of 0.35 mg/kg IV, diltiazem appears to be equivalent to verapamil. A continuous infusion of 5 to 15 mg/h may be used to control the ventricular rate in atrial fibrillation. It has the advantage of causing less myocardial depression.[135,136]

Verapamil, as well as other calcium channel blockers (nifedipine, diltiazem), is also used in the treatment of hypertension and angina.

BETA-ADRENERGIC BLOCKING AGENTS: PROPRANOLOL AND METOPROLOL

Propranolol and metoprolol are beta-adrenergic antagonists (class II antiarrhythmic agents) whose structures are shown in Figures 7–9 and 7–10, respectively. Propranolol hydrochloride is chemically designated 1-(isopropylamino)-3-(1-napthyloxy)-2-propanol hydrochloride, while metoprolol tartrate is chemically designated 1-(isopropylamino)-3-[p-(2-methoxyethyl)phenoxy]-2-propanol (2:1) dextro tartrate. Beta-blocking agents diminish the effects of catecholamines by inhibiting their ability to bind beta receptors. Propranolol is nonselective, affecting both beta-1 and beta-2 receptors equally. It has no sym-

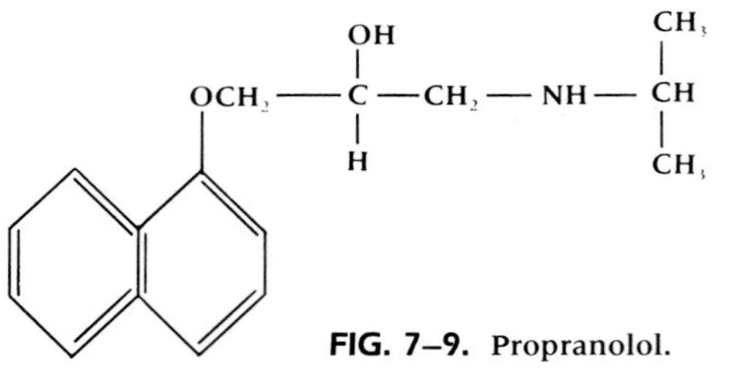

FIG. 7–9. Propranolol.

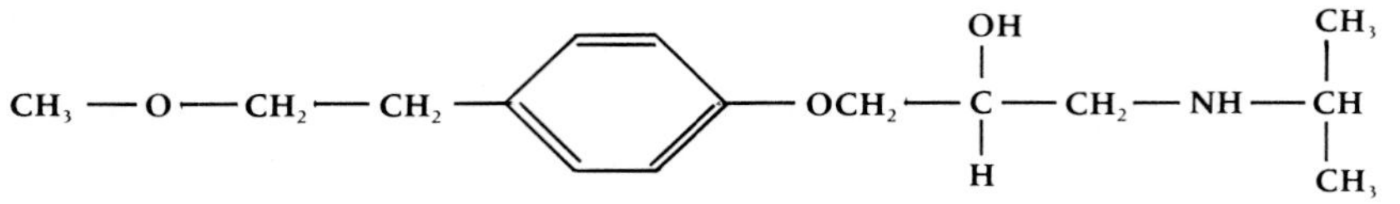

FIG. 7–10. Metoprolol.

pathomimetic activity and does not act at alpha-adrenergic receptors.[126] Metoprolol is a beta-1 selective drug. At lower doses, it preferentially inhibits beta-1 receptors. However, at higher doses, the selective agents lose much of their selectivity.[127,128] Beta-blocking drugs decrease heart rate and blood pressure. In the heart, inhibition of the effects of circulating catecholamines decreases the rate of spontaneous phase 4 depolarization and the rate of sinoatrial discharge. In addition, beta blockers increase the refractory period of the AV node. This also decreases myocardial oxygen consumption. These effects make beta blockers useful in the treatment of hypertension and angina pectoris.

Furthermore, propranolol is useful in the treatment of arrhythmias as well as to decrease the incidence of sudden death in patients after myocardial infarction. Beta blockers are more effective in situations where the arrhythmia is related to increased adrenergic stimulation. Metoprolol decreases the incidence of death in post-myocardial infarction patients. The major indication for beta-adrenergic blockers in an emergency situation is to control recurrent ventricular tachycardia or fibrillation or for rapid supraventricular arrhythmias unresponsive to other therapy.

Propranolol and metoprolol are highly lipid soluble. They are well absorbed and have a relatively short elimination half-life.[129] Propranolol undergoes significant and variable first-pass metabolism in the liver. Only about 25 percent of propranolol reaches the circulation after oral administration, and plasma concentrations may vary by 20-fold between patients. Propranolol has a volume of distribution of 4 liters/kg. Approximately 90 percent of the drug is bound to plasma proteins.[126]

Propranolol may be administered by slow IV push in a dose of 1 to 3 mg (to a total dose of 0.1 mg/kg). The rate of administration should not be faster than 1 mg/min. Metoprolol may be given in doses of 5 to 10 mg by slow IV push every 5 min to a total of 15 mg. Problems associated with administration of beta blockers include bradycardia, hypotension, and AV conduction delays. They also should be avoided in patients with congestive heart failure, second- or third-degree heart block, and bronchospastic lung disease.

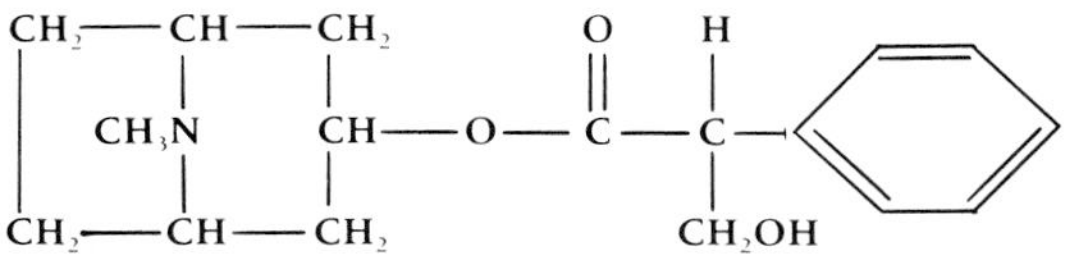

$$CH_2—CH—CH_2 \qquad O \quad H$$
$$CH_3N \qquad CH—O—C—C—\langle\rangle$$
$$CH_2—CH—CH_2 \qquad CH_2OH$$

FIG. 7–11. Atropine.

ATROPINE SULFATE

Atropine is a parasympatholytic agent that is indicated as an initial treatment for symptomatic bradycardia. This includes conditions where bradycardia is associated with myocardial ischemia or hypotension.[131] Atropine enhances sinus node automaticity as well as AV conduction through its vagolytic actions. It may restore normal AV node conduction and initiate electrical activity during asystole.[133] It also may be beneficial in the presence of nodal AV block.[134]

Atropine is a naturally occurring tertiary amine (Fig. 7–11). It is an alkaloid derived from the belladonna plant. The clinical preparation contains equal parts of dextrorotatory and levorotatory isomers. The anticholinergic effects are almost completely due to the levorotatory form. Like other anticholinergic drugs, atropine combines, in a competitive fashion, with muscarinic cholinergic receptors, preventing binding with the neurotransmitter acetylcholine. There is also evidence to support the fact that anticholinergic drugs are not pure muscarinic cholinergic receptor antagonists because small doses of these agents may cause a slowing of the heart rate, even after bilateral vagotomy. This demonstrates a weak peripheral muscarinic cholinergic receptor agonist effect.[137]

Atropine is not indicated and may produce adverse reactions when the bradycardia is not accompanied by hemodynamic compromise or ventricular ischemia.[132] It should be used cautiously in the presence of myocardial ischemia, since excessive increases in heart rate may worsen the ischemia or increase the size of the area of infarction.

The recommended dose of atropine for asystole or slow, pulseless electrical activity is 1.0 mg intravenously, with repeat doses every 3 to 5 min if the asystole persists. In the presence of bradycardia, a dose of 0.5 to 1.0 mg IV may be used. The maximum dose is 0.04 mg/kg, which is approximately 3 mg in an adult. At this level, total vagal blockade is achieved.[138] Doses less than 0.5 mg should be avoided because parasympathomimetic effects may cause further slowing of the heart rate.[131,139] If IV access has not yet been established, atropine may be administered through the endotracheal tube. When given endotracheally, atropine produces a rapid onset of action similar to that observed with an IV injection. For endotracheal administration, 1 to 2 mg may be diluted in 10 ml sterile water or saline.[141–143]

ADENOSINE

Adenosine is an endogenous purine nucleotide (Fig. 7–12) which became available as a pharmacologic agent in the United States in 1990. It is present in all cells in the body. In high doses, it depresses sinus and AV node activity. It is also a potent vasodilator. It can be used as an antiarrhythmic agent or to produce

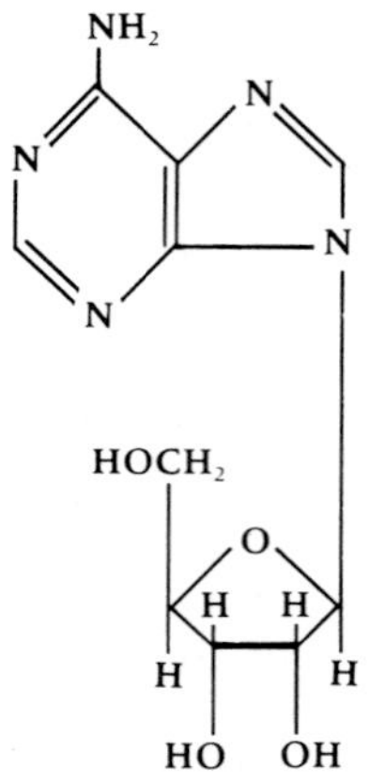

NH$_2$

N

N

N

N

N

HOCH$_2$

O

H   H

H   H

HO   OH   **FIG. 7–12.** Adenosine.

controlled hypotension. As an antiarrhythmatic agent, it is used in the treatment of paroxysmal supraventricular tachycardia involving a reentry pathway through the AV node, including that associated with WPW syndrome. If the arrhythmia does not involve the AV or sinus node, such as atrial flutter, atrial fibrillation, or atrial or ventricular tachycardia, adenosine will not be helpful in terminating the arrhythmia.[146] It should not be used in the presence of a second- or third-degree heart block or in patients with sick sinus syndrome.[144]

Adenosine is rapidly metabolized by enzymes in the blood and tissues. It has a half-life of approximately 5 seconds. Adenosine is competitively antagonized by methylxanthines such as theophylline, while its effects are potentiated by nucleoside transport blockers such as dipyridamole.[145]

Initially, adenosine may be administered in a dose of 6 mg IV. If the response is not satisfactory, a second dose of 12 mg IV should be administered 1 to 2 min later. Sinus bradycardia and ventricular ectopy may occur after termination of supraventricular tachycardia with adenosine, and because of the very short half-life, the arrhythmias may recur. Significant hemodynamic effects are unlikely because of the short duration of action of adenosine.

VASODILATORS: NITROGLYCERIN AND SODIUM NITROPRUSSIDE

Vasodilators may be used in the treatment of hypertension, angina pectoris, for controlled hypotension, and to improve forward stroke volume in patients with regurgitant valve disease or acute cardiac failure. These agents lower blood pressure by decreasing systemic vascular resistance (arterial vasodilation) or through venous dilation causing a decrease in venous return and cardiac output. Nitroglycerin acts principally on venous capacitance vessels to cause pooling of blood, a decrease in the size of the heart, and decrease in myocardial wall tension. As the dose of nitroglycerin is increased, arterial vascular smooth muscle is also relaxed. Nitroprusside is a nonselective, direct-acting vasodilator that causes relaxation of arterial and venous vascular smooth muscle. It does not have significant effects on cardiac or other types of smooth muscle.[147–150]

Organic nitrates such as nitroglycerin (Fig. 7–13) and nitroprusside (Fig. 7–14) produce nitric oxide, which activates guanylate cyclase. This increases the concentration of cyclic guanosine monophosphate in smooth muscle, which causes vasodilation. The smooth muscle relaxation produced by increases in guanosine monophosphate may be secondary to either decreases in calcium ion entry into muscle cells or increased calcium uptake by the sarcoplasmic reticulum.[150]

Nitroglycerin is effective in treating angina pectoris; it dilates large coronary arteries, antagonizing vasospasm and increasing blood flow to ischemic myocardium.[151,152] In patients with congestive heart failure, IV nitroglycerin reduces left ventricular filling pressure and systemic vascular resistance. This decrease in ventricular volume and wall tension decreases the myocardial oxygen requirements and thereby the ischemia.[153] Although nitroglycerin reduces ischemia, it must be used carefully in the setting of an acute myocardial infarction because it may cause hypotension. Hypotension may decrease coronary artery perfusion and increase ischemia. This type of hypotension responds well to fluid replacement.

Nitroglycerin has an elimination half-life of approximately 1.5 min. It has a large volume of distribution, reflecting tissue uptake. Metabolism occurs in the

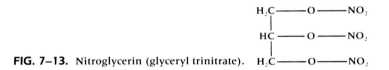

FIG. 7–13. Nitroglycerin (glyceryl trinitrate).

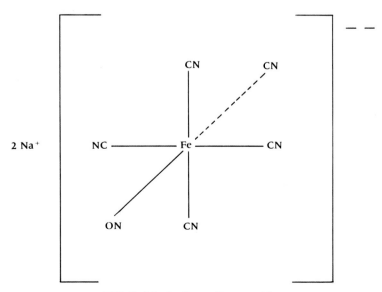

FIG. 7–14. Sodium nitroprusside.

liver by nitrate reductase. It is metabolized to nitrate and glycerol dinitrate, which are excreted in the urine. The nitrate metabolite can convert the ferrous ion of hemoglobin to the ferric state, causing methemoglobinemia. This is unlikely to occur if the nitroglycerin doses are less than 5 mg/kg. Methemoglobinemia may be treated with methylene blue should it occur.[148,150]

Nitroglycerin is administered sublingually (0.3 to 0.4 mg) to treat angina pectoris. It may be repeated at 3- to 5-min intervals if chest pain persists. If there is no relief after administration of three tablets, additional therapy is required. IV administration of nitroglycerin provides more control in patients with unstable angina or congestive heart failure. For continuous IV infusion, nitroglycerin is started at a rate of 10 to 20 μg/min and increased by 5 to 10 μg/min until the desired response is achieved. Most patients will respond to infusion rates between 50 and 200 μg/min. Lower doses (30 to 40 μg/min) produce venodilatation, while higher infusion rates (150 to 500 μg/min) provide arteriolar dilatation as well. A combination of nitroglycerin infusion and dobutamine infusion has been shown to provide hemodynamic improvement while reducing the risk of ischemia.[52]

Sodium nitroprusside acts immediately and has an extremely short duration of action. It is administered by continuous IV infusion, and because of its potency, careful and frequent blood pressure monitoring is essential. It is used to terminate hypertensive crises, to decrease afterload in heart failure, or to provide controlled hypotension. Nitroprusside reduces wall stress and myocardial work in patients with hypertension or ischemia.[154] However, nitroglycerin is less likely than nitroprusside to produce coronary artery steal syndrome. Nitroglycerin is preferred during an acute myocardial infarction because it has been shown to decrease mortality to a greater degree than nitroprusside. Nitroprusside is indicated when elevated blood pressure is present during an acute myocardial infarction with congestive heart failure.[52]

Nitroprusside is metabolized in red blood cells to methemoglobin and nitroprusside radicals. When the nitroprusside radical breaks down, it releases five cyanide ions, one of which forms a cyanmethemoglobin complex. The other four cyanide ions are converted to thiocyanate by the enzyme rhodanase in the liver and kidneys. Any remaining free cyanide may react with the cytochrome oxidase enzyme system, affecting aerobic respiration. The amount of cyanide obtained depends on the total dose of the drug administered. There is a linear relationship between the plasma concentration of cyanide and the total dose of nitroprusside administered.[155] Nitroprusside solutions also react with light to produce cyanide in vitro; therefore, solution containers should be wrapped to prevent light exposure.

The toxic range for sodium nitroprusside is not firmly established. Maximum dosage recommendations vary from 3 to 10 μg/kg/min. Other reports conclude that the maximum continuous infusion rate should not exceed 8 μg/kg/min intravenously for a 1- to 3-h period or 0.5 mg/kg/h for a chronic infusion.[156] Cyanide toxicity should be suspected in a patient who becomes resistant to the hypotensive effects of the drug despite adequate infusion rates. In addition, mixed venous oxygen partial pressures will rise, suggesting inhibition of the cytochrome oxidase system, and arterial blood gases will demonstrate a metabolic acidosis due to anaerobic metabolism. Treatment of cyanide toxicity in-

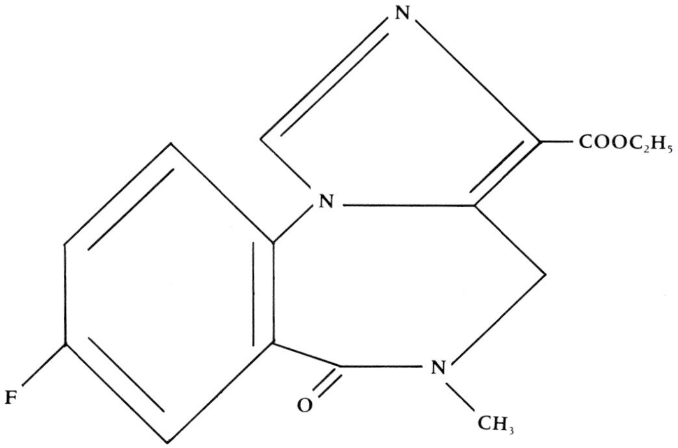

FIG. 7–17. Flumazenil (RO 15-1788).

FIG. 7–15. Furosemide.

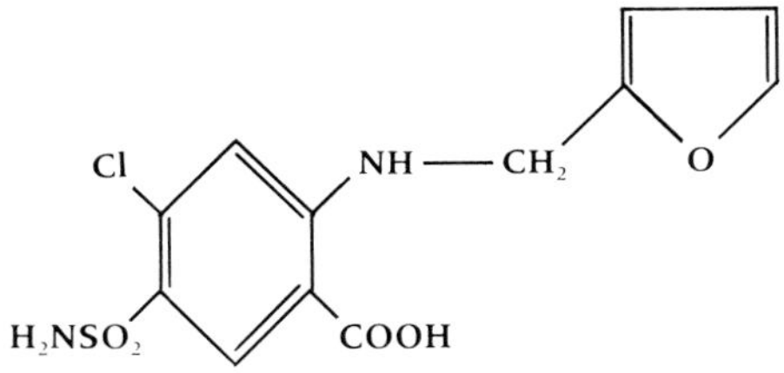

FIG. 7–16. Naloxone.

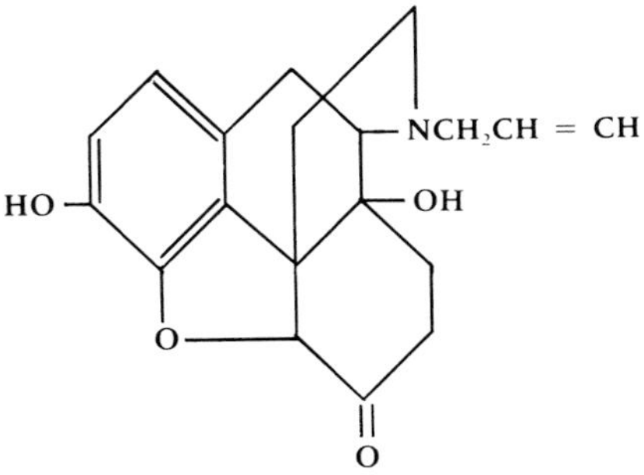

cludes (1) discontinuation of the nitroprusside infusion, (2) inhalation of amyl nitrate every 2 min, (3) IV infusion of sodium nitrate in a dose of 5 mg/kg in 20 ml water over 3 to 4 min, (4) IV infusion of sodium thiosulfate 150 mg/kg in 50 ml water over 15 min, or (5) IV infusion of hydroxycobalamin 12.5 mg over 30 min.[147]

TABLE 7–5. Summary: Drugs Used in Resuscitation in Adults

Drug	Dosage/Route	Indication(s)
Epinephrine	0.5–1.0 mg IV push (7.5–15 µg/kg) every 5 min 15 µg/kg via endotracheal tube	Cardiac arrest
	1–4 µg/min infusion	Inotropic/pressor support
Norepinephrine	2–12 µg/min IV infusion	Refractory hypotension
Dopamine	2–20 µg/kg/min IV infusion	Hypotension
Dobutamine	2.5–20 µg/kg/min IV infusion	Right ventricular failure Low cardiac output Pulmonary congestion
Isoproterenol	2–10 µg/min IV infusion	Refractory bradycardia, torsades de pointes
Amrinone	2–20 µg/kg/min IV infusion	Refractory congestive heart failure
Lidocaine	1 mg/kg IV push 1–4 mg/min IV infusion	Ventricular dysrhythmias (VT, VF, PVCs)
Bretylium	5 mg/kg IV push 2 mg/min IV infusion	Refractory ventricular tachycardia, ventricular fibrillation
Procainamide	100 mg IV (20 mg/min) 1–4 mg/min IV infusion	PVCs and ventricular tachycardia refractory to lidocaine and supraventricular arrhythmias
Atropine	1 mg IV push	Asystole
	0.5 mg IV push	Symptomatic bradycardia
Nitroglycerin	0.3–0.4 mg sublingual	Angina pectoris
Sodium nitroprusside	0.5–8 µg/kg/min IV infusion	Hypertensive emergency
Propranolol	1–3 mg IV push	Recurrent ventricular tachycardia or recurrent ventricular fibrillation or refractory supraventricular arrhythmias

Metoprolol	5 mg IV push every 5 min to a maximum of 15 mg	Same as propranolol
Verapamil	0.075–0.15 mg/kg (max 10 mg), IV push (over 1 min)	Paroxysmal supraventricular tachycardia
Diltiazem	0.25 mg/kg IV push, second dose 0.35 mg/kg IV push or IV infusion of 5–15 mg/h	Paroxysmal supraventricular tachycardia
Adenosine	6 mg IV push, second dose of 12 mg IV push	Paroxysmal supraventricular tachycardia
Calcium chloride	10 ml 10% soln. 2–4 mg/kg, repeat every 10 min as needed	Acute hyperkalemia, hypocalcemia, Ca channel blocker toxicity, hypermagnesemia
Bicarbonate	1 mg/kg, repeat as needed, 0.5 mg/kg but not more frequently than every 10 min	Metabolic acidosis
Magnesium sulfate	1–2 g (8–16 mEq) in 100 ml D_5W, IV infusion over 5 min, then 0.5–1.0 g (4–8 mEq/h) IV infusion for 24 h	Refractory ventricular fibrillation or ventricular tachycardia, torsades de pointes Hypomagnesemia
Furosemide	20–40 mg IV push 0.25–0.75 mg/kg/h IV infusion	Pulmonary congestion/left ventricular dysfunction
Naloxone	1 to 4 µg/kg IV push or 5 µg/kg/h continuous IV infusion	Narcotic overdose (respiratory depression)
Flumazenil	0.2 mg IV over 15 s (up to 1 mg in 5 min)	Benzodiazepine overdose (sedation)

Source: Adapted from Chernow B: *The Pharmacologic Approach to the Critically Ill Patient,* 2d ed. Baltimore, Williams & Wilkins, 1988; *Textbook of Advanced Cardiac Life Support,* 2d ed. Chicago, American Heart Association, 1987; Guidelines for cardiopulmonary resuscitation and emergency cardiac care III: Adult advanced cardiac life support. *JAMA* 268:2199, 1992, with permission.

TABLE 7–6. Drugs Recommended and not Recommended for Endotracheal Administration

Drug	Initial Adult Dose	Volume	Pediatric Dose	Comments
Epinephrine	1 mg	10 ml	0.01 mg/kg 0.1 ml of 1:10,000 (1 mg/10 ml)/kg body weight Dilution may not be required in infants	Endotracheal administration Requires less frequent dosing than the IV route
Atropine	0.5–1.0 mg	5–10 ml	0.01 mg/kg	Less frequent dosing as above
Naloxone	0.4–0.8 mg	1–2 ml	0.01 mg/kg 0.5 ml of 0.02 mg/ml preparation/kg body weight	May be further diluted to enhance delivery to the airways
Lidocaine	50–100 mg	5–10 ml	1.0 mg/kg 0.1 ml of 1% (10 mg/ml) or 0.05 ml of 2% (20 mg/ml)/kg body weight	Effectiveness not determined
Bretylium tosylate	Endotracheal administration is *not* recommended			
Calcium	Endotracheal administration is *not* recommended			
Isoproterenol	Endotracheal administration is *not* recommended			
Norepinephrine	Endotracheal administration is *not* recommended			
Sodium bicarbonate	Endotracheal administration is *not* recommended			

Source: Adapted from Hasegawa EAJ: The endotracheal use of drugs. *Heart Lung,* 15:60, 1986, with permission.

TABLE 7–7. Pediatric Resuscitation: Drugs, Dosages, and Routes of Administration

Drug	Dose
Adenosine	0.1–0.2 mg/kg; maximum single dose 12 mg
Atropine sulfate	0.02 mg/kg per dose; maximum dose 0.1 mg, maximum dose 0.5 mg in child, maximum dose 1.0 mg in adolescent
Bretylium	5 mg/kg IV, up to 10 mg/kg IV
Calcium chloride 10%	20 mg/kg per dose, slowly IV
Dopamine	2–20 μg/kg/min
Dobutamine	2–20 μg/kg/min
Epinephrine (for bradycardia)	IV or IO, 0.01 mg/kg (1:10,000) ET, 0.1 mg/kg (1:1000)
Epinephrine (for asystole or pulseless arrest)	First dose IV/IO, 0.01 mg/kg (1:10,000) ET, 0.1 mg/kg (1:1000) Subsequent doses IV/IO/ET, 0.1 mg/kg (1:1000) Doses as high as 0.2 mg/kg may be effective
Epinephrine intravenous infusion	Start at 0.1 μg/kg/min (range 0.1 to 1.0 μg/kg/min)
Lidocaine	1 mg/kg per dose, IV infusion rate 20–50 μg/kg/min
Sodium bicarbonate	1 mEq/kg per dose or 0.3 × weight (kg) × base deficit

Note: IV = intravenous route; IO = intraosseous route; ET = administered through the endotracheal tube.

Source: Adapted from American Heart Association: Guidelines for cardiopulmonary resuscitation and emergency cardiac care, VI: Pediatric advanced life support. *JAMA,* 268:2262, 1992, with permission.

The recommended dosage range for sodium nitroprusside is 0.1 to 5 μg/kg/min, but infusions as high as 10 μg/kg/min may be required. The usual therapeutic doses range from 0.5 to 8.0 μg/kg/min.[1,52] Side effects include headache, nausea, vomiting, and abdominal cramps. In addition, elevation of cyanide or thiocyanate levels may occur. These toxic side effects must be treated promptly. Blood pressure must be monitored closely, and the nitroprusside infusion must be delivered with a delivery system that ensures a precise flow rate.

CALCIUM (CALCIUM CHLORIDE)

Calcium ions play a pivotal role in myocardial contractile performance. During electrical stimulation of the muscle, calcium ions enter the sarcoplasm from the extracellular space and are transferred to the sites of interaction between the actin and myosin muscle filaments to initiate shortening of the myofibrils.[161] Calcium has positive inotropic effects. Despite this, calcium has not been demonstrated to be beneficial in the setting of cardiac arrest. In addition, high concentrations of calcium may be detrimental.[157–160] These detrimental effects include reperfusion injury and adverse effects on neurologic outcome.

In the setting of hyperkalemia, hypermagnesemia, hypocalcemia (such as that which may occur after massive blood transfusions), or an overdose of a calcium

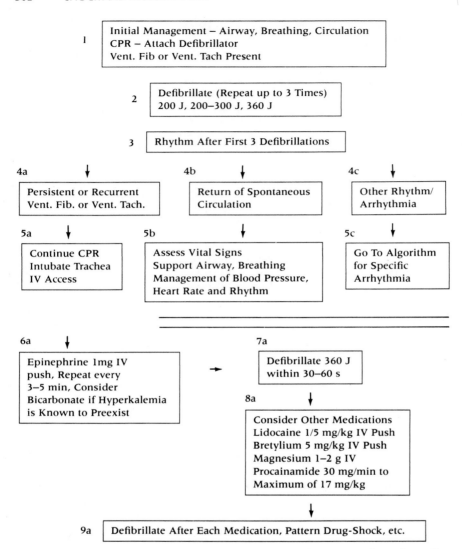

FIG. 7–18. Algorithm for ventricular fibrillation or pulseless ventricular tachycardia. (*Adapted from Adult advanced cardiac life support. JAMA 268:2199, 1992, with permission.*)

channel blocking agent, the administration of calcium may be useful. Otherwise, calcium is not routinely indicated in cardiopulmonary resuscitation.

When needed, calcium chloride solution (10%) may be administered in a dose of 2 to 4 mg/kg and repeated as needed every 10 min. If a calcium gluconate solution is used, the dose is 5 to 8 ml.[52] Calcium chloride is the preferred solution because it produces higher and more predictable levels of ionized plasma calcium.[162]

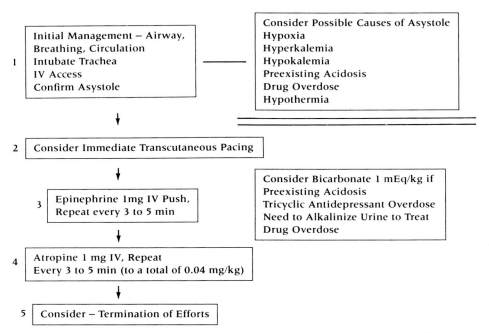

FIG. 7–19. Asystole treatment algorithm. (*Adapted from Adult advanced cardiac life support. JAMA 268:2199, 1992, with permission.*)

SODIUM BICARBONATE

Sodium bicarbonate ($NaHCO_3$) is used to treat the acidosis that develops during states of hypoxemia and hypoperfusion which occur during cardiopulmonary arrest. Hypoxemia or hypoxia results in the production of lactic acid and metabolic acidosis, while hypoventilation leads to carbon dioxide retention and respiratory acidosis. The primary treatment of acidosis during cardiac arrest is tracheal intubation, restoring oxygenation and ventilation, coupled with restoration of tissue perfusion. Initially, this is achieved through chest compressions and, hopefully, rapid restoration of spontaneous circulation.

Sodium bicarbonate reacts with hydrogen ions to form water and carbon dioxide, buffering metabolic acidosis. However, this increases the carbon dioxide content. Since carbon dioxide crosses into cells more quickly than bicarbonate, this causes a transient worsening of acidosis inside the cells.

In situations such as preexisting metabolic acidosis, hyperkalemia, and tricyclic antidepressant or phenobarbital overdose, bicarbonate administration is beneficial. However, there is no evidence to suggest that therapy with bicarbonate improves outcome, and other evidence suggests that (1) it does not improve the ability to defibrillate, (2) it causes a shift of the oxyhemoglobin saturation curve, thereby inhibiting the release of oxygen from hemoglobin to tissues, (3) it causes hyperosmolarity and hypernatremia, and (4) it may inactivate simultaneously administered catecholamines in addition to other adverse effects.[52,163–166]

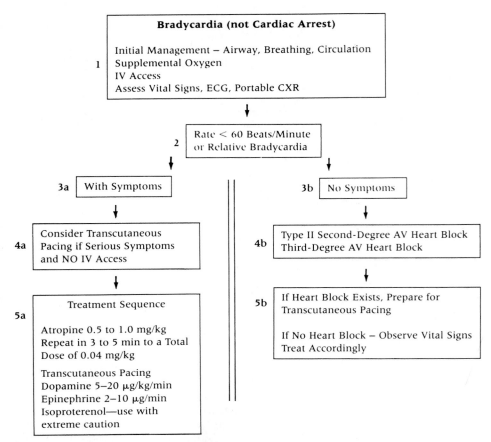

FIG. 7–20. Bradycardia treatment algorithm. (*Adapted from Adult advanced cardiac life support. JAMA 268:2199, 1992, with permission.*)

The recommended dose of bicarbonate is 1 mg/kg intravenously, followed by 0.5 mg/kg every 10 min afterwards. If possible, blood gases should be obtained, and bicarbonate replacement should be guided by the calculated base deficit to minimize the risk of completely correcting, or worse, overcorrecting and iatrogenically inducing alkalosis.[52]

MAGNESIUM SULFATE

Magnesium is an obligatory cofactor in the actions of adenosine triphosphate (ATP). The membrane-bound sodium-potassium–dependent ATPase, which maintains the normal intracellular levels of potassium, requires magnesium to function. The production of adenosine monophosphate by adenylate cyclase is magnesium-dependent, as is the presynaptic release of acetylcholine from nerve endings.

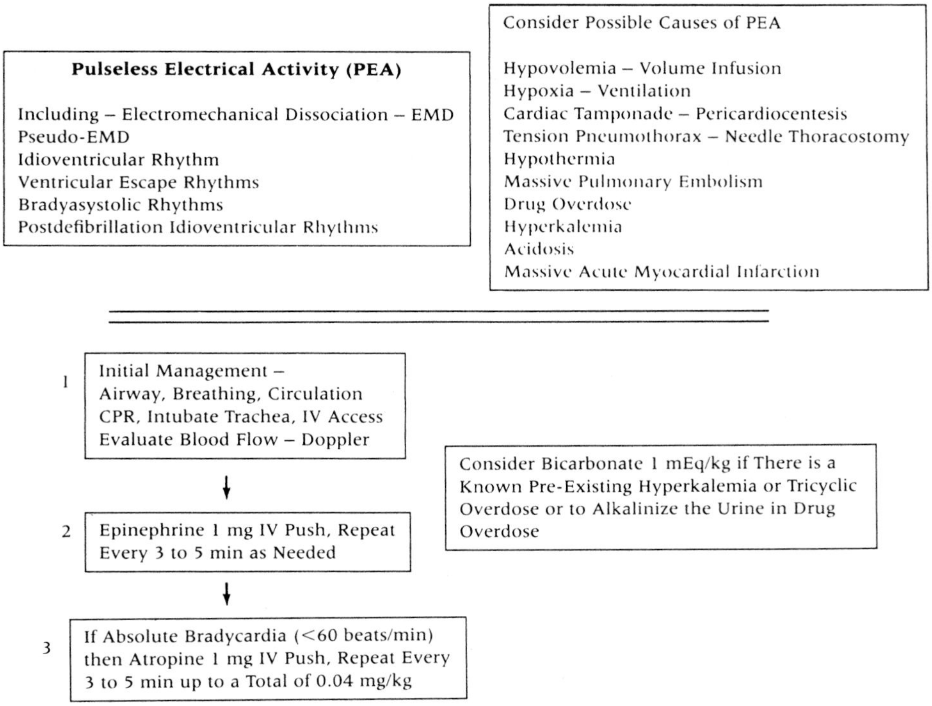

| **Pulseless Electrical Activity (PEA)** |
| Including – Electromechanical Dissociation – EMD Pseudo-EMD
Idioventricular Rhythm
Ventricular Escape Rhythms
Bradyasystolic Rhythms
Postdefibrillation Idioventricular Rhythms |

| Consider Possible Causes of PEA |
| Hypovolemia – Volume Infusion
Hypoxia – Ventilation
Cardiac Tamponade – Pericardiocentesis
Tension Pneumothorax – Needle Thoracostomy
Hypothermia
Massive Pulmonary Embolism
Drug Overdose
Hyperkalemia
Acidosis
Massive Acute Myocardial Infarction |

1 Initial Management –
Airway, Breathing, Circulation
CPR, Intubate Trachea, IV Access
Evaluate Blood Flow – Doppler

↓

2 Epinephrine 1 mg IV Push, Repeat
Every 3 to 5 min as Needed

Consider Bicarbonate 1 mEq/kg if There is a
Known Pre-Existing Hyperkalemia or Tricyclic
Overdose or to Alkalinize the Urine in Drug
Overdose

↓

3 If Absolute Bradycardia (<60 beats/min)
then Atropine 1 mg IV Push, Repeat Every
3 to 5 min up to a Total of 0.04 mg/kg

FIG. 7–21. Algorithm for pulseless electrical activity (PEA). (*Adapted from Adult advanced cardiac life support. JAMA 268:2199, 1992, with permission.*)

Magnesium deficiency (serum levels less than 1.6 mEq/liter) is probably the most common unrecognized electrolyte abnormality.[167] Patients who are at an increased risk for hypomagnesemia include chronic alcoholics and those receiving hyperalimentation. Malabsorption syndromes also may predispose to hypomagnesemia. Manifestations of hypomagnesemia on the electrocardiogram are nonspecific. Magnesium deficiency is associated with ventricular arrhythmias, and it may precipitate ventricular fibrillation which may be refractory to other therapy.

Magnesium is considered the treatment of choice in patients with torsades de pointes (polymorphous ventricular tachycardia with prolonged QT interval). The mechanism of action of magnesium in terminating torsades de pointes is not understood.[130] A loading dose of magnesium sulfate is 1 to 2 g (8 to 16 mEq) infused IV over 5 to 60 min. Subsequently, an infusion of 0.5 to 1.0 g is given for up to 24 h. Serum magnesium levels should be determined to guide replacement therapy.[52]

FUROSEMIDE

Furosemide (Fig. 7–15) is a potent diuretic that acts rapidly in the ascending loop of Henle to inhibit reabsorption of sodium and chloride ions. Furosemide

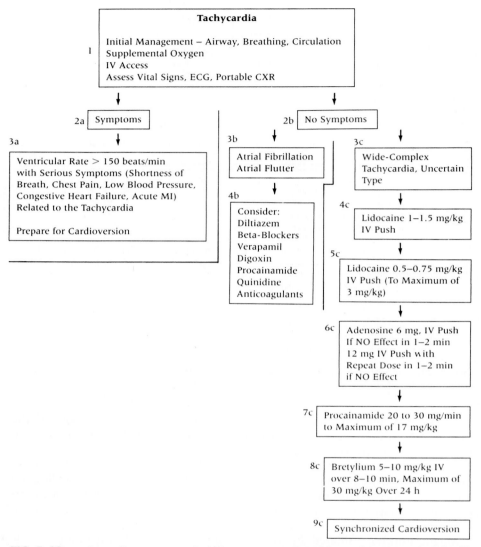

FIG. 7–22. Tachycardia treatment algorithm, part 1. (*Adapted from Adult advanced cardiac life support. JAMA 268:2199, 1992, with permission.*)

is used to mobilize edema fluid secondary to renal, hepatic, or cardiac dysfunction or to decrease intracranial pressure. It also may be used in the differential diagnosis of acute oliguria. In the emergency setting, furosemide is used to treat pulmonary edema during acute myocardial infarction or other conditions associated with left ventricular dysfunction. It has venodilating effects that reduce the venous return and central venous pressure. Reductions in central volume secondary to diuresis causes a decrease in cardiac output.[168]

The most frequent side effects of loop diuretics are electrolyte abnormalities. Sodium, potassium, calcium, and magnesium deficiencies occur commonly and

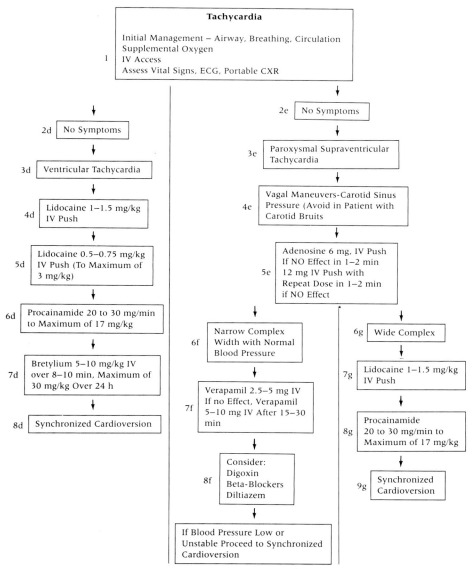

FIG. 7–23. Tachycardia treatment algorithm, part 2. (*Adapted from Adult advanced cardiac life support. JAMA 268:2199, 1992, with permission.*)

can pose serious problems, particularly in those receiving digitalis. Furosemide may elevate concentrations of aminoglycoside antibiotics, enhancing their nephrotoxic effects, and may demonstrate cross-reactivity in patients who are allergic to sulfonamide-containing drugs. In addition, use of furosemide with ethacrynic acid (also a loop diuretic) may produce either transient or permanent deafness.[169]

The dose of furosemide for emergent treatment of pulmonary congestion associated with left ventricular dysfunction is 20 to 40 mg IV, or 0.5 mg/kg (up to

2 mg/kg) as an initial dose given IV over 1 to 2 min. For patients who do not respond, a continuous IV infusion of 0.25 to 0.75 mg/kg/h may be used to promote diuresis.[170–173]

NALOXONE AND FLUMAZENIL

Although naloxone and flumazenil are not used in cardiac resuscitation per se, however, in the emergency or trauma setting, a drug overdose may be a component in the clinical picture, as well as the cause of the traumatic event. Naloxone and flumazenil represent specific narcotic and benzodiazepine antagonists, respectively. They may prove useful in antagonizing unwanted effects of narcotics or benzodiazepines which may complicate the clinical picture.

Naloxone (Fig. 7–16) is a pure opioid antagonist with no agonist activity. Naloxone has a high affinity for mu, delta, and kappa receptors, displacing opioid agonists from receptor binding sites. It is used to treat opioid-induced ventilatory depression. It is metabolized in the liver, having a half-life of 20 min.[178] Close observation of the patient is required because respiratory depression associated with renarcotization may occur.

Naloxone must be used with caution because it also can antagonize opioid analgesia, leading to pain and sympathetic stimulation causing increases in heart rate, blood pressure, and possibly cardiac arrhythmias.[174–176] Furthermore, naloxone improves myocardial contractility and survival in an animal model of hypovolemic shock and hemorrhagic shock and may be beneficial in the treatment of septic shock.[140,177]

Naloxone given IV at a dose of 1 to 4 μg/kg antagonizes opioid-induced analgesia and respiratory depression. A continuous IV infusion of 5 μg/kg/h can antagonize respiratory depression without affecting opioid analgesia.[179]

Flumazenil is a competitive benzodiazepine receptor antagonist that has recently been approved for use in the United States. It has been demonstrated to antagonize the sedation associated with benzodiazepine administration. It seems to have minimal hemodynamic effects. Unfortunately, it is not particularly effective in antagonizing benzodiazepine-induced respiratory depression. In the emergency situation, it will be useful to antagonize benzodiazepine effects when urgent evaluation is necessary or benzodiazepine overdose is part of the clinical situation.

Flumazenil (RO 15-1788) is an imidazobenzodiazepine (ethyl-8-fluoro-5, 6-dihydro-5-methyl-6-oxo-4H-imidazol (1,5a) benzodiazepine-3-carboxylate), shown in Fig. 7–17, that blocks the central effects of benzodiazepines.[180] It acts through competitive inhibition of the benzodiazepine receptor [gamma-aminobutyric acid (GABA) benzodiazepine receptor complex in the central nervous system], antagonizing benzodiazepine-induced sedation within minutes. Flumazenil is rapidly and extensively distributed in the body, with an apparent volume of distribution of 1.06 liters/kg. It is eliminated rapidly by hepatic metabolism and a high plasma clearance (1.14 liters/min). Less than 1 percent of the administered dose is eliminated unchanged in the urine. It has a half-life of about 53 min.[181,182] As a receptor antagonist, flumazenil does not alter the bioavailability of diazepam.[183]

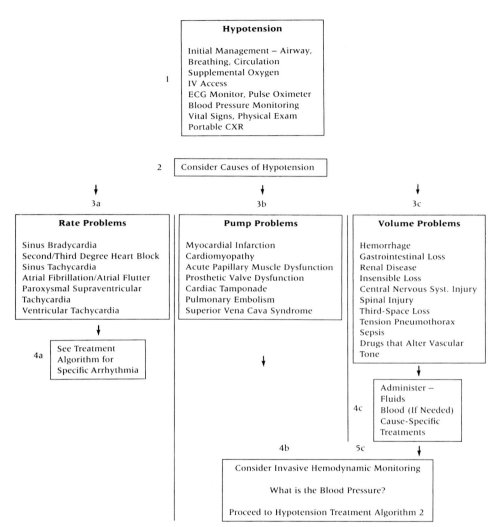

FIG. 7–24. Hypotension treatment algorithm 1. (*Adapted from Adult advanced cardiac life support. JAMA 268:2199, 1992, with permission.*)

Prior to the introduction of flumazenil, nonspecific methods of antagonizing benzodiazepines were used. Physostigmine (Antilirium), an anticholinesterase, crosses the blood-brain barrier. Although diazepam has no known central anticholinergic effects, several reports[184] have suggested that it may antagonize the central effects of diazepam. Using physostigmine to reverse diazepam-induced sedation has met with mixed results.[180,184,185] There also has been evidence that aminophylline partly antagonized diazepam-induced sedation and psychomotor impairment.[180,186] Aminophylline is not a specific benzodiazepine receptor antagonist. There have been no reports of aminophylline causing withdrawal

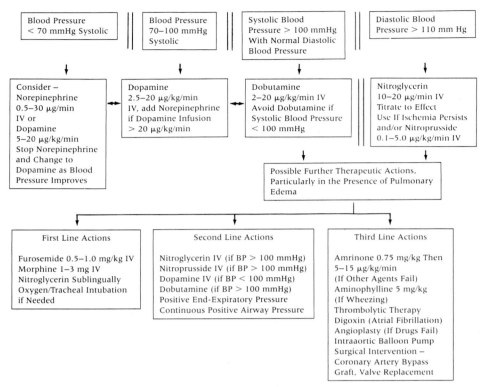

FIG. 7–25. Hypotension treatment algorithm 2. (*Adapted from Adult advanced cardiac life support. JAMA 268:2199, 1992, with permission.*)

symptoms in patients treated with or dependent on benzodiazepines. Other non-specific benzodiazepine antagonists have included opioid antagonists (naloxone) and other analeptics (doxapram). Flumazenil has been shown to antagonize the anxiolytic, muscle-relaxant, sedative, ataxic, anticonvulsant, amnestic, and respiratory depressant effects of benzodiazepines.[187] Despite these reports, flumazenil has not been established as an effective treatment for benzodiazepine-induced hypoventilation.[188–190]

Flumazenil is administered intravenously. The recommended initial dose of flumazenil for antagonism of benzodiazepine-induced sedation is 0.2 mg administered over 15 s. If the desired effect is not seen within 45 s, another 0.2 mg may be administered. Injections can be repeated at 60-s intervals to a maximum dose of 1.0 mg. Then, flumazenil should not be given more frequently than every 20 min. The maximum dose of flumazenil is 3 mg within 1 h. The titration method is advocated to control awakening to the desired end point. A large single bolus may result in confusion and agitation upon awakening. Flumazenil should be used with caution in patients dependent on benzodiazepines. Benzodiazepine withdrawal may occur. In this situation, lower doses of flumazenil are recommended. In addition, seizures have been reported after administration of flumazenil to benzodiazepine overdose patients. In addition, all patients should be observed for at least 2 h after the administration of flumazenil for signs of resedation, respiratory depression, or other residual benzodiazepine effects.[188]

A summary of the drugs used for resuscitation in the adult, doses, and indications is presented in Table 7–5. A summary of agents and dosages that may be given through an endotracheal tube is presented in Table 7–6. Dosages and indications for use in pediatric patients are presented in Table 7–7.

TREATMENT ALGORITHMS

To incorporate the use of pharmacologic agents into the clinical picture of cardiac resuscitation, simplified algorithms for treatment of various arrhythmias are presented. The treatment algorithms presented in Figs. 7–18 to 7–25 are adapted from those provided by the American Heart Association as part of their advanced cardiac life support guidelines.[52] The reader is referred to this source for the complete treatment algorithms and other recommendations. The algorithms should provide a guide to management of various emergency cardiac care situations; however, the practitioner should always consider the entire clinical picture, particularly in the trauma setting, where other factors must be considered.

REFERENCES

1. *Textbook of Advanced Cardiac Life Support*, 2d ed. Chicago, American Heart Association, 1987.
2. Stoelting RK: *Pharmacology and Physiology in Anesthetic Practice*, 2d ed. Philadelphia, Lippincott, 1991, pp 264–284.
3. Paradis NA, Koscove EM: Epinephrine in cardiac arrest: A critical review. *Ann Emerg Med* 19(11):1288, 1990.
4. Hoffman BB, Lefkowitz RJ: Catecholamines and sympathomimetic drugs. In Gilman AG, Rall TW, Nies AS, Paylor P (eds): *Goodman and Gilman's Pharmacological Basis of Therapeutics*, 8th ed. New York, Pergamon Press, 1990, pp 187–220.
5. Lands AM, Arnold A, McAuliff JP, et al: Differentiation of receptor systems activated by sympathomimetic amines. *Nature* 214:597, 1967.
6. Ahlquist RP: A study of the adrenotropic receptors. *Am J Physiol* 153:586, 1948.
7. Langer SZ: Presynaptic regulation of catecholamine release. *Biochem Pharmacol* 23:1793, 1974.
8. Pearson JW, Redding JS: Influence of peripheral vascular tone on cardiac resuscitation. *Anesth Analg* 44(6):746, 1965.
9. Otto CW, Yakaitis RW: The role of epinephrine in CPR: A reappraisal. *Ann Emerg Med* 13:840, 1984.
10. Otto CW: Cardiovascular pharmacology: II. The use of catecholamines, pressor agents, digitalis, and corticosteroids in CPR and emergency cardiac care. *Circulation* 74(suppl 4):IV80, 1986.
11. Niemann JT, Haynes KS, Garner D, et al: Postcountershock pulseless rhythms: Response to CPR, artificial cardiac pacing, and adrenergic agonists. *Ann Emerg Med* 15:112, 1986.
12. Todd GL, Baroldi G, Pieper GM, et al: Experimental catecholamine-induced myocardial

necrosis: I. Morphology, quantification and regional distribution of acute contraction band lesions. *J Mol Cell Cardiol* 17:317, 1985.

13. Haft JI: Cardiovascular injury induced by sympathetic catecholamines. *Prog Cardiovasc Dis* 17:73, 1974.

14. Waters LL, deSuto-Nagy GI: Lesions of the coronary arteries and great vessels of the dog following injection of adrenalin: Their prevention with dibenamine. *Science* 111:634, 1950.

15. Berk JL, Hagen JF, Koo R: Effect of alpha and beta adrenergic blockade on epinephrine induced pulmonary insufficiency. *Ann Surg* 183(4):369, 1976.

16. Martin GB, Gentile NT, Moeggenberg J, et al: End-tidal CO_2 monitoring fails to reflect changes in coronary perfusion pressure after epinephrine. *Ann Emerg Med* 18:916, 1989.

17. Martin GB, Gentile NT, Paradis NA, et al: Effect of epinephrine on end-tidal carbon dioxide monitoring during CPR. *Ann Emerg Med* 19(4):396, 1990.

18. Tang W, Weil MH, Sun S, et al: Epinephrine produces both hypoxemia and hypercarbia during CPR. *Crit Care Med* 18:S276, 1990.

19. Allen WJ, Barcroft H, Edholm OG: On the action of adrenaline on the blood vessels in human skeletal muscle. *J Physiol* 105:255, 1946.

20. Skinner SL, Whelan RF: The circulation in forearm skin and muscle during adrenaline infusions. *Aust J Exp Biol* 40:163, 1962.

21. Holmes HR, Babbs CF, Voorhees WD, et al: Influence of adrenergic drugs upon vital organ perfusion during CPR. *Crit Care Med* 8:137, 1980.

22. Michael JR, Guerci AD, Koehler RC, et al: Mechanisms by which epinephrine augments cerebral and myocardial perfusion during cardiopulmonary resuscitation in dogs. *Circulation* 69:822, 1984.

23. Koehler RC, Michael JR, Guerci AD, et al: Beneficial effect of epinephrine infusion on cerebral and myocardial blood flows during CPR. *Ann Emerg Med* 14:744, 1985.

24. Otto CW, Yakaitis RW, Ewy GA: Spontaneous ischemic ventricular fibrillation in dogs: A new model for the study of cardiopulmonary resuscitation. *Crit Care Med* 11(11):883, 1983.

25. Weiner N: Norepinephrine, epinephrine, and the sympathomimetic amines. In Gilman AG, Goodman LS, Rall TW, Murad F (eds): *Goodman and Gilman's Pharmacological Basis of Therapeutics.* New York, Macmillan, 1985, pp 145–180.

26. Anderson JL: Bretylium tosylate: Profile of the only available class III antiarrhythmic agent. *Clin Ther* 7(2):205, 1985.

27. Leier CV, Unverferth DV: Dobutamine. *Ann Intern Med* 99:490, 1983.

28. Ruffolo RR, Spradlin TA, Pollock GD, et al: Alpha and beta adrenergic effects of the stereoisomers of dobutamine. *J Pharmacol Exp Ther* 219:447, 1981.

29. Ruffolo RR: Review: The pharmacology of dobutamine. *Am J Med Sci* 294(4):244, 1987.

30. Stoner JD III, Bolen JL, Harrison DC: Comparison of dobutamine and dopamine in the treatment of severe heart failure. *Br Heart J* 39:536, 1977.

31. Keung ECH, Siskind SJ, Sonneblick EH, et al: Dobutamine therapy in acute myocardial infarction. *JAMA* 245:144, 1981.

32. Standards and guidelines for cardiopulmonary resuscitation and emergency cardiac care. *JAMA* 255:2905, 1986.

33. Schleien CL, Dean JM, Koehler RC, et al: Effect of epinephrine on cerebral and myocardial perfusion in an infant animal preparation of cardiopulmonary resuscitation. *Circulation* 73(4):809, 1986.

34. Rosetti VA, Thompson BM, Miller J, et al: Intraosseous infusion: An alternative route of pediatric intravascular access. *Ann Emerg Med* 14:885, 1985.

35. Newton DW, Fung EYY, Williams DA: Stability of five catecholamines and terbutaline sulfate in 5% dextrose injection in the absence and presence of aminophylline. *Am J Hosp Pharm* 38:1314, 1981.

36. Ward JT: Endotracheal drug therapy. *Am J Emerg Med* 1:71, 1983.

37. Ralston SH, Tacker WA, Showen L, et al: Endotracheal versus intravenous epinephrine during electromechanical dissociation with CPR in dogs. *Ann Emerg Med* 14:1044, 1985.

38. Zaritsky AL, Jaffe AS: Resuscitation pharmacology. In Chernow B (ed): *The Pharmacologic Approach to the Critically Ill Patient,* 2d ed. Baltimore, Williams & Wilkins, 1988, pp 184–197.

39. Goldberg LI, Rajfer SI: Dopamine receptors: Applications in clinical cardiology. *Circulation* 72:245, 1985.

40. Greenway CV, Stark RD: Hepatic vascular bed. *Physiol Rev* 51:23, 1971.

41. Zaritsky AL, Chernow B: Catecholamines and other inotropes. In Chernow B (ed): *The Pharmacologic Approach to the Critically Ill Patient,* 2d ed. Baltimore, Williams & Wilkins, 1988, pp 584–602.

42. Chernow B, Holbrook P, D'Angona DS Jr, et al: Epinephrine absorption after intratracheal administration. *Anesth Analg* 63:829, 1984.

43. Gombos EA, Hulet WH, Bopp P, et al: Reactivity of renal and systemic circulations to vasoconstrictor agents in normotensive and hypertensive subjects. *J Clin Invest* 41(2):203, 1962.

44. Coffin LH Jr, Ankeney JL, Beheler EM: Experimental study and clinical use of epinephrine for treatment of low cardiac output syndrome. *Circulation* 33-34(suppl 1):I-78, 1966.

45. Schaer GL, Fink MP, Parrillo JE: Norepinephrine alone versus norepinephrine plus low-dose dopamine: Enhanced renal blood flow with combination pressor therapy. *Crit Care Med* 13(6):492, 1985.

46. Douglass HO Jr: Levarterenol irrigation: Control of massive gastrointestinal bleeding in poor-risk patients. *JAMA* 230:1653, 1974.

47. Driscoll DJ, Gillette PC, Ezailson EG, Schwartz A: Inotropic responses of the neonatal canine myocardium to dopamine. *Pediatr Res* 12:42, 1978.

48. Kho TL, Henquet JW, Punt R, et al: Influence of dobutamine and dopamine on hemodynamics and plasma concentrations of noradrenaline and renin in patients with low cardiac output following acute myocardial infarction. *Eur J Clin Pharmacol* 18:213, 1980.

49. Richard C, Ricome JL, Rimailho A, et al: Combined hemodynamic effects of dopamine and dobutamine in cardiogenic shock. *Circulation* 67(3):620, 1983.

50. Jardin F, Sportiche M, Bazil M, et al: Dobutamine: A hemodynamic evaluation in human septic shock. *Crit Care Med* 9(4):329, 1981.

51. Leier CV, Hebran PT, Huss P, et al: Comparative systemic and regional hemodynamic effects of dopamine and dobutamine in patients with cardiomyopathic heart failure. *Circulation* 58(3):466, 1978.

52. Adult advanced cardiac life support. *JAMA* 268:2199, 1992.

53. DellItalia LJ, Starling MR, Blumhardt R, et al: Comparative effects of volume loading, dobutamine, and nitroprusside in patients with predominant right ventricular infarction. *Circulation* 72:1327, 1985.

54. Driscoll DJ, Gillette PC, Fukushige J, et al: Comparison of the cardiovascular action of isoproterenol, dopamine and dobutamine in the neonatal and mature dog. *Pediatr Cardiol* 1:307, 1980.

55. Halloway EL, Stinson EB, Derby GC, Harrison DC: Action of drugs in patients early after cardiac surgery: I. Comparison of isoproterenol and dopamine. *Am J Cardiol* 35:656, 1975.

56. Mueller H, Ayres SM, Gregory JJ, et al: Hemodynamics, coronary blood flow and myocardial metabolism in coronary shock: Response to L-norepinephrine and isoproterenol. *J Clin Invest* 49:1885, 1970.

57. Downes JJ, Wood DW, Harwood I, et al: Intravenous isoproterenol infusion in children with severe hypercapnia due to status asthmaticus: Effects on ventilation, circulation, and clinical score. *Crit Care Med* 1:63, 1973.

58. Mentzer RM Jr, Alegre CA, Nolan SP: The effects of dopamine and isoproterenol on the pulmonary circulation. *J Thorac Cardiovasc Surg* 71:807, 1976.

59. Goldberg IF, Cohn JN: New inotropic drugs for heart failure. *JAMA* 258:493, 1987.

60. Alousi AA, Canter JM, Montenaro MJ, et al: Cardiotonic activity of milrinone, a new and potent cardiac bipyridine, on the normal and failing heart of experimental animals. *J Cardiovasc Pharmacol* 5(5):792, 1983.

61. Alousi AA, Farah AE, Lescher GY, Opalka CJ: Cardiotonic activity of amrinone-Win 40680 [5-amino-3,4'-bipyridin-6(1H)-one]. *Circ Res* 45:666, 1979.

62. Mancini D, LeJemtel T, Sonnenblick E: Intravenous amrinone for the treatment of the failing heart. *Am J Cardiol* 56:8b, 1985.

63. LeJemtel TH, Keung E, Ribner HS, et al: Sustained beneficial effects of oral amrinone on cardiac and renal function in patients with severe congestive heart failure. *Am J Cardiol* 45:123, 1980.

64. Wynn J, Malacoff RF, Benotti JR, et al: Oral amrinone in refractory congestive heart failure. *Am J Cardiol* 45:1245, 1980.

65. Benotti JR, Grossman W, Braunwald E, Carabello BA: Effects of amrinone on myocardial energy metabolism and hemodynamics in patients with severe congestive heart failure due to coronary disease. *Circulation* 62:28, 1980.

66. Edelson J, LeJemtel TH, Alousi AA, et al: Relationship between amrinone plasma concentration and cardiac index. *Clin Pharmacol Ther* 29:723, 1981.

67. Edelson J, Stroshane R, Benziger DP, et al: Pharmacokinetics of the bipyridines amrinone and milrinone. *Circulation* 73(suppl 3):III-145, 1986.

68. Kullberg MP, Freeman GB, Biddlecome C, et al: Amrinone metabolism. *Clin Pharmacol Ther* 29(3):394, 1981.

69. Alousi AA, Johnson DC: Pharmacology of the bipyridines: Amrinone and milrinone. *Circulation* 73(suppl 3, pt 2):10, 1986.

70. Benotti JR, Grossman W, Braunwald E, et al: Hemodynamic assessment of amrinone: A new inotropic agent. *N Engl J Med* 299:1373, 1978.

71. Vaughn-Williams EM: A classification of antiarrhythmic actions reassessed after a decade of new drugs. *J Clin Pharmacol* 24:129, 1984.

72. Collinsworth KA, Kalman SM, Harrison DC: The clinical pharmacology of lidocaine as an anti-arrhythmic drug. *Circulation* 50:1217, 1974.

73. Spear JF, Moore EN, Gerstenblith G: Effect of lidocaine on the ventricular fibrillation threshold in the dog during acute ischemia and premature ventricular contractions. *Circulation* 46:65, 1972.

74. Allen JD, Brennan FJ, Wit AL: Actions of lidocaine on transmembrane potentials of subendocardial purkinje fibers surviving in infarcted canine hearts. *Circ Res* 43:470, 1978.

75. Sanchez-Chapula J, Tsuda Y, Josephson IR: Voltage and use-dependent effects of lidocaine on sodium current and rat single ventricular cells. *Circ Res* 52:557, 1983.

76. Lie KI, Wellens HJ, van Capelle FJ, Durrer D: Lidocaine in the prevention of primary ventricular fibrillation: A double-blind, randomized study of 212 consecutive patients. *N Engl J Med* 291:1324, 1974.

77. DeSilva RA, Hennekens CH, Lown B, Casscells W: Lignocaine prophylaxis in acute myocardial infarction: An evaluation of randomised trials. *Lancet* October 17:855, 1981.

78. Koster RW, Dunning AJ: Intramuscular lidocaine for prevention of lethal arrhythmias in the prehospitalization phase of acute myocardial infarction. *N Engl J Med* 313:1105, 1985.

79. Thomson PD, Melmon KL, Richardson JA, et al: Lidocaine pharmacokinetics in advanced heart failure, liver disease, and renal failure in humans. *Ann Intern Med* 78:499, 1973.

80. Thomson PD, Rowland M, Melmon KL: The influence of heart failure, liver disease, and renal failure on the disposition of lidocaine in man. *Am Heart J* 82:417, 1971.

81. Benowitz NL: Clinical applications of the pharmacokinetics of lidocaine. In Melmon KL (ed): *Cardiovascular Drug Therapy.* Philadelphia, FA Davis, 1974, pp 77–101.

82. Benowitz N, Forsyth RP, Melmon KL, Rowland M: Lidocaine disposition kinetics in monkey and man: I. Prediction of a perfusion model. *Clin Pharmacol Ther* 16:87, 1974.

83. Pfeifer HJ, Greenblatt DJ, Koch-Weser J: Clinical use and toxicity of intravenous lidocaine: A report from the Boston collaborative drug surveillance program. *Am Heart J* 92:168, 1976.

84. Carruth JE, Silverman ME: Ventricular fibrillation complicating acute myocardial infarction: Reasons against the routine use of lidocaine. *Am Heart J* 104:545, 1982.

85. Dunn HM, McComb JM, Kinney CD, et al: Prophylactic lidocaine in the early phase of suspected myocardial infarction. *Am Heart J* 110:353, 1985.

86. Giardina EGV, Heissenbuttel RH, Bigger JT Jr: Intermittent intravenous procainamide to treat ventricular arrhythmias. *Ann Intern Med* 78:183, 1973.

87. Lima JJ, Goldfarb AL, Conti DR, et al: Safety and efficacy of procainamide infusions. *Am J Cardiol* 43:98, 1979.

88. Harrison DC, Sprouse JH, Morrow AG: The antiarrhythmic properties of lidocaine and procaine amide: Clinical and physiologic studies of their cardiovascular effects in man. *Circulation* 28:486, 1963.

89. Woosley RL, Drayer DE, Reidenberg MM, et al: Effect of acetylator phenotype on the rate at which procainamide induces antinuclear antibodies and the lupus syndrome. *N Engl J Med* 298:1157, 1978.

90. Markis JE, Koch-Weser J: Characteristics and mechanisms of inotropic and chronotropic actions of bretylium tosylate. *J Pharmacol Exp Ther* 178:94, 1971.

91. Patterson E, Lucchesi BR: Bretylium: A prototype for future development of antidysrhythmic agents. *Am Heart J* 106:426, 1983.

92. Heissenbuttel RH, Bigger JT Jr: Bretylium tosylate: A newly available antiarrhythmic drug for ventricular arrhythmias. *Ann Intern Med* 91:229, 1979.

93. Sasyniuk BI: Symposium on the management of ventricular dysrhythmias: Concept of reentry versus automaticity. *Am J Cardiol* 54:1A, 1984.

94. Anderson JL: Symposium on the management of ventricular dysrhythmias: Antifibrillatory versus antiectopic therapy. *Am J Cardiol* 54:7A, 1984.

95. Kerber RE, Pandian NG, Jensen SR, et al: Effect of lidocaine and bretylium on energy requirement for transthoracic defibrillation: Experimental studies. *J Am Coll Cardiol* 7:397, 1986.

96. Chow MSS, Kluger J, DiPersio DM, et al: Antifibrillatory effects of lidocaine and bretylium immediately postcardiopulmonary resuscitation. *Am Heart J* 110:938, 1985.

97. Dorian P, Fain ES, Davy JM, Winkle RA: Lidocaine causes a reversible, concentration-dependent increase in defibrillation energy requirements. *J Am Coll Cardiol* 8:327, 1986.

98. Koch-Weser J: Drug therapy: Bretylium. *N Engl J Med* 300:473, 1979.

99. Anderson JL, Patterson E, Wagner JG, et al: Clinical pharmacokinetics of intravenous and oral bretylium tosylate in survivors of ventricular tachycardia or fibrillation: Clinical application of a new assay for bretylium. *J Cardiovasc Pharmacol* 3:485, 1981.

100. Duff HJ, Roden DM, Yacobi A, et al: Bretylium: Relations between plasma concentrations and pharmacologic actions in high-frequency ventricular arrhythmias. *Am J Cardiol* 55:395, 1985.

101. Haynes RE, Chinn TL, Copass MK, Cobb LA: Comparison of bretylium tosylate and lidocaine in management of out of hospital ventricular fibrillation: A randomized clinical trial. *Am J Cardiol* 48:353, 1981.

102. Holder DA, Sniderman AD, Fraser G, Fallen EL: Experience with bretylium tosylate by a hospital cardiac arrest team. *Circulation* 55:541, 1977.

103. Ideker RE, Klein GJ, Harrison L, et al: Epicardial mapping of the initiation of ventricular

fibrillation induced by reperfusion following acute ischemia. *Circulation* 57 and 58(suppl 2):64, 1978.

104. Leveque PE: Antiarrhythmic action of bretylium. *Nature* 207:203, 1965.

105. Singh BN, Ellrodt G, Peter CT: Verapamil: A review of its pharmacological properties and therapeutic use. *Drugs* 15:169, 1978.

106. Rosen MR, Wit AL, Hoffman BF: Electrophysiology and pharmacology of cardiac arrhythmias: VI. Cardiac effects of verapamil. *Am Heart J* 89:665, 1975.

107. McGoon MD, Vlietstra RE, Holmes DR, Osborn JE: The clinical use of verapamil. *Mayo Clin Proc* 57:495, 1982.

108. Waxman HL, Myerburg RJ, Appel R, Sung RJ: Verapamil for control of ventricular rate in paroxysmal supraventricular tachycardia and atrial fibrillation or flutter: A double-blind, randomized cross-over study. *Ann Intern Med* 94:1, 1981.

109. Hwang MH, Danoviz J, Pacold I, et al: Double-blind crossover randomized trial of intravenously administered verapamil: Its use for atrial fibrillation and flutter following open heart surgery. *Arch Intern Med* 144:491, 1984.

110. Plumb VJ, Karp RB, Kouchoukos NT, et al: Verapamil therapy of atrial fibrillation and atrial flutter following cardiac operation. *J Thorac Cardiovasc Surg* 83:590, 1982.

111. Singh BN, Collett JT, Chew CYC: New perspectives in the pharmacologic therapy of cardiac arrhythmias. *Prog Cardiovasc Dis* 22:243, 1980.

112. Weiss AT, Lewis BS, Halon DA, et al: The use of calcium with verapamil in the management of supraventricular tachyarrhythmias. *Int J Cardiol* 4:275, 1983.

113. Sung RJ, Elser B, McAllister RG Jr: Intravenous verapamil for termination of re-entrant supraventricular tachycardias. *Ann Intern Med* 93:682, 1980.

114. Kates RE: Calcium antagonists: Pharmacokinetic properties. *Drugs* 25:113, 1983.

115. McAllister RG Jr: Clinical pharmacology of slow channel blocking agents. *Prog Cardiovasc Dis* 25:83, 1982.

116. Spurrell RA, Krikler DM, Sowton E: Effects of verapamil on electrophysiological properties of anomalous atrioventricular connexion in Wolff-Parkinson-White syndrome. *Br Heart J* 36:256, 1974.

117. Gulamhusein S, Ko P, Carruthers SG, Klein GJ: Acceleration of the ventricular response during atrial fibrillation in the Wolff-Parkinson-White syndrome after verapamil. *Circulation* 65:348, 1982.

118. Harper RW, Whitford E, Middlebrook R, et al: Effects of verapamil on the electrophysiologic properties of the accessory pathway in patients with the Wolff-Parkinson-White syndrome. *Am J Cardiol* 50:1323, 1982.

119. McGovern B, Garan H, Ruskin JN: Precipitation of cardiac arrest by verapamil in patients with Wolff-Parkinson-White syndrome. *Ann Intern Med* 104:791, 1986.

120. Gulamhusein S, Ko P, Klein GJ: Ventricular fibrillation following verapamil in the Wolff-Parkinson-White syndrome. *Am Heart J* 106:145, 1983.

121. Jacob AS, Nielsen DW, Gianelly RE: Fatal ventricular fibrillation following verapamil in Wolff-Parkinson-White syndrome with atrial fibrillation. *Ann Emerg Med* 14:159, 1985.

122. Klein GJ, Bashore TM, Sellers TD, et al: Ventricular fibrillation in the Wolff-Parkinson-White syndrome. *N Engl J Med* 301:1080, 1979.

123. Stewart RB, Bardy GH, Greene HL: Wide complex tachycardia: Misdiagnosis and outcome after emergent therapy. *Ann Intern Med* 104:766, 1986.

124. Morady F, Baerman JM, DiCarlo LA, et al: A prevalent misconception regarding wide-complex tachycardias. *JAMA* 254:2790, 1985.

125. Schamroth L, Krikler DM, Garrett C: Immediate effects of intravenous verapamil in cardiac arrhythmias. *Br Med J* 11:660, 1972.

126. Shand DG: Drug therapy: Propranolol. *N Engl J Med* 293:280, 1975.

127. Koch-Weser J: Drug therapy: Metoprolol. *N Engl J Med* 301:698, 1979.

128. Prichard BNC: Beta-adrenergic receptor blockade in hypertension: Past, present and future. *Br J Clin Pharmacol* 5:379, 1978.

129. Frishman WH, Teicher M: Beta-adrenergic blockade: An update. *Cardiology* 72:280, 1985.

130. Tzivoni D, Banai S, Schuger C, et al: Treatment of torsade de pointes with magnesium sulfate. *Circulation* 77:392, 1988.

131. Dauchot P, Gravenstein JS: Bradycardia after myocardial ischemia and its treatment with atropine. *Anesthesiology* 44:501, 1976.

132. Epstein SE, Goldstein RD, Redwood DR, et al: The early phase of acute myocardial infarction: Pharmacologic aspects of therapy (NIH conference). *Ann Intern Med* 78:918, 1973.

133. Brown DC, Lewis AJ, Criley JM: Asystole and its treatment: The possible role of the parasympathetic nervous system in cardiac arrest. *J Am Coll Emerg Physicians* 8(11):448, 1979.

134. Scheinman MM, Thorburn D, Abbott JA: Use of atropine in patients with acute myocardial infarction and sinus bradycardia. *Circulation* 52:627, 1975.

135. Salerno DM, Dias VC, Kleiger RE, et al: Efficacy and safety of intravenous diltiazem for treatment of atrial fibrillation and atrial flutter. *Am J Cardiol* 63:1046, 1989.

136. Ellenbogen KA, Dias VC, Plumb VJ, et al: A placebo-controlled trial of continuous intravenous diltiazem infusion for 24-hour heart rate control during atrial fibrillation and atrial flutter: A multicenter study. *J Am Coll Cardiol* 18:891, 1991.

137. Stoelting RK: Anticholinergic drugs. In *Pharmacology and Physiology in Anesthetic Practice,* 2d ed. Philadelphia, Lippincott, 1991, pp 242–251.

138. Chamberlain DA, Turner P, Sneddon JM: Effects of atropine on heart-rate in healthy man. *Lancet* 2:12, 1967.

139. Kottmeier CA, Gravenstein JS: The parasympathomimetic activity of atropine and atropine methylbromide. *Anesthesiology* 29:1125, 1968.

140. Rothstein RJ, Neimann JT, Rennie CJ, Suddath WO: Use of naloxone during cardiac arrest and CPR: Potential adjunct for postcountershock electrical-mechanical dissociation. *Ann Emerg Med* 14:198, 1985.

141. Hasegawa EAJ: The endotracheal use of drugs. *Heart Lung* 15:60, 1986.

142. Prete MR, Hannan CJ, Burkle FM: Plasma atropine concentrations via the intravenous, endotracheal, and intraosseous routes of administration (abstract). *Ann Emerg Med* 15:644, 1986.

143. Greenberg MI, Mayeda DV, Chrzanowski R, et al: Endotracheal administration of atropine sulfate. *Ann Emerg Med* 11:546, 1982.

144. DiMarco JP, Sellers TD, Berne RM, et al: Adenosine: Electrophysiologic effects and therapeutic use for terminating paroxysmal supraventricular tachycardia. *Circulation* 68:1254, 1983.

145. Parker RB, McCollam PL: Adenosine in the episodic treatment of paroxysmal supraventricular tachycardia. *Clin Pharmacol* 9:261, 1990.

146. DiMarco JP, Sellers TD, Lerman BB, et al: Diagnostic and therapeutic use of adenosine in patients with supraventricular tachyarrhythmias. *J Am Coll Cardiol* 6:417, 1985.

147. Fyman PN, Cottrell JR, Kushins L, Casthely PA: Vasodilator therapy in the perioperative period. *Can Anaesth Soc J* 33:629, 1986.

148. Kaplan JA, Finlayson DC, Woodward S: Vasodilator therapy after cardiac surgery: A review of the efficacy and toxicity of nitroglycerin and nitroprusside. *Can Anaesth Soc J* 27:254, 1980.

149. Tinker JH, Michenfelder JD: Sodium nitroprusside: Pharmacology, toxicity and therapeutics. *Anesthesiology* 45:340, 1976.

150. Parker JO: Nitrate therapy in stable angina pectoris. *N Engl J Med* 316:1635, 1987.

151. Cohen MV, Downey JM, Sonnenblick EH, Kirk ES: The effects of nitroglycerin on coronary collaterals and myocardial contractility. *J Clin Invest* 52:2836, 1973.

152. Malindzak GS, Green HD, Stagg PL: Effects of nitroglycerin on flow after partial constriction of the coronary artery. *J Appl Physiol* 29:17, 1970.

153. Greenberg H, Dwyer EM Jr, Jameson AG, Pinkernell BH: Effects of nitroglycerin on the major determinants of myocardial oxygen consumption: An angiographic and hemodynamic assessment. *Am J Cardiol* 36:426, 1975.

154. Durrer JD, Lie KI, van Capelle FJL, Durrer D: Effect of sodium nitroprusside on mortality in acute myocardial infarction. *N Engl J Med* 306:1121, 1982.

155. Vesey CJ, Cole PV, Simpson PJ: Cyanide and thiocyanate concentrations following sodium nitroprusside infusion in man. *Br J Anaesth* 48:651, 1976.

156. Michenfelder JD, Tinker JH: Cyanide toxicity and thiosulfate protection during chronic administration of sodium nitroprusside in the dog: Correlation with a human case. *Anesthesiology* 47:441, 1977.

157. Stueven HA, Thompson BM, Aprahamian C, Tonsfeldt DJ: Calcium chloride: Reassessment of use in asystole. *Ann Emerg Med* 13:820, 1984.

158. Harrison EE, Amey BD: Use of calcium in electromechanical dissociation. *Ann Emerg Med* 13:844, 1984.

159. Dembo DH: Calcium in advanced life support. *Crit Care Med* 9:358, 1981.

160. Carlon GC, Howland WS, Kahn RC, Schweizer O: Calcium chloride administration in normocalcemic critically ill patients. *Crit Care Med* 8:209, 1980.

161. Legato MJ: The myocardial cell: New concepts for the clinical cardiologist, editorial. *Circulation* 45:731, 1972.

162. White RD, Goldsmith RS, Rodriquez R, et al: Plasma ionic calcium levels following injection of chloride, gluconate and gluceptate salts of calcium. *J Thorac Cardiovasc Surg* 71:609, 1976.

163. Redding JS, Pearson JW: Resuscitation from ventricular fibrillation: Drug therapy. *JAMA* 203:255, 1968.

164. Telivuo L, Maamies T, Siltanen P, Tala P: Comparison of alkalizing agents in resuscitation of the heart after ventricular fibrillation. *Ann Chir Gynaecol Fenn* 57:221, 1968.

165. Minuck M, Sharma GP: Comparison of THAM and sodium bicarbonate in resuscitation of the heart after ventricular fibrillation in dogs. *Anesth Analg* 56:38, 1977.

166. Mattar JA, Weil MH, Shubin H, Stein L: Cardiac arrest in the critically ill: II. Hyperosmolal states following cardiac arrest. *Am J Med* 56:162, 1974.

167. Gambling DR, Birmingham CL, Jenkins LC: Magnesium and the anaesthetist. *Can J Anaesth* 35:644, 1988.

168. Biddle TL, Yu PN: Effect of furosemide on hemodynamics and lung water in acute pulmonary edema secondary to myocardial infarction. *Am J Cardiol* 43:86, 1979.

169. Stoelting RK: *Pharmacology and Physiology in Anesthetic Practice,* 2d ed. Philadelphia, Lippincott, 1991, pp 445–450.

170. Lawson DH, Gray JM, Henry DA, Tilstone WJ: Continuous infusion of frusemide in refractory oedema. *Br Med J* 2(6135):476, 1978.

171. Copeland JG, Campbell DW, Plachetka JR, et al: Diuresis with continuous infusion of furosemide after cardiac surgery. *Am J Surg* 146:796, 1983.

172. Amiel SA, Blackburn AM, Rubens RD: Intravenous infusion of frusemide as treatment for ascites in malignant disease. *Br Med J* 288(6423):1041, 1984.

173. Krasna MJ, Scott GE, Scholz PM, et al: Postoperative enhancement of urinary output in patients with acute renal failure using continuous furosemide therapy. *Chest* 89:294, 1986.

174. Flacke JW, Flacke WE, Williams GD: Acute pulmonary edema following naloxone reversal of high-dose morphine anesthesia. *Anesthesiology* 47:376, 1977.

175. Michaelis LL, Hickey PR, Clark TA, Dixon WM: Ventricular irritability associated with the use of naloxone hydrochloride. *Ann Thorac Surg* 18:608, 1974.

176. Tanaka GY: Hypertensive reaction to naloxone. *JAMA* 228:25, 1974.

177. Faden AI: Opiate antagonists and thyrotropin-releasing hormone: I. Potential role in the treatment of shock. *JAMA* 252:1177, 1984.

178. Anderson R, Dobloug I, Refstad S: Postanaesthetic use of naloxone hydrochloride after moderate doses of fentanyl. *Acta Anaesth Scand* 20:255, 1976.

179. Rawal N, Schott U, Dahlstrom B, et al: Influence of naloxone infusion on analgesia and respiratory depression following epidural morphine. *Anesthesiology* 64:194, 1986.

180. Klotz U, Ziegler G, Ludwig L, Reimann IW: Pharmacodynamic interaction between midazolam and a specific benzodiazepine antagonist in humans. *J Clin Pharmacol* 25:400, 1985.

181. Bartelsman JFWM, Sars PRA, Tytgat GNJ: Flumazenil used for reversal of midazolam-induced sedation in endoscopy outpatients. *Gastrointest Endosc* 36(3):S9, 1990.

182. Roncari G, Ziegler WH, Guentert TW: Pharmacokinetics of the new benzodiazepine antagonist RO 15-1788 in man following intravenous and oral administration. *Br J Clin Pharmacol* 22:421, 1986.

183. Darragh A, Lambe R, Kenny M, et al: RO 15-1788 antagonises the central effects of diazepam in man without altering diazepam bioavailability. *Br J Clin Pharmacol* 14:677, 1982.

184. Avant GR, Speeg KV, Freemon FR, et al: Physostigmine reversal of diazepam-induced hypnosis. *Ann Intern Med* 91:53, 1979.

185. Garber JG, Ominsky AJ, Orkin FK, Quinn P: Physostigmine-atropine solution fails to reverse diazepam sedation. *Anesth Analg* 59(1):58, 1980.

186. Hoegholm A, Steptoe P, Fogh B, et al: Benzodiazepine antagonism by aminophylline. *Acta Anaesthesiol Scand* 33:164, 1989.

187. Ochs MW, Tucker MR, Owsley TG, Anderson JA: The effectiveness of flumazenil in reversing the sedation and amnesia produced by intravenous midazolam. *J Oral Maxillofac Surg* 48:240, 1990.

188. Roche Laboratories: Mazicon (flumazenil) Product Monograph. Hoffmann-LaRoche, Inc., 1992, ISBN 444-01431-4.

189. Mora CT, Torjman M, DiGiorgio K: Sedative and ventilatory effects of midazolam and flumazenil. *Anesthesiology* 67:A534, 1987.

190. Mora CT, Torjman M, White PF: Effects of diazepam and flumazenil on sedation and hypoxic ventilatory response. *Anesth Analg* 68(4):473, 1989.

191. Grose R, Strain J, Greenberg M, LeJemtel TH: Systemic and coronary effects of intravenous milrinone and dobutamine in congestive heart failure. *J Am Coll Cardiol* 7:1007, 1986.

192. Monrad ES, Baim DS, Smith HS, Lanoue AS: Milrinone, dobutamine, and nitroprusside: Comparative effects on hemodynamics and myocardial energetics in patients with severe congestive heart failure. *Circulation* 73(suppl III):III–168, 1986.

8

HYPOVOLEMIC AND TRAUMATIC SHOCK

Donald Trunkey

In his classic book on traumatic shock, Cannon[1] was the first to express dismay that there was no clear definition of shock. He further concluded that the definition of shock was not a "prime requisite." He thought it more important to do careful clinical descriptions and to treat on the basis of this clinical observation. Cannon made two additional very important observations. Although he was not the first to describe traumatic shock, his observations of World War I battlefield casualties led him to make the classic description:

> Wound shock occurs as a consequence of physical injury. It is characterized by low venous pressure, a low, or falling, arterial pressure, a rapid, thready pulse, a diminished blood volume, a normal or increased erythrocyte count and hemoglobin percentage in peripheral blood (thereby differing from simple hemorrhage), a leukocytosis, an increased blood nitrogen, a reduced blood alkali, a lowered metabolism, a subnormal temperature, a cold skin moist with sweat, a pallid or grayish or slightly cyanotic appearance, also by thirst, by shallow and rapid respiration, often by vomiting and restlessness, by anxiety changing usually to mental illness and by lessened sensitivity. Many of these features may appear at once or as soon after the reception of the wound as observations can be made, or they may develop only after the lapse of several hours.

Another important observation by Cannon was the emergency-induced discharge of the noradrenergic nervous system, which he termed "the preparation for flight or fight."

Samuel Gross, another pioneer in the observations of shock, was first credited as defining shock as a "manifestation of the rude unhinging of the machinery of life."[2] However, in his *System of Surgery,* he described shock as "a depression of the vital powers, induced suddenly by external injury, and essentially dependent upon a loss of innervation."[3] Gross, like his contemporaries, linked shock to collapse of the central nervous system. More recently, surgeons, including myself, have tried to define shock in simpler terms. One of the more simple definitions is that shock represents inadequate tissue perfusion. Implied in this definition is a failure of oxygen transport and the delivery of substrate to the cells. A further implication is that waste products from the cell are no longer being removed from the tissue bed and excreted from the lungs or kidneys or detoxified by the liver.

One of the dilemmas in our attempt to understand the pathophysiology and treatment of shock is our inability to neatly classify the various forms of shock either by anatomic or physiologic mechanisms. Such is the case with hypovolemic shock. I will try to make an argument that hypovolemic shock is uncommon and that what most surgeons deal with on a far more frequent basis is traumatic shock.

HYPOVOLEMIC SHOCK VERSUS TRAUMATIC SHOCK

Is it important to make a distinction between hypovolemic shock and traumatic shock? The answer is clearly yes. It is my contention that traumatic shock, which represents both hypovolemia and tissue injury, is worse than simple hypovolemia. Tissue injury is a potent stimulus of the inflammatory cascade. This is not a new concept, and its importance cannot be understated. Hunter[4] recognized the importance of inflammation in his *Treatise on Wounds* and stated, "This operation of the body, termed inflammation, requires our greatest attention, for it is one of the most common and most extensive in its effects of any in the animal body; it is both very extensive in its causes, and it becomes itself the cause of many local effects, both salutary and diseased." Dr. Benjamin Travers,[5] senior surgeon to St. Thomas' Hospital, also recognized the importance of inflammation: "The irritation which arises from injury or inflammation, when it passes from local to constitutional, becomes imminently hazardous; constitutional irritation being as much more dangerous than local, as the disorder of the whole is of graver importance than the disorder of a part." This is made even more poignant by Malcolm,[6] who stated, "It may be argued that the direct effects of an injury—the devitalization of tissue which Lister has called the 'primary lesion in inflammatory congestion,' the blood stasis, and the excitations into the affected and neighboring parts—constitute the pathological condition in an inflammation; and that the general disturbance which accompanies an inflammation—the traumatic fever—is the result of reflex nervous changes—is caused by physiologic 'reactions,' necessarily induced by the healthy body by the local abnormal conditions."

It can be appreciated from the preceding that trauma is associated with tissue injury which then causes the initiation of inflammation. Once the inflammatory cascade has been set in motion, a severe injury or prolonged course may cause dyshomeostasis within the inflammatory cascade, which then contributes to the pathophysiology of the original insult. Pure hypovolemic shock, which is only occasionally seen in such patients as those suffering a bleeding duodenal ulcer or a ruptured abdominal aortic aneurysm, *is not* associated with extensive tissue injury. Similarly, gastrointestinal obstruction or dehydration is not usually associated with significant tissue injury, and the insult is not nearly as harmful to the organism as a crush syndrome, burn, or polytrauma. It is these latter injuries that have great potential for subsequent multiple organ failure.

Hypovolemic shock may in itself be a stimulus to flight and fight mechanisms and inflammation, but probably not nearly as much of a stimulus as tissue injury. Thus it seems that there are at least three components to the pathophysiology of traumatic shock: volume loss, tissue injury, and subsequent dyshomeostasis if the trauma insult is severe or prolonged in time. Stated another way, volume loss and tissue injury are powerful stimulants to the fight and flight mechanisms and the inflammatory system. It is the imbalance or disruption of these protective mechanisms that leads to dyshomeostasis.

What is dyshomeostasis? During evolution the predator-prey relationship and threat of injury from any cause led to complex "flight and fight" mechanisms.[1] Tissue injury or wounds led to the biologic necessity of repair (inflammation). This phylogenetic development can be appreciated by briefly looking at two species. The earthworm white cell is the colemocyte, which is capable of chemotaxis, phagocytosis, encapsulation, and primitive wound healing. The same white cell can cause rejection and limited humoral responses (histamine, kinins, agglutinins, and lysins). In contrast, the white cell for the lizard is the azurophil granulocyte, which is more complex. It is capable of metamorphosis to a macrophage neutrophil. It functions similarly to a heterophil and eosinophil. This white cell contains peroxidase-positive granules and can generate caseous pus. Human white cells are even more complex, and we can hypothesize that the more complex the organism, the more complex is that organism's immune system. The more complex the immune system, the greater is the potential for major disruption once dyshomeostasis takes place.

The purpose of "flight and fight" is to protect the organism and to increase survivability. The purpose of inflammation is to repair wounds and restore tissue integrity. The combined effects of these protective mechanisms result in a limited ability to preserve life and restore function after injury. In general, humans can withstand and compensate for a 25 percent blood volume depletion, a 30 percent partial-thickness burn, and an injury of modest degree (ISS < 25). However, modern surgery and injury treatment allow survival with greater injury than previously possible. Thus modern treatment creates the opportunity for disruption of the inflammatory cascade and dyshomeostasis.

After severe injury (traumatic shock), the flight and fight mechanism and the inflammatory process become either abnormal or imbalanced and contribute to the original injury insult. This dyshomeostasis affects metabolism, wound healing, and immune function and is caused by loss of regulation, disruption of normal servo mechanisms, and production of mediators, cytokines, and other inflammatory agents in abnormal amounts (Table 8–1). I wish to emphasize that no single factor or substance causes dyshomeostasis and subsequent organ dysfunction. Conversely, no single factor, substance, or antibiotic will protect against dyshomeostasis or prevent organ failure.

PATHOGENESIS

In the fall of 1916, a committee on physiology was established in the National Research Council, which had been organized to aid the U.S. government in case of need (World War I).[1] One of the subcommittees was on traumatic shock, and

TABLE 8–1. Cytokines and Growth Factors

Name	Major Cell Source*	Major Target Cell
Interleukins		
IL-1α and β	MO, Fb, many other cells	T, B, Fb, Hc, and many others
IL-2	T	T, B, NK, LAK
IL-3	T	Early hemopoietic cells
IL-4	T, MC	T, B, MO, MC
IL-5	T	B, Eo
IL-6	MO, T, Fb, Ed, many other cells	T, B, Nu, and many others
IL-7	BSC	B
IL-8	MO	Nu
Interferons		
IFNα	MO	Many cell types
IFNβ	Fb	Many cell types
IFN	T, NK	MO and many others
Colony Stimulating Factors		
GM-CSF	T, Fb, ED	Eo, Nu, other hemopoietic cells
G-CSF	MO, Fb, ED	Nu
M-CSF	MO, Fb, ED	MO
Tumor Necrosis Factors		
TNFα	MO, FB, T	Many cell types
TNFβ	T, B	Many cell types
Growth Factors		
Fibroblast GF	MO, Ed, P	Many cell types
Platelet-derived GF	MO, Ed, P	Connective tissue cells
Epidermal GF	MO	Connective tissue cells
Insulin-like-GF I and II	MO	Connective tissue cells
Transforming GF	MO, T	Many cell types

*T = T lymphocyte; B = B lymphocyte; MO = macrophage/monocyte; Ed = endothelial cell; P = platelet; Fb = fibroblast; Hc = hepatocyte; NK = natural killer cell; LAK = lymphokine-activated killer cells; Eo = eosinophils; Nu = neutrophil; MC = mast cell; BSC = bone marrow stomal cell.

Walter B. Cannon was a member. He went to Europe with a number of other physiologists, including Bayliss, Richards, Dale, and Cowell. Some of these men were surgeons and were involved directly in the care of casualties. Many attempts were made to classify shock, and Cowell proposed two groups: primary and secondary wound shock. *Primary wound shock* was seen when the damage sustained by the body is so great that death will occur unless surgical intervention is soon available. *Secondary wound shock* occurred in the seriously wounded after the lapse of some hours. The French working with the Americans divided shock into hemorrhagic and nonhemorrhagic types. *Hemorrhagic shock* was seen in those in which patients had suffered significant vascular injuries with loss of blood but also had tissue injury. *Nonhemorrhagic shock* was seen only among the severely wounded, those patients with extensive injury of limbs or severe lesions of the viscera. These attempts at classification and the desire to find an explanation for the onset of delayed or secondary shock fell far short according to Cannon.[1] In his classic treatise on traumatic shock, he examines the various theories of shock that were prevalent at that time, including many that are still actively considered.

The first theory was that of inhibition.[1] This theory, which was championed by Meltzer, stated that "the various injuries which are capable of bringing on shock do so by favoring the development of the inhibitory side of all the functions of the body." Although these investigators did not know about monokines and cytokines, it was clear to them that there were certain agents within the circulation that inhibited essential body functions. Cannon did not subscribe to this theory. Another popular theory was one of vasomotor paralysis. It was thought that a large quantity of blood became stagnant in the relaxed vessels, particularly in the splanchnic bed, and that the heart received only a small quantity of blood, and therefore, its output was meager. Again, Cannon did not believe that this could explain the entire phenomenon of secondary shock.

The theory of exhaustion also was explored by Cannon. This theory stated that there was a failure or destruction of the vasomotor centers, which then accounted for the shock state. Considerable experimental evidence from Wiggers, Guthrie, and Crile supported this theory. Based on observations of battlefield casualties, Cannon and Cowell concluded that vasomotor exhaustion was not the pathogenesis of traumatic shock.

As early as 1885, Groeningen stated that fat from long bones and subcutaneous connective tissue could be taken up in the bloodstream after injury and be trapped in the pulmonary microvasculature, leading to severe dyspnea and acute edema of the lung. This theory of fat embolism gained support from a number of investigators, including Wiggers. Cannon recognized that fat emboli could occur in some patients, but not all. Thus fat embolism also failed as a sole cause of traumatic shock. Other investigators thought there was an adrenal factor that caused shock, while still others felt that acidosis was the shock factor. The theory of acapnia was proposed by Henderson in 1908, and there were other theories of vasoconstriction and capillary congestion which seemed to fit also with the morphologic picture seen in patients following extensive trauma.

After considering these various theories, Cannon, working with Bayliss, dismissed them and thought the pathogenesis of traumatic shock was the result of a toxin. There was considerable support during World War I for this theory from other physiologists. None of the investigators was able to find a single factor, and Cannon eventually concluded that the factor was "exemia," a term that he borrowed from Hippocrates. Cannon felt that patients in severe shock from trauma were drained of blood above and beyond the blood loss either externally or internally. He could not explain where this "lost blood" was, thus the term *exemia*. It must be emphasized that the essential observation that all the physiologists in World War I made was that pure hemorrhage was uncommon and that tissue injury in combination with blood loss was the most common injury seen in the battlefield casualty. The depth of shock and time following injury seemed to aggravate the pathologic condition, leading to worsening of the patient's symptoms and eventual death if left untreated. Some patients, no matter how vigorous or aggressive the treatment, still died as a consequence of this traumatic toxemia. Cannon was unable to measure monokines, cytokines, and other mediators of inflammation, yet his term *exemia* is descriptive of the dyshomeostasis that takes place after severe injury.

PATHOPHYSIOLOGY

The human organism is somewhat limited in its compensatory reactions to trauma. These compensatory reactions can be broadly categorized into three groups: redistribution of blood flow, alterations of the components of oxygen supply (transport), and plasma refill. Redistribution of blood flow is achieved by vasoconstriction, venoconstriction, and increased secretion of norepinephrine and epinephrine, the causal agents of "flight and fight." It is the redistribution of blood flow that gives us our classic clinical signs of shock.

The components of oxygen supply are pulmonary gas exchange, blood flow, hemoglobin concentration, and hemoglobin affinity for oxygen.[7] Following traumatic shock, some of these oxygen supply components are unavailable as compensatory mechanisms. The final compensatory mechanism is plasma refill, which is initiated by the reduction in hydrostatic pressure in the capillary bed and hormonal action in the kidney and splanchnic bed. Based on these compensatory mechanisms, we can broadly categorize the pathophysiology of shock into four phases. It also should be appreciated that from a therapeutic standpoint, the clinician should try to augment or supplement these compensatory mechanisms whenever possible during the acute resuscitation.

COMPENSATION PHASE

The first response of the circulation to hypovolemia is contraction of precapillary arterial sphincters; this causes the filtration pressure in the capillaries to fall. Since osmotic pressure remains the same, fluid moves into the vascular space from the interstitium with a corresponding increase in plasma volume. If this compensatory mechanism is adequate to return circulation volume to normal, the capillary sphincters relax and microcirculatory flow returns to normal. If shock is prolonged and profound, the next phase of shock is entered.

During the compensation phase, the initial reaction in oxygen transport is for tachypnea to occur. This may be one of the easiest ways for the human organism to increase oxygen flow to the tissue. This will be impaired if there has been injury to the upper torso, particularly to the chest wall. Blood flow is dependent on cardiac output and the microcirculation. For purposes of this discussion, I will confine my remarks to cardiac output, which is the product of stroke volume and heart rate. One of the early compensatory mechanisms is tachycardia. This may be offset, however, by the reduction in stroke volume as volume to the heart is reduced. In most studies on pure hypovolemic shock, cardiac output falls from the inception of the shock insult. Hemoglobin concentration will fall as red cell mass is lost due to hemorrhage. This is greatly affected by resuscitation and hemodilution during the resuscitation efforts. The affinity of hemoglobin to oxygen will be altered depending on the patient's temperature and the presence or absence of acidosis. If the patient becomes acidotic during shock, this tends to enhance oxygen release from hemoglobin. However, acidosis inhibits red cell glycolysis through a decrease in activity of phosphofructokinase and results in a fall of 2,3-diphosphoglycerate, a ligand that will counterbalance the effect of acidosis.

Redistribution of blood volume is an important compensatory mechanism. One can think of it as "robbing from Peter to pay Paul." Nature is trying to preserve blood flow to the brain and heart at the expense of all other organs. Thus early in shock blood is diverted from skeletal muscle and skin and eventually, as the shock progresses, from the viscera. As mentioned previously, it is this redistribution of blood flow that gives us our classic clinical signs of shock.

CELL DISTRESS PHASE

If the shock insult becomes worse or vascular volume is not restored, the precapillary sphincters remain closed, and arteriovenous shunts open up to divert arterial blood directly back into the venous system, thus maintaining circulation to more important organs—the heart and brain. This continued redistribution of blood volume in the skeletal muscle, skin, and viscera leads to anaerobic metabolism for energy. The amount of glucose and oxygen available for the cell decreases, since there is no delivery, and metabolic waste products such as lactate accumulate. Histamine is released, resulting in closure of the postcapillary sphincters, and this mechanism serves to slow the remaining capillary flow and hold the red blood cells and nutrients in the capillaries longer. The empty capillary bed constricts almost completely; very few capillaries remain open. It is during this stage of shock that cells begin to take up water from the interstitium as well as sodium and calcium. Potassium is released from the cell, and free radicals start to accumulate, setting the stage for further cell destruction.

Oxygen transport becomes severely impaired. The patient often has a ventilatory rate greater than 30 breaths per minute, provided there is no chest wall or neurologic injury. Blood flow is grossly impaired due to reduced venous return if the previously undiseased heart does not fail. Hemoglobin content continues to fall, affecting oxygen delivery.

Plasma refill during this period of time becomes inoperative because the interstitium has been reduced by as much as 60 percent due to the initial plasma refill and shift of fluid into the cell as a consequence of cell distress.

DECOMPENSATION PHASE

If severe shock is left untreated, the patient will approach a preagonal state. Just before cell death, local reflexes (probably initiated by acidosis and accumulated metabolites) reopen the precapillary sphincters while the postcapillary sphincters stay closed. Prolonged vasoconstriction of the capillary bed damages endothelial cells and results in increased capillary permeability. When capillaries finally reopen, fluid and protein are leaked into the interstitial space. Capillaries distend with red blood cells, and sludging occurs. White cells begin to marginate, and platelets are activated. Cells become swollen, are unable to utilize oxygen, and begin to die.

All components of oxygen transport become deranged. Abnormal breathing patterns begin as the brain becomes hypoxic. Cardiac function is impaired, and arrhythmias may occur. Oxygen delivery to the brain is grossly impaired, and the patient progresses from agitation through obtundation, stupor, and finally coma just prior to death.

RECOVERY PHASE

The recovery phase can contribute significantly to the overall pathophysiology depending on the degree of shock and the amount of tissue injury. If blood volume is restored at some point during the compensation phase, the effects on the microcirculation may still be reversible. Badly damaged cells may recover, and capillary integrity may be regained over time. The "sludge" in the microcirculation is swept into the venous circulation and eventually into the lungs, where these platelet and white cell aggregates are filtered out and contribute to postinjury pulmonary failure. Other capillaries may be so badly damaged and filled with sludge that they remain permanently closed; cells dependent on these capillaries die.

Normal distribution of blood flow may not recover for hours after injury. The patient may remain vasoconstricted and cool until core temperature rises and full volume restoration has occurred. This return to normal may be impaired if dopanergic and adrenergic drugs are administered in the postinjury period.

It is the oxygen transport components that may be most adversely affected in the immediate recovery phase. Pulmonary gas exchange can be impaired by a number of factors. These include chest wall injury and injuries to the lung parenchyma, including pulmonary contusion and aspiration. Analgesics and inappropriate ventilatory support also may contribute to impaired pulmonary gas exchange. In general, the heart is very resilient and recovers quickly, except in the elderly. Most patients retain a tachycardia in the immediate postinjury period, and as long as volume status has been restored, stroke volume is more than adequate. Exceptions to this would include patients with myocardial contusions, right ventricular failure secondary to pulmonary hypertension, and microemboli within the pulmonary capillary beds. Left ventricular failure is uncommon and usually implies antecedent heart disease or severe right-sided heart failure, which can then impair left ventricular function.[8,9] The heart is not a protected organ and may become edematous in the postinjury period. Cardiac output is usually supranormal, reflecting increased oxygen consumption and demand in the tissue beds as the counterregulatory hormones and hypermetabolism manifest in the postinjury period. Systemic vascular resistance is initially high, but as core temperature rises and the volume status is restored, there can actually be a fall below normal levels unless adrenergic drugs are used.

After a mild or moderate traumatic shock insult, there is usually a rapid restoration of plasma volume, and red cells are rapidly repleted with the increased formation of erythropoietin. Plasma protein synthesis is increased, vasopressin levels fall, glucocorticoid levels fall, and renin and aldosterone secretion returns towards normal. If the traumatic shock insult is severe, many of these counter-regulatory hormones remain elevated. Cytokines and monokines may be abnormally secreted or depleted, and dyshomeostasis takes place. The patient becomes catabolic, and this is further aggravated if sepsis intervenes.

DIAGNOSIS AND TREATMENT

The great majority of patients with injuries do not present in shock. It has been estimated that 85 percent of patients have moderate or minor injuries.[12] Of the remaining 15 percent of patients with major injury, almost two-thirds are life-threatened, and most of these patients have some form of shock. It is this group of patients that we will discuss regarding diagnosis and the first 4 h of treatment. It has been determined from the American College of Surgeons Committee on Trauma Multiple Outcome study that 62 percent of all in-hospital trauma deaths occur within the first 4 h. The primary causes of death in these patients are hemorrhage and primary or secondary injuries to the central nervous system.

Diagnosis and treatment cannot be separated in the resuscitation of the trauma patient, since they are simultaneous events. The first physician to treat a severely injured patient must begin resuscitation immediately and collect as much information as possible. In addition to the patient's symptoms, essential information includes the mechanism of injury and the presence of any preexisting medical conditions that may influence critical decisions. Gathering information, unfortunately, requires time, and the evaluation of a critically injured patient often must be rushed. In order to help physicians maximize their resuscitative efforts and avoid missing life-threatening injuries, various protocols for resuscitation have been developed, of which the advanced trauma life support (ATLS) course is a model.[13] In the following discussion, I shall use the ATLS course as a paradigm for assessment, resuscitation, and the establishment of priorities in treating the patient's injuries.

Before discussing the hospital diagnosis and resuscitation, it is worthwhile to mention briefly the care provided in the prehospital setting. In modern emergency medical systems (EMS), advanced life support (ALS) is a critical and important feature of prehospital care. In communities where there is a trauma system, the prehospital care is usually provided by highly skilled paramedics and nurses. After responding to the scene, their primary priorities are to extricate the patient and at the same time protect the spine and begin resuscitation. The skills that have proven efficacy in the prehospital system include endotracheal intubation of the severely shocked patient or the patient who has a Glasgow coma scale of 8 or less.[14] The other ALS technique that has withstood scientific scrutiny is the application of splints to long bone fractures.[15] This reduces hemorrhage and prevents further neurovascular damage. In some communities the paramedics and nurses also have been trained to perform surgical airways (cricothyrotomy) and tube thoracostomy. Both these ALS skills are important to a small subset of critically injured patients. The ALS techniques that have not withstood scientific scrutiny to date are application of the pneumatic antishock garment and intravenous fluid resuscitation. However, most surgeons feel that placement of an intravenous line enroute to the hospital is helpful and may save time for the resuscitating team in the hospital.

Another important feature of prehospital care in a modern EMS system is the warning provided to the receiving hospital and the resuscitation team. This prehospital warning allows the trauma team to assemble and be present when the patient arrives. It also allows the team to set up special procedures if the patient warrants them. An example would be a patient who is in shock and it is anticipated that hypothermia may be an issue with multiple transfusions. The thermostat in the resuscitation room can be set to 85 to 90°F, which will minimize heat loss from the patient. Autotransfusers can be readied, and often, type-specific or O-negative blood can be brought to the emergency room to await the patient. Only rarely are such efforts wasted.

PRIMARY SURVEY AND INITIAL RESUSCITATION

Resuscitation has two components: the primary survey and initial resuscitation and the secondary survey with continuing resuscitation. All patients undergo the primary survey of airway, breathing, circulation, and assessment of neurologic status. Only patients who become hemodynamically stable will progress to the secondary survey, which focuses on a complete physical examination that directs further diagnostic studies. The great majority of patients who remain hemodynamically unstable require operative intervention immediately.

In keeping with the patient's own compensatory mechanisms, the goals of the primary survey are, in order, to establish a patent airway and adequate ventilation, to maintain the circulation (including cardiac function and intravascular volume), and to assess the global neurologic status.

AIRWAY ASSESSMENT

Almost immediately upon arrival, on going up to assess the airway, I feel the patient's lower extremity in order to get some assessment of the patient's circulatory status. The second thing that I note is the status of the neck veins. These two critical pieces of information allow me to proceed to immediately assess and treat airway and breathing. These first two pieces of information, however, are critical, and I will return to discuss them in subsequent sections. As noted above, in a community with a trauma system, the critically injured patient will often arrive with an airway already in place. If an airway has not been placed and the patient is severely shocked or comatose, a bag-mask should be instituted immediately in preparation for endotracheal intubation.[16] If the patient has obvious airway obstruction, high-flow nasal oxygen may help during attempts at oral tracheal intubation or while a surgical airway is being established. The question always arises as to what takes priority, airway or spinal cord injury. It must be emphasized that airway always takes priority. To prevent injury to the spinal cord, the cervical spine must not be excessively flexed or extended during intubation. This is best achieved by having a fellow physician, nurse, or paramedic hold the patient in an axial orientation. Traction should not be done until after the initial cervical spine x-rays. Oral endotracheal intubation is successful in the majority of injured patients. Although there are many advantages to nasotracheal intubation in a patient with potential neck injury, it also has a major disadvantage in that it usually requires a more experienced physician. During all endotracheal intubations, firm compression of the cricoid cartilage against the cervical spine occludes the esophagus and reduces the risk of aspirating vomitus.

A few patients will have bleeding, deformity, or edema from maxillofacial injuries that will necessitate placement of a surgical airway (Fig. 8–1). A skilled surgeon should be able to perform a tracheostomy rapidly. If the resuscitating physician does not feel facile in doing a prompt tracheostomy, an alternative is cricothyrotomy. In 90 percent of patients, it makes no difference which procedure is performed, but in the 10 percent who have blunt laryngeal injuries, particularly class IV or V injuries,[17] tracheostomy will be required, since cricothyrotomy may be impossible to perform because of the injury. Blunt laryngeal trauma should be suspected in all patients who have difficulty phonating, have upper airway stridor, have crepitance over their anterior neck, or have cyanosis with associated external evidence of blunt trauma to the neck. Blunt laryngeal trauma also should be suspect when routine lateral C-spine films reveal subcutaneous air in the anterior neck, retropharyngeal air in the deep cervical space, or the hyoid bone is above a line drawn parallel to the top of C3.

Once the patient has been intubated, a bag is connected to the endotracheal tube, and high-flow oxygen is administered by hand ventilation. In my opinion, there is never an indication for a ventilator in the emergency room for critically

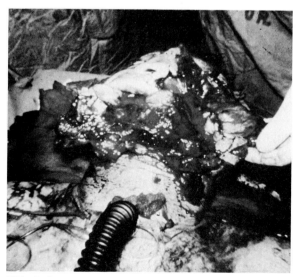

FIG. 8–1. This patient sustained a gunshot wound to his face causing a severe airway problem. The only way to access the trachea was by performing tracheostomy. Cricothyroidotomy would have been an acceptable alternative.

injured patients, since time in the emergency room should be kept to a bare minimum. Patients are more appropriately monitored and ventilated in an intensive care unit or operating room.

To summarize, the priorities with respect to the airway are to clear the upper airway, to administer high-flow oxygen initially with a bag-mask, and to proceed immediately to endotracheal intubation in most cases and surgical airway in a few. Once an airway has been established, hand ventilation with a mask and high-flow oxygen is all that is necessary to assist breathing. Although the preceding procedures tend to maximize certain components of pulmonary gas exchange, they do not totally negate the effects of aspiration, pulmonary contusion, or direct tracheobronchial injury.

CIRCULATION

As noted earlier, just prior to assessing and treating the airway, a quick assessment of the patient is made to determine whether or not shock is present and what its etiology might be. Shock is a clinical diagnosis and should be readily apparent. Traumatic shock has at least two primary causes, hemorrhage and obstructed venous return. This emphasizes the importance of feeling the patient's extremity to ascertain whether or not shock is present and then to assess the neck veins to see whether it is due to hypovolemia or obstructed venous return (Fig. 8–2). A cool, pale extremity with decreased venous filling is clinical shock until proven otherwise. A patient who is in shock with flat neck veins is assumed to have hypovolemic shock. If the neck veins are distended, there are at least five possibilities: tension pneumothorax, pericardial tamponade, air embolism, myocardial contusion, and myocardial infarction. In my experience, myocardial contusion is a rare cause of cardiac failure in patients with trauma in the first 4 h following injury. I have seen only two patients in the emergency room who had cardiogenic shock secondary to myocardial contusion. In contrast, myocardial infarction is not uncommon in elderly persons. There are two

CIRCULATION PRIORITIES

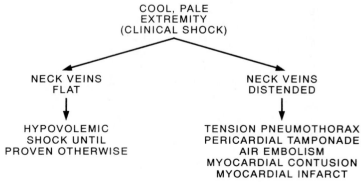

FIG. 8–2. The circulatory priorities based on clinical examination are shown in this algorithm.

possibilities: The patient may have suffered a myocardial infarct and then had his or her accident and sustained injuries, or an elderly patient may have had an accident, sustained minor or modest blood losses, and suffered a myocardial infarct consequent to this hemorrhage. It is prudent in the elderly patient to do a full 12-lead ECG early in the course of assessment and resuscitation.

Tension pneumothorax should always come first in the physician's differential diagnosis of shock caused by obstructed venous obstruction, since it is the easiest life-threatening injury to treat in the emergency department. These patients have percussion tympany and absence of breath sounds on the ipsilateral hemithorax. Because of the mediastinal shift, venous inflow to the heart is occluded from mechanical kinking of the great veins. The same shift may cause the trachea to be shifted from the midline to the contralateral side. A simple tube thoracostomy is the definitive method of management. It is not necessary to obtain an x-ray prior to placement of the chest tube if the diagnosis is clinically obvious. Sometimes, in the preagonal patient, tension pneumothorax may not be obvious, and bilateral tube thoracostomies are warranted. It is necessary to obtain an x-ray after placement of the tube thoracostomy to make sure of its proper position.

Air embolism has come to be appreciated as an important complication in injured patients.[18,19] It consists of air in the systemic circulation and is caused by a bronchopulmonary venous fistula. Air embolus occurs in 4 percent of all patients with major thoracic injuries. In approximately one-third of such patients, air embolism is a result of blunt trauma, usually a laceration of the pulmonary parenchyma by a fractured rib. In the remaining two-thirds, air embolism is a result of gunshot or stab wounds. Unfortunately, the diagnosis is difficult to make. Thus the surgeon must have a high index of suspicion of air embolism whenever thoracic injury has occurred. Any patient who has no obvious head injury but has focal or lateralizing neurologic signs may have air bubbles occluding the cerebral circulation. This can sometimes be confirmed by doing funduscopic examination, where air will be observed in the retinal vessels. Normally, the pressure differential between the pulmonary circulation and the airway is from the pulmonary vein to the bronchus. Not surprisingly, 25 percent of patients with subsequent air embolism have hemoptysis in the emergency room. During resuscitation, the patient may become agitated, grunt, or forcibly expire air against a closed glottis or airway obstruction. This will reverse the pressure differential from the bronchus to the pulmonary vein. Similarly, the patient who is intubated and has positive-pressure ventilation also will have reverse of the pressure differential, allowing air to enter the pulmonary venous circulation. Thus any patient who has a sudden cardiovascular collapse after oral tracheal intubation should be presumed to have air embolism with air in the coronary circulation. Doppler monitoring of an artery has been a useful aid in detecting air embolism. A continuous machinery-like murmur will be heard.

Approximately two-thirds of affected patients have signs or symptoms of air embolism on or shortly after presentation to the emergency room. The remaining one-third usually manifest their symptoms within the first 24 h of admission, although symptoms may occur as late as several days after injury. Those patients who present with signs and symptoms may quickly become agonal, particularly if the air is in the cerebral or coronary circulation. Definitive treatment is immediate thoracotomy, clamping of the hilum of the injured lung to prevent further embolism, and expansion of the intravascular volume. If the patient has already lost spontaneous cardiac activity, the pericardium should be opened immediately and the coronary arteries examined for air. If it is present, internal cardiac massage is started with one hand, and with the other the ascending aorta is grasped with a thumb and index finger for two or three cardiac contractions. This will tend to drive the air out of the coronary vessels. At the same time, the anesthesiologist should administer 1 mg in a 1:10,000 dilution epinephrine down the endotracheal tube in order to achieve systemic hypertension. This will further aid removal of air from the coronary circulation and also help in removing air from the cerebral circulation. It is also prudent to vent the left side of the heart with a needle to remove any residual air that may be in the left atrium or left ventricle. Once resuscitation has been achieved, the pulmonary injury is definitively treated by oversewing of the laceration or resection.

Although pericardial tamponade can occur after blunt trauma, it is encountered most commonly in patients with penetrating injuries to the torso. Approximately 25 percent of all patients with penetrating cardiac injuries reach the emergency room alive. The diagnosis is often obvious. The patient has poor peripheral perfusion (shock) and distended neck veins. A few will have pulsus paradoxus. The great majority will require immediate thoracotomy, preferably in the operating room. In a few patients with penetrating trauma and many patients with blunt trauma, there may be equivocal physical findings. Ultrasonography may help in establishing the diagnosis, and pericardiocentesis is occasionally useful as a diagnostic and therapeutic aid.

Let us return to the other side of the decision tree, where the patient arrives in clinical shock with flat neck veins. In a small percentage of these patients, once volume has been restored, they may manifest one of the diseases causing venous obstruction. However, the great majority will have major hemorrhage as the cause of their shock. I would like to amplify on the signs and symptoms of shock, since it is a clinical diagnosis and dependent on one of the compensatory mechanisms for shock (the redistribution of blood flow). In Fig. 8–3, the signs and symptoms of shock are plotted, showing a progression of depth of shock over time. It should be emphasized that these signs and symptoms do not necessarily occur in a rigid temporal sequence. This will depend on the time in shock and the severity of bleeding.

Seventy percent of our blood volume is stored in capacitance vessels. It is thus easily explained why one of the earliest signs of volume depletion is decreased venous filling in superficial arm and leg veins. The easiest veins to examine are those on the dorsum of the foot or on the back of the hand. I will often strip these veins to see how rapidly they refill. Associated with this finding is early redistribution of blood from skin and muscle to the viscera and vital organs. This will lead to a pale, cool extremity with decreased capillary refill. If the autonomic nervous system is intact, the skin will be clammy. Often these are the only findings in a patient with up to a 20 percent blood volume depletion. As the patient progresses in shock, visceral blood flow is impaired. The first sign of such impairment is the development of oliguria. This emphasizes the need for rapid placement of a Foley catheter early in the course of the resuscitation of trauma patients. Once the bladder has been emptied, urine output should be monitored carefully. Obviously, the urine should be examined for blood and a sample kept for other urinalysis, including toxicology. Between 20 and 40 percent blood volume depletion, not only is oliguria a good sign, but the patient now develops

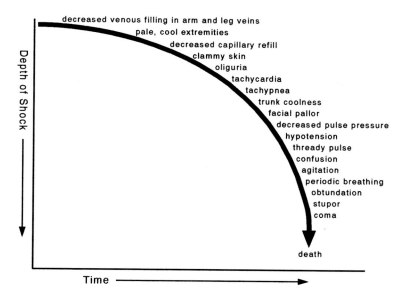

Depth of Shock

decreased venous filling in arm and leg veins
pale, cool extremities
decreased capillary refill
clammy skin
oliguria
tachycardia
tachypnea
trunk coolness
facial pallor
decreased pulse pressure
hypotension
thready pulse
confusion
agitation
periodic breathing
obtundation
stupor
coma

death

Time

DIAGNOSIS OF SHOCK

FIG. 8–3. The redistribution of blood flow causes the major clinical signs of shock. Further compensatory changes in oxygen transport help the clinical assessment.

tachycardia and tachypnea. Blood is diverted from the skin and muscle of the trunk with resulting trunk coolness. Facial pallor is common, and there is decreased pulse pressure. Somewhere between 35 and 45 percent blood volume depletion, depending on whether the patient is a child or adult, hypotension develops. Pulses are thready, and we see the first signs of brain hypoxemia. Plum and Posner,[20] in their classic book, *The Diagnosis of Stupor and Coma,* describe three states of altered consciousness. The first is *clouding of consciousness,* which most often in the trauma patient is manifest by agitation. Although *delirium* is described as an incipient alteration of consciousness, this is most often seen in the trauma patient who is recovering from unconsciousness. *Obtundation* means mental blunting or torpidity. This is common in deep shock and is followed shortly thereafter by *stupor,* which is deep sleep or a patient that can only be aroused by vigorous and repeated stimuli. Just prior to death, the patient lapses into *coma.*

Once hemorrhage has been established as the primary cause of shock, there are four treatment priorities: Gain access to the circulation, obtain a blood sample from the patient, determine where volume loss is occurring, and give fluids for resuscitation. The fastest and most reliable way to gain access to the circulation is by a surgical cutdown on the saphenous vein at the ankle. An incision is made 1 cm above the medial malleolus. Using sharp and blunt technique, longitudinal dissection is carried out along the vein, and a hemostat is rapidly passed around the vein and a silk suture is used to tie the vein distally. An incision is made with a no. 11 blade through the anterior one-third of the vein, the cephalad lip of the incision is then grasped with the hemostat, and a diagonally cut piece of IV tubing is inserted into the vein. If the vein is too small to accept the venous IV tubing, a no. 8 French or no. 5 French feeding tube is cut off diagonally and inserted. A final 4-0 silk tie is then placed on the cephalad part of the vein, securing the tube. The inner diameter of intravenous tubing is approximately 3/16 in, and this allows rapid fluid resuscitation. Alternatively, the resuscitating physician can perform bilateral percutaneous femoral vein cannulation with a large-bore catheter or a no. 8 French introducer, more commonly used for passing a pulmonary artery catheter. Some experienced physicians prefer to gain access through the subclavian or internal jugular vein, but this approach is associated with a higher frequency of pneumothorax. I prefer to start my resuscitation with a peripheral line, and after 2 liters of Ringer's lactate have been infused, a central line is placed to monitor further resuscitation. The line size and incision may be modified for younger patients. A surgical cutdown of the saphenous vein at the groin ensures access with a large tube in the child or neonate.

As soon as the first intravenous line has been established, baseline blood work should be undertaken; it should include the hematocrit, toxicologic screening, blood typing and crossmatching, and a screening battery of laboratory tests if the patient is elderly or has premorbid conditions. An arterial blood gas determination should be performed at approximately the same time, and this not only will give baseline information but also will serve as a guide for subsequent resuscitation, including necessary correction of acidosis.

The third priority is to determine where occult blood loss is occurring. Many times the blood loss is obvious, and paramedics or family can be of great assistance in documenting how much blood was at the scene or if there was active arterial bleeding from an extremity or facial wound. In many instances, however, the blood loss is occult. The three sites of hidden blood loss are the pleural cavities, the thigh, and the abdomen, including the retroperitoneum and pelvis. Rapid chest radiography will quickly eliminate either pleural cavity as a source of hidden blood loss (Figs. 8–4 and 8–5). A fractured femur should be clinically obvious. In contrast, assessment of the abdomen on the basis of physical findings can be extremely misleading. Fifty percent of patients with substantial hemoperitoneum have no clinical signs.[21,22] Common sense dictates that if the patient's chest film is normal and the femur is not fractured, the patient who remains in shock must be suspected of having ongoing hemorrhage in the abdomen or pelvis. Most such patients require immediate celiotomy if death from hemorrhage is to be averted. If the patient is hemodynamically unstable, they should not be taken to CT scan. Diagnostic peritoneal lavage is a test that can be performed to determine intraperitoneal hemorrhage, but it may not help with retroperitoneal hemorrhage. The fourth and final volume priority for the resuscitating physician is to administer fluids for resuscitation, beginning with balanced salt solution and adding type-specific whole blood as soon as possible.[23,24] Type O blood should be given to the patient with exsanguination, whereas in the case of a stable patient, it is more prudent to wait for either type-specific or typed and crossmatched blood.

Although whole blood is preferable, it is difficult to obtain from modern blood banks; thus the use of blood components may be the only choice. In patients with limited blood loss, the infusion of balanced salt solution and packed red

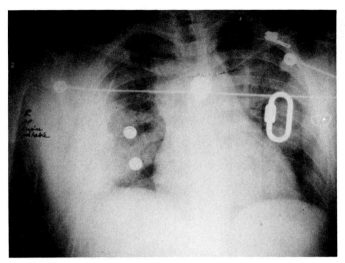

FIG. 8–4. This young man was involved in a high-speed motor vehicle accident. When he arrived in the emergency room, he was in clinical shock with flat neck veins. There were no femur fractures. The chest radiograph shows significant right chest injuries (multiple rib fractures, pulmonary contusion, extrapleural blood) but not enough intrapleural blood to explain his shock. Thus the most likely source of hidden blood loss is within the abdominal cavity, and the most likely organ injured is the liver because of the right-sided chest injury. This was confirmed at immediate celiotomy.

cells is all that is required. In those patients with extensive hemorrhage who require massive transfusion (more than 1 blood volume), administration of blood components must be guided by monitoring of specific defects such as thrombocytopenia, hypofibrinogenemia, and factor V or factor VIII deficiency.

The criteria for adequate resuscitation are simple and straightforward: Keep atrial filling pressure at normal levels, give sufficient fluid to achieve adequate urinary output (0.5 ml/kg/h per body weight in adults, 1.0 ml/kg/h in children), and maintain peripheral perfusion. The only practical way to measure atrial filling pressure in the emergency room and immediately in the operating room is by monitoring central venous pressure. In elderly patients with extensive traumatic injuries, it may be prudent to place a pulmonary artery catheter immediately, since it can be used to direct a sophisticated, multifactorial resuscitation effort in the operating room or in the intensive care unit. Resuscitation should be directed toward achieving adequate delivery and consumption of oxygen. An important caveat is not to delay necessary therapeutic interventions or lifesaving surgery to obtain noncritical diagnostic tests. Urinary output is a good index of visceral blood flow, provided there is no antecedent renal disease or administration of drugs that would alter urinary output, such as osmotic diuretics (sugar, mannitol) or diagnostic intravenous contrast agents. Although good peripheral

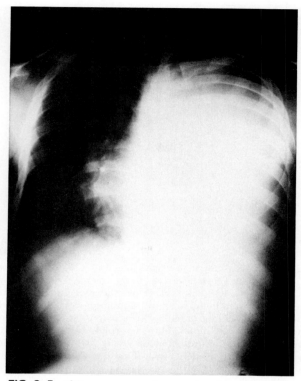

FIG. 8–5. This young man also was involved in a motor vehicle accident and was in clinical shock with flat neck veins. The chest radiograph shows significant blood loss into the left pleural cavity. This blood should be considered for autotransfusion. The pitfall in the management of this patient is to proceed immediately to left thoracotomy. Prior to thoracotomy, a quick exploratory celiotomy should be done to rule out ruptured left hemidiaphragm with blood in the left pleural cavity coming from the abdomen. If the celiotomy is negative, a left anterolateral thoracotomy can be done promptly.

perfusion is desirable, it may take several hours to achieve optimal resuscitation, since venoconstriction may persist and be aggravated by hypothermia or repeated hypotensive episodes.

There has been continuous controversy as to whether or not acellular colloids such as albumin, dextran, or starch have any role in the resuscitation of the acutely injured patient. In my opinion, they do not. I am led to this conclusion by simply examining the forces that make up Starling's law of the capillary. Some of the values for Starling's equation have not been measured directly; however, estimates are available. These are shown in Fig. 8–6. When there is normal permeability, a reflection coefficient is equal to 0.8 to 0.9. One can appreciate that if hydrostatic force is increased to supranormal levels, this will cause a fluid shift into the extravascular space. If one were to give acellular

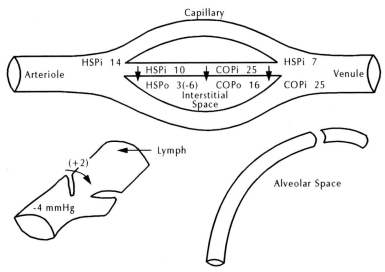

FIG. 8–6. Starling's law of the capillary is illustrated. HSP$_i$ is hydrostatic pressure inside the capillary. HSP$_o$ is hydrostatic pressure outside the capillary; COP$_i$ is colloid pressure inside the capillary; COP$_o$ is colloid pressure outside the capillary. The actual or estimated values are shown. Estimates for HSP$_o$ vary from 3 to -6 mmHg.

colloid when permeability is normal, it still has a measured escape rate from the vascular space, which would then increase pulmonary lymphatic flow. In a healthy individual, giving acellular colloid solutions has minimal, if any, benefit. If there is an increased permeability, the reflection coefficient is usually 0.5. Under these circumstances, any attempt at giving acellular colloid will simply aggravate the escape rate and increase extravascular fluid. If the patient has pulmonary contusion or aspiration, pulmonary lymphatics may be damaged, which will increase extravascular fluid accumulation. One can also appreciate that by treating the patient with positive end-expiratory pressure, the resuscitating physician may have to compensate for the change in intrathoracic pressure by increasing the hydrostatic force within the capillaries.

Another controversy that arises during fluid resuscitation is the amount of blood that needs to be given. Arguments for not giving or minimizing the amount of blood include (1) the risk of viral transmission of disease, (2) transfusion reactions, (3) an immunosuppressive effect of homologous transfusions, and (4) a lower hematocrit is associated with reduced viscosity and improved flow in the microcirculation. The risk of transmission of disease by blood-borne viruses is truly a concern, and all surgeons will weigh this risk in determining the need for transfusion following shock. The risk of transfusion reaction should be minimal if a hospital has modern blood banking and established procedures for transfusions. The immunosuppressive effect of homologous blood is probably minimal compared with the benefits in almost all shock situations. The benefit from reduction in viscosity achieved by hemodilution during shock resuscitation is probably more theoretical than practical.

It is my opinion that the overriding concern in blood replacement is achieving the optimal hemoglobin concentration for the *individual* patient. There is a linear relationship between hemoglobin concentration [Hgb] and O_2 delivery. An increase in [Hgb] from 10 to 15 g/dl increases the oxygen transported when the [Hgb] is fully saturated by 50 percent. During acute resuscitation, it is more practical to measure the hematocrit, and in a previously healthy young person, it is relatively safe to allow the hematocrit to approach 25. However, one must be cognizant of other oxygen transport factors that may be damaged or impaired. In the older patient or patients with depressed cardiopulmonary function, it is prudent to keep the hematocrit as close to normal as possible. Once the patient reaches the intensive care unit, more sophisticated monitoring may be initiated, such as O_2 delivery or on-line venous oximetry.

NEUROLOGIC ASSESSMENT

The final priority during primary assessment and initial resuscitation is to assess neurologic status and to initiate diagnostic and therapeutic procedures. There are six key components to a rapid neurologic evaluation: level of consciousness, size and reactivity of the pupils, eye movements and oculovestibular responses, skeletal muscle motor responses, pattern of breathing, and peripheral sensory function. In most trauma systems, prehospital personnel, emergency room physicians, and nurses use the Glasgow coma scale so that comparisons can be made of neurologic function in the prehospital and hospital settings. The major disadvantages of the Glasgow coma scale are the inability to take into consideration lateral and focal neurologic findings and to more precisely determine the level of consciousness and the contribution made by drugs and alcohol. Nevertheless, the Glasgow coma scale is an easy and reproducible scale that can be determined from the six components mentioned above.

The assessment of neurologic status is important for two fundamental reasons. A resuscitating surgeon must determine whether or not the patient has a mass lesion, since this will immediately direct the treatment priorities. A corollary to this primary assessment is to determine the contribution of secondary injury from hypoxia or hypovolemia. There have been two studies in the past 10 years that have emphasized the importance of secondary injury.[25,26] The first study, in 1982 from the Medical College of Virginia, showed that 50 percent of patients diagnosed as having closed head injury in fact had either hypoxia or hypotension as an explanation for their neurologic symptoms.[25] A more recent study, in 1989, showed that 43 percent of patients with a diagnosis of closed head injury had either hypoxia or hypovolemia as the cause of their neurologic injury.[26]

A decreasing level of consciousness is the single most reliable indication that the patient has had a serious head injury or secondary insult (usually hypoxic or hypotensive) to the brain. Consciousness has two components—awareness and arousal. *Awareness* is manifested by goal-directed or purposeful behavior. The use of language is an indication of functioning cerebral hemispheres. If the patient attempts to protect himself or herself from a painful insult, this also implies cortical function. *Arousal* is a crude function equivalent to simple wakefulness. Opening the eyes, either spontaneously or in response to stimuli, is indicative of arousal and is a brainstem function. In coma, both awareness and arousal are absent; eye opening does not occur, there is no comprehensible speech, and the extremities move neither on command nor appropriately in response to noxious stimuli.

The size and reactivity of the pupils are extremely important because they may be the first clue the examining physician can obtain that there are lateral or focal neurologic findings. Pupil size and reactivity in combination with the skeletal muscle motor response are important signs to determine if a mass lesion is present. The oculovestibular response is assessed by the cold caloric test, since "dolls eyes" would be inappropriate in the trauma patient. Pattern of breathing and peripheral sensory function are also useful findings in this minineurologic examination. The physician must assess all six components of neurologic status and make sure the four primary reflexes (ankle, bone, biceps, and triceps) are assessed, and this examination should be repeated at frequent intervals. In this way it is possible to both diagnose and monitor the neurologic status in the emergency department. An improving neurologic status reassures the physician that resuscitation is improving cerebral blood flow. Neurologic deterioration is strong presumptive evidence of either a mass lesion or important neurologic injury. Computed tomographic (CT) scanning of the head is the preferred technique for diagnosing head injury and should be performed as soon as possible.[27] In the patient who is hemorrhaging to death without focal or lateralizing neurologic signs, it is more important to take the patient immediately to surgery and stop the hemorrhage. Further neurologic assessment, including CT examination, can be performed after the lifesaving surgery for hemorrhage. If the patient has exsanguinating hemorrhage and has focal or lateralizing neurologic signs, an option is for the general surgeon to do the lifesaving surgery on the torso at the same time the neurosurgeon performs exploratory burr holes based on the neurologic examination.

There are certain minimal diagnostic studies that should be considered when the patient is hemodynamically unstable during the primary survey and initial resuscitation. These diagnostic studies include the chest x-ray, lateral film of the cervical spine, plain film of the pelvis, and a single-shot intravenous pyelogram. The chest x-ray is extremely important, and the only time it is not performed is when the patient has had an emergency thoracotomy in the emergency department. The chest x-ray gives the resuscitating surgeon tremendous information regarding volume status and undetected intrathoracic injuries, including hemothorax, pneumothorax, and pulmonary contusion. The lateral cervical spine film is not necessary in every patient, since it is only effective in diagnosing approximately 89 percent of cervical injuries. A negative lateral cervical spine film does not allow the physician to remove protective collars or sandbags during lifesaving surgery. One could argue that if it takes too much time to obtain the film, it is better just to leave the patient protected and to make the necessary diagnostic studies after lifesaving surgery. A plain film of the pelvis can be helpful, particularly when the abdomen is the source of life-threatening hemorrhage. When the patient is explored, if there is a huge retroperitoneal pelvic hematoma, this may be best left unopened until after assessment by arteriogram and/or placement of external fixation devices. A single-shot intravenous pyelogram during the resuscitation adds very little to the time in the emergency department. The information obtained, however, can be extremely helpful once the abdomen is explored. For example, if the patient has a retroperitoneal hematoma in association with one of the kidneys and no contrast material has been seen on that side, one would suspect a renal vascular injury. It must be emphasized that resuscitation should not cease during these films, and the resuscitation team must wear protective lead aprons. Optimally, the x-ray facilities will be close to the emergency department; if necessary, however, the basic x-rays can be obtained with a portable machine. Some hospitals have already installed rapid CT machines either in the resuscitation area or near it in order to facilitate and expedite diagnostic studies, particularly CT scans of the brain. It must be emphasized that if a hemodynamically unstable patient arrives and fails to stabilize during the primary assessment and initial resuscitation, further diagnostic studies and resuscitation must be carried out in the operating room during or after lifesaving surgery.

SECONDARY SURVEY AND CONTINUING RESUSCITATION

If the patient becomes hemodynamically stable during the initial phase of assessment and resuscitation, it is then appropriate to perform diagnostic studies as indicated to determine surgical priorities. The first few minutes of the secondary survey should be devoted to doing a complete physical examination beginning with the top of the patient and proceeding caudal to the lower extremities. Starting with the head, the patient's neurologic examination should be repeated, checking for pupillary signs and any lateralizing signs. Eye injuries should be looked for, including lens dislocation or penetrating injuries involving the canthus or lacrimal apparatus. A quick check for visual acuity should be performed. The patient should be asked to bite down for malocclusion. The facial bones should be palpated, including gently lifting up on the anterior maxilla using the front teeth as a fulcrum. If a nasogastric tube is indicated and there are associated maxillofacial fractures, the safest route is through the oropharynx.

A more thorough examination of the cervical spine, palpating the spinous processes or having the patient gently lift his or her head off the table or move the chin laterally against pressure, will determine if there is pain. None of these procedures should be performed if the patient is under the influence of drugs or alcohol. If the patient has a penetrating wound to the neck, this may direct the surgeon to perform other diagnostic studies, including arteriography, bronchoscopy, esophagoscopy, and esophagography.

A thorough examination of the chest includes log-rolling the patient to completely examine the back for open wounds and to palpate the spinous processes and the paraspinous muscles. Complete auscultation should be carried out, and the chest wall gently palpated, checking for evidence of rib fractures or sternal injury. As mentioned earlier, patients who present with hypovolemia and undergo successful resuscitation may then manifest evidence of venous obstruction which could be due to tension pneumothorax or pericardial tamponade. Changes in the status of the neck veins or auscultatory findings will often be the first clue that such injuries exist.

Examination of the abdomen can be extremely difficult, and as mentioned earlier, approximately 50 percent of occult bleeding into the peritoneal cavity is missed on physical examination. Most often the examiner is looking for associated findings such as rib tenderness on the left side, which has an approximately 20 percent incidence of associated rupture to the spleen. Fractured ribs on the lower right chest have an incidence of approximately 10 percent associated injury to the liver. Similarly, pelvic fractures are often the only clue that there is injury to the bladder or bowel. Seatbelt marks are very presumptive evidence that significant visceral injury has taken place. Repeated examination of the abdomen, including serial hematocrits, white blood counts, amylase determinations, and special diagnostic studies, should be carried out during this period of the secondary survey. If a rectal examination has not already been done, it should be done at this time. This includes testing stool for the presence of blood and checking the location of the prostate. The quality of the sphincter tone should be noted and may be the first clue in the unconscious patient that there is associated paralysis.

All four extremities should next be evaluated for contusions and deformity, and their pulses should be assessed. Particular attention should be paid to the joints and whether or not dislocation has taken place. Tenderness, crepitation, or abnormal movements along the shaft of the bone help identify fractures. The iliac wings of the pelvis should be compressed, checking for pain and crepitence. Soft tissue injuries, including those in proximity to major vessels, should be noted and may warrant further diagnostic studies.

The six components of the neurologic examination should be checked and rechecked during the stay in the emergency department. If there has been any history of loss of consciousness, this may direct the physician to do further diagnostic studies[27] or consider admission to a monitored ward for observation.

Penetrating injuries to the upper torso that have a normal chest x-ray will usually be observed for a period of time. Injuries to the lower torso (nipple to pubis) will require either celiotomy or observation. Wounds in the flank can be assessed by celiotomy or double-contrast CT examination. Posterior wounds do not have a high incidence of entering the peritoneum or causing other visceral injury. Nevertheless, these patients may require observation, double-contrast CT examination, or celiotomy if there are clear indications of visceral damage. Laparoscopy may prove useful in ruling out intraperitoneal injury.

For patients with blunt torso trauma, there are certain special diagnostic studies that must be considered while the patient is in the emergency room. These are listed in Table 8–2. In general, I favor doing contrast studies of the genitourinary tract from distal to proximal (Fig. 8–7). If the patient has gross urethral meatus blood, hematoma within the scrotum, perineal wounds, anterior pelvic

TABLE 8–2. Torso Trauma: Special Diagnostic Studies

Urethrogram
Cystogram—2 views
Pyelogram
Gastrograffin swallow
Arteriogram
CT

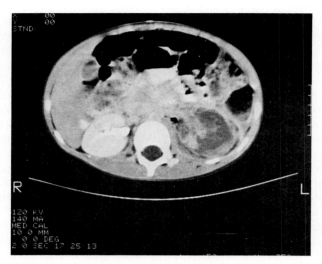

FIG. 8–7. This patient was involved in a motor vehicle accident with significant torso trauma. The CT scan shows a renovascular injury with minimal perfusion of the parenchyma of the left kidney. This was confirmed at exploratory celiotomy.

fractures, or a dislocated prostate, a retrograde urethrogram is indicated. If resistance is met when passing the Foley catheter, then leave it in place and perform a urethrogram. If the Foley catheter passes with ease and the first urine sample is grossly bloody, I would perform a two-view cystogram. This might include an anteroposterior lateral, anteroposterior oblique, or anteroposterior voiding urethrogram. If one obtains only one view, 40 percent of bladder ruptures will be missed. It also should be noted that CT scan is not sensitive for ruptured bladder. If the urethrogram and cystogram are normal and microscopic or gross hematuria exists, the next test would either be an intravenous pyelogram or CT examination of the kidney. Increasingly, I have relied on the CT scan because of its ability to pick up parenchymal defects as well as renal vascular injuries.

If the patient presents with blunt torso trauma and a history of epigastric pain either from assault or the steering column, the minimum test that I will perform is a gastrograffin swallow. The purpose of this swallow is to evaluate the duodenum and whether or not there is swelling in the head of the pancreas. A better diagnostic study is a CT scan, which will give more information and will allow the surgeon to make decisions as to whether or not operation is indicated.

CT scan has become my procedure of choice in evaluation of the abdomen in the hemodynamically stable patient. In many ways, CT fulfills some of the criteria of an ideal diagnostic modality. Not only does it assess intraperitoneal structures, but it also may diagnose retroperitoneal and intrathoracic injuries. This study is qualitative and quantitative. It demonstrates which organ is injured, and it also gives a rough estimate of the amount of blood within the peritoneal cavity, retroperitoneal area, and pelvic space (Fig. 8–8). In addition, CT has made

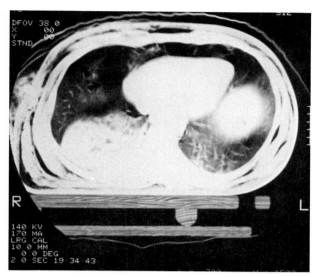

FIG. 8–8. This CT scan was obtained in a young man following epigastric trauma from a steering wheel. The CT shows a significant pneumothorax that was not present on plain chest radiograph. Plain x-rays of the chest miss approximately 10 percent of all pneumothoraces.

grading of injuries possible, particularly those of the liver, spleen, and kidney (Fig. 8–9).

CT is not without its problems. Early experience showed that the resolution of the various scanners was fairly disparate. It has become evident that fast-sequencing machines are necessary and, probably most important of all, that the presence of a senior radiologist is required. In many of the studies currently cited in the literature, a senior radiologist was not present to help perform the CT studies and interpret the results, a problem that usually occurred late at night.[28] This situation has led to a number of misdiagnoses and inadequate studies. One could argue that if CT is so dependent on a nonsurgical specialist, it is not worthwhile to have CT in a busy trauma center. The counterargument is that a general surgeon with experience can become at least 90 percent accurate. The fact that CT has varying sensitivity, specificity, and accuracy with various intraabdominal and retroperitoneal organs is also now appreciated. For example, CT of the pancreas has only an 85 percent sensitivity rate, partly because of the time it takes for the pancreas to manifest injury, particularly periglandular edema. This lower sensitivity rate is not too dissimilar from that of the brain, in which approximately 12 to 15 percent of the injuries may take 6 to 12 h to manifest signs on a CT scan. Diaphragmatic and urinary bladder injuries also may be missed on CT examination. Considerable controversy exists about the diagnostic accuracy and sensitivity of CT for hollow viscus injury such as may occur in the small bowel or colon. Some studies report high sensitivity and accuracy, and others report only modest results.[29] In many instances, the enthusiasm and support provided by senior radiologists are what make the difference. If the surgeon feels uncomfortable with CT in his or her hospital, an alternative is to continue doing

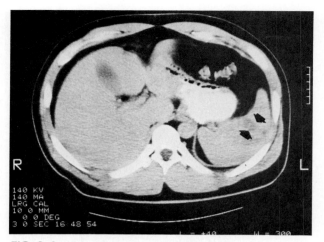

FIG. 8–9. This CT scan of the abdomen was obtained in a young man after a motor vehicle accident. The arrows show a transverse fracture through the spleen (grade 2), and further views showed less than 300 cc of blood (estimated) in the abdomen. Nonoperative management was successful.

diagnostic peritoneal lavage. It must be recognized, however, that diagnostic peritoneal lavage will not diagnose retroperitoneal injuries, and the sensitivity may lead to nontherapeutic celiotomy in 5 to 20 percent of patients. Ultrasonography has become very popular in Europe as a substitute for diagnostic peritoneal lavage.

The final diagnostic study to be considered in torso injury is the arteriogram. This is indicated primarily in patients with a widened mediastinum. This will be discussed further in the next section. Arteriograms also may be indicated if the renovascular injury is suspected and in patients with extensive hemorrhage from pelvic trauma. In this latter instance, the pelvic arteriogram is not only diagnostic but also may be therapeutic in that embolization may be employed.

SURGICAL PRIORITIES

Patients who need lifesaving surgery immediately after their primary assessment and initial resuscitation have priorities no different from those in a hemodynamically stable patient.[30] Brain injury always takes first priority. As pointed out earlier, the critical decision is whether the patient has a mass lesion. Sometimes the trauma surgeon has a strong clinical suspicion. A classic example is the patient who arrives at the hospital unconscious, with a blown pupil, eighth nerve intact, and an associated contralateral hemiparesis. This leads to a strong presumptive clinical diagnosis of uncal herniation. A minority of neurosurgeons would advocate taking such a patient to the operating room immediately to make a burr hole on the side of the dilated pupil to decompress the mass lesion if found. The general surgeon would simultaneously operate on life-threatening torso hemorrhage. If the neurosurgeons do not find a mass lesion on the side of the blown pupil, the procedure is repeated on the opposite side. If still no lesion is found, after the torso surgery the patient is sent for a CT scan (under the same anesthetic) to look for an intracerebral hematoma, which would then have to be decompressed in the operating room. If no mass lesion is found, an intracerebral pressure monitor is placed. The rationale for immediate operative intervention is that time is critical, and diagnostic studies would delay the operation for hemorrhage. However, the majority of neurosurgeons would send such a patient for a CT scan before operating. If no mass lesion shows on CT, they would place an intracerebral ICP monitor and repeat the scan in 6 to 8 h to pick up that minority of patients in whom the injury takes time to show on the CT scan. If a mass lesion appears on the initial CT scan, the patient needs immediate decompression. Deterioration of neurologic signs during resuscitation is also presumptive evidence of a mass lesion. It cannot be overemphasized that during the initial resuscitation the surgeon is responsible for preventing secondary injury to the brain from hypoxia or hypovolemia.

Patients do not usually present with single-organ injuries. Head injury is usually accompanied by torso, maxillofacial, or extremity trauma. Thus some injuries may have to be managed simultaneously and require two and sometimes even three surgical teams. In the case of head injury and torso trauma, mass lesions still take priority. At the same time that neurosurgical decompression is being carried out, the trauma to the torso can be addressed by the general surgeon. A chest x-ray can determine in which torso cavity the blood loss is occurring. In general, lower torso injuries take priority over upper torso injuries, since upper torso injuries are often low-pressure vascular injuries (lung parenchyma). Aggressive bleeding invariably takes place in the abdomen. If the chest x-ray shows a massive hemothorax, one caution must be exercised. This sometimes represents rupture of the diaphragm with decompression of blood from the abdomen into the pleural cavity. In no instance should a patient be placed in a position other than the supine position prior to ruling out intraabdominal injury.

In patients with multiple injuries and a widened mediastinum, mass lesion is still the number one priority. If the patient arrives in shock, the shock is not due to the widened mediastinum, and other causes must be sought. Most often the bleeding is into the peritoneal or retroperitoneal space. Therefore, exploratory celiotomy is indicated prior to performing the arteriogram. The anesthesiologist has an important role during the celiotomy and subsequent arteriogram, since the patient must not be allowed to become hypertensive. Once life-threatening hemorrhage has been controlled, the patient is taken to the arteriogram suite under the same anesthetic, and the arteriogram is obtained. If there is a contained rupture of the thoracic aorta, the patient is returned to the operating room, and the injury is repaired through a posterolateral thoracotomy. If the patient arrives in the emergency room with multiple injuries and a widened mediastinum but not in shock, an arteriogram is obtained after the initial resuscitation. If this confirms a contained rupture, repair should not be carried out until abdominal bleeding has been ruled out. This requires either diagnostic peritoneal lavage, CT scan, or celiotomy prior to the thoracotomy.

The timing of repair of orthopedic injuries is one of the most important concepts introduced to trauma management in the last 10 years.[30] In general, all orthopedic injuries should be fixed at the first operation after head and torso injuries have been addressed. Exceptions to this general rule are those patients who develop hypothermia or coagulopathy or who are hemodynamically unstable after the torso and head injuries have been addressed. In this instance, the patient should be taken to the intensive care unit, the coagulopathy corrected, and the patient warmed and returned to the operating room as soon as possible to correct the orthopedic injuries. This concept is extremely important, since it has been shown that early mobilization of the multiply injured patient reduces pulmonary complications and the incidence of other organ failure.[31] This concept also illustrates the importance of the entire trauma team and particularly of the anesthesiologist. During prolonged operations to correct head, torso, and orthopedic injuries, the anesthesiologist must continue the resuscitation, ventilation, blood replacement, and monitoring equivalent to what is provided in an intensive care setting.

Patients with multiple injuries and pelvic fractures can be particularly vexing. Mass lesions still take priority. Control of other hemorrhage within the torso is the number two priority. Pelvic hemorrhage can be massive and must be addressed almost simultaneously with other torso hemorrhage, such as liver or spleen. In some instances this also may require early temporary external fixation of the anterior pelvis and consideration for a posterior plate or percutaneous lag screw of the sacroiliac joint in order to minimize venous hemorrhage. At the same time, it is imperative that the surgeon rule out significant pelvic arterial bleeding, which occurs in approximately 15 percent of pelvic fractures. This arterial hemorrhage can only be ruled out by performing an arteriogram as soon as possible following the initial resuscitation. If an arterial bleeder is found, it is usually found off the branches of the internal iliac artery. By far the great majority of these can be treated with embolization, and only 2 to 5 percent require operative intervention. Operative intervention is indicated if there are larger branches of the iliac system involved with a laceration. Internal fixation of pelvic fractures is usually delayed for 3 to 4 days following the injury. It must be emphasized that associated genitourinary injuries must be ruled out prior to operative intervention, since approximately one-third of patients with significant pelvic fractures have an associated genitourinary injury.

Compound pelvic fractures are particularly problematic. Strong consideration should be given to diversion of the fecal stream in order to minimize soiling of the pelvic wound by stool in the postinjury period. The presence of an associated genitourinary injury or a compound pelvic fracture can make decision making easier for the surgeon. Both these associated injuries usually require celiotomy. Thus the surgeon does not need to do additional diagnostic studies to rule out intraperitoneal bleeding once a compound fracture or genitourinary injury is appreciated.

In patients with multiple injuries who also have a peripheral vascular injury, the priorities are mass lesion, torso trauma, and then peripheral vascular injury. Often, however, the patient must be assigned double teams, with one surgical team repairing the neurologic injury and the other team working on the peripheral vascular injury or one team handling the torso injury and the other team handling the peripheral vascular injury. Some surgeons feel that orthopedic stabilization takes priority over peripheral vascular repair; however, I feel that the peripheral vascular injury takes priority over the orthopedic injury. It has been my experience that the peripheral vascular repair will not be disrupted by a careful orthopedic surgeon.

Maxillofacial injuries usually take last priority in operative management. Many maxillofacial surgeons want to wait 3 to 5 days following injury to minimize the amount of edema within the tissue, thus making operative repair easier. The only maxillofacial injury that takes immediate priority is the associated airway problem.

SUMMARY

Hypovolemic shock is uncommon compared with traumatic shock. A ruptured aneurysm or bleeding duodenal ulcer does represent "pure" hypovolemic shock. More commonly, the surgeon encounters patients with multiple injuries in whom hemorrhage is the underlying problem made worse by the tissue injury. It is the combination of tissue injury and shock that activates the inflammatory cascade and wound healing which may lead to the problems in the postinjury period of sequential or multiple organ failure. Diagnosis and treatment of traumatic shock are complex and require fairly rigid adherence to a protocol such as ATLS in order not to miss occult injuries and to establish priorities in the surgical management of these multiply injured patients.

REFERENCES

1. Cannon WB: *Traumatic Shock.* New York, D Appleton, 1923.
2. Wiggers CJ: The present status of the shock problem. *Physiol Rev* 22:74, 1942.
3. Gross SD: *A System of Surgery: Pathological, Diagnostic, Therapeutic, and Operative,* vol 1, 5th ed. Philadelphia, Henry C Lea, 1872, p 426.
4. Hunter J: *Treatise on the Blood, Inflammation, in Gunshot Wounds.* Birmingham, Classics of Surgery Library, 1985, p 249.
5. Travers B: *An Inquiry Concerning that Disturbed State of the Vital Functions Usually Denominated Constitutional Irritation.* New York, H Stevenson, 1826, p 38.
6. Malcolm AD: *The Physiology of Death from Traumatic Fever.* London, J & A Churchill, 1893, p 20.
7. Finch CA, Lenfant C: Oxygen transport in man. *N Engl J Med* 286:407, 1972.
8. Glantz SA, Misbach GA, Moores WY, et al: The pericardium substantially affects the left ventricular diastolic pressure volume relationship in the dog. *Circ Res* 42:433, 1978.
9. Hoffman MJ, Greenfield LJ, Sugarman HJ, et al: Unsuspected right ventricular dysfunction in shock and sepsis. *Ann Surg* 198:307, 1983.
10. Stürm JA, Lewis FR, Trentz O, et al: Cardiopulmonary parameters and prognosis after severe multiple trauma. *J Trauma* 19:305, 1979.
11. Lucas CE: Renal considerations in the injured patient. *Surg Clin North Am* 62:133, 1982.
12. Eastman AB, West JG: Field triage. In EE Moore, KL Mattox, DV Feliciano (eds): *Trauma* Norwalk, CT, Appleton & Lange, 1991, pp 67–79.
13. *Advanced Trauma Life Support Program.* Chicago, American College of Surgeons, 1989.
14. Jacobs LM, Berrizbeitia LD, Bennett B, Madigan C: Endotracheal intubation in the prehospital phase of emergency medical care. *JAMA* 250:2175, 1983.

15. Bone LB, Johnson KD, Weigelt J, et al: Early vs delayed stabilization of femoral fractures: A prospective, randomized trial. *J Bone Joint Surg* 71A:336, 1989.

16. Taryle DA, Chandler JE, Good JT Jr, et al: Emergency room intubations: Complications and survival. *Chest* 75:541, 1979.

17. Myers EM, Iko BO: Management of acute laryngeal trauma. *J Trauma* 27:448, 1987.

18. Thomas AN, Stevens BG: Air embolism: A cause of morbidity and death after penetrating chest trauma. *J Trauma* 14:633, 1974.

19. Yee ES, Verrier ED, Thomas AN: Management of air embolism in blunt and penetrating thoracic trauma. *J Thorac Cardiovasc Surg* 85:661, 1983.

20. Plum F, Posner JB: *The Diagnosis of Stupor and Coma*, 3d ed. Philadelphia, FA Davis, 1985.

21. Bivins BA, Sachatello CR, Daugherty ME, et al: Diagnostic peritoneal lavage is superior to clinical evaluation in blunt abdominal trauma. *Am Surg* 44:637, 1978.

22. Olson WR, Hildreth DH: Abdominal pericentesis and peritoneal lavage in blunt abdominal trauma. *J Trauma* 11:824, 1971.

23. Loong ED, Law PR, Healey JN: Fresh blood by direct transfusion for hemostatic failure in massive hemorrhage. *Anesth Intensive Care* 9:371, 1981.

24. Shapiro M: Blood transfusion practice: Facts and fallacies. *S Afr Med J* 50:105, 1976.

25. Gildenberg PL, Makela M: Effect of early intubation and ventilation on outcome following head injury. In Dacy RG (ed): *Trauma of the Nervous System*. New York, Raven Press, 1985, pp 79–90.

26. Shackford SR, Mackersie RC, Davis JW, et al: Epidemiology and pathology of traumatic deaths occurring at a level I trauma center in a regionalized system: The importance of secondary brain injury. *J Trauma* 29:1392, 1989.

27. Stein SC, Ross SE: Mild head injury: A plea for routine early CT scanning. *J Trauma* 33:11, 1992.

28. Trunkey DD, Federle MP: Computed tomography in perspective. *J Trauma* 26:660, 1986.

29. Donohue JH, Federle MP, Griffiths VG, Trunkey DD: Computed tomography and the diagnosis of blunt intestinal and mesenteric injuries. *J Trauma* 27:11, 1987.

30. Trunkey D: Initial treatment of patients with extensive trauma. *N Engl J Med* 324:1259, 1991.

31. Seibel R, LaDuca J, Hassett JM, et al: Blunt multiple trauma (ISS 36), femur traction, and the pulmonary failure septic state. *Ann Surg* 202:283, 1985.

9

CARDIOGENIC SHOCK

Alan R. Hartman
Wayne Lipson

Cardiogenic shock may be defined as insufficient blood flow to vital organs caused by inadequate cardiac output. Impaired cardiac function can follow impaired filling (cardiac compressive shock) or impaired cardiac pump function (cardiogenic shock). Both types of shock lead to insufficient blood flow to vital organs. This may result in hypotension, ischemia, organ failure, and eventually, death. Cardiogenic shock has as its common denominator inadequate cardiac output despite normal filling pressures. Clearly, adequate blood flow needs to be separately defined for individual patients, but generally, it is the flow of blood that will prevent organ ischemia and allow for normal organ function. Similarly, adequate filling pressures vary but may be defined generally as the pressure generated by a volume of blood sufficient to cause adequate stretch of the myocardial fibers. Optimal pressures are related to those volumes of blood which cause the degree of myocardial stretch that maximizes cardiac output.

Cardiogenic shock can be defined as a primary abnormality of the heart resulting in impairment of cardiac function. Etiologies include arrhythmia, myocardial failure, valvular or septal defects, cardiomyopathy, and trauma. *Cardiac compressive shock* can be defined as compression of the heart or great veins which decreases ventricular end diastolic volumes. Etiologies include pericardial tamponade, tension pneumothorax, mechanical ventilation, and increased intra-abdominal pressure (Table 9–1).

Although both these types of shock may produce hypotension and inadequate tissue perfusion, there are clinical signs that can immediately aid in differentiating one etiology from another and consequently guide therapy. This chapter will focus on shock caused by (1) primary impairment of the heart and (2) compression of the heart or great veins, each leading to insufficient cardiac output.

TABLE 9–1. Cardiac Derangements that Result in Shock

Type of Shock	Cardiac Derangement	Pathophysiology

Cardiogenic	Arrhythmias
	Heart failure
	   Primary myocardial disease
	   Coronary insufficiency
	   Air embolus
	Valvular dysfunction
	Elevated systemic or
	   pulmonary arterial
	   resistance
		Ineffective pumping of blood because of intrinsic abnormality of heart or vasculature; poor cardiac index and inadequate delivery of oxygen to the tissues

Cardiac compressive	Cardiac tamponade
	Tension pneumothorax
	Positive pressure ventilation
	Ruptured diaphragm with
	   direct compression of heart
	   by abdominal viscera
	Elevated diaphragm
	Ascites
	Abdominal bleeding
	External compression of
	   abdomen (e.g., by inflation
	   of pneumatic antishock
	   garment)
		Compression of interior and superior venae cavae, with limitation of ventricular filling, diminution of end-diastolic volumes and decreased stroke volume
		Compression of atria and right ventricle, with diminution of end-diastolic volumes
		
		Compression of pulmonary vasculature (except in pure cardiac tamponade), with hindrance of right ventricular emptying.

Source: From Harken AH: Cardiac arrhythmias, in Willmore DW, Brennan MF, Harken AH, et al (eds): *Care of the Surgical Patient, vol 1: Critical Care: A Publication of the Committee on Pre- and Postoperative Care, American College of Surgeons.* New York, Scientific American, 1989.

CLINICAL CIRCUMSTANCES

Although the heart is a single organ, the various components, including the myocardium, valves, conduction system, associated great vessels, and surrounding pericardial cavity, can all produce a shock syndrome when pathology is present. The first priority is to recognize the presence of shock. The clinical signs produced by adrenergic discharge and high plasma levels of angiotensin are reflected as pallor of the skin, clamminess, and tachycardia—all common signs of shock, cardiogenic or otherwise. Historical information relating to symptoms, trauma, and profound hypovolemia is of primary importance in directing further investigation and treatment. A critical differentiating clinical sign is the determination of neck vein distension. If neck vein distension is present, then a primary cardiac, pericardial, or cardiac compressive syndrome is likely. Since patients with cardiogenic shock have poor cardiac output despite adequate diastolic and venous pressures, the veins in the neck will bulge from overdistension with blood. Once the presence of neck vein distension has been determined, then the differentiation of a cardiac compressive syndrome versus a primary cardiogenic etiology is imperative. Although chest x-ray, electrocardiogram, and echocardiogram may be useful, physical examination and key historical information are the cornerstones of diagnosis.

CARDIOGENIC SHOCK

Myocardial infarction is the most common cause of cardiogenic shock.[1-9] It is expected that 5 million Americans will suffer myocardial infarction in the coming year. Although the exact incidence of pump failure after infarction is difficult to ascertain, this complication can vary from 10 to 30 percent depending on the criteria used and the time period examined. Large regions of myocardial necrosis are more likely to cause cardiogenic shock.[1-10] Smaller infarcts can result in severe global left ventricular dysfunction if coexisting left main coronary artery disease or triple vessel disease results in generalized ischemia. Of patients with acute infarcts, it is estimated that 10 percent may have left main disease and another 30 percent may have triple vessel disease or the equivalent.[10,11] Cardiac indices of less than 2 liters/m^2 are generally inadequate to provide organ perfusion without detrimental consequences. This usually correlates with a significantly depressed left ventricular ejection fraction and elevated left ventricular end-diastolic or pulmonary wedge pressure.

In addition to myocardial failure, there are several postinfarction sequelae that can cause profound shock. These complications usually have a mechanical basis.[3,12] Specifically, these sequelae are postinfarction ventricular septal defect (VSD), mitral valve incompetence, and rupture of the left ventricle. The postinfarction VSD is secondary to necrosis and breakdown of the muscular septum (Fig. 9–1), causing shunting of blood from the left ventricle to the right ventricle (Fig. 9–2). Mitral incompetence is frequently related to papillary muscle necrosis with secondary avulsion of the muscle from the ventricular wall (Fig. 9–3). Rupture of the left ventricle usually results from transmural infarction and necrosis of the left ventricle with complete loss of structural integrity[13] (Fig. 9–4).

Each of these sequelae is considered an unusual complication of myocardial infarction, with the incidence of each varying between 1 and 5 percent. They typically occur 3 to 7 days after infarction, when liquefication necrosis of the muscle has resulted in loss of structural integrity. The acute shunting of blood in VSD and the acute mitral regurgitation of papillary muscle necrosis are hemodynamically debilitating lesions that cause acute compromise of the patient. Cardiogenic shock ensues rapidly, and urgent treatment is required. Shock from free rupture of the ventricular wall is a mixed picture, with cardiac compression from blood in the pericardium as the major component.

Arrhythmias may be secondarily related to ongoing cardiac ischemia and may or may not contribute to the shock syndrome. Certainly, life-threatening arrhythmias can exist independent of infarction or ischemia and be the sole cause of cardiogenic shock. Less severe arrhythmias, however, also may contribute to the shock state. These arrhythmias may be either preexisting or secondary to acute ischemia or irritability of the myocardium. Tachyarrhythmias or rhythms precluding proper atrial function may adversely affect an already compromised cardiac output, contributing to cardiogenic shock.

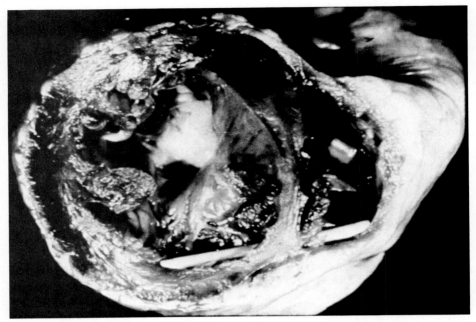

FIG. 9–1. Postinfarction ventricular septal defect. Note the probe demonstrating communication between the right and left ventricles.

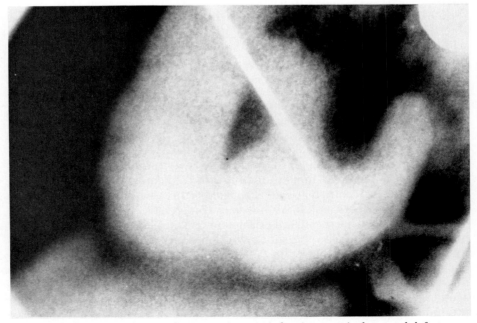

FIG. 9–2. Ventriculogram demonstrating postinfarction ventricular septal defect.

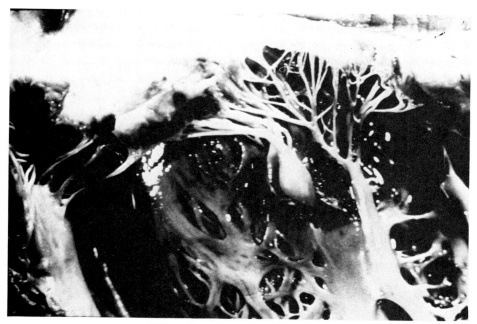

FIG. 9–3. Papillary muscle rupture.

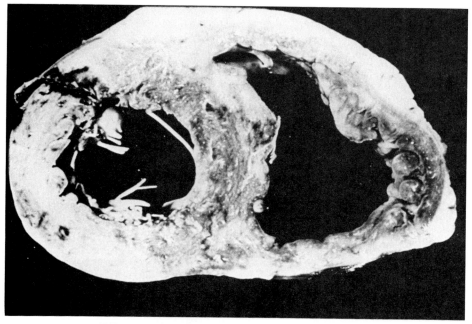

FIG. 9–4. Myocardial rupture secondary to infarction.

Injury to the heart caused by penetrating trauma or, rarely, blunt trauma can produce cardiogenic shock. Penetrating injuries can damage the myocardium, valves, or coronary arteries. Blunt trauma to the heart also has been described to rarely cause valvular pathology, and this, in turn, can be responsible for cardiogenic shock. However, blunt trauma to the heart may lead to consequences as diverse as arrhythmia or cardiac rupture that is immediately fatal or produce no injury of clinical consequence.[14]

Acute pulmonary embolism, specifically a large saddle embolus situated in the main pulmonary artery (Fig. 9–5), can cause right-sided heart failure and cor pulmonale severe enough to cause cardiogenic shock. Severe right ventricular distension with impaired left ventricular filling will rapidly result in shock and death.[15]

Myocardial infiltration by malignant and benign processes also can cause cardiac failure and shock.[16] Tumors of the heart are frequently metastatic but can cause extensive infiltration and dysfunction. Benign processes include amyloidosis, hemochromatosis, and sarcoidosis. Löeffler's disease is associated with marked eosinophilic myocardial infiltration and likewise can cause severe myocardial failure.

More commonly, many of today's antianginal regimens include beta blockers and calcium channel blockers. Both these agents can cause myocardial depression. Overdosage resulting from prescribing or dispensing errors may lead to cardiogenic shock. Suicide attempts with these agents also have been reported.[17,18]

Valvular etiologies for cardiogenic shock result predominantly from dysfunction of the aortic or mitral valves. The lesions most likely to cause acute hemodynamic compromise and shock include acute insufficiency of either valve. Pa-

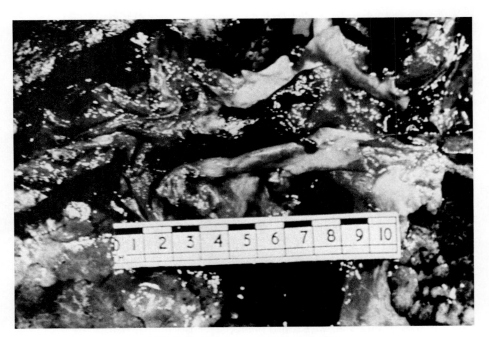

FIG. 9–5. Pulmonary saddle embolus.

thology includes myxomatous degeneration, endocarditis, ascending aortic dissection involving the aortic valve, and papillary muscle necrosis affecting the mitral valve. Stenotic lesions of these valves may cause shock, but because of the chronicity of presentation, intervention usually occurs before shock sets in.[19,20] Similarly, ventricular aneurysm may cause serious compromise of left ventricular function, but chronicity usually allows intervention prior to shock.

Complications of percutaneous angioplasty may cause shock. Acute thrombosis or dissection of a coronary vessel can lead to myocardial infarction or ischemia. Perfusion catheters, intraaortic balloon pumping, and early surgery are frequently required. Rarely, catheter perforation may cause shock of the cardiac compressive nature secondary to pericardial tamponade.[21,22]

CARDIAC COMPRESSIVE SHOCK

The most common cardiac compressive syndromes include tension pneumothorax and cardiac tamponade from pericardial effusion. Tension pneumothorax is frequently caused by trauma, with blunt and penetrating injuries being common etiologies. Iatrogenic tension pneumothorax may result from central line placement or thoracentesis. Spontaneous pneumothorax leading to mediastinal displacement also occurs in positive-pressure–ventilated patients, as well as in young patients from juvenile idiopathic bullous rupture. Cardiac tamponade also can be caused by trauma if penetrating or blunt injury leads to pericardial effusion. Iatrogenic causes include left heart catheterization, endomyocardial biopsies, and placement of temporary and permanent pacing wires. Many medical etiologies may be cause for massive pericardial effusion and subsequent cardiac compression. These include uremic pericarditis, tuberculosis, collagen vascular disorders, and malignant involvement of the pericardium.

Other causes of cardiac compressive shock include compression of the heart by bowel that has eviscerated through a ruptured diaphragm and compression caused by any process associated with high abdominal pressures such as ascites, abdominal bleeding, or the inflation of the abdominal portion of the pneumatic antishock garment.[23]

CLINICAL PRESENTATION AND DIAGNOSIS

The clinical symptoms relating to cardiogenic shock generally are related to pulmonary congestion and poor peripheral perfusion. Thus dyspnea is quite profound and is often associated with cool and diaphoretic skin. The air hunger associated with cardiac compressive syndromes frequently is even more striking, associated with extreme restlessness and agitation. Associated historical information and careful questioning relating to prior illnesses, medication, and prodromal symptoms are key.

SIGNS

Many of the overt signs of cardiogenic shock and cardiac compressive syndromes are similar to those of other shock presentations, namely hypotension

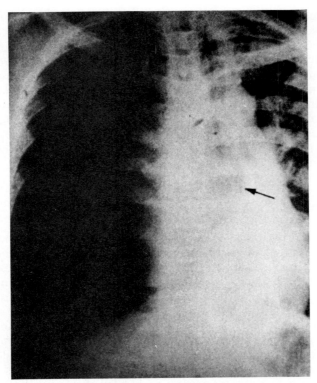

FIG. 9–6. Tension pneumothorax. Arrow indicates leftward deviation of the trachea.

and tachycardia. Therefore, a careful physical examination is as important as obtaining an adequate and thorough history. Vital signs, mental status, skin perfusion, and urine output must be noted. It is important to note that hypotension is not an early sign of shock and need not be present. The skin changes of pallor and clamminess, oliguria, and tachycardia all may be present significantly before blood pressure deteriorates. In fact, some patients can produce intense peripheral vasoconstriction to maintain normal blood pressure, even in the face of a severely depressed cardiac output. A priority in the physical examination is assessment of the neck veins. This will enable the clinician to distinguish cardiogenic and cardiac compressive shock syndromes from other shock states. In the early stages of shock, the clinical finding of neck vein distension can be valuable in directing the diagnostic options and the ultimate therapy.

The auscultation of cardiac and lung sounds is of obvious importance. Assessments for murmurs, the quality of S_1 and S_2, the presence of an S_3 or S_4 gallop, and the clarity of the sounds all provide relevant information. The presence of rales at the lung bases or absence of lung sounds likewise lends support to the presence of heart failure or pneumothorax, respectively. Percussion of the chest, determination of the point of maximal impulse of the heart, or the presence or absence of dullness at the lung bases may yield telltale information regarding heart failure. The position of the trachea is of critical importance when considering the diagnosis of tension pneumothorax (Fig. 9–6).

The abdominal examination, with emphasis on palpation of hepatomegaly, is valuable in assessing the presence of right-sided heart failure.[11,24] Finally, palpation of peripheral pulses will yield information on the severity of shock and the capability of instituting femoral artery cannulation if needed for intraaortic balloon insertion or even cardiopulmonary bypass.

STUDIES

A plain film of the chest is quite valuable in differentiating cardiogenic from cardiac compressive syndromes. A cardiogenic etiology is likely to show congested lung fields with increased pulmonary vascular markings, notably toward the apices (Fig. 9–7). The presence of an effusion may be evident, the right side being more likely than the left. Calcification of either the aortic or mitral valves may be seen, lending support to a diagnosis of aortic or mitral stenosis.

Tension pneumothorax should ideally be diagnosed and treated prior to obtaining a chest x-ray. A chest x-ray may be helpful, however, in diagnosing cardiac tamponade, especially if it has been slow in developing. A large, globular

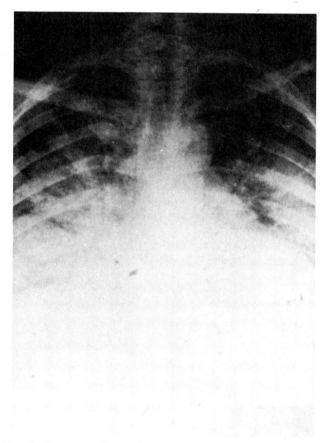

FIG. 9–7. Chest radiograph demonstrating pulmonary edema.

cardiac silhouette would be expected in a patient with a slow accumulation of pericardial fluid, whereas in acute tamponade the pericardium is less distensible and the silhouette may not be enlarged.

Careful inspection of the lung fields to eliminate the possibility of pneumothorax is imperative, and tension pneumothorax with contralateral shift of the mediastinum is usually quite evident.

Cardiac echocardiogram and right catheterization (Swan-Ganz catheter) are usually pursued for patients diagnosed with cardiogenic or cardiac compressive shock. The information gathered from the pulmonary arterial, wedge, and central venous pressures and cardiac output measurements will give baseline data from which improvement or deterioration can be gauged. Additional diagnostic information is available from the Swan-Ganz catheter, including waveforms indicative of mitral valvular incompetence and pulmonary arterial O_2 measurements suggestive of postinfarction ventricular septal defects. The echocardiogram also will yield information on right and left ventricular septal defects. The echocardiogram will yield additional information on right and left ventricular contractility, the presence or absence of valve pathology, as well as the presence of pleural fluid. Emergency cardiac catheterization detailing left ventricular pressures and coronary anatomy is imperative in patients who are considered potential candidates for open-heart surgery or those in whom emergency percutaneous angioplasty is to be considered.[3,14,25,26]

CARDIAC COMPRESSIVE SYNDROMES

The presence of distended neck veins in cardiac compressive and cardiogenic shock is the hallmark diagnostic sign, but clinical circumstances usually help differentiate cardiac compressive shock from myocardial failure. The presence of neck vein distension in an upright position bears more significance than that seen in a supine position. If neck veins become more distended with deep inspiration, this is pathognomonic for cardiac compression and is the sign described by Kussmaul. Although these signs are helpful, if hypovolemia coexists with cardiac compression, the vein distension may not necessarily be present. Therefore, a fluid bolus should be given to any patient in whom there is a question of cardiac compressive shock and a mechanism of injury has occurred such that hypovolemia may be present. Regardless of the mechanism of injury, however, administration of fluid is appropriate treatment in cardiac compressive shock.

The conditions that result in cardiac compressive shock can be differentiated by clinical characteristics. Patients with tension pneumothorax have a deviation of the trachea to the side opposite that of the pneumothorax, absent breath sounds on the side of the pneumothorax, normal or quiet heart sounds, and distended neck veins. The skin is pale, cool, and clammy secondary to adrenergic discharge, although the superficial veins may be distended because of high venous pressures.[27] The diagnosis becomes obvious if time allows a chest x-ray to be obtained. The process of a tension pneumothorax is caused by the failure of a pneumothorax to seal spontaneously, allowing air to continue to enter the pleural space. As air accumulates through a flap-valve type mechanism that allows air to enter but not to leave the pleural space, the lung is compressed.

Continual positive pressure in the pleural space compromises ventilation. The increasing pressure of the pleural space also impinges on the mediastinal structures, raising intrathoracic pressure and obstructing venous return, thereby reducing cardiac output and producing hypotension.

Patients with pericardial tamponade present with signs of shock similar to those observed in cardiac compressive shock, namely pale, cool, clammy skin, oliguria, hypotension, and distended neck veins. Differential diagnosis of pericardial tamponade versus that in tension pneumothorax is found in Table 9–2.

The process of tamponade is caused by fluid accumulation into the rigid pericardial sac. Restriction of myocardial function results from increased pericardial pressure which causes elevation of intracardiac pressures, impaired ventricular filling, and reduced cardiac output. This results in a rise of the central venous pressure, equalization of right and left filling and diastolic pressures, and pulsus paradoxus of more than 10 to 15 mmHg. Pulsus paradoxus can only be diagnosed if a decrease of more than 10 mmHg in systolic pressure occurs during inspiration.[28] Normally, there is a small decrease in systolic blood pressure during inspiration. The exaggerated fall in pressure found in pulsus paradoxus is thought to occur by at least two mechanisms: First, on inspiration, pressures in the thoracic cavity diminish and venous return increases. The right ventricle enlarges and impinges on the left ventricle. Ordinarily, this causes only a slight decrease in the ejection volume of the left ventricle. Patients with tamponade, however, have a tight pericardium and an exaggerated inspiratory increase in venous return because of elevated venous pressures. There is not enough room for the left ventricle to fill normally at the same time that the right ventricle is filling. Thus the left ventricular ejection fraction is diminished significantly. Second, the decrease in the intrathoracic pressure caused by inspiration is transmitted to the myocardium but not to the extrathoracic arteries. This effect raises the arterial afterload on the heart and makes it more difficult for the myocardium to empty.[29]

Other diagnostic signs include diminished voltage on the electrocardiogram and the possibility of a large globular cardiac silhouette on the chest film. Caution must be exercised when the situation is acute, since the cardiac shadow may not be enlarged. The diagnosis can be established with an echocardiogram.

TREATMENT OF CARDIAC COMPRESSIVE SHOCK

Chest tube decompression in tension pneumothorax should be done without delay. If this is not possible, then needle aspiration can be performed until a

TABLE 9–2. Differential Diagnosis of Cardiac Compressive Shock

	Trachea	Breath Sounds	Heart Sounds
Cardiac tamponade	Midline	Normal	Muffled
Tension pneumothorax	Deviated to side opposite pneumothorax	Absent on side of pneumothorax	Normal or quiet

chest tube is ready to be inserted. Chest tubes for air need not be very large, with sizes 20 to 26 French more than adequate. It is imperative that the chest tube be directed to the apex of the chest, preferably inserted in the anterior axillary line and in the fourth or fifth intercostal space.

The treatment for pericardial effusion is rapid decompression of the pericardial sac to allow restoration of normal hemodynamics. This can be done initially with needle or catheter pericardiocentesis. Most pericardial effusions are best drained in the operating room. If unexpected pathology is found, this setting allows for flexibility in surgical treatment. Approaches include subxyphoid, anterolateral, median sternotomy, or thoracoscopy. Whichever approach is used, a drain is usually positioned to effect continued drainage for 24 to 48 h. Pericardial windows are usually only temporary and seal rapidly by compression from adjacent organs or structures. Only complete pericardiectomy extending from phrenic nerve to phrenic nerve is considered a definitive method of preventing recurrent pericardial effusion.

Mechanical ventilation is becoming one of the most prevalent causes of cardiac compressive shock. Impairment of cardiac function from mechanical ventilation is usually the result of three mechanisms: (1) compression of the superior and inferior vena cava as they enter the chest, with the consequence of impaired filling of the right side of the heart, (2) direct compression of the right atrium, right ventricle, and left atrium resulting in decreased end-diastolic and stroke volumes, and (3) compression of the pulmonary vasculature resulting in increased pulmonary vascular resistance and hinderance of right ventricular emptying.[30] Treatment goals are judicious volume loading and keeping airway pressures to a minimum, as well as setting the inspiratory/expiratory ratio to as short a time as possible.

CARDIOGENIC SHOCK

As one can see, the causes of cardiac or cardiac compressive shock are varied, but they all have one sign in common other than shock itself—*neck vein distension*. In the early stages of clinical presentation, this finding can be valuable in directing the employment of diagnostic options and ultimate therapy.

Despite the variety of pathology, there are some common hemodynamic abnormalities which are found in cardiogenic shock. The systolic blood pressure is likely less than 80 mmHg. The cardiac index is less than 2.1 liters/min/m². Additionally, the peripheral vascular resistance is usually elevated. Objectives include the diagnosis of the underlying pathology, correction of mechanical problems and improving perfusion pressure, raising cardiac output while reducing cardiac work, and improving coronary blood flow. Since cardiac output is the product of the stroke volume and heart rate, both these variables can be treated to maximize performance. Stroke volume, in turn, is influenced by preload, afterload, and contractility of the myocardium. Preload is the volume of blood required to stretch myocardial fibers to maximize contractility. Since volume cannot be measured easily, pressure is utilized instead. The pulmonary artery wedge pressure, which under ideal conditions approximates the left atrial pressure, indirectly approximates the left ventricular end-diastolic pressure. These pressures may vary between 8 and 10 mmHg, but the desirable level is that which maximizes the cardiac output. This is the Frank-Starling relationship (Fig. 9–8).

Optimization of ventricular end-diastolic pressures, and hence volume, is critical in the treatment of cardiogenic shock. Although the Swan-Ganz catheter gives reasonably accurate information regarding intracardiac pressure, there are situations that make the readings inaccurate. The atrial pressures measured, i.e., right atrial pressure (CVP) and the left atrial pressure (PCW), are not good representations of the end-diastolic ventricular pressures in the presence of mitral and tricuspid stenosis. Additionally, pressure exerted on the heart by the lungs or by the pericardium also may falsely elevate atrial pressures, thus not truly reflecting adequate intracavitary volume.

The contractility developed by myocardial fibers, as mentioned, is stretch related. If stretch alone does not improve cardiac output, contractility can be increased pharmacologically and mechanically. Examples of pharmacologic support include inotropic agents such as dobutamine, epinephrine, amrinone, and dopamine. Examples of mechanical support include institution of intraaortic balloon pump assistance or myocardial revascularization, which through the augmentation of coronary blood flow can increase myocardial contractility. Myocardial revascularization can be surgical or by percutaneous technique. Intraaortic balloon pumping also decreases peripheral vascular resistance, which is another way of improving cardiac output and hence reversing cardiogenic shock.

Afterload is the peripheral vascular resistance which determines the amount of tension required by the left ventricle to open the aortic valve and eject blood. As peripheral vascular resistance increases, so does the amount of left ventricular wall tension, which ultimately causes an increased utilization of myocardial oxygen. Therefore, increased afterload may contribute to myocardial ischemia. Pharmacologic or balloon pump treatment may improve cardiac output by effectively reducing cardiac afterload. Pharmacologic agents useful for afterload reduction include nitroprusside and ACE inhibitors. These agents must be utilized cautiously and with continuous monitoring of cardiac filling pressure and systolic blood pressure, since inappropriate dosage may exacerbate shock. Cardiogenic shock caused by muscle necrosis may be treated aggressively, providing

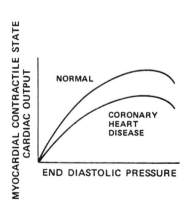

FIG. 9–8. Frank-Starling curve.

TABLE 9–3. Treatment of Cardiogenic Shock

▼

Maintain adequate arterial oxygen saturation (>90%)
Initiate monitoring:
PA catheter
Arterial line
Assess CO, SVR, V_{O_2}, PAWP
Measure blood gases and lactate levels

▼

Restore MAP to >60 mmHg
To maintain coronary flow:
This may require use of careful fluid challenge and/or
pressor agents for short term

▼

If low perfusion persists

▼	▼	▼	▼
Inotropic support avoid tachycardia	Consider IABP Consider surgery	Fluid challenge	Vasodilator if tolerated

Source: From Demling RH, Wilson RF: *Decision Making in Surgical Critical Care.* Philadelphia, Decker, 1988, with permission.

that no more than 40 percent of the left ventricle is involved in the infarct. Either emergency surgical myocardial revascularization or placement of an intraaortic balloon pump, or both, can be done to treat this form of cardiogenic shock. An algorithm outlining general treatment for cardiogenic shock is presented in Table 9–3.

ARRHYTHMIAS

Arrhythmia must be considered as a possible cause of cardiogenic shock. This is rapidly diagnosed by assessing the pulse and placing the patient on a cardiac monitor. Arrhythmias responsible for cardiogenic shock can cover the spectrum from tachyarrhythmias to bradyarrhythmias and heart block. One needs to bear in mind that the arrhythmia may be exacerbating another primary cardiac impairment, such as valvular or atherosclerotic coronary disease, but this should become apparent as diagnostic options are pursued. Examples of tachyarrhythmias causing cardiogenic shock include ventricular tachycardia, paroxysmal atrial tachycardia, nodal tachycardia, atrial flutter, and atrial fibrillation (Figs. 9–9 and 9–10). Generally, ventricular rates greater than 130 beats per minute need to be treated aggressively. Indeed, ventricular tachycardia and other arrhythmias with rates greater than 180 beats per minute may need immediate cardioversion. Any patient with sustained ventricular fibrillation will require cardiopulmonary resuscitation and immediate defibrillation. As always, securing an airway and maintaining ventilation are fundamental. Additional therapy may

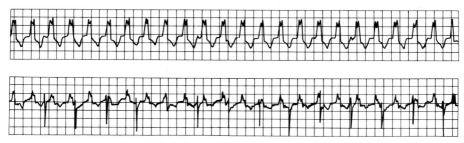

FIG. 9–9. Ventricular tachycardia.

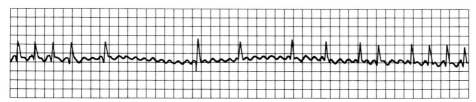

FIG. 9–10. Atrial flutter with variable block.

require antiarrhythmic medication, including lidocaine or bretylium, digoxin, tensilon, calcium channel or beta-blocking agents.

Bradyarrhythmias, including heart block, may be an etiology of cardiogenic shock. These include sinus arrest, sick sinus syndromes, and third-degree heart block (Figs. 9–11 and 9–12). Usually, heart rates of less than 40 beats per minute or pauses of greater than 4 to 6 s are required to produce symptoms. Therapy usually includes institution of temporary pacing as an interim measure pending placement of a permanent pacemaker. Pharmacologic agents may be utilized until a temporary wire is placed. These agents include atropine, isoproterenol, and dopamine.

There are many abnormal rhythms that occur in the absence of hemodynamic compromise and therefore require little or no treatment. However, rhythms that impair mechanical activity are life-threatening and therefore demand immediate attention and treatment. Treatment options will depend on the type of rhythm and the condition of the patient. The first issue that needs to be ascertained is whether the rhythm is asystole. If it is not asystole but it causes severe hemodynamic compromise, then cardioversion is in order. It is recommended to start with at least 100 J of energy, and if there is no result, one should rapidly proceed to 400 J. If asystole is present, then use of steady cardiopulmonary resuscitation is appropriate, with reassessment of the rhythm at periodic intervals. Appropriate attempts at cardioversion can be done if coarse ventricular fibrillation is present. If asystole persists, then placement of a temporary transvenous pacing wire is reasonable, or external pacing can be used if available.

For bradycardia in stable patients, temporary internal or external pacing needs to be considered. For unstable patients, atropine is administered until the rate responds, and then pacing is instituted. For rapid arrhythmias, diagnosis by ECG rhythm strip is imperative to differentiate between ventricular and atrial origin. Ventricular tachycardia should be treated with cardioversion and lidocaine.

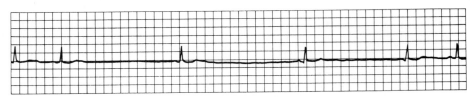

FIG. 9–11. Bradycardia.

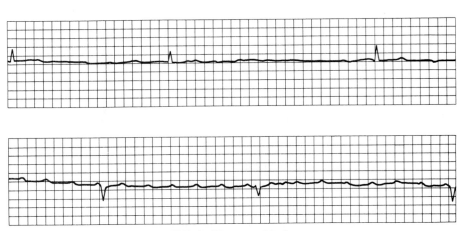

FIG. 9–12. Heart block.

Atrial tachyarrhythmias can be treated with a combination of digoxin, calcium channel blockers, or beta blockers. Chapter 7 provides an algorithm for treatment of arrhythmias.

MYOCARDIAL MUSCLE DYSFUNCTION

There are various diseases of the heart muscle, acute and chronic, that can cause cardiogenic shock. The most common is acute myocardial infarction. Large infarctions (greater than 30 to 40 percent of muscle mass) or infarctions associated with global ischemia can cause cardiogenic shock. Primary treatment of ischemia is mandatory and may include thrombolytic agents, nitrates, intraaortic balloon counterpulsation, or myocardial revascularization by angioplasty or surgery.[1–6,11,21,22,25,31–34] Two other situations that are associated with acute myocardial infarction and frequently cause profound cardiogenic shock are postinfarction ventricular septal defect and rupture of the papillary muscle of the mitral valve. These classically complicate 1 to 2 percent of myocardial infarctions and occur 3 to 7 days after the acute event. They are usually marked by sudden clinical deterioration with hypotension and pulmonary edema. A new murmur is often noticeable, and diagnosis can be confirmed by Swan-Ganz catheterization with a detectable oxygen stepup in the pulmonary artery port for ventricular septal defects or a significant *v* wave on the wedge tracing for papillary muscle necrosis. Institution of immediate intraaortic balloon counterpulsation, followed by a diagnostic catheterization, is necessary. Surgery is undertaken immediately in most cases.

There are a multitude of primary myocardial problems classified as cardiomyopathies that can cause cardiogenic shock. A few can be acute, such as viral or peripartum myopathy, but the majority are chronic and gradual in presentation. These include familial, alcoholic, diabetic, neuromuscular, and hypertrophic cardiomyopathies. Endomyocardial fibrosis also may lead to cardiogenic shock. The acute viral syndromes are usually classified as myocarditis and are commonly caused by coxsackie A and B viruses. Toxoplasmosis in newborns may be associated with cardiac failure. Chagas' disease, caused by *Trypanosoma cruzi* and encountered in Central and South America, is also an etiology. Finally, radiation therapy for lymphoma, Hodgkin's disease, lung disease, or breast carcinoma can cause acute and chronic myocarditis, as well as myocardial fibrosis.

Diagnosis of a primary muscle problem is usually made by right and left heart catheterization, determination of end-diastolic pressure, calculation of cardiac output, and exclusion of valvular heart disease. Additional evidence is usually gleaned from echocardiography, which will confirm wall motion abnormalities, determine myocardial wall thickness, document systolic and diastolic ventricular dimensions, and exclude valvular heart disease. Nuclear-gated ventriculography will add information regarding left and right heart ejection fractions. Endomyocardial biopsy may be diagnostic and helpful in long-term planning. Options for treatment of cardiomyopathy are limited and may include expectant therapy, inotropic support, steroids, or heart transplant if appropriate.

In the face of muscle failure, the maintenance of adequate filling pressure is essential. Although the pulmonary wedge pressure tends to reflect end-diastolic left ventricular pressure, this will not be true in mitral stenosis. Additionally, the pulmonary catheter measurements reflect both intracardiac pressures and the pressure exerted on the heart from the pericardium and the lungs. Recognizing these limitations, the goal is to obtain the maximum cardiac output associated with the lowest end-diastolic pressure. The treating physician seeks the maximum cardiac output at the lowest energy expenditure and the lowest rate of oxygen consumption. Optimization of filling pressure may require volume loading, manipulation of peripheral vascular resistance with a vasodilator agent, reduction of preload with nitroglycerin, or the use of inotropic support to increase myocardial contractility.

VALVULAR DYSFUNCTION

Valvular causes of cardiogenic shock primarily involve either the mitral or aortic valve. Tricuspid disease may be present but rarely is the dominant lesion, except for drug addiction–associated endocarditis. This entity is rarely associated with cardiogenic shock but can present as septic shock.

Acute mitral valve prolapse associated with papillary muscle necrosis has already been discussed. Other causes of cardiogenic shock caused by mitral valve pathology include mitral chordae rupture (Fig. 9–13) and mitral leaflet perforation from endocarditis. Both these lesions can result in acute exacerbation of

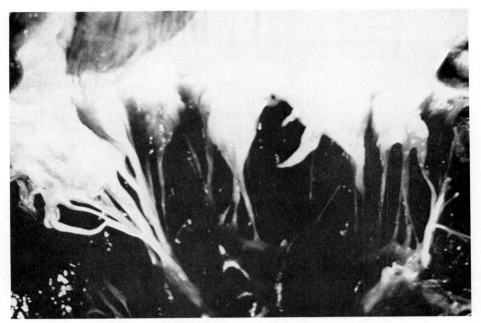

FIG. 9–13. Ruptured chordae tendinae of the mitral valve.

mitral regurgitation and may rapidly lead to acute pulmonary hypertension and biventricular failure (Fig. 9–14). Again, early and aggressive efforts at diagnosis are mandatory, with institution of intraaortic balloon counterpulsation as a bridge to urgent surgical valve repair or replacement.

Aortic valve pathology includes regurgitant and stenotic lesions. It is the sudden onset of aortic valvular insufficiency that is most likely to present as cardiogenic shock. The sudden regurgitant volume is poorly tolerated by the unprepared ventricle, leading to biventricular failure. Causes for sudden aortic valvular insufficiency include either acute perforation from a fulminant septic endocarditis or acute leaflet prolapse from aortic dissection. In both instances, rapid diagnosis, usually with the aid of echocardiography and root aortography, is crucial. Diagnosis is followed by urgent cardiac surgery. There is *no* role for intraaortic balloon pumping in lesions associated with aortic valvular insufficiency. In fact, it is contraindicated, for it will exacerbate the diastolic volume overload of the left ventricle.

Aortic stenosis, like mitral stenosis, is generally gradual in onset. However, it may remain clinically silent for many years before it becomes critically stenotic as valve areas reach less than 0.8 cm². The onset of heart failure, syncope, or angina may in fact be the initial symptom. Cardiogenic shock may soon follow if operative intervention is not undertaken. Etiologies of aortic stenosis include congenital bicuspid aortic stenosis (Fig. 9–15), the most common cause presenting in the adult, followed in incidence by senile calcific aortic stenosis in the elderly. Rheumatic heart disease is now an infrequent third cause (Fig. 9–16).

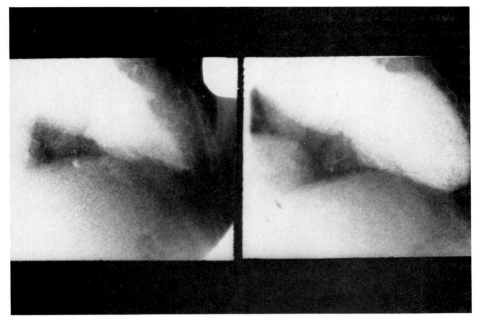

FIG. 9–14. Ventriculogram demonstrating acute mitral regurgitation.

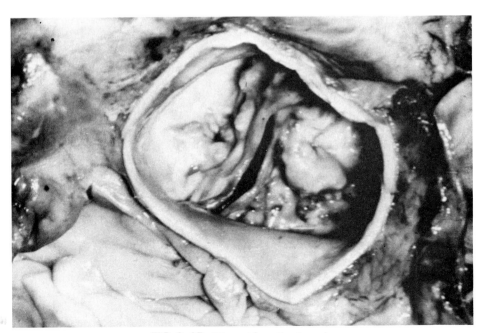

FIG. 9–15. Bicuspid aortic stenosis.

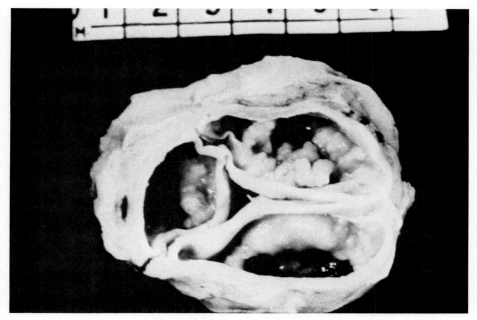

FIG. 9–16. Acquired calcific aortic stenosis.

Pulmonary valve pathology is unusual in the adult, but main pulmonary artery embolization is another important cause of cardiogenic shock.[15] This event is frequently marked by profound hypoxemia and predominantly right-sided heart failure. As with all diagnoses, the presenting history and clinical setting are critical. Clinical signs include tachycardia, cyanosis, respiratory distress, and prominent second heart sound. If hypotension is present, then a massive saddle embolus is likely. Rapid diagnosis is imperative, with simultaneous institution of heparin therapy or vena cava filter placement and inotropic support. If hypotension persists for more than 2 h despite maximal inotropic support in the setting of a large defect seen on angiography in the main, left, or right pulmonary arteries, then surgical intervention is justified for extraction of the embolus (Fig. 9–17).

GREAT VESSELS DISEASE

The most common great vessel catastrophe that will lead to cardiogenic shock is that of a type 1 (type A) aortic dissection of the ascending aorta. Aortic dissections are classified as either type I, II, or III (Debakey classification) or as type A or B (Stanford classification) (Fig. 9–18). An ascending aortic tear may cause acute prolapse of the aortic valve leaflet, resulting in massive aortic insufficiency and heart failure. Additional mechanisms leading to cardiogenic shock from aortic dissections include a tear into the coronary ostium, leading to an acute myo-

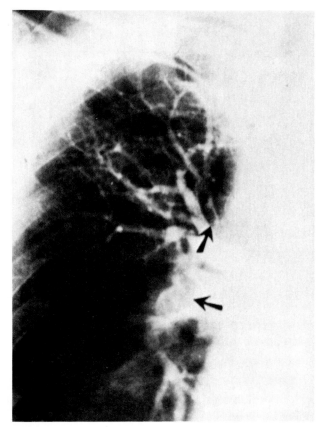

FIG. 9–17. Pulmonary angiography demonstrating emboli within the branches of the right pulmonary artery.

cardial infarction or global ischemia. Finally, the dissection may rupture into the pericardial cavity, causing cardiac tamponade and shock (Figs. 9–19 and 9–20).

Because Debakey types I and II (Stanford type A) are the types most likely to cause proximal extension involving the valve, coronary ostium, or pericardium, these must be considered surgical emergencies. Diagnosis is frequently made on clinical grounds and confirmed with echocardiography and cardiac catheterization. Transesophageal echocardiography can be very reliable and is sufficient to confirm the diagnosis and mandate surgery. Surgery always involves cardiopulmonary bypass, addressing both the primary aortic dissection and the secondary effects.

The other ascending aorta pathology that can present as fulminant cardiogenic shock is a rupture of a sinus of Valsalva aneurysm into the right ventricle or right atrium. This aneurysm is usually congenital but slowly enlarges with time. It may remain silent until it ruptures into the right side of the heart, causing an acute left-to-right shunt. This may be poorly tolerated, and cardiogenic shock may ensue. Rapid diagnosis, usually by means of echocardiography and root aortography, is followed by urgent cardiac surgery.

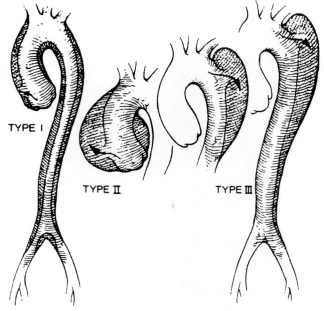

FIG. 9–18. Classification of aortic dissections.

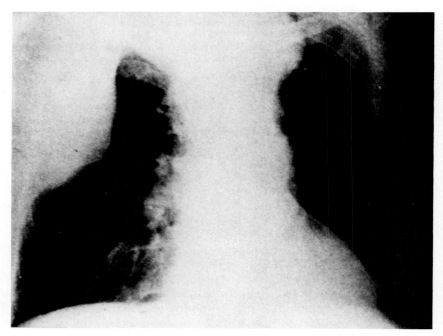

FIG. 9–19. Chest radiograph demonstrating aortic dissection.

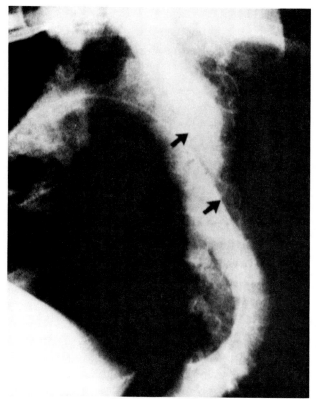

FIG. 9–20. Aortogram demonstrating aortic dissection.

SUMMARY

Cardiogenic shock may result from either pump failure or cardiac compressive effects. Diagnosis depends on an accurate history and the appreciation of salient physical signs. Jugular venous distension is a key feature in the differentiation of this etiology from other causes of shock. Once identified, treatment of cardiac compressive shock is directed toward relief of the cause of increased intrathoracic pressure, either tension pneumothorax or pericardial tamponade. If primary pump failure is determined to be the cause of shock, it is necessary to determine whether the etiology is related to myocardial dysfunction, valvular disease, or arrhythmia. Appropriate pharmacologic and mechanical interventions are then directed toward the primary cause of inadequate cardiac output. In all cases, the goal is to maximize cardiac output at the minimum cost of myocardial work.

REFERENCES

1. Scholz KH, Hering JP, Schroder T, et al: Protective effects of the Hemopump left ventricular assist device in experimental cardiogenic shock. *Eur J Cardiothorac Surg* 6(4):209, 1992.
2. Dresdale AR, Paone G: Surgical treatment of acute myocardial infarction. *Henry Ford Hosp Med J* 39(3–4):245, 1991.
3. Moosvi AR, Gheorghiade M, Goldstein S, Khaja F: Management of cardiogenic shock complicating acute myocardial infarction: The Henry Ford Hospital experience and review of the literature. *Henry Ford Hosp Med J* 39(3–4):240, 1991.
4. Mueller HS, Cohen LS, Braunwald E, et al: Predictors of early morbidity and mortality after thrombolytic therapy of acute myocardial infarction: Analyses of patient subgroups in the Thrombolysis in Myocardial Infarction (TIMI) Trial, phase II. *Circulation* 85(4):1254, 1992.
5. Oneill WW: Angioplasty therapy of cardiogenic shock: Are randomized trials necessary? (editorial). *J Am Coll Cardiol* 19(5):915, 1992.
6. Moosvi AR, Khaja F, Villaneuva L, et al: Early revascularization improves survival in cardiogenic shock complicating acute myocardial infarction. *J Am Coll Cardiol* 19(5):907, 1992.
7. Corain FI, Owen A, Trubel W, et al: Regulatory effect of neurotransmitter by hemofiltration in cardiogenic shock patients after open heart surgery. *Contrib Nephrol* 93:90, 1991.
8. Coraim F, Trubel W, Ebermann R, Werner T: Isolation of low-molecular-weight peptides in hemofiltrated patients with cardiogenic shock: A new aspect of myocardial depressant substances. *Contrib Nephrol* 93:237, 1991.
9. Lee TH, Ting HH, Shammash JB, et al: Long-term survival of emergency department patients with acute chest pain. *Am J Cardiol* 69(3):145, 1992.
10. Hedberg PA: Congestive heart failure in acute myocardial infarction: Treating the spectrum from mild failure to cardiogenic shock. *Postgrad Med* 90(6):99, 1991.
11. Rock SM: Right ventricular myocardial infarction. *J Cardiovasc Nurs* 6(1):44, 1991.
12. Violaris AG, Angelini GD: Congenital ventricular septal defect presenting as rupture of the ventricular septum subsequent to myocardial infarction. *Int J Cardiol* 34(1):97, 1992.
13. Vassal T, Porte JM, Archambaud F, et al: Fortuitous discovery of the association of true and false left ventricular aneurysm in a patient in cardiogenic shock (letter). *Intensive Care Med* 17(4):243, 1991.
14. Wisner DH, Read WH, Riddick RS: Suspected myocardial contusion: Triage and indications for monitoring. *Ann Surg* 212:82, 1990.
15. Kieny R, Charpentier A, Kieny MT: What is the place of pulmonary embolectomy today? *R Cardiovasc Surg (Torino)* 32(5):549, 1991.
16. Mansur A-de-P, Ramires JA, de-Oliveira-Filho JL: Cardiogenic shock due to neoplastic infiltration of cardiac muscle. *Int J Cardiol* 33(2):320, 1991.
17. Frierson J, Bailly D, Schultz T, et al: Refractory cardiogenic shock and complete heart block after unsuspected verapamil SR and atenolol overdose. *Clin Cardiol* 14(11):933, 1991.
18. Hantson P, Ronveau JL, DeConinck B, et al: Amrinone for refractory cardiogenic shock following chloroquine poisoning. *Intensive Care Med* 17(7):430, 1991.
19. Kirschner E, Berger M, Goldberg E: Hypertrophic obstructive cardiomyopathy presenting with profound hypotension: Role of two-dimensional and Doppler echocardiography in diagnosis and management. *Chest* 101(3):711, 1992.
20. Cribier A, Remadi F, Konig R, et al: Emergency balloon valvuloplasty as initial treatment of patients with aortic stenosis and cardiogenic shock (letter). *N Engl J Med* 326(9):646, 1992.
21. Beyersdorf F, Sarai K, Maul FD, et al: Immediate functional benefits after controlled reperfusion during surgical revascularization for acute coronary occlusion. *J Thorac Cardiovasc Surg* 102(6):856, 1991.

22. Applebaum R, House R, Rademaker A, et al: Coronary artery bypass grafting within thirty days of acute myocardial infarction: Early and late results in 406 patients. *J Thorac Cardiovasc Surg* 102(5):745, 1991.

23. Rankins JS, Olsen CO, Arentzen CE, et al: The effects of airway pressure on cardiac function in intact dogs and man. *Circulation* 66:108, 1982.

24. Risoe C, Hall C, Smiseth OA: Blood volume changes in liver and spleen during cardiogenic shock in dogs. *Am J Physiol* 261(6):H1763, 1991.

25. Gacioch GM, Ellis SG, Lee L, et al: Cardiogenic shock complicating acute myocardial infarction: The use of coronary angioplasty and the integration of the new support devices into patient management. *J Am Coll Cardiol* 19(3):647, 1992.

26. Hibbard MD, Holmes DR Jr, Bailey KR, et al: Percutaneous transluminal coronary angioplasty in patients with cardiogenic shock. *J Am Coll Cardiol* 19(3):639, 1992.

27. Holcroft JW, Blaisdell FW: Shock—Causes and management of circulatory collapse, in Sabiston DC (ed): *Textbook of Surgery: The Biological Basis of Modern Surgical Practice.* Philadelphia, Saunders, 1992.

28. Demling RH, Wilson RF: *Decision Making in Surgical Critical Care.* Philadelphia, Decker, 1988.

29. Fowler NO: Physiology of cardiac tamponade and pulsus paradoxus. *Mod Concepts Cardiovasc Dis* 12:109, 1978.

30. Holcroft JW, Robinson MK: Shock, in Wilmore DW, Brennan MF, Harken AH, et al (eds): *Care of the Surgical Patient,* vol 1: *Critical Care: A Publication of the Committee on Pre- and Postoperative Care, American College of Surgeons.* New York, Scientific American, 1989.

31. Klein LW: Optimal therapy for cardiogenic shock: The emerging role of coronary angioplasty (editorial). *J Am Coll Cardiol* 19(3):654, 1992.

32. McKendall GR, Attubatoi MJ, Drew TM, et al: Safety and efficacy of a new regimen of intravenous recombinant tissue-type plasminogen activator potentially suitable for either prehospital or in-hospital administration. *J Am Coll Cardiol* 18(7):1774, 1991.

33. Setaro JF, Cabin HS: Right ventricular infarction. *Cardiol Clin* 10(1):69, 1992.

34. Seydoux C, Goy JJ, Beuret P, Stauffer JC, et al: Effectiveness of percutaneous transluminal coronary angioplasty in cardiogenic shock during acute myocardial infarction. *Am J Cardiol* 69(9):968, 1992.

10

SEPTIC SHOCK

Donald E. Fry

Septic shock has traditionally been viewed as clinical hypotension secondary to severe and uncontrolled infection. However, as in many areas of medicine and surgery today, septic shock as a concept is undergoing a rapid conceptual change. Septic shock occurs at a cellular level at a much earlier period of time than the simple clinical identification of hypotension. Indeed, hypotension occurs after the microcirculatory shock state may have existed for hours to days. Whereas septic shock has traditionally been viewed as being a consequence of severe infection, it is now apparent that septic shock may in some cases be secondary to endogenous microorganisms *not* associated with an infectious source or may be seen even in the absence of microorganisms altogether.

Septic shock is an end phase of the septic response. The septic response represents the nonspecific host response to inflammation that is unleashed at a systemic level. The septic response is the consequence of a biologic stimulus that activates systemic inflammation. This chapter will discuss the natural history and biology of the human septic response. The interrelationships among the septic response, septic shock, and multiple organ failure will be addressed. The currently defined management of the septic state will be discussed, and future management options also will be suggested.

THE SEPTIC RESPONSE

The septic shock syndrome begins with the septic response. The literature on the subject of the septic response is confusing, primarily because standardized definitions are lacking. Clinicians use the terms *septic, septicemia, sepsis, septic syndrome,* and many others, but each term means different things to different people. Often these terms are used synonymously to imply that systemic manifestations of severe infection are present. These terms imply that infection has reached a severe level that is no longer contained at the primary site of infection.

When a patient is deemed to be *septic*, it is understood that failure to reverse the patient's clinical course will result in the septic shock syndrome and subsequent death. *Septic shock* in this setting refers to the reduction in arterial blood pressure that is the extreme consequence of the septic response.

The natural history of the septic state in humans has been described by Siegel and associates.[1] These authors defined four states of human sepsis that were identified among numerous physiologic and biochemical observations of critically ill patients (Table 10–1).

The first stage of the process is state A. State A represents the classic stress response. This state is characterized by a modest elevation of cardiac output and a slight reduction in systemic peripheral vascular resistance. Arterial blood pressure is unchanged. The patient will usually have a mild tachycardia, which is reflective of the neuroendocrine response to injury, major operation, and pain. Oxygen consumption is increased, and lactate concentration is normal. Patients will usually have mild hyperglycemia from accelerated gluconeogenesis secondary to increased glucagon concentrations.[2] The increased rate of gluconeogenesis requires alanine to provide the carbon skeleton necessary to synthesize new sugar. The increased rate of gluconeogenesis requires increased protein intake because amino acids will have become a preferred fuel for purposes other than protein synthesis. State A is usually a short-term process that will complete its course in 3 to 4 days for most patients in the absence of an intercurrent stress event (e.g., reoperation, postoperative hemorrhage, etc.).

State B represents the exaggerated stress response. It is an exaggerated response by virtue of the profound and sustained nature of the physiologic changes. State B is characterized by marked elevations of cardiac output to levels that may be 100 percent or more above normal values. These patients have a severe decline in systemic vascular resistance. This loss of systemic vascular resistance reduces left ventricular afterload and is the principal force which drives the elevated cardiac output. The reduction of systemic vascular resistance to levels less than 800 dyn-cm/s[5] defines the septic response. During state B, a narrowing of peripheral arteriovenous oxygen difference is identified as being representative of a peripheral defect in oxygen metabolism. Narrowing of the arteriovenous oxygen difference heralds the emergence of increased serum lactate concentration. The magnitude of the serum lactate elevation appears to correlate with the probability of patient mortality.[3] Patients that are in state B have a reduced mean arterial pressure but are not clinically hypotensive. Such patients have a profound tachycardia of 120 beats per minute or more. The in-

TABLE 10–1. The Four States of the Septic Response

State	Cardiac Output	Peripheral Vascular Resistance	Arterial Pressure	Lactate
A	Slightly increased	Slightly reduced	Normal	Normal
B	Markedly increased	Markedly reduced	Normal	Increased
C	Normal/slightly increased	Markedly reduced	Shock	Markedly increased
D	Reduced	Increased	Shock	Markedly increased

ability to extract oxygen in the periphery is evidence that a shock state exists at the level of the cell, though arterial hypotension may not be manifest.

State C represents the progression of state B to the point where the patient is no longer able to generate a cardiac output sufficient to meet the demands of the profound loss of systemic vascular resistance. Even though cardiac output is at a level that would customarily be viewed as normal or slightly elevated, clinical hypotension is present because of the loss of resistance. Patients in state C are commonly described as having "hot" shock in that they are warm to the touch and are flushed in appearance. Inadequate perfusion pressure has the deleterious effect of further compounding the peripheral defect of oxidative metabolism in the septic response. Lactate accumulation in the serum is now further exacerbated. The patient in state C represents the classic septic shock patient.

While it is implied in this discussion that the transition from state B to state C would likely occur in all severely infected patients, this may, in fact, not be true. State B requires that the patient has sufficient cardiac reserve to mount the hyperdynamic response. Patients with significant coronary artery disease or impaired ventricular function may not be able to generate the cardiac output necessary to maintain arterial pressure in the face of the profound reduction of systemic vascular resistance. These latter patients may clinically enter directly into state C with the onset of the septic response. This clinical scenario is commonly identified in older patients, in whom the absence of cardiac reserve results in "septic shock" as an early manifestation of severe infection.

State D represents the evolution of frank congestive heart failure from the fundamental septic process. The state D patient has a reduced cardiac output and peripheral vasoconstriction. The patient is now in "cold" shock, with a cool touch and an ashen or dusky appearance. State D is generally viewed as a preterminal event and is very difficult to manage. The patient has arterial hypotension, inadequate cardiac output, and peripheral vasoconstriction superimposed on defective peripheral oxygen utilization. Elevation of cardiac output and afterload reduction become major objectives in this stage of patient management.

THE SEPTIC RESPONSE: AMPLIFICATION OF A NORMAL PROCESS

The biologic events which ultimately result in septic shock and its sequelae are actually accentuated normal physiologic responses. When the septic response is viewed as a systemic event, it must be considered deleterious. However, when the same process is viewed from a local or regional perspective, it may be perceived as a positive reaction. Both the systemic and local responses have their foundation in the human inflammatory response.

Cell-to-cell signaling processes are an important part of our inflammatory response. Cell responses and cell-to-cell signals are initiated by stimuli, mediators, and effectors. There are numerous stimulators of the inflammatory response (Table 10–2). Endotoxins, whole bacteria, exotoxins, foreign debris, and necrotic tissue all represent potential stimuli of inflammation. In transplantation immunology, foreign antigen represents a potential stimulus to inflammation.

TABLE 10–2. Stimuli Responsible for Activation of the Septic Response

---

Infections Secondary to Microorganisms

Intraabdominal infection
  Peritonitis
  Abscess
  Infarcted intestine
Pneumonitis
  Non-ventilator-associated
  Ventilator-associated
  Aspiration-associated
Wound infections
  Necrotizing fasciitis
  Clostridial myonecrosis
Pleural space/chest infections
  Mediastinitis
  Empyema
Urinary tract infections
  Perinephric abscess
  Obstructed urinary tract
  Cystitis in the elderly
Intravascular device infections
  Central catheters
  Peripheral catheters
  Swan-Ganz catheters
  Arterial lines

Microorganisms without Infection

Bacterial translocation
  Staphylococcus epidermidis
  Enterococcus sp.
  Other enteric aerobic species
Fungal translocation
  Candida albicans
  Other *Candida* sp.

No Microorganisms and No Infection

Necrotic tissue
  Large soft tissue injuries
  Long bone fractures
Sterile inflammatory foci
  Pancreatitis
  Acute aspiration pneumonitis
  Inhalation injuries
Nonspecific activation of the complement cascade
  Cardiac surgery following membrane oxygenation
  Hemodialysis
  Antigen/antibody interactions (e.g., acute graft rejection
    in transplantation, antibiotic hypersensitivity)

The stimulus may activate protein mediators directly or may activate cells which then synthesize and release mediators that stimulate other cells to produce secondary responses. The response of the cell that has been stimulated by a mediator then has an effector response. The effector response may be a terminal effect or another mediator designed to signal another cell population.

Mediators may be endocrine, paracrine, or autocrine in scope (Table 10–3). *Endocrine* mediators are released by one cell population and then travel some distance via the bloodstream or lymphatic circulation to effect responses from remote receptor cells. The hypothalamic release of adrenocorticotropic hormone (ACTH), which then stimulates the adrenal cortex, is a classic example of an endocrine mediator. The effector signal from the adrenal cortex (i.e., cortisol) is itself another mediator, since it signals a second-order response from additional cell populations.

Paracrine mediators are released by one cell population and stimulate effector cells within the immediate environment. Thus interactions between Kupffer cells via interleukin 6 (IL-6) with adjacent hepatocytes would be an example of a paracrine interaction. Vascular endothelial cells that regulate contraction or relaxation of adjacent smooth muscle cells would be a second example. The differences between endocrine and paracrine responses are actually technical in terms of the distance traveled by the chemical mediator.

An *autocrine* mediator is a chemical messenger that is released by a cell and stimulates itself to a secondary action. Tumor necrosis factor (TNF) and IL-1 are mediators released by macrophages which stimulate macrophages to a second response. Autocrine responses are potentially internal and external in domain. Tumor necrosis factor is released outside the macrophage cell and, by binding to TNF receptors on the macrophage, stimulates second-order effects. Internal autocrine mediators would be illustrated by the effect of PgE compounds on skeletal muscle. IL-1 is an endocrine signal that binds to skeletal muscle membrane. This binding results in the release of arachidonic acid substrate, which through the cyclooxygenase pathway results in PgE synthesis. The PgE effector signal from the IL-1 mediator now becomes the intracellular autocrine mediator that

TABLE 10–3. The Three Types of Mediator Systems that Typify Cell-to-Cell Interactions

Class of Mediator	Example	Description
Endocrine	Cortisol release by the adrenal gland Interleukin 1 release by activated macrophages	An endocrine mediator is one in which the chemical signal is released remote from the target cell population that is to receive signal; the chemical messenger must travel some distance via the bloodstream.
Paracrine	Prostacyclin or nitric oxide released by endothelial cell to affect adjacent vascular smooth muscle	A paracrine mediator is released adjacent to the target population of cells and needs to diffuse only a biologically short distance.
Autocrine	Tumor necrosis factor (TNF) release activates the same cell population that produced it Prostaglandin E_2 released within the cell activates lysosomal enzymes for proteolysis	An autocrine mediator is released by a cell and has the same cell or the same cell type as the target; this type of mediator may be released into the external environment (e.g., TNF) or internally within the cell (PgE).

activates lysosomal enzyme–stimulated muscle proteolysis. PgE is synthesized intracellularly and has its autocrine receptor target within the same cell of synthesis.

Cell-to-cell signals are important in the normal inflammatory response. For example, one may examine the normal events that follow a soft tissue injury. A stab wound or puncture of the tissues of the thigh occurs. Collagen is disrupted, capillaries are injured, and red cells extravasate into the area of injury. Exposed collagen and extravasated elements of blood then activate platelets, the clotting cascade, and the complement cascade. Complement cleavage products activate mast cells, which then release inflammatory proteins. This provokes local vasodilation and increased capillary permeability of uninjured microcirculatory components to increase perfusion of the injured area.[4] Vascular permeability changes result in soft tissue edema about the injury site. For those segments of the microvasculature which were disrupted by the injury, platelet aggregation is activated by the exposed collagen. Platelet activation causes the release of thromboxane A_2, one of the many metabolites of the prostaglandin metabolic pathway (Table 10–4). This further activates platelets and vasoconstricts the vas-

TABLE 10–4. The Five Groups of Prostaglandin Metabolites and Their Biologic Function

Prostaglandin Group	Synthetic Enzyme	Biologic Function
PgD	Prostaglandin endoperoxide D isomerase	1. Inhibits ADP-induced platelet aggregation 2. Inhibition of lymphocyte activation 3. Contraction of longitudinal muscle in small bowel 4. Bronchoconstrictor
PgE	Prostaglandin endoperoxide E isomerase	1. Inhibition of lymphoid mitogenesis 2. Inhibition of antibody production 3. Inhibition of cytolysis 4. Inhibition of gastric acid secretion 5. Increases gastric blood flow 6. Increases gastric motility 7. Cytoprotective 8. Vasodilatation
PgF	Prostaglandin F reductase	1. Potent bronchoconstrictor 2. Uterine contraction 3. Venoconstriction
PgI	Prostacyclin synthetase	1. Inhibition of platelet aggregation 2. Vasodilation
Thromboxane	Thromboxane synthetase	1. Platelet aggregation 2. Vasoconstrictor

cular unit leading to and around the injured blood vessel.[5] A platelet-clot plug obliterates the site of the injured vessel and effects hemostasis.

The microenvironment of tissue injury with activated complement cleavage products is now invaded by neutrophils[6] (Table 10–5). The *chemotactic* signals that diffuse from the site of injury now become beacons to neutrophils that injury has occurred. The mediator signal of the complement cleavage products binds to the neutrophils and stimulates *margination* of the neutrophils to the endothelial cells adjacent to the injured area. The neutrophils follow the diffused signal of complement cleavage products to the area of injury by the process of *diapedesis*. The process of *phagocytosis* is then initiated to eliminate bacteria, foreign debris, and dead tissue. *Intracellular killing* and *digestion* complete elimination of the internalized contaminants as the neutrophils secrete reactive oxygen intermediates and lysosomal enzymes into the phagosome, which contains the ingested particles.

Injuries with minimal contamination, minimal foreign debris, and minimal necrotic tissue result in a minimal inflammatory response. The elective surgical wound should fulfill these criteria and accordingly should result in minimal edema and inflammation. When the wound is created under controlled circumstances, the inflammation is reduced in intensity and very short lived.

However, with traumatic wounds, the initial infiltration of the injured area by neutrophils is followed in 24 to 48 h by the infiltration of the area by macrophage cells. Stimulation of macrophage cells by a critical threshold of summed complement cleavage products, endotoxins, foreign debris, and other stimuli results in the fully activated macrophage. When fully activated, the macrophage then releases an array of cytokines which serve as paracrine and autocrine signals in the environment of the injury. TNF is released by the activated macrophage, which activates neutrophils to a frenzied level of activity. The fully activated neutrophils may release reactive oxygen intermediates into the injury environment as a consequence of the maximally activated state. Extracellular killing of bacteria may occur, as well as autolysis of necrotic tissue in the area.

TABLE 10–5. The Current Components of Neutrophil Function

Function	Description
Margination	This is the process whereby the neutrophil binds to the endothelial cell within the microcirculation. Margination represents the first phase of neutrophil migration toward an area of injury or infection.
Diapedesis	This is the method of locomotion for neutrophils as they migrate toward the area of infection.
Chemotaxis	This reflects the responsiveness of neutrophils to chemical signals that direct diapedesis toward an epicenter of injury or infection.
Phagocytosis	This is the process of internalization of a particle or microorganism by the creation of an intracytoplamic sphere of invaginated plasma membrane.
Intracellular killing and digestion	This process represents the secretion of lysosomal enzymes and reactive oxygen intermediates into the phagosome after phagocytosis to either kill or digest particles.

The neutrophils themselves are commonly killed by this indiscriminate and generalized release of toxic reactive intermediates. Inflammation begets more inflammation, and complement activation is further accelerated. Neutrophils are recruited into this area of inflammation by virtue of the endocrine release of IL-1. The resultant neutrophilia results in massive margination of neutrophils around the area of injury. Microvascular thrombosis occurs from margination of neutrophils that are fully activated within the microcirculation prior to diapedesis into the area of injury itself. Necrotic tissue and extracellular tissue digestion by lysosomal enzymes and reactive oxygen intermediates, combined with thrombosis of the surrounding nutrient microcirculation, result in the formation of pus. External drainage or systematic phagocytosis of all nonviable tissue and bacteria then completes a marvelously intricate and complex system of nonspecific host defense mediated by the inflammatory response.

THE SEPTIC RESPONSE: A PATHOLOGIC EVENT

The systemic septic response is simply the normal and appropriate local inflammatory response that is activated at a systemic level. In essence, normal autocrine and paracrine signals become endocrine mediators, with resultant systemic inflammation. The normal local response becomes a pathophysiologic systemic septic response.

For purposes of discussion, examine the natural course of events in a patient with gram-negative bacteremia. Circulating gram-negative organisms and cell wall endotoxins now become systemic in distribution. Dissemination of gram-negative organisms results in neutrophil activation. The activated neutrophils are the product of the same process described above in the example of the soft tissue wound. First, endotoxin is a very potent activator of the complement cascade through the alternative pathway.[7] This results in systemic release of complement cleavage products. As noted above, the complement cleavage products serve as chemotactic or directional signals to draw neutrophils into an area of injury and contamination. If complement activation is generalized, one has fully activated neutrophils, but in a nondirected fashion. Second, endotoxin activates macrophages by two mechanisms. Endotoxins directly bind to the macrophages, which, in turn, stimulate the activated macrophages to synthesize and release TNF and an array of other cytokines.[8] Complement cleavage products also activate macrophages to release cytokines. Finally, it now appears that endotoxin will directly activate neutrophils through the CD14 membrane receptor.[9] The aggregate effects of complement cleavage products, macrophage-derived cytokines, and direct stimulation from endotoxins are nondirected, diffusely activated neutrophils.

Given full activation of neutrophils without direction, the neutrophils indiscriminately bind to endothelial cells through the CD18 receptor site.[10] Why the neutrophils bind to certain endothelial cells and not others remains unexplained. Those organs which have increased levels of oxygen consumption appear most vulnerable, while the endothelial cells of the resting skeletal muscle mass appear relatively unaffected until very late in the process. Neutrophil localization tends to occur in those endothelial cells within organs known to fail in the multiple organ failure (MOF) syndrome.

The activated neutrophils are marginated to the endothelial cells but still have no chemotactic signal to direct them into the soft tissue. The influence of full activation, as occurred in the soft tissue wound analogy noted earlier, results in release of toxic reactive oxygen intermediates normally employed to kill bacteria or digest necrotic tissue in a local inflammatory focus. The inflammatory damage of reactive oxygen intermediates results in endothelial cell injury, platelet activation, and activation of the coagulation mechanism. The summed effects of the endothelial cell–neutrophil–platelet–fibrin aggregate is a biomechanical plug that now becomes a component of the microcirculatory ischemic injury of the nutrient circulation of critical visceral structures.[11] The biomechanical plug increases the vascular resistance of the splanchnic circulation, which results in the redistribution of cardiac output to the uninvolved periphery (e.g., skeletal muscle).

A second important event attends the activation of platelets at the site of the neutrophil–endothelial cell aggregate. The platelet release of thromboxane A_2 results in microvasoconstriction and further promotes the aggregation of platelets. Selective inhibition of thromboxane synthetase appears to protect the microcirculation in rats with severe sepsis.[12,13] It would appear that thromboxane A_2 is of significance in addition to the microaggregate in the resultant microcirculatory arrest. Thus progressive increases in cardiac output result in increased perfusion to the low-resistance, low-metabolic-demand tissues (e.g., skeletal muscle), while the high-resistance, high-metabolic-demand tissues of the splanchnic circulation are ischemic.[14] This increased cardiac output is accompanied by a narrowed arteriovenous difference, because cardiac output is distributed to tissues that already have more than ample oxygen delivery. Septic shock is present in the state B septic response patient even though systemic measurements of arterial pressure would give the clinical appearance of adequate tissue perfusion.

Microcirculatory arrest results in focal ischemic necrosis. Focal necrosis now results in a new inflammatory lesion. The area of necrosis now becomes the stimulus to recycle the entire process. Inflammation begets necrosis, which begets additional inflammation. The process is a self-energizing, recycled wheel of inflammation. If systemic blood pressure is maintained by various therapeutic measures, the patient remains in state B and develops multiple organ failure. If the severity of the process exceeds a certain threshold or the patient's cardiac reserve is inadequate, then state C or state D evolves with "septic shock." Multiple organ failure and septic shock are end stages of the systemic septic response and are terminal expressions of the same pathophysiologic process.

THE SEPTIC RESPONSE: COMPONENT PARTS

How is the diagnosis of septic shock made? How is *septic shock* even defined? The pathophysiologic definition of septic shock is the ineffective oxygenation of critical tissues secondary to the systemic manifestations of the septic response. This definition would consider the state B patient as being in shock, even though arterial blood pressure is deemed to be normal. If purists must have arterial hypotension as a requirement for the septic shock definition, then one could amend the definition to be a hypotensive state secondary to the consequences of the systemic septic response.

Diagnosis of the septic response can be somewhat more complex than might first appear to be the case. Fever and leukocytosis are commonly identified as components of the septic response, but both can be identified in simple local infections when no other sequelae or systemic manifestation of sepsis can be recognized. Fever and leukocytosis are consequences of the macrophage release of IL-1.[15] TNF and IL-6 also have endogenous pyrogen effects.[16,17] Fever and leukocytosis are not self-destructive components of the septic response but are integral parts of the state A stress response.

Other nonspecific signs of the septic response include gastrointestinal ileus and hyperglycemia. Postoperative and postinjury patients may have an ileus response for reasons other than sepsis. Exogenous glucose administration and the increased gluconeogenesis of the state A stress response make modest hyperglycemia up to 200 mg/dl a very commonplace observation.

The septic response has four component parts that establish this diagnosis. These four components include (1) reduced peripheral vascular resistance, (2) elevated cardiac output, (3) narrowed arteriovenous oxygen difference, and (4) serum accumulation of lactate.

REDUCED SYSTEMIC VASCULAR RESISTANCE

The loss of systemic peripheral vascular resistance is the sine qua non of the septic response. Other forms of shock and shock states (e.g., hypovolemia, cardiogenic failure) are associated with increased systemic vascular resistance. The loss of vascular resistance is obviously the total effect summed from all peripheral vascular beds. Inflammatory aggregate formation within the microcirculation, as described above, would be associated with increased vascular resistance if sufficient vascular units were affected.

The paradox of reduced systemic vascular resistance is further underscored by the increased catecholamine concentrations that are identified in the septic patient. Increased concentrations of epinephrine have been consistently identified, with catecholamines identified as part of the counterregulatory hormonal environment of the neuroendocrine response to injury and stress.[18,19] The alpha-adrenergic effects of the catecholamines are overridden by other mechanisms.

One hypothesis to explain the loss of systemic vascular resistance has been the production of false neurotransmitters by the liver during the stress response. Aromatic amino acids are part of the circulating pool of amino acids present from either dietary intake or muscle proteolysis and are oxidized by the liver. The liver during the septic response does not completely oxidize the aromatic amino acids but rather produces incomplete metabolites. One such metabolite is octopamine, which is the product of the incomplete oxidation of phenylalanine.[20] Octopamine may then act as a false neurotransmitter and compete for catecholamine receptors in the periphery. Sufficiently high concentrations of octopamine or other competitive products may functionally create alpha-adrenergic blockade and vasodilation. Since cirrhotic patients, like septic patients, lack the ability to completely oxidize aromatic amino acids in the liver, and since cirrhotics also have reduced peripheral vascular resistance and high octopamine concentrations in blood, it would appear that the false neurotransmitter theory of reduced systemic vascular resistance has some credibility.[21]

Vascular resistance would appear to be under some degree of paracrine control, mediated by cyclooxygenase metabolites from endothelial cells and platelets.[22,23] Septic patients have been identified as having elevated concentrations of thromboxane B_2[24] and 6-keto-PgF$_1$-alpha,[25] which are the respective stable metabolites of thromboxane A_2 and prostacyclin (PgI). Thromboxane A_2 is a potent constrictor of vascular smooth muscle, while prostacyclin is a vasodilator by virtue of causing relaxation of vascular smooth muscle. Both are derived via the prostaglandin cascade.[26] They can be viewed as having a yin-yang relationship, with the net effects of the two opposing forces dictating smooth muscle and hence vascular tone.[23] A marked prostacyclin effect in uninjured endothelial cells competes with a thromboxane A_2 effect from aggregated platelets in those microcirculatory units with endothelial cell–neutrophil–platelet aggregates. This phenomenon would potentially explain the summed vasodilatory effects of the septic response. Since both prostacyclin and thromboxane A_2 are paracrine signals, systemic measurements of stable circulating metabolites may not reflect biologic effects at the microenvironmental level.

Recently, a new mediator of relaxation of vascular smooth muscle has been more fully characterized. Endothelial-derived relaxing factor (EDRF) has been a described but chemically undefined mediator of the relaxation of vascular smooth muscle. EDRF was initially identified as being produced by endothelial cells even in the presence of cyclooxygenase inhibitors, thus differentiating it from prostacyclin or other known cyclooxygenase-derived relaxing metabolites (e.g., PgE).

The evidence now supports EDRF as being nitric oxide.[27,28] Certain metabolites of nitric oxide also may have smooth muscle effects. These have given rise to a whole new group of mediators termed *reactive nitrogen intermediates*. Nitric oxide is produced by endothelial cell metabolism of the amino acid arginine to citrulline. Nitric oxide appears to be produced on an constituitive basis; i.e., it is produced at a constant baseline level in the absence of specific stimulatory events. Nitric oxide is also esterified and stored within lysosomal bodies for induced acute release when appropriate membrane stimulation occurs. Endothelial cells have binding sites for kinins and acetylcholine, each of which provokes the acute release of nitric oxide and results in the relaxation of vascular smooth muscle. Endothelial cells have receptor sites for endotoxin, which also produces nitric oxide release. Nitric oxide is a potent paracrine signal that may assume a major role in the profound reduction of systemic vascular resistance during the septic response. The presence of receptor sites for endotoxin and inflammatory proteins such as kinins would certainly support this speculation. If this hypothesis proves to be valid, then the nutritional manipulation of arginine, which serves many important functions (e.g., hepatic ureagenesis), will become an area of special interest.

Thus the paradigm is presented that vascular tone in the septic response has a vasoconstrictive component in the splanchnic area, while vasodilatation predominates in the skeletal muscle and cutaneous areas. The flushed, warm, and diaphoretic feel of the skin that is recognized in "septic" patients confirms this observation. To use an analogy from the physics of electricity, current will flow in a parallel circuit to those pathways with least resistance. Low-resistance tissue beds will receive the predominant volume of cardiac output, while high-resistance tissue beds will receive less flow. Summed resistance in the parallel circuit of the state B and state C septic response patient yields a low calculated systemic vascular resistance.

The discussion to this point has implied the simple hypothesis that each organ has a defined vascular resistance that is either low or high in a quantitative sense. Reality is likely more complex than this model. Studies utilizing flow probes have examined gross *bulk flow* to organs like the liver. These studies have consistently demonstrated that summed liver flow from both the portal and arterial circulations increases with cardiac output.[29,30] However, our studies with indicator clearance techniques have consistently shown a reduced *nutrient flow*.[31-35] Indeed, tissue flow within an organ may well be autoregulated so that redistribution of flow occurs to those microcirculatory units without inflammatory lesions and altered flow exists in units with microaggregation injury. Perfusion through the liver should be viewed as a multichanneled parallel circuit. Hence normal hepatocyte units are identified in immediate proximity to histologically identified areas of necrosis.

ELEVATED CARDIAC OUTPUT

An elevated cardiac output is an obligatory response of the left ventricle when afterload reduction occurs. Vasodilatation of an experimental animal by progressive alpha blockade at the same time that intravascular volume is administered to meet the increased capacitance of the vasodilated state results in a reflex increase in cardiac output. The requirements for an elevated cardiac output with afterload reduction are both adequate volume administration and the physiologic reserve of the myocardium to increase stroke volume. If either of these requirements is not met, then clinical hypotension is the result.

The transition of the patient from the normal state through state A and then to state B requires an expanded volume and ventricular reserve. The state B patient will become hypotensive in the face of inadequate volume; this can be reversed by volume expansion. If coronary artery disease or severe left ventricular myopathy is present, then the patient will have a state A to state C transition even with adequate volume expansion. The sustained state B patient may develop ventricular fatigue or exhaustion, which then results in evolution of the state C or classic septic shock state.

Therefore, for most patients with the septic response and an acceptable systemic arterial blood pressure, an elevated cardiac output is the anticipated physiologic response in the face of extreme afterload reduction. The inverse relationship of changes between resistance and cardiac output is necessary for arterial pressure to be maintained.

Much discussion has surrounded the subject of myocardial depression and circulating factors that mediate reduced ventricular performance in septic patients.[36-39] Measurement of ventricular contractility even in state B hyperdynamic patients appears to demonstrate reduced ventricular wall compliance and increased end-diastolic volume. Ventricular performance would appear to be less efficient than might be the case with pure afterload reduction. Impaired ventricular performance may indicate that cardiac and skeletal muscle are not immune to the inflammatory pathology of the septic response. Indeed, inflammatory histologic lesions of the myocardium can be seen in extreme challenges with endotoxin[40] or live gram-negative bacteria.[41] The afterload reduction and tachycardia of the septic state appear to be important compensatory mechanisms that sustain cardiac output in the face of an inefficient left ventricle. These compensatory mechanisms maintain adequate oxygen delivery to the peripheral tissues. However, the progression of the microcirculatory injury within even the myocardium may reach such a level of severity as to become a major variable in the state B to state C transition. The responsiveness of the myocardium to inotropic support may reflect the severity of the microcirculatory injury within the myocardium itself. Nevertheless, it would appear that the myocardium, like skeletal muscle, is less vulnerable to the development of the microcirculatory injury of the septic response.

NARROWED ARTERIOVENOUS OXYGEN DIFFERENCE

The patient with the state B septic response, while hypermetabolic, does not appear to have a total level of oxygen consumption consistent with the hyperdynamic state.[42,43] While having an increased concentration of lactate in serum, further elevations of cardiac output with inotropic support only seem to narrow the arteriovenous oxygen content differences. When venous phlebotomy is undertaken for purposes of laboratory studies in the "septic" patient, bright red blood is identified that has a high venous oxygen saturation.

Hyperperfusion of low-resistance microcirculatory units results in relatively constant total oxygen extraction per unit of time but less extraction per volume of blood passing through the microvasculature. High-resistance microcirculatory units receive no increased perfusion by increasing oxygen delivery from the hyperdynamic state because flow favors the low-resistance units. Hence oxygen-starved tissue beds have no appreciable improvement in oxygen consumption with increased delivery, while already hyperperfused tissue beds further reduce the extraction coefficient.

INCREASED SERUM LACTATE CONCENTRATIONS

Cellular production of lactate is the consequence of anaerobic glycolysis. Under normal circumstances of adequate cellular oxygenation, glucose is metabolized to pyruvate via the Embden-Myerhof pathway within the cytoplasm of the cell. This is an oxygen-independent event that produces limited useful energy for the cell. Pyruvate is then transported into the mitochondrion for oxidation into CO_2, water, and the aerobic production of adenosine triphosphate (ATP).

When the cell is in an oxygen-deprived state, such as shock or hypoxemia, the cytochrome complexes within the mitochondrion become fully reduced, and no additional pyruvate can be transported into the mitochondrion. Energy demands by the cell may remain unchanged or increased and have only anaerobic glycolysis as a means for ATP generation. Because anaerobic glycolysis requires the reduction of NAD^+ to $NADH^+$, anaerobic glycolysis without oxidation of pyruvate to acetyl-CoA results in the saturation of all available NAD^+. Without available NAD^+, even anaerobic glycolysis will cease, and cellular death will rapidly ensue.

The physiologic mechanism which allows cell populations to withstand transient episodes of hypoxemia is the production of lactate. The oxidation of $NADH^+$ to NAD^+ by the enzyme lactate dehydrogenase produces lactate from the pyruvate that cannot enter into oxidation within the mitochondrion and regenerates NAD^+ to permit sustained anaerobic glycolysis. The lactate that is generated by this process then diffuses out of the cell and can be measured in the systemic circulation. Lactate can then become an energy substrate for other cell populations which have both the oxygen and the enzyme systems for lactate-to-pyruvate oxidation. Measurements of increased lactate in the sera of patients and experimental animals implies that tissue beds are present which are producing lactate at rates that exceed lactate oxidation by perfused or oxygenated tissues. Obviously, if systemic hypoxemia or profound arterial hypotension is present, then lactate production will be great and lactate oxidation will be minimal. This results in very high concentrations of lactate within the circulation. If only a region of the body is ischemic or hypoxic, lactate production may not exceed its oxidation by other tissues, and no concentration increase will be seen in circulating blood. The synthesis and oxidation of lactate as a dynamic process must be carefully considered.

From the preceding discussion it should be apparent that the molar ratio of [lactate]/[pyruvate] is equal to $[NADH^+]/[NAD^+]$ ratio. Thus the [lactate]/[pyruvate] ratio of a cell reflects the oxidation-reduction state within the cytoplasm of that cell. Similarly, the [lactate]/[pyruvate] ratio of a tissue represents the summed oxidation-reduction states of all cells within that tissue. Some could be well oxygenated and others could be ischemic, but a composite sampling such as might be done by measuring the lactate and pyruvate from the venous drainage would reflect the biologic summation of all component cells. Furthermore, the measurement of [lactate]/[pyruvate] ratios in the systemic circulation may then represent the summed cytoplasmic oxidation-reduction states of all contributing and actively metabolizing cells.

In the state B septic response patient, lactate concentrations in the systemic circulation are increased, but they are increased in an equimolar relationship with circulating pyruvate. This equimolar increase in lactate and pyruvate has been used as a rationale for implicating a primary cellular metabolic abnormality as being responsible for the defective oxygen metabolism of the septic response. Such a line of reasoning concludes that the unchanged [lactate]/[pyruvate] ratio reflects a normal cytoplasmic oxidation-reduction state and that the increased lactate and pyruvate concentrations in blood represent a mitochondrial transport defect, wherein substrate cannot enter the mitochondrion. Defective pyruvate dehydrogenase complex has been hypothesized as the enzyme system responsible for the cellular abnormality of oxygen consumption.[44,45]

Why such an explanation is even plausible remains obscure. Inability of pyruvate to enter the mitochondrion via pyruvate dehydrogenase still leaves the fundamental problem of a lack of recycled NAD^+ to support glycolysis. Such a defect should still require pyruvate reduction to lactate to facilitate the regeneration of NAD$^+$ and sustain glycolysis. A more plausible explanation is that the systemic oxidation-reduction potential within the cytoplasm as a summation of the entire organism is reflected by the skeletal muscle, which is well oxygated and well perfused. Lactate is consumed by the muscle cell, and the [lactate]/[pyruvate] ratio within the muscle cell is normal equilibrium. Excess pyruvate production from the abundant lactate, which is derived from the ischemic cells of the splanchnic and visceral compartments, exceeds the needs of the resting muscle cell and diffuses into the extracellular space. Thus *lactate production is from ischemic visceral cells, but systemic oxidation-reduction ratios are dictated by the well-oxygenated, hyperperfused skeletal muscle mass.* Our experimental data comparing liver tissue [lactate]/[pyruvate] ratios, when compared with concurrent serum concentrations, clearly support this hypothesis.[14]

THE SEPTIC RESPONSE: MANAGEMENT

Management of the septic response patient is as complex as the process itself. Management requires careful monitoring, control of the stimulus during the septic response, and supportive care of the organ systems that are the targets of the autodestructive systemic inflammatory response. As more information about the basic mechanism of the septic response is learned, newer therapies will hopefully improve the results of management.

MONITORING

Monitoring systems represent an important component of the management of the septic response patient. Monitoring systems are important for continuous assessment of the dynamic and rapid changes that can occur during sepsis. Monitoring is primarily directed at the assessment of oxygenation and support of cardiac performance.

The adequacy of systemic oxygenation is important. The emergence of tachypnea and respiratory distress means that arterial oxygenation needs to be monitored by arterial blood gas determinations. Blood gases become important tools after ventilator support has been initiated to ensure that the pO$_2$ and hemoglobin oxygen saturation are maintained. Blood gas determinations also remain important in the process of monitoring patients who are being weaned from ventilator support. Pulse oximetry has become very popular and has allowed a continuous on-line assessment of hemoglobin saturation. Refinements in this technology should permit a reduction in the use of blood gases for monitoring patients. Confidence has not yet been achieved with pulse oximetry as the exclusive means of monitoring the adequacy of diffusible oxygen in blood.

Blood pressure monitoring remains an important tool in the management of septic response patients. Traditional cuff measurements of blood pressure are labor intensive and suffer from a lack of precision needed in critically ill patients. However, the continuous cuff measurement techniques which display the pressure information on a monitor have become practical for use in many patients. When inotropic or vasoactive therapy is employed, or when large volumes of fluids are anticipated as being necessary components of the patient's management, the arterial line remains the most accurate and rapidly responsive blood pressure monitoring method.

The Foley catheter is an important monitoring device. Urine output remains a useful method for assessing renal perfusion. In general, oliguria (<20 cc urine per h) indicates that renal perfusion is inadequate because of hypovolemia, and polyuria (>100 cc urine per h) means that the patient is having a diuresis because of excessive renal preload. The oliguric state requires expansion of intravascular volume with administration of crystalloid solutions or blood component therapy. A relative polyuric state means that volume administration can be restricted during the period where diuresis of excess sodium and water is occurring. However, certain precautions must be exercised in the interpretation of urinary output.

The patient may have a polyuric syndrome seen in the septic response.[46] The polyuric syndrome of the septic state may represent the corticomedullary redistribution of renal blood flow which "washes out" the countercurrent concentrating system of the kidney. The subsequent loss of concentrating ability may result in an inappropriately large volume urinary output, even though the patient is hypovolemic. Occasional comparisons of urinary and plasma osmolarity may be helpful in avoiding this pitfall. Additionally, patients with the septic response demonstrate a relative insulin resistance and accelerated gluconeogenesis and receive exogenous glucose as part of their nutritional support efforts. These patients may have increased urine output because of glycosuria. Periodic measurement of urinary glucose level can be useful in validating the urine output as a monitor of renal perfusion.

Use of the Swan-Ganz catheter has become routine for the management of the septic response patient during the past 10 years.[47] This balloon-tipped pulmonary artery catheter can be placed within the intensive care unit and does not require fluoroscopic support. The pulmonary capillary wedge pressure can be a very sensitive method to optimize left ventricular preload. Thermistor-equipped catheters allow accurate cardiac outputs to be determined. A proximal port on the catheter may allow the measurement of central venous pressure, which can be important for calculation of systemic vascular resistance. Some catheters are equipped with an oximeter so that the mixed venous oxygen saturation can be monitored continuously. Although adopted by cardiac surgeons in many areas of the country, the oximetric Swan-Ganz catheter has not been quite so popular for use in the septic response patient. While some interest has focused on use of thoracic impedance monitoring as a noninvasive means of monitoring cardiac output,[48] this method has not yet been shown to have the reliability needed to replace the Swan-Ganz catheter.

The metabolic cart has now become the newest monitoring device for the septic patient.[49] Oxygen consumption and caloric expenditure can be determined. Computation of caloric expenditure is now adding new sophistication to the design and management of nutritional support.

The use of monitoring devices has proliferated to the point that conventional physical examination and bedside observations of the patient are not fully utilized or are simply ignored. All monitoring devices will have potential mechanical or calibration failures that will lead to false information. The clinician must maintain the perspective that the monitored information is interpreted on the basis of the clinical appearance of the patient. Inconsistencies between the monitored information and clinical appearance must be reconciled by the physician. An alert and responsive patient that is deemed to be profoundly hypotensive on the arterial line monitor may indeed not need heroic volume resuscitation or inotropic support but may simply need to have the transducer for the arterial line recalibrated. Monitors do not replace competent and concurrent clinical examination of the patient's condition.

CONTROL OF THE STIMULUS

The most important feature of managing the septic response patient is to achieve control of the stimulus that is driving the systemic inflammatory response. As has been emphasized in the preceding discussions, the septic response is a nonspecific response of the host to any number of biologic stimuli. While the septic response and septic shock have traditionally been viewed as being the consequences of bacteria arising from an infectious focus, neither microorganisms nor infection is necessary to provoke the process (see Table 10–2). Thus the septic response may occur as a result of (1) microorganisms secondary to infection, (2) microorganisms *not* secondary to infection, or (3) sterile inflammation *without* microorganisms or infection.

MICROORGANISMS SECONDARY TO INFECTION

Infection is defined as clinical inflammation that is the consequence of microorganisms as the inciting stimulus. The clinical inflammation arises from defined anatomic sites. Such sites include the visceral compartments, lung, urinary tract, surgical or traumatic wounds, and intravascular devices. These anatomic sites will account for over 95 percent of septic responses in patients.

   Intraabdominal infection remains the prototype infection associated with the septic response, multiple organ failure, and septic shock. The peritoneal surface represents the equivalent of 40 percent of total body surface area in the adult. Accordingly, infection within the peritoneal cavity becomes the biologic analogue of a large burn wound that can result in the dissemination of bacteria, bacterial cell products, and inflammatory mediators.

   Peritonitis begins with bacterial seeding of the peritoneal cavity. Peritonitis is usually secondary to another disease process leading to bacterial contamination of the peritoneal space. Perforation of the intestine, transmural inflammation of the gut with secondary bacterial contamination of the peritoneal cavity, and perforation of the biliary tract represent the usual processes that result in peritonitis. Peritonitis may be a primary infection without a biliary-enteric source when hematogenous or lymphatic seeding of the peritoneal cavity occurs.[50,51] This latter event of primary, or spontaneous, peritonitis is quite uncommon and is usually seen in the contemporary clinical setting among patients with ascites secondary to hepatic cirrhosis.

   With contamination of the peritoneal cavity, dissemination is a natural consequence as the normal movement of peritoneal fluid facilitates movement of the bacterial organisms away from the primary site of soilage. Peritoneal fluid is normally produced within the peritoneal cavity as the result of extracellular fluid accumulation from physiologic hydrostatic pressures within the mesentery. Clearance of peritoneal fluid is normally through the numerous lymphatic fenestrations present on the diaphragmatic surface of the peritoneal cavity.[52–54] When the patient is in a recumbent position, the relatively negative pressure beneath the diaphragm with each expired breath results in movement of the peritoneal fluid toward the fenestrations. The fluid passes through the fenestrations and then into the lymphatic system and subsequently into the thoracic duct. In essence, the peritoneal cavity is a large lymphocele that directly communicates into the lymphatic system.

Dissemination of the bacterial contaminants within the peritoneal cavity increases the interface between the host and the potential pathogens. Dissemination also diminishes the density of bacteria at the site of contamination, and in this sense, it represents a nonspecific host defense mechanism.

Bacterial lodgment into the peritoneal tissues initiates an inflammatory response in much the same way that any injury provokes inflammation. Neutrophils become the primary phagocytic cells to infiltrate the areas of contamination, followed by the macrophage cells. As noted earlier in this discussion, the inflammatory response is initiated to effect containment of the bacteria. Host defense is primarily the phagocytic response and phagocytic elimination of the bacteria. When the density of bacteria exceeds the phagocytic capability of the host, loculation of the contaminant becomes the secondary line of defense to contain the infectious process.

Since host response is generic, characteristics of the bacterial inoculum and certain adjuvant factors dictate whether infection is contained or systemic activation of the inflammatory cascade occurs. First, the number of bacteria within the peritoneal contaminant is important. With a perforated peptic ulcer in a young patient with considerable gastric acidity, the number of actual bacteria introduced into the peritoneal cavity is quite small. The inflammatory process is basically chemical in nature, and resolution of the peritonitis, assuming repair of the perforation responsible for initiating the process, occurs by normal physiologic processes.

The bacteria present may have their virulence greatly enhanced by the presence of adjuvant factors in the microenvironment of the infectious process. Hemoglobin is a very potent adjuvant for bacterial virulence. Hemoglobin may increase the virulence of bacteria by increasing the availability of iron for bacterial proliferation, or the metabolism of hemoglobin by bacteria may actually produce a leukotoxin that poisons the phagocytic response.[55,56] Regardless of mechanism, hemoglobin within the peritoneal cavity makes containment of the bacterial inoculum by host defense mechanisms less likely. Necrotic tissue and foreign bodies are potent adjuvant variables as well. While the mechanism responsible for the adjuvant effects of necrotic tissue and foreign bodies remains uncertain, they likely make bacterial contaminants less accessible to phagocytic cells.

Thus the natural history of peritonitis can have three potential outcomes. The summed effects of a small bacterial inoculum plus minimal contributions from adjuvant factors result in resolution of the peritonitis, assuming that the primary biliary-enteric defect (e.g., perforated peptic ulcer) has been repaired. On the other hand, the magnitude of bacterial contamination plus adjuvant factors (e.g., necrotic intestine) may be biologically overwhelming and result in fulminant peritonitis with death of the host. A third potential outcome can occur, wherein a relative standoff develops between the inflammatory response and the bacterial pathogens, with abdominal abscess being the result. In general, if the abscess state within the peritoneal cavity is not drained, host defense mechanisms will ultimately fail, and the patient will die from the septic response and its sequelae.

The diagnosis of acute peritonitis is primarily a clinical one. The patient history will usually identify a sudden event that characterizes the perforation. With acute peritonitis, the abdominal examination will usually demonstrate diffuse tenderness that may involve the entire abdomen depending on the magnitude of contamination, the duration of time since perforation, and the degree of dissemination that has occurred. Rebound tenderness is the characteristic sign of peritonitis. Boardlike rigidity may be present, reflecting the muscular spasm of the abdominal wall in patients with severe peritoneal inflammation. Fever and leukocytosis are usually present in these patients and are nonspecific findings for the septic response, regardless of the source. Flat and upright abdominal roentgenograms are commonly obtained on these patients, although frequently the study is of little value. The one notable exception is when free air can be identified underneath the diaphragm as evidence that perforation of the gastrointestinal tract has indeed occurred.

The diagnosis of abdominal abscess is much more difficult. Many of these patients will have already undergone a recent laparotomy for peritonitis or trauma. The recent surgical wound severely compromises findings of abdominal tenderness even in the patient with significant purulent collections in the abdominal cavity. Rectal examinations may be of use in selected cases (e.g., perforated appendix) in the identification of postoperative abscess. Routine abdominal roentgenograms are of little value.[57] Ultrasound examinations are commonly done and are only rarely of diagnostic merit. Seldom would a surgeon base a decision for reoperation on results of an ultrasound examination alone.

The computed tomographic (CT) scan has become the diagnostic method of choice for intraabdominal abscess. The CT scan provides remarkable anatomic detail. The use of oral and intravascular contrast agents can be very helpful in separating artifacts of normal intraluminal contents from pathologic collections within the peritoneal cavity. The accuracy afforded by the CT scan may even permit percutaneous drainage of the purulent collection.[58,59]

When peritonitis or abdominal abscess is established as the diagnosis, the treatment regimens follow the same sequence of events. First, the biliary-enteric source of bacterial contamination must be controlled. Repair, resection, or exteriorization of the perforated structure must be achieved to eliminate the ongoing soilage of the peritoneal cavity. Second, all purulent drainage must be evacuated and necrotic tissue debrided. Finally, antibiotic therapy appropriate for the likely pathogens responsible for the infection needs to be initiated.

When abdominal abscess is established as the diagnosis, the clinician will be confronted with the issue of percutaneous drainage versus open drainage. Percutaneous drainage avoids the potential morbidity of the reoperative event but may not be as effective in specific circumstances. Percutaneous drainage is appropriate when precise anatomic localization of the abscess can be achieved with the CT scan, when drainage can be achieved without traversing another luminal structure within the abdomen, and when the patient is not demonstrating evidence of the septic response. Open drainage is preferred for complex and multiloculated abscess collections. The open method is favored if the patient has an uncontrolled perforation of the gastrointestinal tract or leakage of a failed suture line from a previous operation. When patients are demonstrating evidence of a severe septic response, early organ failure, or septic shock, the urgency to effect complete and total control of the septic focus mandates an open drainage effort.

While antibiotic therapy is an important adjunctive treatment for the patient with suppurative peritonitis and abscess, it is important to emphasize that drug therapy cannot replace mechanical drainage of the primary focus. The environment of an abscess prevents antibiotic efficacy. The inoculum of the bacteria is very great, the pH of the environment is low, and there is a very low oxidation-reduction potential, a condition that is deleterious for certain antibiotic choices (e.g., aminoglycosides). The protein-rich milieu of an abscess tends to bind antibiotics and neutralize activity. Pus still must be drained.

With the advent of CT scans, a certain reluctance to pursue empirical reoperation for abdominal abscess has developed.[60,61] This attitude is in counterdistinction to aggressive attitudes about reoperation that were present about 10 years ago.[57,62,63] While the CT scan has dramatically improved the diagnostic accuracy for abdominal abscess, it still remains falsely negative or equivocal in about 10 percent of cases. Empirical reoperation must still be considered when patients have considerable evidence to favor the intraabdominal compartment as the source for a continued septic response. For example, the patient who has previously undergone an abdominal exploration for a perforated sigmoid colon from a gunshot wound and who is experiencing a septic response on the seventh postinjury day must be strongly considered for reoperation, even if the CT scan does not clearly define an abscess.

The selection of antibiotic coverage for the patient with peritonitis or abdominal abscess remains controversial.[64] There is general agreement that both aerobic gram-negative rods (*E. coli*) and anaerobic *Bacteroides fragilis* should be covered. Including the *Enterococcus* sp. within the antibiotic spectrum of coverage is advocated by some but remains highly debatable. With the introduction of the expanded-spectrum beta-lactam group of antibiotics, one can now identify both aerobic and anaerobic spectrums of activity in a single drug. Some clinicians have advocated these single antibiotic drugs for patients with intraabdominal infection. Double or triple antibiotic combinations continue to be the choice of others. Many of the commonly chosen antibiotic regimens for the treatment of intraabdominal infection are listed in Table 10–6.

Pleural space infection can be another infectious focus that provokes the septic response. These infections commonly occur after thoracic operations or after the placement of a chest tube into the pleural space for any number of indications. Pleural space infection may occasionally be a complication of subdiaphragmatic infection.

The pathophysiology of infection in the pleural space shares many common characteristics with infection in the peritoneal cavity. The parietal and visceral pleura are histologically similar to the peritoneum. Contaminants within the pleural space doubtlessly elicit the same series of inflammatory responses iden-

TABLE 10–6. The Advantages and Disadvantages of Potential Antibiotic Choices for the Treatment of Intraabdominal Infection

Antibiotic Choice	Advantages	Disadvantages
Cefoxitin	Monotherapy Activity against anticipated pathogens	Short half-life (45 min) Some *B. fragilis* resistance reported
Cefotetan	Monotherapy Longer half-life (3.5 h) *B. fragilis* activity	Poor non-*fragilis Bacteroides* coverage ? Coagulopathy problems
Ampicillin/sulbactam	Reasonable coverage of likely pathogens, including *Bacteroides*	Penicillin hypersensitivity Short half-life (1 h) ? *E. coli* resistance
Ticarcillin/ clavulanate	Good coverage of anticipated pathogens	Short half-life (1 h) Penicillin hypersensitivity
Cefotaxime	Monotherapy Excellent coverage of Enterobacteriacea	Short half-life (1 h) ? *B. fragilis* coverage
Ceftizoxime	Monotherapy Excellent coverage of Enterobacteriacea	Adequacy of *B. fragilis* remains controversial
Ceftriaxone	Monotherapy Excellent coverage of Enterobacteriacea Long half-life (8 h)	Weak *B. fragilis* coverage
Imipenem	Monotherapy Coverage of all proven and suspected pathogens	Short half-life Overly broad coverage
Aminoglycoside/ clindamycin	Good coverage of anaerobes and Enterobacteriacea	Combination therapy Aminoglycosides require pharmacokinetic dosing Toxicity of aminoglycoside
Aminoglycoside/ metronidazole	Good coverage of anticipated pathogens	Combination therapy Aminoglycoside toxicity and pharmacokinetic dosing
Ampicillin/ aminoglycoside/ clindamycin or metronidazole	Coverage of all proven and suspected pathogens	Cost of administration of triple-drug therapy is enormous; no proven value over lesser choices Aminoglycoside toxicity

tified within the peritoneal cavity. Fluid accumulation is in response to the bacterial contamination, and loculated infection seems to occur very early in the pleural space.

Pleural space infections following thoracotomy or chest tube placement are not easily defined by physical examination. Chest roentgenograms will usually show obliteration of the costophrenic angle or other extrapleural collections of fluid within the chest. CT scans are commonly used to provide better anatomic localization of the empyema. Drainage is achieved by chest tube placement into the area or may be achieved by CT-directed methods. Occasionally, more extensive marsupialization of the abscess cavity or even decortication may be required. For the patient with a septic response, simple external drainage by whatever method is all that is required to blunt the process.

Antibiotics are commonly employed but are only secondary considerations to drainage of the empyema from the pleural space. Postoperative and postthoracostomy infections will commonly have *Staphylococcus aureus* as the principal pathogen. Antibiotic therapy must be directed to cover this organism. Because of the increasing frequency of methicillin-resistant *Staphylococcus* sp., vancomycin is employed until specific sensitivities are available. If empyema is the consequence of infection arising from a subdiaphragmatic process, then the bacteria will likely be similar to intraabdominal pathogens. Thus a broader spectrum of antibiotic therapy that includes aerobic and anaerobic coverage will be necessary.

Pulmonary infection is a significant cause of the septic response. Pulmonary infection may arise via three separate mechanisms to cause the septic response. First, pulmonary infection may occur secondary to atelectasis. In postoperative or injured patients, normal tidal volumes may be compromised because of painful abdominal incisions or injuries of the chest wall. A reduced tidal volume often leads to atelectasis. Atelectasis is the collapse of segments of small airways and alveoli, often with entrapment of bacteria within the collapsed segment. Bacterial proliferation occurs within the collapsed alveolar segments of the lung, which, in turn, provokes an inflammatory response. The pulmonary inflammatory response is somewhat different from that in other areas of the body in that the lung is normally populated by resident macrophages. The release of inflammatory cytokines by resident macrophages then recruits systemic neutrophils into the area. If the atelectasis is uncorrected, the bacterial proliferation and resultant inflammatory response will extend into other uninvolved segments of the lung, resulting in more edema, phagocytic cell infiltration, and increasing inflammation. Pneumonia is the result. The escape of bacteria, bacterial cell products, and inflammatory mediators from the area of infection then precipitates the systemic septic response.

The diagnosis of atelectasis is a clinical decision. The usual scenario involves a patient who has undergone a major abdominal operation. Incisional pain leads to splinting of the patient's normal breathing pattern, resulting in reduced tidal volume and atelectasis. The patient will usually have modest tachypnea and a febrile response on the first night following the operative procedure. Chest roentgenograms at this stage will not be helpful, unless the threshold for pneumonia has already been reached. Coughing, deep breathing, and ambulation of the patient at this point will reexpand the collapsed segments of airway units and prevent pneumonia from developing. Antibiotics are not indicated for the treatment of atelectasis.

The diagnosis of clinical pneumonia is usually quite evident for these patients. Persistent fever and leukocytosis are present. Infiltration is readily identified on chest roentgenogram. The patients will commonly expectorate purulent sputum. Sputum cultures will be necessary to document the offending bacterial pathogen (Table 10–7).

The bacteria responsible for pulmonary infection in non-ventilator-associated pneumonia can be highly variable. If the patient had a minimal preoperative hospitalization and did not receive a course of antibiotics prior to the operative procedure, then the offending pathogen will be one of the bacteria that are nor-

TABLE 10–7. The Likely Pathogens to Be Identified in Patients with Postoperative Pneumonia

Organism	Frequency of Isolation
Pseudomonas sp.	41
Klebsiella sp.	29
Staphylococcus sp.	25
Escherichia coli	24
Proteus sp.	18
Enterobacter sp.	16
Pneumococcus	13
Serratia sp.	10
Streptococcus sp. (group A)	5
Hemophilus influenzae	4
Other gram-negative organisms	9

SOURCE: From Martin LF, Asher EF, Casey JM, Fry DE: Postoperative pneumonia: Determinants of mortality. *Arch Surg* 119:379, 1984, with permission.

mal colonists of the tracheobronchial tree. This will usually be *Streptococcus pneumoniae* or *Hemophilus influenzae*. However, if the patient has had a prolonged preoperative hospitalization or a prior course of antibiotics, then the airways will usually be colonized with hospital-acquired bacteria. Pulmonary infection in this setting will commonly be with *Pseudomonas* sp., *Serratia* sp., or resistant *Enterobacter* sp. Antibiotic choices in this latter situation can be difficult (Table 10–8).

A second mechanism for pulmonary infection is ventilator-associated pneumonitis. Many patients require ventilator support because of the inability to maintain normal oxygenation. Prolonged anesthesia, massive volume resuscitation, and direct chest injury with pulmonary contusion will require ventilator support. The common denominator for all these patients is that the lung has sustained an acute injury. Some patients may have a degree of pulmonary compromise prior to the acute injury, from either tobacco use or other reasons, with the underlying disease amplifying the need for ventilator support to maintain oxygenation.

When the patient is placed on the ventilator, the endotracheal tube breeches the normally protective effects of the glottis. The ventilator apparatus thus becomes a potential source for direct airway contamination. The exogenous contamination into the compromised and commonly edematous lung tissue sets the stage for invasive lung infection. Contamination of the small airways, proliferation of bacteria, and an inflammatory response by the resident macrophage cells result in pneumonia. The already compromised lung now becomes a fertile tissue for extension of the infection, with a septic response as the consequence.

The diagnosis of ventilator-associated pneumonia can be very difficult. All patients who have been on a ventilator for 48 to 72 h will have culturable bacteria in the airway, but this finding alone does not constitute infection. Chest roentgenograms only become positive for new or expanding infiltrates very late in the process. Quantitative culture of the tracheal aspirate has been advocated

TABLE 10-8. Potential Antibiotic Choices for the Treatment of Postoperative Pneumonia

Antibiotic	Advantages	Disadvantages
Gentamycin	*Pseudomonas* coverage	Toxicity Pharmacokinetic dosing
Tobramycin	*Pseudomonas* coverage	Toxicity Pharmacokinetic dosing
Amikacin	Best resistant gram-negative coverage	Toxicity Pharmacokinetic dosing
Mezlocillin	Does not require pharmacokinetic dosing	Short half-life (1 h) *Pseudomonas* resistance
Piperacillin	Reasonable gram-negative coverage; no pharmacokinetic dosing	Short half-life (1 h) *Pseudomonas* resistance
Ticarcillin/clavulanate	Reasonable gram-negative coverage	Short half-life (1 h) *Pseudomonas* resistance
Aminoglycoside/expanded-spectrum penicillin	Comprehensive coverage Antibiotic synergism	Combination therapy Toxicity and pharmacokinetic dosing of the aminoglycoside
Ceftaxidime	Low toxicity	Some *Pseudomonas*/gram-negative resistance
Imipenem	Comprehensive bacterial coverage	Short half-life (1 h) Fungal overgrowth Expense
Aztreonam	Low toxicity	*Pseudomonas* coverage is suspect
Ciprofloxacin	Low toxicity	*Pseudomonas* coverage is suspect

but represents a practical problem in the rapid processing of the aspirated specimen. Also, it is controversial whether tracheal concentrations of bacteria truly reflect tissue level concentrations of bacteria at the site of infection.[65,66] Elastin fibers on Gram's stain can be used for diagnosis of pneumonia but reflect necrosis of tissue and are necessarily a late finding of severe pulmonary infection.[67] The collection of specimens by bronchoscopy, via either the protected-brush technique[68] or bronchoalveolar lavage,[69] remains attractive but relatively untested in postoperative ventilator-supported patients. In the final analysis, a Gram's stain of the tracheal aspirate that demonstrates bacteria within polymorphonuclear cells in a patient with clinical evidence of infection is probably as good as any technique in establishing the diagnosis.

Cultured bacteria from the lung in the patient with a ventilator-associated pneumonia will usually reflect hospital-acquired organisms. *Pseudomonas* sp., *Serratia* sp., and resistant *Enterobacter* sp. are commonly encountered. *Staphylococcus* sp. may be found and potentially represent airway contamination by intensive care unit personnel. Antibiotic therapy must be directed accordingly.

A third mechanism for pulmonary infection is aspiration. Aspiration may be a clinically evident event, from vomiting and direct entry of gastrointestinal contents into the airway, or it can be a more subtle process. Gross clinical aspiration is initially a chemical pneumonitis as particulate matter or gastric acid provokes an inflammatory response from the lung. This chemical pneumonitis results in the need for ventilator support, which then subjects the patient to all the risks of secondary ventilator-associated pulmonary infection.

When gross aspiration events are suspected, bronchoscopy can be of both diagnostic and therapeutic value. Bronchoscopic evaluation can identify foreign material within the airway and also afford the opportunity to evacuate aspirated particles. A baseline culture can be obtained at this time. Antibiotics should be withheld as a preventive measure, since institution of such treatment will not prevent a subsequent infection from occurring but will adversely influence the subsequent pathogen. The diagnosis and management of pneumonia induced by an aspiration event become very similar to those of the patient with a ventilator-associated pneumonia.

Aspiration can be a chronic and subtle process for the critically ill patient. Recent evidence suggests increased nosocomial pneumonitis rates in patients who have received stress bleeding prophylaxis with antacids and H_2 antihistamine agents.[70,71] These agents are alleged to cause alkalinization of the upper aerodigestive tract, promote colonization of this area with hospital-acquired gram-negative bacteria, and because of subtle chronic aspiration events, result in infection. While this conclusion has been reached by several authors, the data really only demonstrate that antacids are associated with increased pneumonia rates. Liquid antacids introduced via the nasogastric tube create an increased volume reservoir within the stomach of critically ill patients. These patients do not have normal gastric motility. The nasogastric tube compromises the functional integrity of the cardioesophageal sphincter. Reflux of the pooled fluids from within the gastric reservoir of these patients results in aspiration and pneumonia. Clinical differentiation of these subtle aspiration pneumonias from other ventilator-associated or non-ventilator-associated pneumonias in the intensive care unit patient can be very difficult. Establishment of a clinical basis for the diagnosis of pneumonia and prudent use of antibiotics become the hallmarks for care regardless of the mechanism responsible for the development of the infection.

Urinary tract infection is a common community-acquired infectious disease. In hospitalized patients, it can be the cause of the septic response. Hospital-acquired urinary tract infections usually are the consequence of bladder catheterization.[72] The indwelling Foley catheter provides a direct conduit from the external world into the urinary bladder. Bacteria colonize the urethra along the catheter and within the pericatheter space and then migrate proximally into the bladder. The Foley catheter balloon compresses and erodes the bladder epithelium in and about the trigone area so that bladder colonization may result in bacterial invasion of the soft tissues and invasive infection.

While infections of the urinary bladder are fairly common after a period of catheterization, a severe septic response or clinical septic shock from the well-drained urinary tract is quite uncommon. Dissemination of bacteria and bacterial cell products from the urinary tract reservoir usually requires both infection and urinary stasis. Infections within the urinary bladder, even with culturable bacteria that are present at concentrations greater than 10^5 organisms per milliliter, generally will not be responsible for a septic response in surgical patients if there is a free flow of urine without obstruction.

A major issue in establishing the significance of the urinary tract as a source of the septic response is the nebulous nature of making the diagnosis of post-catheterization urinary tract infection. The traditional teaching in clinical infectious disease has been that an infection exists within the urinary tract when the number of bacteria exceed the threshold of 10^5 organisms per milliliter in the voided urine.[73] Unfortunately, these studies were performed on patients with community-acquired infections rather than those with Foley catheters in place. It has been assumed that the same criteria should apply to catheter-related infection. This latter assumption may not be valid. My published experience would indicate that most Foley catheter infections resolve simply by removal of the catheter and establishment of normal urine flow.[72]

The urinary tract should be strongly considered as the source of the septic response in very specific circumstances. In the patient who has had a Foley catheter removed within the preceding several hours, an acute febrile and septic response must make the clinician suspect that urinary retention from the colonized urinary tract is now the inciting factor. Male patients with underlying prostatic disease are well known to have urinary retention after a period of catheterization. The treatment for these septic events is to replace the Foley catheter and reestablish adequate drainage of the bladder. The clinical response after catheter replacement is usually quite dramatic. Antibiotic therapy is recommended but serves a relatively minor role compared with bladder drainage. Gram-negative hospital-acquired bacteria are the usual pathogens identified in these patients.

The complex intensive care unit patient will commonly have febrile and septic events that are difficult to diagnose. The common practice in the management of these difficult patients is to culture everything. The urinary tract culture will frequently be positive. For surgical patients, it is rare for a urinary tract infection to be the ultimate explanation for the septic response. It is not uncommon for the clinician to initially ascribe the clinical events to the urinary tract only to subsequently identify the more significant, and usually occult, real cause of sepsis.

Intravascular devices have become a more frequently recognized source of septic events in hospitalized patients. The number of indwelling devices within the venous and arterial vasculature of seriously ill patients seems to be increasing every day. Central lines, arterial lines, and Swan-Ganz catheters, as well as large numbers of peripheral intravenous catheters, all become potential ports for pathogens to gain access to the intravascular compartment and become disseminated.

Catheter infections begin with colonization of bacteria about the skin of the entrance site for the line. Proliferation and migration of the potential pathogens progress down the barrel of the line and into the intravascular compartment. Embolization of bacteria from the device into the circulation then establishes a bacteremia (or fungemia). These patients will then demonstrate an acute septic response.

Diagnosis requires a keen sense of awareness for this diagnosis. Intravascular device bacteremias are usually identified with the precipitous onset of a septic response. Evidence of inflammation or induration about the site of catheter placement is unusual. Removal of the catheter and semiquantitative culture of the catheter tip is essential for documentation of the disease.[74] Removal of the catheter will usually prove both diagnostic and therapeutic.

For most patients who have an intravascular device as the cause of the septic event, removal will be associated with rapid defervescence. Antibiotic therapy is usually initiated and continued until the culture data are returned from the laboratory. An S. aureus isolate from the catheter and blood will require at least 7 days of intravenous antibiotics because of the risk of metastatic infection to the patient's heart valves. Gram-negative infections will usually resolve quite rapidly with removal of the device, and antibiotic therapy for longer than 48 h is usually unnecessary in the patient who has had an appropriate clinical response.

Several considerations should be borne in mind for the patient with a suspected or proven intravascular device infection who does not respond to removal of the catheter. First, the catheter may not have been the cause of the septic response. A patient who is in the intensive care unit with multiple intravascular lines in place will usually have numerous other potential sites for infection. The clinician must examine these other potential sites. Second, such a patient may have suppurative thrombophlebitis and still have pus residing within the infected vein. A careful examination of the site of device placement is very important, particularly in the patient who has had a staphylococcal bacteremia. The primary site of catheter placement may require local drainage or even excision of the segment of infected vein.[75] Patients will continue to have bacteremia from the infected vein in many cases even after removal of the device. The site therefore must be managed as an abscess.

Soft tissue infections can be a source of the septic response. Simple skin and skin structure infections usually are well contained by normal host defense mechanisms. However, traumatic injuries and surgical wounds can lead to necrotizing infections that can lead to the septic response and septic shock. Acute hemolytic streptococcal gangrene can follow any cutaneous injury and become a rapidly dissecting infection of the skin and skin structures. These virulent infections are the consequence of a rapidly proliferating streptococcal pathogen that invades along the subdermal tissues and progressively creates thrombosis of the blood supply to the skin. The diagnosis is made by identification of rapidly advancing hemorrhagic necrosis of the skin. At the time of clinical presentation, one may not be able to identify the small puncture wound that resulted in the virulent infection. Skin blebs are commonly present and permit aspiration so that Gram's stains can be performed and the characteristic gram-positive chains of cocci can be identified. Treatment is radical debridement of the area of infection and antistreptococcal antibiotic therapy.

Staphylococcal infections of traumatic and surgical wounds can lead to a septic response. Unlike streptococcal infections, pathogenic staphylococci are commonly coagulase-producing organisms. These infections will usually produce pyogenic infections, although they are sometimes associated with lymphangiitis and lymphadenitis. The pyogenic character of these infections means that culture of the primary suppuration is possible, and Gram's stains that identify gram-positive cocci in clusters afford an immediate presumptive diagnosis. Drainage of the pus and debridement of fibrin and necrotic tissue remain the critical means to eliminate this stimulus to the septic response. In severe staphylococcal infections of surgical wounds, it is important to remove suture material within the wound as part of the debridement. Antibiotic therapy is adjunctive to surgical management. Because of the increasing incidence of methicillin-resistant staphylococci, vancomycin therapy often will be required until specific microbial sensitivity data are available.

Clostridial soft tissue infections remain an infrequent but important complication of traumatic and even surgical wounds. *Clostridium perfringens* produces a potent toxin that causes a fulminant necrosis of tissue. This necrosis permits proliferation of bacteria. Classic clostridial gangrene occurs when the infection results in myonecrosis beneath the fascia, leading to rapid dissection of the infection into adjacent areas. These patients have a severe septic response with shock. Clinical evidence of the infection at the site of the wound can be quite subtle. A brown discharge may be seen at the site of the wound. Some crepitance is palpable around the sight of the injury, but because the infection dissects beneath the fascia, this may not be readily identified at any distance from the primary sight. Roentgenograms of the area will usually show the extensive distribution of gas deep to the fascia.

The treatment of clostridial soft tissue infection requires prompt recognition and aggressive surgical debridement. All necrotic tissue must be excised. The extent of the infection will be underestimated by the inexperienced clinician. Muscle must be excised until viable, bleeding tissue is clearly present. High-dose penicillin therapy remains the antibiotic of choice. Some enthusiasts have advocated hyperbaric oxygen for the treatment of these clostridial infections, but no convincing evidence is presently available to support this therapeutic modality.

Necrotizing fasciitis is probably the most common of the soft tissue infections to cause the septic response. Penetrating injuries or major operations within the abdomen for frankly infected or contaminated intraabdominal processes will result in polymicrobial contamination of the soft tissues. Infection begins along the relatively avascular plane of the fascia overlying the muscle and beneath the subcutaneous tissue. The fascia then becomes progressively necrotic as the infection invades this plane of tissue. Necrotizing fasciitis is common secondary to gram-negative and anaerobic bacteria combined in a mixed synergistic infection. The stimulus for the septic response is controlled by surgical debridement of the necrotic fascia and adjacent necrotic tissues. As was noted in the treatment of clostridial infections, the extent of the necrotizing process can be easily underestimated. Debridement needs to be extensive. Antibiotic therapy must address the enteric gram-negative rods and anaerobic bacteria. Frequent reoperation for additional debridement of nonviable tissue is often necessary.

The preceding infections represent the overwhelming majority of sites that will be responsible for the septic response and septic shock. Others that can occur include meningitis following injuries of the central nervous system or basilar skull fractures. Septic joints and even suppurative sinusitis can provoke a septic response. Indeed, infection of any potential space or tissue can lead to the septic response. The common denominator for management of these infections is surgical drainage and debridement of the focus responsible for triggering the septic response. In surgical and trauma patients, it is always advisable to look where the "human hands" have been when searching for a focus of infection.

MICROORGANISMS WITHOUT INFECTION

Can microorganisms be responsible for stimulation of the septic response without infection? Infection is the provocation of the local inflammatory response in tissue secondary to microorganisms or the cell products of microorganisms. Thus infections of the peritoneal cavity and lung are the consequence of microorganisms that initiated a local inflammatory response. If the magnitude of bacterial contamination, the rapidity of bacterial proliferation, or the inability of host defense results in bacterial access to the systemic circulation, then a systemic septic response occurs.

In the late 1950s, Jacob Fine and associates[76] developed the hypothesis that endotoxin, and perhaps even whole viable bacteria, was a significant pathophysiologic participant in hemorrhagic shock. Basically, these authors suggested that the low-flow state of hypovolemic shock resulted in splanchnic ischemia, which, in turn, resulted in failure of the gastrointestinal barrier function, permitting the leakage of endotoxin or viable gastrointestinal bacteria into the portal circulation. Dissemination of bacteria or endotoxin resulted in a septic component to the hemorrhagic shock state. In essence, the host's own normal bacterial colonization was no longer contained within the gut and gained systemic access because of the biologic stress from the hypovolemic shock state. Bacteria became systemic provocateurs, but without causing any inflammatory event at the site of entrance into the circulation; i.e., the septic response was activated by bacteria but without infection.

The original hypothesis of Fine et al. was discredited at the time of its formulation. The theory laid dormant for nearly 30 years before returning to favor at the present time. Bacterial translocation has now been shown experimentally to occur with hemorrhage, burns, and other forms of biologic stress.[77–80] Bacteria have been identified in the circulation of shocked and seriously ill patients, and the bacteria are ascribed to bacterial translocation.[81,82] Considerable evidence now supports the hypothesis that the gastrointestinal tract reservoir is a major source for the dissemination of *Candida* sp., and that candidemia may be for many patients an expression of failed host defense rather than infection in the classical sense of the term.[83,84]

The critical requirement for the translocation of potentially offensive microorganisms into the host's circulation is failure of the barrier function of the gastrointestinal tract. The gut barrier function has numerous components, all of which play a contributory role in keeping the microorganisms that colonize the luminal compartment contained. The principal mechanisms function by preventing binding of potentially translocating microorganisms to the endothelial cells of the gut.

Gut motility is a simple but very effective component of the gastrointestinal barrier. Normal intestinal peristalsis minimizes the period of time that bacteria have to bind to the epithelial cells of the intestine. Fiber and bulk in the gut lumen are a stimulus to peristalsis and facilitate transit time, which also prevents bacterial binding. When rapid transit of contents through the gut is viewed as a nonspecific positive host defense, it is perfectly understandable why diarrhea becomes the host response to inflammatory events affecting the gut mucosa. Rapid transit prohibits bacterial penetration. The loss of gut motility, such as is seen in the ileus following injury, operation, and critical illness, may favor the binding of microorganisms to the gut epithelial cells and consequent translocation.

Gut mucins and secretory IgA antibodies within the intestinal lumen also prevent bacterial (or fungal) binding to epithelial cells. The glycoprotein mucins provide a barrier film between the luminal contents and the epithelial cell binding sites for microorganisms.[85] Nonspecific IgA antibodies, perhaps from the submucosal resident lymphocytes of the intestine, bind to the intraluminal bacteria and also prevent adhesion to epithelial cells.[86] Under circumstances of severe biologic stress of either an acute (e.g., hemorrhage) or chronic (e.g., protein-calorie malnutrition) nature, the production of mucins and IgA appears to be impaired. When combined with impaired motility, the setting for epithelial binding and movement of bacteria across the gut mucosal barrier is facilitated.

The bacterial composition within the gut also would appear to be a significant issue in translocation phenomena. The concentration of bacteria within the gut lumen progressively increases from essentially no culturable bacteria within the normally acidified stomach to 10^9 to 10^{10} bacteria per gram of fecal material in the distal colon. As the concentration of bacteria increases, so does the concentration and relative proportion of anaerobic species. Anaerobic bacteria are part of the gut barrier function. These organisms bind to epithelial cells and prevent the binding of potentially unfriendly aerobic species. Gut anaerobes are rarely identified in either experimental studies or the few clinical studies as being organisms of translocation. However, the eradication of gut anaerobes by broad-spectrum antibiotic therapy is thought to eliminate a major component of the barrier function and permit the proliferation of unfriendly microorganisms.[87] Anaerobes that are part of the contamination of the peritoneal cavity with gut perforations and are found in necrotizing infections of the soft tissues are pathologic and require antibiotic treatment. Anaerobes within the lumen of the human gut are likely to be positive components of our gut barrier. Antibiotic therapy that includes anaerobic coverage may be a double-edged sword and must be selected prudently.

A final consideration in the gut barrier involves the physical integrity of the cell barricade between the luminal bacteria and the submucosal space where blood and lymphatic channels are present. The physical mucosal barrier consists of epithelial cells and the intercellular matrix. Atrophy of cells and/or degradation of the intercellular matrix means that physical defects will permit the direct access of microorganisms into the submucosal space, with resultant dissemination of whole microbial cells or cell products. Thus protein-calorie malnutrition and severe catabolic states will result in atrophy of the epithelial cells of the gut and loss of the intercellular matrix, leading to the creation of a physically porous barrier.

Since the true biologic significance of translocation continues to be debated, the diagnosis of a translocation event is quite problematic. In general, when the clinician is confronted with a patient who has a septic response but without a clear site of bacterial infection, then microbial translocation is a consideration. All the usual sites of bacterial infection must be systematically evaluated and conclusively determined not to be the stimulus to the patient's septic behavior. Positive blood cultures without a source of infection constitute a presumptive diagnosis, but obviously, a positive blood culture is not a requirement for the process to be fully active. Since most of these patients will be on extensive antibiotic therapy, the probability of a positive blood culture is small. Most of the time, the diagnosis is one of exclusion and assumption.

I have used the recovery of certain bacteria from blood as being presumptive evidence of translocation. The trilogy of translocation includes *S. epidermidis, Enterococcus* sp., and *Candida* sp. as presumptive evidence of the gut as the reservoir for the septic response and even clinical septic shock. Since both *Candida* sp. and *S. epidermidis* are identified pathogens from intravascular devices, all devices must be ruled out as sources of the bacteremia. *Enterococcus* sp. are normal colonists of the biliary tract and the human colon and may well be participants in polymicrobial infections that are secondary to either biliary tract sepsis or intraabdominal infection secondary to colonic perforation; thus infection from these sources must be ruled out conclusively. Since these three microbes are consistently resistant to commonly employed antibiotic combinations used in empirical therapy, they will be most commonly identified as markers of the translocation phenomenon. Unfortunately, for most patients with the septic syndrome without infection, translocation remains an assumed diagnosis by the clinician with a high index of suspicion.

The treatment of translocation requires that the clinician attempt to reinforce gut barrier function in an effort to eliminate the stimulus that is driving the engine of the septic response. The major treatment modality would appear to be nutritional support of the host. Nutritional support will hopefully restore the production of mucins and IgA antibody. Appropriate protein and calorie support will permit reconstitution of the physical barrier within the gut by support of the epithelial cells and restoration of the intercellular matrix.

There are currently two major areas of controversy in the nutritional management of critically ill patients. First, the route of protein-calorie delivery has become a source of considerable discussion. Traditional nutritional support over the last 20 years has focused primarily on parenteral support. Refinements in intravenous preparations and comfort with central venous delivery have made parenteral nutrition the standard support route. However, when one is focusing on nutritional support of the gut, it would appear that much of the protein and calorie support actually is derived by gut epithelial cells from the luminal compartment. The absence of intraluminal nutrients when the patient is supported by parenteral nutrition has raised concern that the gut mucosa, and hence the physical barrier, is being inadequately supported. This has been supported by experimental data in burned animals, where enteral nutritional support appeared to be superior to isocaloric, isonitrogenous support delivered via the intravenous route.[88] A prospective study by Moore and associates[89] has demonstrated fewer septic complications when trauma patients are supported by enteral as opposed to parenteral protein-calorie delivery. Enteral delivery of nutritional support also stimulates gastrointestinal motility and may foster a more normal bacterial microflora within the gut. Thus considerable enthusiasm presently exists for use of the enteral route of nutritional delivery if possible. Severe ileus and intolerance to enteral nutrition may make this impossible in critically ill patients.

A second area of evolving interest surrounds the composition of nutrients provided for injured and severely ill patients. The stress response is clearly associated with changes in the energy substrates that are required by selected cell populations. Liver cells prefer alanine and glycine as glucogenic amino acids to preferentially support the accelerated gluconeogenesis of the stress state. Skeletal muscle cells prefer branched-chain amino acids. It appears that the enterocyte of the small intestine prefers glutamine as a substrate during the stress state. Atrophy of intestinal mucosa and hence loss of gut barrier function may be the consequence of selective enterocyte malnutrition secondary to inadequate glutamine administration.[90] Similarly, the colonocyte appears to prefer short-chain fatty acids as a fuel substrate.[91] Thus a new area of support for the patient at risk for translocation will be specially designed nutritional preparations. Since conventional parenteral solutions for nutritional support have essentially no glutamine content, the enteral route of nutritional support appears to also offer a more efficient route for the delivery of glutamine.

Earlier ambulation and mobilization have been advocated to prevent the "gut origin" septic state. The enforced recumbent position of the injured or critically ill patient supports the quiescent state of the gut. Border and associates[92,93] have advocated rapid mobilization of injured patients to stimulate a return of gastrointestinal function. They have been enthusiastic advocates of early fixation of extremity fractures in severely injured patients in order to enable earlier mobilization and prevention of the septic state, which they have concluded is derived, at least in part, from the absence of gut motility.

A final but very problematic area of management of the patient with a suspected septic response from microbial translocation is antibiotic therapy. Antibiotic therapy with broad-spectrum agents designed to comprehensively cover all suspected pathogens dramatically alters the microbial flora of the gut. Patients with established severe infections, such as polymicrobial intraabdominal infection, require antibiotic therapy that addresses both aerobic and anaerobic species. However, sustained antibiotic therapy results in the elimination of normal gut microflora and overgrowth of those organisms particularly known to be associated with translocation. Therefore, prolonged antibiotic therapy may allow the initial inciting stimulus for the septic response to be controlled but creates the clinical circumstances for microbial translocation to be an intercurrent or sustaining cause of the septic response. It is important for systemic antibiotic therapy to be discontinued when the primary infection has been controlled. Since nosocomial infections in intensive care unit patients are seldom secondary to anaerobic bacteria, the empirical use of anaerobic antibiotics in the treatment of suspected nosocomial pathogens should be avoided. Indeed, selective decontamination of the gut with antibiotics for aerobic species with attempts to preserve the anaerobic organisms has become an area of considerable interest as efforts to therapeutically manage the gut barrier are now becoming clinical reality.[87]

Systemic antibiotic therapy for the isolated translocating organism is indicated. *Candida* sp. require antifungal therapy. Enterococcal bacteremia requires an appropriate antibiotic. *S. epidermidis* is commonly methicillin-resistant and often requires vancomycin therapy. When treating these bacteremias, it is important to avoid coverage of the obligate anaerobe unless such an organism is isolated from the blood. Anaerobic bacteremia usually means that the patient has undrained infection at some location that needs surgical attention.[94]

NO MICROORGANISMS AND NO INFECTION

It is now apparent that the septic response, and perhaps even frank septic shock, can be the consequence of events that do not have any participation of microorganisms. In the earlier sections of this chapter, evidence was presented that the septic response is a consequence of systemic activation of the inflammatory response, mediated by a host of cell-derived chemical signals. Any pathophysiologic process that activates an inflammatory response of sufficient magnitude may cause normal autocrine and paracrine signals to become endocrine in scope and provoke a systemic septic response.

Several examples of noninfectious inflammatory stimuli can be provided. Severe *necrotizing pancreatitis* results in a major retroperitoneal inflammatory response that is initially sterile. The severe pancreatitis and autodigestion of the gland results in thrombosis of the blood supply, leading to glandular necrosis and more inflammation. The process doubtlessly activates the complement cascade and macrophages. Systemic activation of complement and the systemic distribution of TNF and other cytokines results in widescale activation of neutrophils and the full-blown septic response without bacteria. Such patients develop hemodynamic parameters (including hypotension) that are totally consistent with the septic response.

Severe *aspiration* or *inhalation injury* causes a dramatic inflammatory response within the lung. Activation of the pulmonary macrophages sets in motion a full inflammatory response that is quite analogous to that seen with invasive infection. Again, the systemic release of inflammatory mediators may, in turn, activate the whole inflammatory process at a systemic level. A similar systemic inflammatory response can be seen on occasion in the patient with *cardiopulmonary bypass,* where, in selected patients, it would appear that the period of extracorporeal membrane oxygenation may have activated the complement cascade and resulted in systemic activation of inflammation.

When the septic response has been activated by these sites of sterile inflammation, the initial management is directed toward the inciting process. Unfortunately, these inciting stimuli are commonly complicated by an intercurrent infectious event. Pancreatitis commonly becomes pancreatic abscess, and aspiration pneumonia frequently becomes nosocomial pneumonia. The inciting and sustaining stimuli to the septic response become very difficult to separate in many of these complex patients.

Thus a given patient may demonstrate all three potential classes of stimuli to the septic response during the course of a difficult illness. Pancreatitis may begin as a sterile septic response, which is then followed by pancreatic abscess and an infectious stimulus, which is then followed by protein-calorie malnutrition, broad-spectrum antibiotics, profound gastrointestinal ileus, and microbial translocation. The sensitivity of our diagnostic acumen in differentiating the primary stimulus is, at best, poor for the present time.

CIRCULATORY MANAGEMENT

When the state C or state D septic response occurs, management requires fundamental supportive care to maintain oxygen delivery to the peripheral tissues.

This management means that oxygenation of the blood is maximized, the circulating volume of the intravascular compartment is optimized, the circulating oxygen-carrying capacity is appropriate for efficient tissue delivery, and finally, the myocardium is supported with inotropic agents to provide an adequate cardiac output.

Alterations in ventilation-perfusion ratios in the lung are characteristic of the septic response. Shunting of blood flow means that aerated segments of lung may not be perfused. Conversely, collapsed segments of lung result in perfused segments that are not aerated. The net effect is arterial hypoxemia in these patients.

When arterial hypoxemia becomes a reality for these patients, adequate oxygenation must be achieved.[95] An increased arterial pO_2 requires increasing the FiO_2 to whatever level is necessary. Positive end-expiratory pressure is added in increments to maintain the pO_2 and hopefully minimize the period of time at which the FiO_2 remains above 0.5. Frequent blood gas determinations are necessary for monitoring these patients during the period of hemodynamic lability, and usually are best achieved by use of an arterial line. An arterial catheter should therefore be a component part of the management.

Maintenance of intravascular volume is essential for a hypotensive patient with a septic response. The systemic inflammatory response results in expansion of the interstitial space and extravasation of plasma volume into the extracellular space. In addition, the septic response results in vasodilatation of the capacitance venules, which results in expansion of the intravascular volume necessary to achieve an adequate circulation. The net effect of these two changes is that hypotension is commonly not a true state C or state D but rather reflects the state B septic response with an inadequate circulating intravascular volume.

Management requires complete expansion of the intravascular volume. Crystalloid administration until the pulmonary capillary wedge pressure is 15 to 18 cm H_2O is necessary. At the peak of the septic response, the use of colloidal solutions will not likely be of value, since the colloid particles will not be retained within the intravascular compartment. If hypotension persists after maximizing the intravascular volume using objective parameters, then inotropic support should be considered for cardiac output.

A critical consideration in both oxygen delivery and intravascular volume expansion is optimization of the red cell mass. Septic patients invariably will demonstrate a declining hematocrit, even though no blood loss has occurred. The physiologic response to progressive hemodilution is for cardiac output to be increased so that total oxygen delivery is maintained. Because the septic patient will have already demonstrated a compensatory elevation of cardiac output to meet the needs of the reduced peripheral vascular resistance, significant anemia is not well tolerated. What degree of anemia is deleterious remains unclear from current clinical information.

There are also legitimate reasons against restoring the patient's hematocrit to levels approaching the normal circumstance of 40 to 45 percent. Studies of the rheologic properties of blood have identified a hematocrit of 30 to 32 percent as providing the optimal flow characteristics of red cells through capillaries. Furthermore, current considerations of viral diseases transmitted through the blood supply, as well as evidence to implicate homologous transfusion as being immunosuppressive, mitigate against potentially excessive transfusion.[96,97] A hematocrit in the range of 30 percent is the desired target in my view, realizing that little data are available to define the optimal hematocrit in the septic response patient.

The use of inotropic agents for the hypotensive septic patient is a necessary support measure (Table 10–9). In the state C patient, the cardiac output may appear to be normal or may even be increased relative to the estimated cardiac output for a given patient. The vasodilated state implies that the observed cardiac output is simply inadequate for peripheral demands. Dobutamine at doses of 5 to 20 μg/kg/min is a useful agent for elevating the cardiac output while causing minimal peripheral vasoconstriction.[98] While vasoconstricting agents may increase arterial blood pressure, they do so by further reducing peripheral microcirculatory flow. A further critical reduction in flow within the splanchnic or

TABLE 10–9. Potential Inotropic Agents for the Management of Septic Shock

Drug	Dosage	Value in Septic Response Patients
Dobutamine	5–20 μg/kg/min	Primarily a beta-adrenergic agent; only shows chronotropic or vasoconstrictive effects at high doses; is the agent of choice for elevation of the cardiac output in the septic patient.
Dopamine	2–4 μg/kg/min	This is the dopaminergic dose; it increases renal blood flow but has no alpha- or beta-adrenergic effects; it is commonly used for improving renal blood flow in septic patients prior to the development of either hypotension or renal dysfunction.
Dopamine	4–12 μg/kg/min	This is the beta-adrenergic dose of this agent; many patients will be refractory to this drug for beta effects; at this dose, the dopaminergic effects are lost.
Dopamine	>12 μg/kg/min	This is primarily an alpha-adrenergic dose and is generally not desirable for the septic patient, even though vasoconstriction might seem appropriate for the vasodilated septic response.
Epinephrine	1–4 μg/min	At all doses, this is a good beta-adrenergic drug, but becomes an alpha constrictor at higher doses; vasoconstrictive effects are undesirable, but this is commonly used as a last resort agent in severe shock patients.
Norepinephrine	2–8 μg/min	This is a potent alpha-adrenergic but only has significant beta effects at higher doses; generally, not a desirable agent for the septic patient.
Isoproterenol	1–4 μg/min	This is a potent beta agent, but it has a marked chronotropic effect; it can also be a vasodilator; it has some arrhythmia potential.

renal circulation in the septic patient may prove fatal by initiating terminal multiple organ failure.

Alternative inotropic agents have been used with less effectiveness. Dopamine is an effective inotropic agent in concentrations yielding the delivery of 4 to 12 μg/kg/min.[99] Concentrations less than 4 μg/kg/min have only a dopaminergic effect and, while potentially beneficial for renal and splanchnic blood flow, do not have any significant inotropic effects. Concentrations of dopamine greater than 12 to 15 μg/kg/min are primarily vasoconstrictive in effect and offer little inotropic benefit.

Isoproterenol is a potent inotropic agent that can raise cardiac output in septic patients.[100] Isoproterenol is associated with a marked tachycardic effect and tachyarrhythmias at doses necessary to raise cardiac output. Isoproterenol also has marked peripheral vasodilatory effects that may prove to be undesirable in certain patients.

In state D patients, the need for afterload reduction may be necessary, in addition to increasing the cardiac output.[101] Nitroprusside, nitroglycerin, and trimethaphan camsylate have been most useful for this indication. Afterload reduction is necessary when some success has been achieved in elevating cardiac output but the patient remains with an elevated peripheral vascular resistance and clinically is not perfusing the periphery. Afterload reduction is highly variable between patients. Continuous arterial monitoring is essential to prevent the catastrophic loss of vascular resistance in a patient with an already compromised left ventricle.

FUTURE MANAGEMENT OF THE SEPTIC RESPONSE AND SEPTIC SHOCK

The current management of the profoundly septic patient is unsatisfactory. Our support systems for central hemodynamics and end-organ function have indeed been symptomatic therapy and have not addressed the fundamental pathology of the disease. Newer treatment modalities will need to focus on the basic mechanism of the systemic inflammatory response and how this response can be down-regulated without impairing the responsiveness of the host to local tissue injury and contamination.

A primary treatment modality to blunt the septic response is to eliminate the stimulus that activates the systemic inflammatory events. An antiendotoxin antibody has had the promise of being effective treatment for patients with gram-negative infection.[102,103] This new monoclonal antiendotoxin antibody appears to have a broad base of activity to the lipid A component of the basic molecule that is common to all endotoxins of gram-negative bacteria.[104] While this is appealing from a conceptual basis, current diagnostic specificity for the identification of a given septic event as being of gram-negative origin is quite inexact. Indeed, even those infections with gram-negative participation are commonly polymicrobial in nature. The present clinical data have demonstrated efficacy for the antiendotoxin monoclonal antibody for gram-negative infections but not for all patients with septic shock and the septic response. This therapy will be extremely costly and, while holding real promise for improved results, will likely be used for large numbers of patients without benefit. Better diagnostic methods for the rapid detection of gram-negative bacteremia or circulating endotoxin appear to be necessary before this new treatment modality can be optimally employed.

Considerable interest in recent years has focused on TNF as the arch villain of the cytokine mediators of the septic response. There are now experimental data that have demonstrated beneficial effects on survival of experimentally infected animals with the use of an anti-TNF monoclonal antibody.[105] However, these animal experiments have been short-term simulations of severe infection. Clinical trials with the anti-TNF antibody are currently underway. As discussed previously, TNF appears to be an adverse mediator when it has an endocrine scope of domain. Its autocrine and paracrine functions are doubtlessly of positive value for the patient's host defense. The potential benefits of anticytokine therapy will need to be examined carefully.

Another form of anticytokine therapy that has been introduced recently is the IL-1 receptor antagonist.[106] Some experimental evidence supports its effectiveness. However, fever, neutrophilia, and the up-regulation of acute phase reactants that are synthesized by the liver are all generally viewed as positive host defense responses. As was noted with anti-TNF monoclonal antibodies, the IL-1 receptor antagonist will need to be scrutinized very carefully.

Platelet-activating factor appears to be an amplification mediator for the activation of complement and its effects. There are experimental data in experimental models to support the use of certain of these antagonists.[107,108] Several of these antagonists are presently available, and all may not demonstrate the same biologic effects. Considerable research will be necessary before these agents can be used in clinical trials.

The adhesion of activated neutrophils to endothelial cells appears to have pathophysiologic significance in mediating the endothelial injury of systemic inflammation. This has led to considerable interest in methods to interfere with the adhesion process. Recent evidence has focused on the use of antibodies to the CD18 receptor site on the neutrophil as a means of inhibiting neutrophil–endothelial cell interaction.[10] The benefits of such potential therapy versus the negative effects of general inhibition of neutrophil margination as an important host defense response will need to be carefully evaluated.

Considerable interest has been focused on the potential utility of various scavengers of reactive oxygen intermediates.[109] Reactive oxygen intermediates may be products of xanthine oxidase via the ischemia-reperfusion mechanism. These toxic reactive intermediates of oxygen may be the products of fully and indiscriminately activated neutrophils. Inhibition of reactive oxygen intermediates has been achieved by either inhibition of xanthine oxidase or by enzymatic neutralization via compounds such as superoxide dismutase (SOD). My previous experiments have not shown xanthine oxidase inhibitors to be of value.[110] Data generally support the idea that positive effects of SOD relate to neutralization of neutrophil-derived reactive oxygen intermediates. Further research in this interesting area is certainly warranted.

Prostaglandin derivatives have been viewed as having both positive and negative effects on the host during the septic response. Thus the administration of PgI as a vasodilator,[111] administration of PgE,[112] or inhibition of thromboxane A_2 have all been areas of research.[113] Considerable data have demonstrated positive effects from inhibition of prostaglandin synthetase with compounds such as indomethacin or ibuprofen.[114,115] My own data have demonstrated potentially adverse consequences of long-term administration of prostaglandin synthetase inhibitors in peritonitis.[116] Rather, selective inhibition of thromboxane synthetase would seem to be a preferred means to eliminating the adverse effects of thromboxane A_2 while preserving the beneficial effects from other derivatives of the prostaglandin cascade.

The search for newer therapies for the septic response and septic shock patient will continue. There appears to be a general consensus that for the severely septic patient, surgical drainage, antibiotics, and supportive care may have achieved a near maximum effect. Newer treatments address the fundamental mechanisms of the disease.

While preliminary data for many of these newer treatments look promising, all appear to be focused on inhibition of specific components of the inflammatory cascade by use of monoclonal antibodies, receptor blockade, or enzymatic inhibition. An area of research that has not been fully explored is that of how our normal responses down-regulate the inflammatory response once it has been activated. Not all patients with the septic response proceed to a hypotensive shock state and death. Down-regulatory mechanisms need to be elucidated. Perhaps by simulation of our natural down-regulatory mechanisms, we can achieve better treatments for the septic response and septic shock.

SUMMARY

The septic response and septic shock are part of the continuum of the systemic inflammatory response. The processes are exaggerated consequences at a systemic level of normal tissue-level mechanisms. Systemic activation of the inflammatory cascade may be the consequence of (1) microorganisms secondary to infection, (2) microorganisms not secondary to infection, or (3) processes that are without either microorganisms or infection. Current management employs aggressive surgical management, antibiotic therapy when appropriate, and supportive care for central hemodynamics and end-organ function. Future treatment will need to address the fundamental mechanisms of the systemic septic response if improved clinical results are to be achieved.

REFERENCES

1. Siegel JH, Cerra FB, Coleman B, et al: Physiologic and metabolic correlations in human sepsis. *Surgery* 86:163, 1979.
2. Wilmore DW, Lindsey CA, Moylan JA, et al: Hyperglucagonemia after burns. *Lancet* 1:73, 1974.
3. MacLean LD, Mulligan WG, McLean AP, et al: Patterns of septic shock in man—A detailed study of 56 patients. *Ann Surg* 166:543, 1967.
4. Johnson AR, Hugli TE, Muller-Eberhard HJ: Release of histamine from rat mast cells by the complement peptides C3a and C5a. *Immunology* 28:1067, 1975.
5. Hamberg M, Svensson J, Samuelsson B: Thromboxanes—A new group of biologically ac-

tive compounds derived from prostaglandin endoperoxides. *Proc Natl Acad Sci USA* 72:2994, 1975.

6. Fry DE, Polk HC Jr: Host defense and organ system failure, in Richardson JD, Polk HC Jr, Flint LM (eds): *Trauma: Clinical Care and Pathophysiology.* Chicago, Year Book Medical Publishers, 1987, pp 41–75.

7. Shin HS, Snyderman R, Friedman E, et al: Chemotactic and anaphylatoxic fragment cleaved from fifth component of guinea pig complement. *Science* 162:361, 1968.

8. Beutler B, Cerami A: Cachectin—More than a tumor necrosis factor. *N Engl J Med* 316:379, 1987.

9. Wright SD, Ramos RA, Tobias PS, et al: CD14 α receptor for complexes of lipopolysaccharide (LPS) and lipopolysaccharide binding protein. *Science* 249:1431, 1990.

10. Carlos TM, Harlan JM: Membrane proteins involved in phagocytic adherence to endothelium. *Immunol Rev* 114:5, 1990.

11. Asher EF, Rowe RL, Garrison RN, et al: Experimental bacteremia and nutrient hepatic blood flow. *Circ Shock* 20:43, 1986.

12. Cook JA, Wise WC, Halushka PV: Elevated thromboxane levels in the rat during endotoxic shock: Protective effects of imidazole, 13-azaprostanoic acid, or essential fatty acid deficiency. *J Clin Invest* 65:227, 1980.

13. Halushka PV, Cook JA, Wise WC: Beneficial effects of UK-37248, a thromboxane synthetase inhibitor, in experimental endotoxic shock in the rat. *Br J Clin Pharmacol* 15:133s, 1983.

14. Townsend MC, Hampton WW, Haybron DM, et al: Effective organ blood flow and bio-energy status in murine peritonitis. *Surgery* 100:205, 1986.

15. Dinarello CA: Interleukin-1. *Rev Infect Dis* 6:51, 1984.

16. Dinarello CA, Cannon JG, Wolff SM, et al: Tumor necrosis factor (cachectin) is an endogenous pyrogen and induces production of interleukin-1. *J Exp Med* 163:1433, 1986.

17. Nijesten MWN, DeGroot ER, Tenduis HJ, et al: Serum levels of interleukin-6 and acute phase responses. *Lancet* 2:921, 1987.

18. Bessey PQ, Watters JM, Aoki TT, et al: Combined hormonal infusion simulates the metabolic response to injury. *Ann Surg* 200:264, 1984.

19. Watters JM, Bessey PQ, Dinarello CA, et al: Both inflammatory and endocrine mediators stimulate host responses to sepsis. *Arch Surg* 121:179, 1986.

20. McMenamy RH, Birkhahn R, Oswald G, et al: Multiple systems organ failure: I. The basal state. *J Trauma* 21:99, 1981.

21. Siegel JH, Giovanni I, Coleman B, et al: A manifestation of a common metabolic defect. *Arch Surg* 117:225, 1982.

22. Moncada S, Vane JR: Pharmacology and endogenous roles of prostaglandin endoperoxides, thromboxane A_2, and prostacyclin. *Pharmacol Rev* 30:293, 1978.

23. Moncada S, Higgs EA, Vane JR: Human arterial and venous tissues generate prostacyclin (prostaglandin-X), a potent inhibitor of platelet-aggregation. *Lancet* 1:18, 1977.

24. Reines HD, Halushka PV, Cook JA, et al: Plasma thromboxane concentrations are raised in patients dying with septic shock. *Lancet* 2:174, 1982.

25. Halushka PV, Reines HD, Barrow SE, et al: Elevated plasma 6-keto-prostaglandin $F_{1\alpha}$ in patients in septic shock. *Crit Care Med* 13:451, 1985.

26. Reines HD, Cook JA: Prostaglandins, in Fry DE (ed): *Multiple System Organ Failure.* Chicago, Mosby Year Book, 1992, pp 123–141.

27. Moncada S, Palmer RMJ, Higgs EA: The discovery of nitric oxide as the endogenous nitro-vasodilator. *Hypertension* 12:365, 1989.

28. Ignarro LJ: Biological actions and properties of endothelium-derived nitric oxide formed and released from artery and vein. *Circ Res* 65:1, 1989.

29. Imamura M, Clowes GHA Jr: Hepatic blood flow and oxygen consumption in starvation, sepsis and septic shock. *Surg Gynecol Obstet* 141:27, 1975.

30. Gump FE, Price JB, Kinney JM: Whole-body and splanchnic blood flow and O_2 consumption measurements in patients with intraperitoneal infection. *Ann Surg* 171:321, 1970.

31. Hampton WA, Townsend MC, Haybron DM, et al: Effective hepatic blood flow and hepatic bioenergy status in murine peritonitis. *J Surg Res* 42:33, 1987.

32. Schirmer WJ, Townsend MC, Schirmer JM, et al: Galactose elimination kinetics in sepsis: Correlations of hepatic blood flow with function. *Arch Surg* 122:349, 1987.

33. Schirmer WJ, Schirmer JM, Naff GB, et al: Complement activation in peritonitis. Association with hepatic and renal perfusion abnormalities. *Am Surg* 53:683, 1987.

34. Haybron DM, Townsend MC, Hampton WW, et al: Alterations in renal perfusion and renal energy charge in murine peritonitis. *Arch Surg* 122:328, 1987.

35. Schirmer WJ, Schirmer JM, Naff GB, et al: Systemic complement activation produces hemodynamic changes characteristic of sepsis. *Arch Surg* 123:316, 1988.

36. Parrillo JE: Cardiovascular dysfunction in septic shock: New insights into a deadly disease. *Int J Cardiol* 7:314, 1985.

37. Ognibene FP, Parker MM, Natanson C, et al: Depressed left ventricular performance: Response to volume infusion in patients with sepsis and septic shock. *Chest* 93:903, 1988.

38. Parrillo JE, Burch C, Shelhamme JH, et al: A circulating myocardial depressant substance in humans with septic shock. *J Clin Invest* 76:1539, 1985.

39. Raymond RM: When does the heart fail during shock? in Fry DE (ed): *Multiple System Organ Failure*. Chicago, Mosby Year Book, 1992, pp 363–372.

40. Bardakhchian EA, Palchikova EI: Ultrastructural evidences of direct endotoxin action on the heart. *Cor Vasa* 29:64, 1987.

41. Coalson JJ, Archer LT, Benjamin BA, et al: Morphologic study of live *Escherichia coli* organism shock in baboons. *Exp Mol Pathol* 31:10, 1979.

42. Siegel JH, Greenspan M, Del Guercio LRM: Abnormal vascular tone, defective oxygen transport, and myocardial failure in human septic shock. *Ann Surg* 165:504, 1967.

43. Siegel JH, Farrell EJ, Miller M, et al: Cardiorespiratory interactions as determinants of survival and the need for respiratory support in human shock states. *J Trauma* 13:602, 1973.

44. Vary TC, Siegel JH, Rivkind AI: Clinical and therapeutic significance of metabolic patterns of lactic acidosis. *Perspect Crit Care* 1:85, 1988.

45. Vary TC, Siegel JH, Nakatani T, et al: Effect of sepsis on activity of pyruvate dehydrogenase complex in skeletal muscle and liver. *Am J Physiol* 250:E634, 1986.

46. Lucas CE: Renal considerations in the injured patient. *Surg Clin North Am* 62:133, 1982.

47. Swan HJC, Ganz W, Forrester JS, et al: Catheterization of the heart in man with use of a flow-directed balloon-tipped catheter. *N Engl J Med* 283:447, 1970.

48. Porter JM, Swain ID: Measurement of cardiac output by electrical impedance plethysmography. *J Biomed Eng* 9:222, 1987.

49. Makk LJK, McClave SA, Creech PW, et al: Clinical application of the metabolic cart to the delivery of total parenteral nutrition. *Crit Care Med* 18:1320, 1990.

50. Conn HO, Fessel JM: Spontaneous bacterial peritonitis in cirrhosis: Variations on a theme. *Medicine* 50:161, 1971.

51. Conn HO: Spontaneous bacterial peritonitis, multiple revisitations. *Gastroenterology* 70:455, 1976.

52. Allen L, Weatherford T: Role of fenestrated basement membrane in lymphatic absorption from the peritoneal cavity. *Am J Physiol* 197:551, 1959.

53. Tsilibary EC, Wissig SL: Absorption from the peritoneal cavity: SEM study of the mesothelium covering the peritoneal surface of the muscular portion of the diaphragm. *Am J Anat* 149:127, 1977.

54. Hau T, Simmons RL: Heparin in the treatment of experimental peritonitis. *Ann Surg* 187:294, 1978.

55. Polk HC Jr, Miles AA: Enhancement of bacterial infection by ferric iron: Kinetics, mechanisms, and surgical significance. *Surgery* 70:71, 1971.

56. Pruett TL, Rotstein OD, Fiegel VD, et al: Mechanisms of the adjuvant effect of hemoglobin in experimental peritonitis: VIII. A leukotoxin is produced by *Escherichia coli* metabolism in hemoglobin. *Surgery* 96:375, 1984.

57. Fry DE, Garrison RN, Heitsch RC, et al: Determinants of death in patients with intraabdominal abscess. *Surgery* 88:517, 1980.

58. Haaga JR, Alfidi RJ, Havrilla TR, et al: CT detection and aspiration of abdominal abscesses. *AJR* 128:465, 1977.

59. Gerzof SG, Johnson WC: Radiologic aspects of diagnosis and treatment of abdominal abscesses. *Surg Clin North Am* 64:53, 1984.

60. Norton LW: Does drainage of intraabdominal pus reverse multiple organ failure. *Am J Surg* 149:347, 1985.

61. Bunt TJ: Urgent relaparotomy: The high-risk, no choice operation. *Surgery* 98:555, 1985.

62. Polk HC Jr, Shields CL: Remote organ failure: A valid sign of occult intraabdominal infection. *Surgery* 81:310, 1977.

63. Hinsdale JG, Jaffe BM: Re-operation for intraabdominal sepsis: Indications and results in modern critical care setting. *Ann Surg* 199:31, 1984.

64. Mosdell DM, Morris DM, Voltura A, et al: Antibiotic treatment for surgical peritonitis. *Ann Surg* 214:543, 1991.

65. Johanson WG, Pierce AK, Sanford JP, et al: Nosocomial respiratory infections with gram-negative bacilli: The significance of colonization of the respiratory tract. *Ann Intern Med* 77:701, 1972.

66. Polk HC Jr: Quantitative tracheal cultures in surgical patients requiring mechanical ventilatory assistance. *Surgery* 78:485, 1975.

67. Salata RA, Lederman MM, Shlaes DM, et al: Diagnosis of nosocomial pneumonia in intubated intensive-care unit patients. *Am Rev Respir Dis* 135:426, 1987.

68. Wimberly N, Faling LJ, Bartlett JG: A fiberoptic bronchoscopy technique to obtain uncontaminated lower airway secretions for bacterial culture. *Am Rev Respir Dis* 119:337, 1979.

69. Stover DE, Zaman MB, Hajdu SI, et al: Bronchoalveolar lavage in the diagnosis of diffuse pulmonary infiltrates in the immunosuppressed host. *Ann Intern Med* 101:1, 1984.

70. Driks MR, Craven DE, Celli BR, et al: Nosocomial pneumonia in intubated patients given sucralfate as compared with antacids or histamine type 2 blockers: The role of gastric colonization. *N Engl J Med* 317:1376, 1987.

71. Tryba M: The risk of acute stress bleeding and nosocomial pneumonia in ventilated ICU patients: Sucralfate vs. antacids. *Am J Med* 83:117, 1987.

72. Asher EF, Oliver BG, Fry DE: Urinary tract infections in the surgical patient. *Am Surg* 54:466, 1988.

73. Kass EH: Bacteriuria and the diagnosis of infections of the urinary tract. *Arch Intern Med* 100:709, 1957.

74. Maki DG, Weise CE, Sarafin HW: A semiquantitative culture method for identifying intravenous-catheter-related infection. *N Engl J Med* 296:1305, 1977.

75. Garrison RN, Richardson JD, Fry DE: Catheter-associated septic thrombophlebitis. *South Med J* 75:917, 1982.

76. Fine J, Frank ED, Ravin HA, et al: The bacterial factor in traumatic shock. *N Engl J Med* 260:214, 1959.

77. Maejima K, Deitch EA, Berg RD: Bacterial translocation from the gastrointestinal tracts of rats receiving thermal injury. *Infect Immun* 43:6, 1984.

78. Baker JW, Deitch EA, Li M, et al: Hemorrhagic shock induces bacterial translocation from the gut. *J Trauma* 28:896, 1988.

79. Deitch EA, Winterton J, Li M, et al: The gut as a portal of entry for bacteremia: Role of protein malnutrition. *Ann Surg* 205:681, 1987.

80. Deitch EA, Berg R, Specian R: Endotoxin promotes the translocation of bacteria from the gut. *Arch Surg* 122:185, 1987.

81. Rush BF, Redan JA, Flanagan JJ, et al: Does the bacteremia observed in hemorrhagic shock have clinical significance? *Ann Surg* 210:342, 1989.

82. Dietch EA: Simple intestinal obstruction causes bacterial translocation in man. *Arch Surg* 124:699, 1989.

83. Stone HH, Kolb LD, Currie CA, et al: *Candida* sepsis: Pathogenesis and principles of treatment. *Ann Surg* 179:697, 1974.

84. Dyess DL, Garrison RN, Fry DE: *Candida* sepsis: Implications of polymicrobial blood-borne infection. *Arch Surg* 120:345, 1985.

85. McNabb PC, Tomasi TB: Host defense mechanisms at mucosal surfaces. *Annu Rev Microbiol* 35:477, 1981.

86. Tomasi TB Jr, Bienenstock J: Secretory immunoglobulins. *Adv Immunol* 9:1, 1968.

87. Vanderwaaij D: Colonization resistance of the digestive tract: Clinical consequences and implications. *J Antimicrob Chemother* 10:263, 1982.

88. Mochizuki H, Trocki O, Dominioni L, et al: Mechanism of prevention of postburn hypermetabolism and catabolism by early enteral feeding. *Ann Surg* 200:297, 1984.

89. Moore FA, Moore EE, Jones TN, et al: TEN versus TPN following major abdominal trauma reduced septic morbidity. *J Trauma* 29:916, 1989.

90. Wilmore DW, Smith RJ, O'Dwyer ST, et al: The gut: A central organ after surgical stress. *Surgery* 104:917, 1988.

91. Rolandelli RH, Koruda MJ, Settle RG, et al: The effect of enteral feedings supplemented with pectin on the healing of colonic anastomoses in the rat. *Surgery* 99:703, 1986.

92. Border JR, Hassett J, LaDuca J, et al: The gut origin septic states in blunt multiple trauma (ISS-40) in the ICU. *Ann Surg* 206:427, 1987.

93. Seibel R, LaDuca J, Hassett JM, et al: Blunt multiple trauma (ISS-36), femur traction, and the pulmonary failure septic state. *Ann Surg* 202:283, 1985.

94. Fry DE, Garrison RN, Polk HC Jr: Clinical implications in *Bacteroides* bacteremia. *Surg Gynecol Obstet* 149:189, 1979.

95. Demling R, Decamp M: Pulmonary management, in Fry DE (ed): *Multiple System Organ Failure.* Chicago, Mosby Year Book, 1992, pp 229–243.

96. Nichols RL, Smith JW, Klein DB, et al: Risk of infection after penetrating abdominal trauma. *N Engl J Med* 311:1065, 1984.

97. Crowe JP Jr, Gordon NH, Fry DE, et al: Breast cancer survival and perioperative blood transfusion. *Surgery* 106:836, 1989.

98. Jewitt D, Birkhead J, Mitchell A, et al: Clinical cardiovascular pharmacology of dobutamine: A selective inotropic catecholamine. *Lancet* 2:363, 1974.

99. MacCannell KL, McNay JL, Meyer MB, et al: Dopamine in the treatment of hypotension and shock. *N Engl J Med* 275:1389, 1966.

100. Tarazi RC: Sympathomimetic agents in the treatment of shock. *Ann Intern Med* 81:364, 1974.

101. Cerra FB, Hassett JM, Siegel JH: Vasodilator therapy in clinical sepsis with low output syndrome. *J Surg Res* 25:180, 1978.

102. Lachman E, Pitsoe SB, Gaffin SL: Anti-lipopolysaccharide immunotherapy in management of septic shock of obstetric and gynecological origin. *Lancet* 1:981, 1984.

103. Baumgartner JD, McCutchan JA, Van Melle G, et al: Prevention of gram-negative shock and death in surgical patients by antibody to endotoxin core glycolipid. *Lancet* 2:59, 1985.

104. Ziegler EJ, Fisher CJ, Sprung CL, et al: Treatment of gram-negative bacteremia and septic shock with HA-1A human monoclonal antibody against endotoxin. *N Engl J Med* 324:429, 1991.

105. Tracey KJ, Fong Y, Hesse DG, et al: Anticachetin/TNF monoclonal antibodies prevent septic shock during lethal bacteremia. *Nature* 330:662, 1987.

106. Wakabayashi G, Gelfand JA, Burke JF, et al: A specific receptor antagonist for interleukin 1 prevents *Escherichia coli*–induced shock in rabbits. *FASEB J* 5:338, 1991.

107. Chang SW, Fernyak S, Voelkel NF: Beneficial effect of a platelet-activating factor antagonist, WEB 2086, on endotoxin-induced lung injury. *Am J Physiol* 258:H153, 1990.

108. Fletcher JR, DiSimone AG, Earnest MA: Platelet-activating factor receptor antagonist improves survival and attenuates eicosanoid release in severe endotoxemia. *Ann Surg* 211:312, 1990.

109. Sussman MS, Schiller HJ, Buchman TG, Bulkley GB: Oxygen free radicals, in Fry DE (ed): *Multiple System Organ Failure.* Chicago, Mosby Year Book, 1992, pp 143–165.

110. Schirmer WJ, Schirmer JM, Naff GB, Fry DE: Allopurinol and Iodoxamide in complement-induced hepatic ischemia. *J Surg Res* 45:28, 1988.

111. Krausz MM, Utsunomiya T, Feuerstein G, et al: Prostacyclin reversal of lethal endotoxemia in dogs. *J Clin Invest* 67:1118, 1981.

112. Holcroft JW, Vassar MJ, Weber CJ: Prostaglandin E_1 and survival in patients with the adult respiratory distress syndrome: A prospective trial. *Ann Surg* 203:371, 1986.

113. Wise WC, Cook JA, Halushka PV, et al: Protective effects of thromboxane synthetase inhibitors in rats in endotoxic shock. *Circ Res* 46:854, 1980.

114. Schirmer WJ, Schirmer JM, Townsend MC, et al: Imidazole and indomethacin improve hepatic perfusion in sepsis. *Circ Shock* 21:253, 1987.

115. Michie HR, Manogue KR, Spriggs DR, et al: Detection of circulating tumor necrosis factor after endotoxin administration. *N Engl J Med* 318:1481, 1988.

116. Schirmer WJ, Schirmer JM, Townsend MC, et al: Effects of ibuprofen, indomethacin, and imidazole on survival in sepsis. *Curr Surg* 44:102, 1987.

11

NEUROGENIC SHOCK

Zelma H. T. Kiss
Charles H. Tator

DEFINITIONS

Despite the many definitions and classifications of shock described over the years, the 1940 classification of Blalock[1] based on the etiology of the shock state remains the most useful. He defined *neurogenic shock* as that caused primarily by nervous influences and their effect on the balance between vasodilator and vasoconstrictor actions on the vascular system. However, as described below, neurogenic shock causes other changes in the cardiovascular system such that the pathophysiology of neurogenic shock may overlap with other types of shock.

Vasovagal syncope, acute spinal cord injury, and severe head injury with increased intracranial pressure are the most common causes of neurogenic shock. While spinal cord injury and head injury have some similar pathophysiologic mechanisms, this chapter will limit discussion to neurogenic shock due to acute spinal cord injury. Neurogenic shock due to increased intracranial pressure is discussed in the following chapter.

It is important to note that some authors have mistakenly used the term *spinal shock* interchangeably with *neurogenic shock due to spinal cord injury.* Spinal shock occurs acutely after spinal cord injury and consists of loss of sensation, flaccid paralysis, and absent reflexes in all voluntary and involuntary muscles below the level of injury. After minor spinal cord injury, spinal shock resolves within minutes or hours of injury; however after major spinal cord injury, it resolves slowly over the ensuing hours to weeks and then evolves into the classic upper motor neuron picture of chronic spinal cord injury. In cases of significant cord injury in the cervical or upper thoracic cord, spinal shock would include neurogenic shock because of the damage to the sympathetic nervous system resulting from interruption of the sympathetic fibers traveling in the spinal cord. In these cases there would be flaccid paralysis of sympathetically innervated muscles of the heart and blood vessels. The ensuing cardiovascular response would be described as "neurogenic shock secondary to spinal cord injury."

The following discussion of neurogenic shock due to spinal cord injury includes a basic overview of the anatomy and physiology of the autonomic nervous system and the pathology, mechanisms, clinical diagnosis, and classification of spinal cord injury. The experimental and clinical studies underlying the elucidation of the various phases of neurogenic shock and, lastly, resuscitation of the patient with neurogenic shock due to acute spinal cord injury are also discussed.

BACKGROUND

ANATOMY AND PHYSIOLOGY INVOLVED IN THE NEURAL MODULATION OF HEMODYNAMICS

Although a discussion of all the neural and humoral factors controlling tissue perfusion is beyond the scope of this chapter, a basic understanding of the neural modulation of blood pressure, heart rate, cardiac output, and systemic vascular resistance is necessary for an understanding of neurogenic shock.

The sympathetic and parasympathetic components of the autonomic nervous system interact to control heart rate, contractility, venous capacitance, and arteriolar tone. The sympathetic nervous system is under the control of hypothalamic nuclei via lateral brainstem pathways to the lateral and ventrolateral funiculi of the spinal cord. The axons in these tracts then synapse with cell bodies situated in the intermediolateral cell column in the central gray matter of the spinal cord from the C8 to L2 spinal cord levels. The sympathetic fibers from these preganglionic cell bodies exit with the anterior roots at the T1 to L2 levels, and each gives a white ramus communicantes to the sympathetic trunk. The myelinated axons of the white rami communicantes then synapse with the postganglionic neurons situated in the ganglia of the sympathetic chain, and the sympathetic fibers travel with blood vessels to the viscera and vascular beds they innervate (Fig. 11–1). Somatic branches of the sympathetic system are vasoconstrictor to arterioles via alpha-adrenergic neurotransmission. The cardiac sympathetic nervous supply arises from the T1 to T4 spinal cord levels and exerts positive chronotropic and inotropic influences via beta-adrenergic neurotransmission. Table 11–1 summarizes the various sympathetic receptors and their physiologic effects.

The parasympathetic system has no somatic distribution and is wholly visceral in its activity. The cardiac parasympathetic fibers travel via the vagus nerves and originate from the dorsal motor nuclei in the medulla oblongata to exert a negative chronotropic effect through cholinergic neurotransmission (Fig. 11–2).

PATHOLOGIC CHANGES IN SPINAL CORD INJURY

Even in the most severe cases of clinically complete spinal cord injury with total absence of voluntary motor or sensory function below the level of the injury, the spinal cord is seldom anatomically transected. Thus every effort must be exerted to preserve the remaining tissue. In these severe cases, the acute pathologic features at the injured and adjacent levels of the cord usually consist of

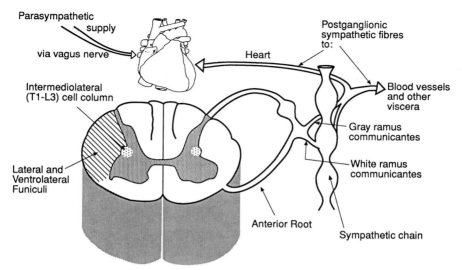

FIG. 11–1. Diagram showing upper thoracic spinal cord segment and sympathetic supply to the heart, blood vessels, and viscera. Parasympathetic supply to the heart via the vagus nerves is also shown.

compression, contusion, partial laceration, edema, and hemorrhage.[2] The hemorrhage is usually much more severe in the gray matter, and if it is very large, it is termed *hematomyelia* (Fig. 11–3). Microscopically, there is extensive axonal interruption and varying degrees of vascular injury consisting of petechial hemorrhages, edema, and vascular stasis. After the acute stage, the injured tissue shows necrosis, infarction, and cavitation.[3]

MECHANISMS OF SPINAL CORD INJURY

Motor vehicle accidents are the most common causes of spinal cord injury in North America and Europe and include pedestrians, bicyclists, and motorists. Other frequent causes are sports and recreational activities, work accidents, and falls at home. Worldwide, diving is probably the most common cause of injury in the sports-recreational category, with rugby, football, and hockey also being common causes. Work accidents are especially frequent in construction, logging, and mining, and falls at home are often falls down stairs in the elderly.

CLINICAL DIAGNOSIS OF SPINAL SHOCK

The clinical manifestations of spinal shock include loss of somatic motor and sensory function and loss of autonomic function. Spinal shock is thought to be due to a temporary pathophysiologic imbalance, such as increased neuronal membrane permeability to potassium ions. Excess potassium accumulates in the extracellular space in the cord and causes conduction block. The loss of somatic

TABLE 11–1. Sympathetic Nervous System Physiologic Effects

Receptor	Location	Action
Alpha-1	Postsynaptic—vascular smooth muscle	Vasoconstriction
Alpha-2	Presynaptic	Stimulation inhibits norepinephrine release, i.e., negative feedback
	Postsynaptic—vascular smooth muscle	Vasoconstriction
Beta-1	Postsynaptic—heart	Stimulation: Positive inotropy Positive chronotropy Increased automaticity Increased conduction velocity
Beta-2	Postsynaptic—vascular smooth muscle	Stimulation—vasodilatation

Source: Adapted from Lawson NW: Use of inotropes and vasopressors, in *Annual Refresher Course in Anesthesia*, Table 412-2, 1988, with permission.

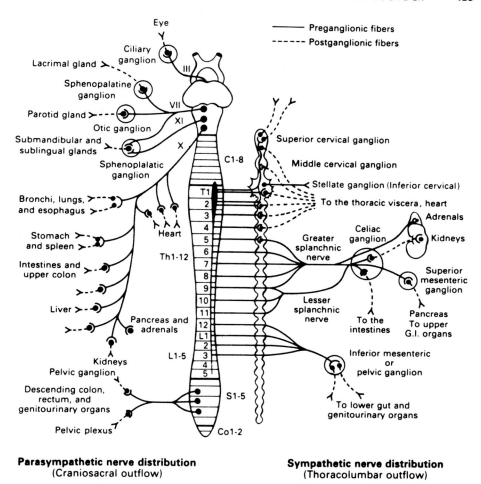

FIG. 11–2. Anatomy of the autonomic nervous system. (*From Durrett LR, Lawson NW: Autonomic nervous system physiology and pharmacology, in Barash PG, Cullen BF, Stoelting RK (eds): Clinical Anesthesia. Philadelphia, Lippincott, 1989, p 168, Fig 7–3, with permission.*)

voluntary motor power in the limbs renders them flaccid, and there is loss of sensation as well, below the level of the lesion. The deep tendon, cutaneous, and other reflexes such as the bulbocavernosus reflex are all absent. The duration of each of these somatic aspects of spinal shock is variable, but in many cases they have largely subsided within an hour of injury. Thus in the emergency department it is safest to attribute all neurologic deficits found in the motor and sensory examination of limbs and trunk to structural spinal cord injury rather than to spinal shock. Conversely, the deep tendon, cutaneous, and other reflexes such as the bulbocavernosus reflex may remain absent for days or weeks. Of importance is the fact that neurogenic shock, which is the autonomic component of spinal shock and includes principally hypotension and bradycardia, may persist for days or weeks.

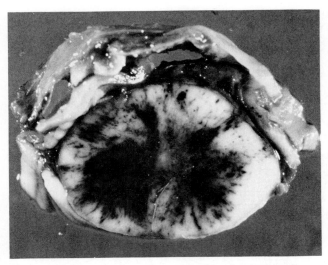

FIG. 11–3. Photograph of acute spinal cord injury in the cervical cord. Both gray and white matter contain numerous hemorrhages. (*Courtesy of Dr. John Deck, Department of Pathology, Toronto Hospital.*)

CLINICAL CLASSIFICATION OF SPINAL CORD INJURY

It is strongly suggested that all physicians and allied medical personnel use the system of classification of spinal cord injuries proposed by the American Spinal Injury Association (ASIA), which is a modification of the Frankel system (Table 11–2). Most important is the establishment of whether a patient is grade A, which is a complete injury, or grade B, in which there is some preservation of sensory function below the injury. Grades C and D refer to patients with increasing motor function, and grade E is normal. Therapeutic efforts at improving cord function should be directed toward all patients with grade A to D injuries because even some grade A patients (although a minority) will show some recovery below the level of the injury. However, the prognosis is much better with incomplete or partial injuries (grades B to D). The definitive assignment of injury severity and grading can only be made in a fully conscious, cooperative patient who is free of alcohol or drugs that might alter brain function. Spinal shock and neurogenic shock can occur in all grades of spinal cord injury. However, they both are more profound and last longer in grades A and B.

PATHOPHYSIOLOGY OF NEUROGENIC SHOCK DUE TO SPINAL CORD INJURY

The cardiovascular changes due to spinal cord injury have been examined in both animal models and human cases. Although investigators have used a number of experimental models of acute spinal cord injury in different species, there has been agreement on most of the hemodynamic changes in acute spinal cord injury. There is little agreement, however, on the mechanisms responsible for these changes.

TABLE 11–2. American Spinal Injury Association (ASIA) Classification of Spinal Cord Injury (Revised 1992)

Grade	Type	Description
A	Complete	No sensory or motor function preserved in the sacral segments S4–5
B	Incomplete	Sensory but no motor function preserved below the neurologic level and extends through the sacral segments S4–5
C	Incomplete	Motor function preserved below the neurologic level, and the majority of key muscles below the neurologic level have a muscle grade less than 3/5
D	Incomplete	Motor function preserved below the neurologic level, and the majority of key muscles below the neurologic level have a muscle grade greater than or equal to 3/5
E	Normal	Sensory and motor function normal

ANIMAL STUDIES

PRESSOR PHASE

The initial stage of the cardiovascular response to spinal cord injury is known as the *pressor response*. This phase is characterized by a brief period of hypertension mediated by alpha-adrenergics and is considered due to a massive sympathetic discharge as a direct result of trauma to the central nervous system. It occurs at all anatomic levels of brain or spinal cord injury. The pressor response is not identified in most human injuries because its onset is within 2 to 6 s of injury and it lasts only 1 to 4 min. Although it is too fleeting to be recorded in most clinical injuries, it has been reported when intraoperative iatrogenic spinal cord injury has occurred.[4]

Animal studies on cats, rats, dogs, and monkeys with injury produced by weight drop, transection, weighted foot compression, balloon compression, or clip compression techniques have identified many aspects of the pressor response. It consistently occurs 2 to 6 s after injury, lasts 4 to 5 min, and involves an increase in systolic, diastolic, and pulse pressures.[5,6] The magnitude of the hypertensive response correlates directly with the degree of injury.[7,8] Alexander and Kerr[8] in 1964 found that it occurred at all levels but was most marked at T3–5. Rawe and Perot[6] in 1978 described it as occurring at all levels. Eidelberg[5] found it to be most dramatic in the cervical cord, moderate at thoracic levels, and minimal in the upper lumbar cord. The hypertensive response persists in decerebrate preparations, and only the thoracolumbar sympathetic efferents are necessary to produce the response.[5,6,8] Bilateral adrenalectomy does not alter the pressor response,[6,8] and it is also not prevented by atropine, hexamethonium, propranolol, or reserpine. The pressor response is prevented, however, by phenoxybenzamine, an alpha-adrenergic blocker.[5,6,9]

More recent experimental work has quantified the parameters involved in these hemodynamic changes. Tibbs et al.[10] found an increase in mean arterial pressure to 145 percent of control values, with a 34 percent increase in systemic vascular resistance and a left ventricular (LV) contractility index of rate of change of LV pressures (*dp/dt*) of 92 percent. The pulse pressure increased by 208 percent, with no significant change in cardiac output. Their data support the hypothesis that both alpha- and beta-adrenergic stimulation occurs via the sympathetic efferents because they found that both increased afterload and contractility contributed to the hypertension (Fig. 11–4). In view of the very short latency of the responses as well as the lack of effect of adrenalectomy on the pressor response, the source of the hypertension must be neural stimulation via the sympathetic nervous system. The only possible mechanism is that the preganglionic cell bodies in the intermediolateral column or the central sympathetic efferents in the lateral and ventrolateral funiculi of the cervical spinal cord are activated by mechanical deformation and produce hypertension.[5,6,8–10]

During the pressor phase, varying effects on heart rate have been described from sinus tachycardia[11] to sinus bradycardia.[7–10] Bradycardia is now generally regarded as the primary cardiac rhythm disturbance, occurring within one heartbeat of cord compression.[9] Subsequent arrhythmias such as rotation of the cardiac axis, premature ventricular contractions,[5] escape rhythms, sinus arrest, junctional capture, and ventricular tachycardia are likely secondary to baroreceptor-mediated vagal activation[10] or beta-adrenergic stimulation.[9] Vagotomy

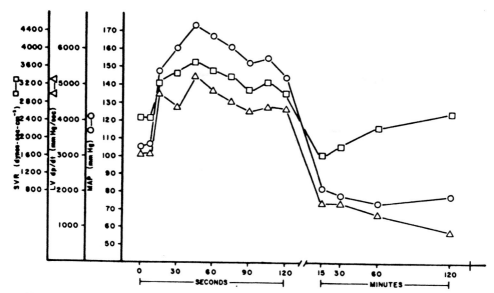

FIG. 11–4. Pathophysiology of neurogenic shock in experimental spinal cord injury: Changes in mean arterial pressure (*circles*), left ventricular *dp/dt* (*triangles*), and systemic vascular resistance (*squares*) over time in acute spinal cord compression. (*From Tibbs PA, Young B, McAllister RG, et al: Studies of experimental cervical spinal cord transection: I. Hemodynamic changes after acute spinal cord transection. J Neurosurg 49:558, 1978, with permission.*)

decreased the bradycardic response in Alexander and Kerr's work[8] and eliminated arrhythmias in Greenhoot and Mauck's.[11] Atropine was used in the study by Evans et al.[9] to eliminate bradycardia, although it was not successful in Eidelberg's preparations.[5] Tibbs et al.[10] believed that the initial bradycardia which occurred immediately after cord sectioning was not baroreceptor-mediated but that other escape dysrhythmias were. Evans et al.[9] were able to prevent the primary arrhythmia with atropine, but later arrhythmias were only prevented by propranolol. This suggests that the beta-adrenergic stimulation in combination with cholinergic stimulation resulted in the later arrhythmias (Fig. 11–5). The sympathetic hyperactivity of the pressor response is easily explained by direct mechanical stimulation of descending sympathetic pathways resulting in diffuse stimulation of the cardiac beta-adrenergics and peripheral alpha-adrenergics. However, the parasympathetic stimulation suggests that spinal cord injury causes direct mechanical stimulation of spinal afferents to the medullary vasomotor centers resulting in vagal activation and immediate bradycardia.[9]

HYPOTENSIVE PHASE

The secondary and more prolonged hemodynamic change following acute spinal cord injury is hypotension. Although this has been regarded as a generalized loss of sympathetic tone, experimental work has shown that it involves more than vasodilatation and may involve an element of cardiogenic shock. Unfortunately, experimental studies of the hemodynamics of spinal cord injury are hampered by variations in the species used, the parameters measured, and the

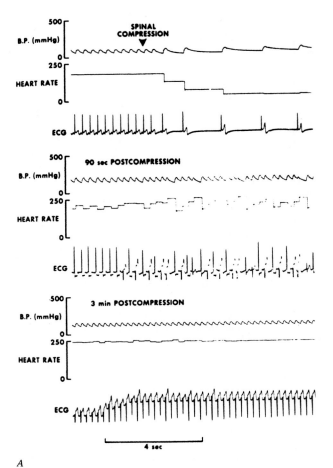

A

FIG. 11–5. Effects of various drugs on neurogenic shock in experimental spinal cord injury. *A.* Effects of spinal cord compression on blood pressure, heart rate, and ECG. *B.* Effects of atropine on cardiovascular response to cord compression. *C.* Effects of atropine and propranolol on cardiovascular response to cord compression. *D.* Effects of phenoxybenzamine and atropine on the cardiovascular response. (*From Evans DE, Kobrine DE, Rizzoli HV: Cardiac arrhythmias accompanying acute compression of the spinal cord. J Neurosurg 52:52, 1980, with permission.*)

methods of injury induction. However, there now appears to be some consensus after decades of study.

Rawe and Perot[6] quantified hypotension at 63 percent of pretrauma levels. They reversed the hypotension with an alpha-adrenergic stimulator such as metaramine and potentiated it with the beta-adrenergic agent isoproterenol, likely due to its vasodilating effect via beta-2 stimulation. In 1978, Tibbs et al.[10] examined more thoroughly the factors contributing to the hypotension by measuring systemic vascular resistance and the change in left ventricular pressure

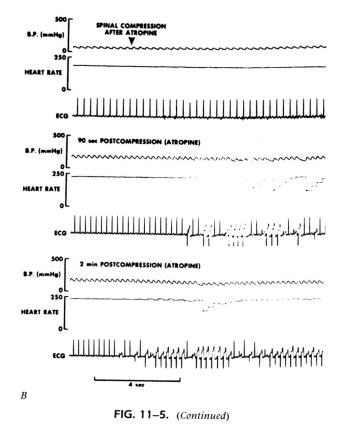

B

FIG. 11–5. (*Continued*)

with respect to time (*dp/dt*). They found a 71 percent decrease in mean arterial pressure but only a 16 percent decrease in systemic vascular resistance, with a 59 percent decrease in the left ventricular pressure curve. There was no change in cardiac output despite the dramatic drop in cardiac contractility, and their findings suggested that the cardiac loss of beta-adrenergic tone contributed more significantly to the hypotension than the loss of alpha-adrenergic vascular tone (see Fig. 11–4). Guha and Tator[7] in 1988 found a marked decrease in cardiac output which persisted in the hypotensive phase while systemic vascular resistance gradually returned to preinjury levels in a rat model of spinal cord injury. These findings suggested a primary myocardial injury that prevented return of contractility. Myocardial injury also has been described by Greenhoot et al.[4] in the context of acute spinal cord injury, although this was not seen in other studies of myocardial blood flow and histology after acute spinal cord injury.[12]

PULMONARY EDEMA

The association between spinal cord injury and pulmonary edema has been known since the last century. However the mechanism by which it occurs remains unknown. Animal studies have suggested that it is due to the catecholamine surge causing a massive left ventricular burden from the sudden increase

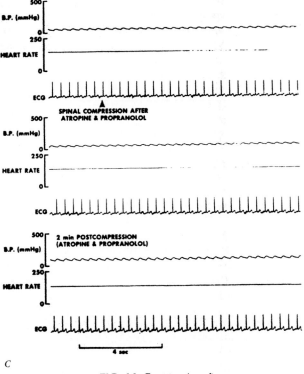

C

FIG. 11–5. (*Continued*)

in afterload as well as the shift of volume from the periphery into the central pulmonary vasculature.[13] If the myocardium is compliant, the increase in left ventricular end-diastolic pressure will result in an increase in cardiac output, but if the myocardium is noncompliant, left ventricular failure will ensue.[14]

The first human study examining this problem was a retrospective review of Vietnam War casualties by Meyer et al.[15] Nine patients were examined within 4 h of acute spinal cord injury, and four developed fulminant pulmonary edema, three of whom died. These investigators suggested that these patients had overreplacement of intravascular volume which contributed to their demise. However, this study only had a small number of patients, and other factors, such as associated chest trauma, could not be controlled. Others have disputed this mechanism, and more recent speculations implicate massive sympathetic discharge with hypertension contributing to the increase in afterload, dysrhythmias, and left ventricular strain, along with disruption of capillary endothelium, thereby setting the stage for either the pulmonary capillary leak syndrome (i.e., low-pressure pulmonary edema or adult respiratory distress syndrome) or high-pressure cardiogenic pulmonary edema.[16]

CLINICAL STUDIES

A number of problems are encountered when one assesses the human studies of the cardiovascular effects of spinal cord injury. First, as noted earlier, the pres-

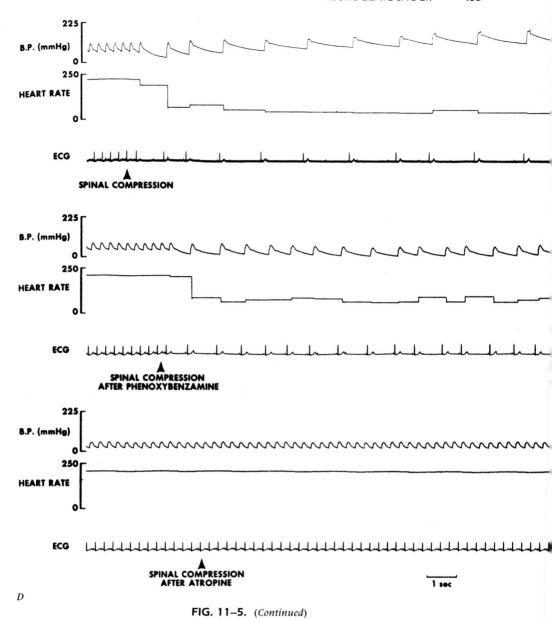

B.P. (mmHg)

HEART RATE

ECG

SPINAL COMPRESSION

B.P. (mmHg)

HEART RATE

ECG

**SPINAL COMPRESSION
AFTER PHENOXYBENZAMINE**

B.P. (mmHg)

HEART RATE

ECG

**SPINAL COMPRESSION
AFTER ATROPINE**

1 sec

D

FIG. 11–5. (*Continued*)

sor phase is not seen because of the delay usually encountered between injury and assessment by a medical team. Also, most clinical studies are limited by the small numbers of cases documented in the acute phase, and in addition, there is the confounding admixture of associated chest or other injuries. Difficulties also have arisen as a result of the inclusion of both complete and incomplete spinal cord lesions in nonstratified studies and the use of varying hemodynamic monitoring parameters.

In general, hypotension and bradycardia have been the most consistent findings in cervical and upper thoracic spinal cord injury. Most observers attribute these findings to a decrease in sympathetic tone resulting in a decrease in systemic vascular resistance, dilatation of capacitance vessels, and a decrease in preload contributing to a further decrease in blood pressure. These effects result in a vicious cycle. The relationship between the cord level of injury and the degree of hemodynamic alteration was examined in a retrospective review of 41 patients with spinal cord injury in 1970 by Meineke et al.,[17] who found that the most marked hypotension occurred in cervical and upper thoracic cord injuries. With respect to heart rate, it was surprising that tachycardia was the most frequent finding within the first few days. However, the numbers were small, included both complete and incomplete lesions, and only 28 patients were seen within the first 24 h of injury.

The study by Meyer et al.[15] described above comprises data from patients at the earliest interval after injury: Nine patients were seen within 4 h of injury and had recordings of central venous pressure, mean arterial pressure, and cardiac output. As indicated, four developed fulminant pulmonary edema, three of whom died. Significant differences in hemodynamic parameters were discovered between the pulmonary edema and non-pulmonary edema groups. Both groups had hypotension with a decrease in diastolic blood pressure and an increase in pulse pressure and cardiac output, but the pulmonary edema group had a significantly higher CVP. The non-pulmonary edema group had significantly more marked bradycardia. The two groups, however, were not controlled for other associated injuries, and the degree of chest trauma suffered by the pulmonary edema group was enough to require a tube thoracostomy in three of the four, while none of the non-pulmonary edema group required a thoracostomy. The authors concluded that the critical level of transection was T2–6 in order to produce arterial hypotension. They warned against overinfusion of blood, which was felt to cause the pulmonary edema, and they speculated about a sudden release of catecholamines in a sympathetically denervated system as the cause of sudden vasoconstriction and acute volume overload.[15]

In 1979, Mathias et al.[18] compared the blood pressure, heart rate, and ratio of plasma norepinephrine to epinephrine in five recent (<2 weeks) quadriplegics, six chronic quadriplegics, and six normal individuals. The recently injured group had lower diastolic blood pressure, heart rate, and ratio of norepinephrine to epinephrine, while those with chronic quadriplegia had the lowest mean arterial pressure. In general, the quadriplegics had lower norepinephrine and epinephrine plasma levels, reflective of decreased sympathetic tone.

In a 1987 study of 71 cord-injured patients of whom 31 were severe (grades A and B), 17 were moderate to mild (grades C and D), and the remaining 23 were thoracolumbar injuries, all the severely injured group had persistent bradycardia. Bradycardia peaked at about postinjury day 4 and then resolved spontaneously within 2 to 6 weeks. Bradyarrhythmias were universal in the severely injured group, who also experienced more supraventricular arrhythmias, cardiac arrest, and marked hypotension. The most common supraventricular arrhythmia was atrial fibrillation in 6 of the 31 patients with severe spinal cord injuries. Isoproterenol completely eliminated sinus pauses and increased the heart rate by 40 percent, while epinephrine, dobutamine, ephedrine, and terbutaline did not (Fig. 11–6). Hypotension was accompanied by a decrease in systemic vascular resistance and an increase in cardiac output, thereby implicating vasodilatation as the primary disturbance. This human study supports the findings in

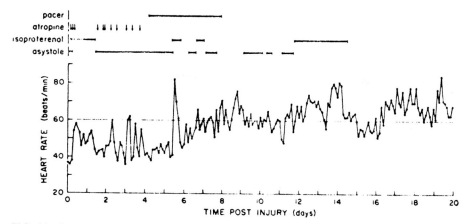

FIG. 11–6. The effects of various drugs on heart rate in the clinial setting of spinal cord injury. *(From Lehman KG, Lane JG, Piepmeier JM, Batsford WP: Cardiovascular abnormalities accompanying acute spinal cord injury in humans: Incidence, time course, and severity. J Am Coll Cardiol 10:46, 1987, with permission.)*

the animal studies in which low-dose sympathomimetics prevented the brady-arrhythmias of acute spinal cord injury.[19]

In 1986, Winslow et al.[20] found that 22 of 83 patients with traumatic quadriplegia had significant bradycardia that resolved within 3 to 5 weeks of injury. Three of the 22 patients suffered asystolic cardiac arrest within 24 h of injury, and the majority of episodes occurred when the patients were prone or during suctioning. Bradycardia was seen only with complete tetraplegia and was felt to be related to the inability to mount an immediate sympathetic response to the cardiovascular effects of vagal stimulation. All responded to vagolytics, but 3 patients required cardiac pacemakers to control hemodynamically significant bradycardia. Two were in patients with preexisting cardiac disease and one in a patient whose pacemaker failed, but he ultimately regained normal spontaneous heart rate.

Two additional case reports show that not all cardiac arrhythmias accompanying spinal cord injury are self-limited. One describes a patient requiring vagolytics for 3.5 months to prevent severe bradycardia,[21] and the other describes a patient with C2 complete quadriplegia related to a birth injury who required a pacemaker insertion at 21 months of age after three episodes of bradycardia leading to cardiac arrest.[22] Theoretically, the sympathetic dysfunction of acute spinal cord injury should resolve as spinal shock resolves. As the chronic stage of spinal cord injury leads to spasticity of the skeletal muscles, the autonomic nervous system becomes hyperactive as well, leading to the stage of autonomic hyperreflexia.

In summary, acute spinal cord injury involves a sudden traumatic injury to the central nervous system resulting in activation of central autonomic pathways. This begins within one heartbeat of injury with bradycardia induced by direct activation of spinal cord afferents stimulating the medullary vasomotor center and inducing vagal initiation of cardiac slowing. A simultaneous stimulation of spinal sympathetic efferents either in the white matter tracts and/or gray matter cell columns causes the pressor response consisting of an increase in systolic and diastolic blood pressure which resolves within a few minutes of injury. This pressor response stimulates a baroreceptor reflex to further activate the vagus and maintain the bradycardia. The secondary vasomotor response is that of hypotension. Sympathetic tone is lost below the level of the injury, and hypotension ensues as a result of the loss of arteriolar tone and an increase in venous capacitance. Cardiac output may increase in an attempt to maintain adequate central nervous system (CNS) blood flow, although this does not occur in a previously damaged myocardium or if the sudden catecholamine surge associated with the initial injury to the CNS damages the myocardium. Only in an entirely noncompromised myocardium will there be adequate recovery to maintain or increase cardiac output to compensate for the decrease in afterload. Cardiac slowing also occurs as a result of the unopposed vagal tone. The only mechanism by which the heart can increase blood pressure is by increasing contractility; preload, afterload, and heart rate are all fixed as a result of the spinal cord injury. Unfortunately, the previously injured myocardium will not be able to increase contractility, and the result may be pulmonary edema, cardiac arrhythmias, and further hypotension. This will exacerbate the spinal cord injury because the injured spinal cord is unable to autoregulate blood flow and is passively dependent on mean arterial pressure for perfusion in the region of injury.[2,26] This cycle must be interrupted to prevent these hemodynamic effects from further worsening the spinal cord damage.

MANAGEMENT

Ideally, treatment of shock associated with acute spinal cord injury should be accomplished by managing each of the accompanying physiologic abnormalities. Obviously, hypoxia must be treated first by managing any airway or breathing abnormalities. In practice, bradyarrhythmias and hypotension are the most clinically relevant, and there are four possible modalities with which to treat them: volume loading, inotropes, chronotropes, and electrical pacing.

Hypotension usually has been managed with both volume loading and vasopressors. Those who advocate inotrope use with volume restriction fear the possibility of pulmonary edema[23] and have based their management plan on the study by Meyer et al.[15] described earlier, who found that pulmonary edema was a complication in four of nine quadriplegics. More recent approaches to management include volume replacement as the primary mode of resuscitation based on the pathophysiology of neurogenic shock as that of relative hypovolemia due to an expanded intravascular space. Thus initial treatment is aimed at replacing volume, ideally with colloid solutions because of their propensity to remain in the intravascular space.[16,24] Use of whole blood and plasma has become obsolete with the availability of albumin and its low risk of transmission of infectious agents. In our practice, we start with volume replacement with crystalloids and colloids to support blood pressure. If volume replacement does not succeed, we insert a Swan-Ganz catheter and initiate inotropic blood pressure support.[19] Dopamine is our preference for a pressor agent, although others have recommended dobutamine.[16] Dobutamine increases cardiac output by decreasing afterload in the patient with myocardial dysfunction, but this clearly does not help the spinal cord–injured patient who already has a low systemic vascular resistance and increased myocardial contractility. Dopamine even in renal doses frequently has an effect on blood pressure and can be increased to alpha levels, which will counteract the loss of peripheral sympathetic tone. Phenylephrine is frequently used in bolus injections for spinal anesthesia. It is a pure alpha agonist, and therefore, it will counteract the vasodilatation that occurs in neurogenic shock and transiently improve venous return. An epinephrine drip is another possibility, and it works by reversing the loss of both alpha- and beta-adrenergic activity to return blood pressure to normal (Table 11–3).

Pulmonary edema may occur in acute spinal cord injury, although it is more frequent in multiply injured patients, especially those with chest injuries. In these complicated cases, early use of invasive monitoring is advocated, which allows therapy to be determined by the hemodynamic abnormality in each case. High-pressure pulmonary edema should be managed with judicious use of fluids, investigation of the cardiac abnormality, and early maximization of left ventricular function. Low-pressure pulmonary edema is usually related to capillary leak from endothelial damage at the time of the catecholamine surge. It should be managed with positive end-expiratory pressure (PEEP) ventilation and inotropes, as well as an adequate intravascular volume. Positive-pressure ventilation will further decrease venous return and compromise cardiac output if intravascular volume is not maintained.

Bradycardia is often a major component of the cardiovascular abnormalities in acute spinal cord injury. Vagolytic drugs can be used to increase heart rate and thus contribute to improving blood pressure. Bradycardia on its own can be a significant cause of morbidity and mortality in the spinal cord–injured patient. Vagolytic therapy with atropine for short-term use[20] and propantheline for longer-term use[21] have been suggested.

Lehman et al.[19] emphasized the self-limited course of the bradyarrhythmias, which last 2 to 6 weeks after the acute injury, and found that the life-threatening arrhythmias occurred only within the first 14 days. They also suggested that sinus arrest can be predicted in patients with the most severe bradyarrhythmias, marked hypotension, supraventricular and ventricular tachycardias, and AV block. They advocate the use of low-dose isoproterenol infusions to counteract the loss of beta-adrenergic tone and prevent some of the life-threatening arrhythmias.

Pacemaker insertion should be considered in patients refractory to medical management of bradyarrhythmias. Patients requiring this aggressive measure are unusual, since most respond to atropine, propantheline, or isoproterenol. However, with the relatively low morbidity associated with pacemaker insertion and the high risk of significant mortality without adequate cardiac rhythm control, pacemakers should be considered earlier in high-risk individuals, especially in those with preexisting heart disease.[25]

Restoration of systemic normotension may help counteract the posttraumatic ischemia that occurs in the spinal cord after acute severe injury.[2,26] Theoretically, the loss of autoregulation in the injured spinal cord causes spinal cord blood flow to become passively dependent on mean systemic arterial pressure. The maintenance of adequate spinal cord blood flow may ultimately influence the extent of secondary cord injury.[7] Unfortunately, animal studies have failed to

TABLE 11–3. Agents Used in the Management of Neurogenic Shock Due to Spinal Cord Injury

Name	Mechanism of Action	Advantages	Disadvantages
Fluids (crystalloid and colloid)	Fill expanded intravascular space, thereby increasing preload	Safe Two-thirds of crystalloid may spill extravascularly	Risk of pulmonary edema
Dopamine	(i) <2 μg/kg/min, dopaminergic effects on renal vasculature (ii) 3–7 μg/kg/min, beta effects on HR/contractility (iii) >7 μg/kg/min, alpha effects with peripheral vasoconstriction	Can be dialed to level at which underlying pathophysiology is corrected	(i) Dopaminergic levels may increase urine output, thereby decreasing effective circulating volume (ii) Beta effects may decrease BP by decreasing SVR (iii) Alpha effects of vasoconstriction may decrease spinal cord blood flow
Dobutamine	Major effect on beta receptors to increase HR/contractility	May be helpful in pulmonary edema to decrease pulmonary vascular resistance	Expense Beta-2 effect will decrease BP by decreasing SVR
Phenylephrine	Alpha agonist	Vasoconstriction of capacitance vessels to increase preload Rapid effect on BP	Vasoconstriction may decrease spinal cord blood flow Usually used intermittently with bolus injections
Epinephrine	Both alpha and beta effects	Counteracts directly the decrease in sympathetic activity	Mild beta-2 effect might decrease SVR to drop diastolic BP
Norepinephrine	Major beta-1 effect, less alpha effects	Less likely to decrease BP by beta-2 effects on SVR	
Atropine	Postganglionic muscarinic cholinergic blocker	Vagolytic with rapid reversal of bradycardia Prevention of sinus arrests with vagal stimulating maneuvers	Short-term bolus use only
Propantheline	Postganglionic anticholinergic	Long-acting vagolytic	
Isoproterenol	Mainly beta-1 agonist	Can increase HR to allow increase in BP	
Pacemaker	Electrical HR modification	Can dial HR up to rate at which BP is better controlled	Invasive Expense

demonstrate conclusively an improvement in neurologic functional recovery after restoration of blood pressure to normal levels following experimental spinal cord injury.[27,28]

In summary, normotension should be achieved in the patient with acute spinal cord injury, initially with volume replacement to fill the relatively expanded intravascular space. If this is unsuccessful, inotropes should be used along with invasive hemodynamic monitoring to assess the physiologic response. If bradycardia is a major component contributing to hypotension or is producing life-threatening arrhythmias independently, vagolytics or beta-adrenergic sympathomimetics should be started. If medical management of the arrhythmias has failed, and if they are severe and life-threatening, consideration should be given to early placement of a cardiac pacemaker for consistent and complete control of cardiac rhythm.

REFERENCES

1. Blalock A: *Principles of Surgical Care: Shock and Other Problems.* St. Louis, Mosby, 1940.
2. Tator CH: Review of experimental spinal cord injury with emphasis on the local and systemic circulatory effects. *Neurochirurgie* 37:291, 1991.
3. Wallace MC, Tator CH, Lewis AJ: Chronic regenerative changes in the spinal cord after cord compression injury in rats. *Surg Neurol* 27:209, 1987.
4. Greenhoot JH, Shiel FOM, Mauck HP: Experimental spinal cord injury: Electrocardiographic abnormalities and fuchsinophilic myocardial degeneration. *Arch Neurol* 26:524, 1972.
5. Eidelberg EE: Cardiovascular response to experimental spinal cord compression. *J Neurosurg* 38:326, 1973.
6. Rawe SE, Perot PL: Pressor response resulting from experimental contusion injury to the spinal cord. *J Neurosurg* 50:52, 1979.
7. Guha A, Tator CH: Acute cardiovascular effects of experimental spinal cord injury. *J Trauma* 28:481, 1988.
8. Alexander S, Kerr FWL: Blood pressure responses in acute compression of the spinal cord. *J Neurosurg* 21:485, 1964.
9. Evans DE, Kobrine DE, Rizzoli HV: Cardiac arrhythmias accompanying acute compression of the spinal cord. *J Neurosurg* 52:52, 1980.
10. Tibbs PA, Young B, McAllister RG, et al: Studies of experimental cervical spinal cord transection: I. Hemodynamic changes after acute spinal cord transection. *J Neurosurg* 49:558, 1978.
11. Greenhoot JH, Mauck HP: The effect of cervical cord injury on cardiac rhythm and conduction. *Am Heart J* 83:659, 1972.
12. Tibbs PA, Young B, Todd EP, et al: Studies of experimental spinal cord transection: IV. Effects of cervical spinal cord transection on myocardial blood flow in anesthetized dogs. *J Neurosurg* 52:197, 1980.
13. Theodore J, Robin ED: Speculations on neurogenic pulmonary edema. *Am Rev Respir Dis* 113:405, 1976.
14. Brisman R, Kovach RM, Johnson DO, et al: Pulmonary edema in acute transection of the cervical spinal cord. *Surg Gynecol Obstet* 139:363, 1974.
15. Meyer GA, Berman IR, Doty DB, et al: Hemodynamic responses to acute quadriplegia with or without chest trauma. *J Neurosurg* 34:168, 1971.

16. Albin MS, Gilbert TS: Acute spinal cord trauma, in Shoemaker W, Ayres S, Grenvik A, et al (eds): *Textbook of Critical Care,* 2d ed. Philadelphia, Saunders, 1989, pp 1277–1285.

17. Meinecke FW, Rosenkranz KA, Kurek CM: Regulation of the cardiovascular system in patients with fresh injuries to the spinal cord: Preliminary report. *Paraplegia* 9:109, 1971.

18. Mathias CJ, Christensen NJ, Frankel HL, Spalding HMJ: Cardiovascular control in recently injured tetraplegics in spinal shock. *Q J Med* 48:273, 1978.

19. Lehman KG, Lane JG, Piepmeier JM, Batsford WP: Cardiovascular abnormalities accompanying acute spinal cord injury in humans: Incidence, time course and severity. *J Am Coll Cardiol* 10:46, 1987.

20. Winslow EBJ, Lesch M, Talano JV, Meyer PR: Spinal cord injuries associated with cardiopulmonary complications. *Spine* 11:809, 1986.

21. Abd AG, Braun NMT: Management of life-threatening bradycardia in spinal cord injury. *Chest* 95:701, 1989.

22. Gilgoff IS, Davidson SL, Hohn AR: Cardiac pacemaker in high spinal cord injury. *Arch Phys Med Rehabil* 72:601, 1991.

23. Luce JM: Medical management of spinal cord injury. *Crit Care Med* 13:126, 1985.

24. Ogilvy CS, Heros RC: Spinal cord compression, in Ropper AH, Kennedy SF (eds): *Neurological and Neurosurgical Intensive Care,* 2d ed. Rockville, Md, Aspen, 1988, pp 309–322.

25. Kiss Z, Tator CH: Cardiac pacing in the management of bradyarrhythmias of acute spinal cord injury (abstract). *Can J Neurol Sci* 19:303, 1992.

26. Tator CH, Fehlings MG: Review of the secondary injury theory of acute spinal cord injury with emphasis on vascular mechanisms. *J Neurosurg* 75:15, 1991.

27. Wallace MC, Tator CH: Failure of blood transfusion or naloxone to improve clinical recovery after experimental spinal cord injury. *Neurosurgery* 19:489, 1986.

28. Dolan EJ, Tator CH: The treatment of hypotension due to acute experimental spinal cord compression injury. *Surg Neurol* 13:380, 1980.

12

HEAD INJURY

Steven R. Shackford
Steven L. Wald

Head injury remains the leading cause of traumatic death in the United States.[1,2] Recent evidence suggests that events occurring after the primary insult play an important role in determining outcome.[3-8] These secondary events are a consequence of the brain's response to injury. They appear to be significantly worse when shock accompanies the primary injury, and they appear to be related to the manner in which the patient with a brain injury is resuscitated.[8,9]

Despite the importance of the brain in determining outcome after injury, there has been very little focused investigation of the response of the injured brain to shock and resuscitation.[10] This chapter will attempt to summarize the current knowledge and recent developments in resuscitation of the patient with a brain injury. We have included a brief summary of transcapillary fluid exchange, as well as a review of relevant cerebral circulatory physiology and the physiologic aberrations produced by brain injury, in order to allow the reader to judge the relative importance of pertinent laboratory and clinical investigations of brain injury with and without associated hypovolemia. The chapter will not address brain resuscitation after either cardiopulmonary arrest or thromboembolic stroke.

THE PROBLEM: SECONDARY BRAIN INJURY

Cerebral trauma can be divided temporally into primary and secondary injury. The *primary injury* is a result of energy absorption by the skull and brain, which can cause immediate neuronal and axonal disruption, shearing or laceration of the brain, and vascular disruption. Of patients dying of head injury, 50 to 90 percent have pathologic evidence of diffuse edema, herniation, or frank necrosis not apparent at the time of the impact injury.[1,3-5] These changes have been grouped under the term *secondary injury* because they appear to occur after the primary impact injury. Secondary injury can be due to ischemia (as a result of systemic hypotension, hypoxia, or loss of cerebral autoregulation), cerebral swelling, or intracranial hypertension.[3-8]

Systemic hypotension and/or hypoxia should be readily treated in trauma systems.[11] Despite advanced prehospital and early hospital care available in trauma systems, 35 percent of patients with severe head injury [Glasgow coma score[12] (GCS) ≤ 8] are hypotensive and/or hypoxic during the early phases of care.[7,8] Of the two, hypotension appears to have the greatest impact on outcome. Chestnut et al.,[7] using data from the National Traumatic Coma Data Bank, examined the effect of hypotension and/or hypoxia on patients with a severe head injury. The mortality of the entire group was 37 percent; in those patients in whom either hypotension or hypoxia was present, the mortality rates were 64 and 50 percent, respectively. In examining each of the factors independently, the mortality rate from hypoxia alone was found to be similar to that of the cohort as a whole. Hypotension alone resulted in a mortality rate of 60 percent, significantly greater than that of the whole cohort. The results of this large study confirmed previous work done by Miller et al.[6] and Eisenberg et al.[13] In rural Vermont, we have made similar observations, noting a doubling of mortality in the presence of hypotension and/or hypoxia.[8] These clinical studies emphasize the vulnerability of the injured brain to even brief periods of hypoperfusion and suggest that rapid treatment of hypovolemia is an important factor in determining the outcome of patients with severe brain injury.

Secondary insults also can occur as a result of increased intracranial pressure (ICP). It is useful to consider ICP as a function of the relative space occupied by the brain, the cerebrospinal fluid (CSF), and the cerebral blood volume (Table 12–1). An increase in the volume of one must be accompanied by a reduction in one or more of the other volumes or there will be an increase in the ICP. For example, the volume of brain tissue can be increased by edema, due to a disruption of the blood-brain barrier, or brain swelling, both of which accompany brain injury. The increased volume of brain will result in intracranial hypertension if there is not a compensatory reduction in either the CSF volume or the cerebral blood volume. ICP also can be increased by expansion of the cerebral blood volume, such as occurs with vasodilatation of capacitance vessels. Ischemia, severe enough to cause a shift from aerobic to anaerobic metabolism, generates lactate, a potent cerebral vasodilator. The resultant increase in cerebral blood volume can increase the ICP. An increase in ICP, in turn, results in diminished cerebral perfusion pressure (CPP = MAP − ICP) and a decrease in cerebral blood flow (CBF), resulting in a further decrease in delivery of both oxygen and glucose (Fig. 12–1).

TABLE 12–1. Determinants of Intracranial Pressure

$$ICP = V_{brain} + V_{blood} + V_{CSF} + V_{ECF} + V_x$$

where ICP = intracranial pressure
V = volume
CSF = cerebrospinal fluid
ECF = extracellular fluid
x = hematoma, edema, swelling (engorged blood vessels)

FIG. 12–1. The increase in intracranial pressure (ICP) after brain injury is thought to be due to a number of factors. The primary impact injury disrupts the blood brain barrier (BBB) resulting in local hemorrhage and edema. The local edema, either through mechanical compressive effects or due to the release of local vasoactive mediators, decreases regional cerebral blood flow (rCBF) leading to local hypoxia/ischemia. This reduction in oxygen delivery leads to anaerobic metabolism and a decrease in pH. This can lead to vasodilation and vasoparesis, which increases the cerebral blood volume and increases the ICP.

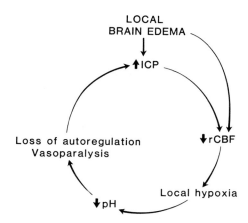

Increased ICP (>20 mmHg) is associated with an increase in poor outcome (death, severely neurologically disabled or vegetative).[14,15] In brain-injured patients without a mass lesion who had slight elevations in the initial ICP (11 to 20 mmHg), Miller et al.[14] showed a significant increase in poor outcome (25 percent mortality, 11 percent severely disabled or vegetative) compared with patients whose initial ICP was 0 to 10 mmHg (8 percent mortality, 7 percent severely disabled or vegetative; $p < 0.02$). In a subsequent series, Miller et al.[15] demonstrated a significant correlation between raised ICP and poor outcome ($p < 0.001$) and observed a universal mortality in those patients in whom the ICP could not be controlled. Controlling intracranial hypertension has historically been the major focus of therapeutic efforts.[16,17]

In order to understand the factors that contribute to raised ICP and, therefore, to rationally resuscitate patients with head injuries, it is important to understand the principles of transcapillary fluid exchange and the factors controlling normal cerebral blood flow and metabolism and to have an appreciation of how this physiology is altered by brain injury.

TRANSCAPILLARY FLUID EXCHANGE

Transcapillary fluid exchange is governed by capillary permeability and the hydrostatic and oncotic pressure gradients that exist between the capillary and the interstitium. The relationship of these forces in determining net fluid movement across the capillary membrane is described by the Starling equation:[18]

$$Q_f = K_f S[P_c - P_t) - r(\pi_c - \pi_t)]$$

where Q_f is net fluid flux across the membrane, K_f is the filtration coefficient of the membrane, S is the surface area of the membrane, P_c is the capillary hydrostatic pressure, P_t is the tissue hydrostatic pressure, r is Staverman's coefficient of reflectance,[19] π_c is the oncotic pressure of plasma proteins, and π_t is the oncotic pressure of the interstitial fluid proteins.

Under normal conditions, edema is prevented by a combination of a low hydrostatic gradient between the capillary and the interstitium and the relatively high reflectance coefficient of albumin, the major colloid in serum and the primary determinant of the colloid osmotic pressure (COP). Normally, these hydrostatic and oncotic gradients favor net fluid movement out of the arterial end of the capillary. Fluid accumulation in the interstitium is prevented by the lymphatics, which have a great capacity for fluid removal.[20]

Based on these normal relationships, one would expect that electrolyte solutions without colloid or protein would result in greater fluid movement out of the capillary (Q_f) at any given hydrostatic pressure (P_c) because they dilute plasma proteins and reduce the COP. Colloids, by raising the albumin concentration (increased π_c), would be expected to sustain the COP, resulting in a lower Q_f at a given P_c.

Interpretation of the Starling equation, as Civetta[18] points out, depends on a number of factors, including the methodologies for measuring both hydrostatic and oncotic pressures, the physiologic state of the organism, and the location of the capillary bed. Cerebral capillary endothelial cells have extremely tight intracellular junctions, are devoid of fenestrae, and contain few microvesicles for transport. These attributes, in the aggregate, constitute the blood-brain barrier (BBB),[21,22] which has an extremely low filtration coefficient (equal to one-thirtieth the filtration coefficient of the muscle capillary). The intact BBB, therefore, has a very low hydraulic conductivity which abrogates, to a large extent, the effects of any changes in either hydrostatic or oncotic pressure. Thus the BBB protects the brain from edema formation which might occur as a result of an increase in mean arterial pressure (MAP) or a decrease in COP. The integrity of the BBB in preventing edema formation is quite important because the brain, unlike muscle or lung, lacks lymphatics.

NORMAL CEREBRAL BLOOD FLOW AND METABOLISM

An in-depth review of normal circulatory physiology is beyond the scope of this chapter and can be found elsewhere,[23–26] but certain points deserve emphasis.

CEREBRAL METABOLIC REQUIREMENTS

The brain, relative to its size, has an immense requirement for energy.[25] To understand this need, recall that the neuron has a large membrane surface area relative to its volume and that axons and dendrites extend for considerable distances away from the cell body.[23] Energy is required by the neuron to maintain ionic gradients for depolarization and volume regulation over the large membrane area, to synthesize phospholipids for maintenance of membrane integrity, and to transport proteins (excitatory and inhibitory transmitters) to axon terminals. Prough and Rogers[25] have suggested that 40 to 50 percent of substrate consumed by the brain is needed to maintain cellular integrity, while the rest is used to perform electrophysiologic work.

It is estimated that the oxygen requirement of the "resting" brain is approximately 3.5 ml/100 g per minute. The average adult brain weighs approximately 1400 g and would, therefore, consume about 50 ml oxygen per minute in the "resting" state, or 20 percent of the oxygen consumed by the entire body. To provide this large amount of substrate, the brain requires a high blood flow (approximately 700 ml/min) and has a high oxygen extraction ratio (approximately 0.35). Because of the large energy requirement and a limited capacity to store substrate, the brain is extremely vulnerable to ischemia or hypoxia.

REGULATION OF CEREBRAL BLOOD FLOW

Regulation of the cerebral blood flow (CBF) occurs through alteration in cerebral vascular resistance (CVR). CVR is influenced by the cerebral perfusion pressure (CPP), the cerebral metabolic rate, and the chemical milieu. There also may be direct neural influences, especially on the larger branches of the cerebral arteries, but these are of relatively little consequence and are not considered to play a major role in controlling CVR.[24,26,27]

PRESSURE AUTOREGULATION

Pressure autoregulation is the normal homeostatic mechanism that maintains a constant CBF as CPP varies. Between a MAP of 50 and 150 mmHg, CBF is relatively constant. Within this range of MAP, CBF is maintained by changes in CVR; as MAP increases, CVR increases (vasoconstriction), and as MAP decreases, CVR decreases (vasodilation). As MAP falls below 50 mmHg, CBF decreases because vasodilatation is maximal; similarly, elevation in MAP above 150 mmHg is accompanied by a corresponding elevation in CBF because vasoconstriction is maximal. It had been thought that alterations in cerebrovascular tone were mediated by effects of stretch on the arterial wall (i.e., "myogenic").[24] Recent work examining the relationship between venous pressure and CBF[28] has shown that increases in CVP result in a decrease in venous return and an increase in CBF. The opposite would have been expected if the myogenic hypothesis were true, since a decrease in venous return would cause vascular congestion and dilatation of the capacitance vessels, thus increasing their "stretch." Increased stretch, in the myogenic hypothesis, should initiate reflexic vasoconstriction and reduced CBF, not increased CBF. Pressure autoregulation, therefore, appears to be mediated by the local concentration of vasodilator metabolites (see below).[26]

METABOLIC REGULATION OF CBF

There is a linear relationship between functional activity of the brain and the regional CBF.[25,26] Any neuronal activity in the brain increases oxygen consumption and results in an increase in CBF. Similarly, systemic motor activity will increase the oxygen requirements of the motor cortex and increase CBF to that area. It is now generally accepted that the cerebral metabolic rate for oxygen (CMRO$_2$) and CBF are directly and positively coupled.

CHEMICAL REGULATION OF CBF

Changes in the arterial blood gases have profound effects on CBF.[23-26] A direct and positive relationship exists between CBF and the carbon dioxide tension of blood (P_{CO_2}) within the range of 20 to 80 mmHg.[29,30] The effects of P_{CO_2} are

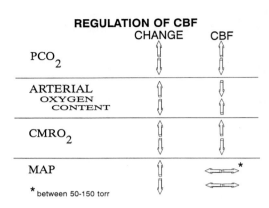

REGULATION OF CBF

FIG. 12–2. Cerebral blood flow (CBF) is regulated by changes in P_{CO_2}, arterial oxygen content, the cerebral metabolic rate ($CMRO_2$), and the mean arterial pressure (MAP). Arrows pointing upward indicate an increase (i.e., an increase in P_{CO_2} will result in an increase in the CBF), arrows pointing downward indicate a decrease (i.e., a decrease in $CMRO_2$ will result in a decrease in CBF), and paired arrows pointing right and left indicate no change [i.e., an increase or a decrease in MAP (in the range of 50 to 150 mmHg) will result in no change in CBF provided pressure autoregulation is intact (see text)].

mediated through changes in the concentration of hydrogen ions in the extracellular fluid.[26]

There is an inverse relationship between the oxygen tension in blood (P_{O_2}) and CBF. This appears to be due, in large part, to the dependency of the hemoglobin saturation on the P_{O_2} and their combined effects on arterial oxygen content. Brown and coworkers[31–33] have elegantly shown that hemodilution, with reduction of the arterial oxygen content, increases CBF. These changes were not explained by changes in blood viscosity. The regulation of CBF is summarized in Fig. 12–2.

CEREBRAL BLOOD FLOW AND METABOLISM AFTER HEAD INJURY

A considerable volume of clinical and experimental information exists about CBF and metabolism after isolated head injury. Much less is known about changes in CBF and metabolism when hypotension or hypoxia accompany head injury.

As previously discussed, the regulation of CBF is a function of both mean arterial pressure and local cerebral metabolism. Severe head injury, however, may lead to ischemia or hyperemia, suggesting that, in some patients, normal regulation of CBF may be lost.[34–38] It is now felt that many patients with severe head injury exhibit an early reduction in CBF. Jaggi et al.[39] conducted acute CBF determinations in 96 patients with severe head injury, 70 percent of whom underwent analysis within 48 h of the injury. Forty-four patients (46 percent) were found to have reduced CBF which was significantly related to adverse outcome. Marion et al.[35] were able to perform CBF studies on 43 percent of a series of 32 patients during the first 24 h. Reduced CBF was evident in the group of patients without mass lesions during the first hours after the injury. By 24 h, however, global blood flow had returned to nearly normal levels. It has been suggested on the basis of these studies and others that the first few minutes to hours after a severe head injury are characterized by a significant reduction of

CBF, both globally and regionally, followed by a period of relative hyperemia.[34,35] Although many investigators have attempted to correlate CBF with outcome following head injury,[40–42] most of these studies have failed to conclusively demonstrate a direct correlation.

Laboratory evaluation would seem like an ideal setting for the observation of acute changes in CBF produced by brain injury. The graded fluid percussion model of head injury has received the widest attention, although few experiments have been done combining shock with this model of head injury. Fluid percussion injury, without shock, produces an abrupt rise of MAP followed by brief periods of hypotension.[43–45] The time course of this immediate rise in blood pressure suggests that it is mediated by both direct neural influences and humoral effects, specifically catecholamine release. DeWitt et al.[45] noted an elevation of CBF 1 min after both high and low levels of impact. Within 30 to 60 min, CBF returned to normal values. Using the same model, Muir et al.[9] recently reported that cortical CBF increased within seconds after injury but dropped to 50 percent of normal 1 h after the injury. These results were similar to those reported by Yuan et al.[46] and Pfenninger et al.[47] using different techniques to measure CBF. These experiments support the concept of impaired control of the cerebral circulation after head injury, although the evidence of early and significant posttraumatic ischemia is not compelling. We believe that these early changes in circulatory control lay the ground work for future ischemic changes to neurons and initiate the complex metabolic and chemical changes that may further damage the brain.

The metabolic events that occur after head injury are complex and have, until recently, been limited by technical restrictions. If cerebral energy requirements for glucose and oxygen cannot be met by compensatory flow or pressure changes, the brain will revert to anaerobic metabolism to meet its energy needs. In temporary ischemia and stroke models, it has been shown that increased production of lactate, the marker for anaerobic metabolism, occurs during both the hypoperfusion period as well as during the reperfusion period. It is assumed that the continued increase in anaerobic metabolism during the reperfusion period, when oxygen and glucose delivery have returned to normal, is due to derangement of aerobic pathways.[48] Elevated levels of lactate in the CSF have been reported in many clinical studies of head injury.[42,49,50] CSF lactate concentration is probably a direct reflection of intracellular lactate accumulation. Lactic acidosis would be expected to result in a lowering of the pH, which may lead to further cell deterioration and edema. Using ^{31}P magnetic resonance spectroscopy, Ishige et al.[51] demonstrated a statistically significant fall in intracellular pH of rats subjected to a cranial impact injury and systemic hypotension compared with groups subjected to only one of these insults. Rango et al.,[52] however, were unable to demonstrate intracellular acidosis in 22 head-injured patients, although the earliest studies were done 36 h after injury.

The information from experimental isolated head injury studies provides an important reference for reviewing results from experimental studies of head injury combined with either shock or hypoxia. It is only logical to speculate that the addition of hypotension would result in further degradation of neuronal function.

Using a porcine model of cryogenic injury and hemorrhagic shock, Schmoker et al.[53] demonstrated a decrease in cerebral oxygen delivery which occurred immediately after shock and persisted for 24 h despite the restoration of cardiac output, MAP, and CVP. This study suggested that the current clinical parameters of resuscitation inadequately represent cerebral oxygen delivery and may account for the significantly worse outcome of patients with combined head injury and hemorrhagic shock. This experimental work is supported by the recent clinical report by Bouma et al.,[54] who found no relationship between cardiac output and CBF in 35 patients with severe head injury, regardless of the status of autoregulation. Jenkins et al.[48] subjected animals to an initial concussive injury followed by a global ischemic insult, neither of which by themselves would have produced cell death. The combination of injuries, however, resulted in an isoelectric EEG and histologic evidence of diffuse neuronal death with early cerebral edema. Ishige et al.[51] studied the effect of hypotension on cerebral metabolism in rats subjected to head injury. Magnetic resonance spectroscopy revealed a marked reduction in high-energy phosphates following head injury and hypotension that was significantly greater than that seen with head injury alone. These data support the concept that the traumatized brain appears to be more vulnerable to hypotension or hypoxia than does the normal brain. The detrimental effect of this combination of events clearly underscores the need for vigorous and active resuscitation after head injury.

RESUSCITATION OF THE PATIENT WITH HEAD INJURY

Based on our knowledge of the metabolic requirements of the brain and what happens to the normal physiology after injury, it is obvious that cerebral resuscitation must be a high priority in the multiply injured patient. Furthermore, the vulnerability of the brain to even brief periods of hypoperfusion suggests that short delays in airway control and volume restitution may result in irreversible neuronal damage with permanent adverse outcome. We will briefly review the basic priorities in resuscitation, especially as they apply to the patient with a head injury. The main thrust of what follows, however, will be on fluid resuscitation and pharmacologic therapy which may be useful in rapidly restoring cerebral perfusion and controlling ICP.

To control ICP, one must reduce the volume of the intracranial contents to accommodate swelling and edema formation. Specific treatment methods aimed at reducing ICP include hyperventilation (to decrease cerebral blood volume, CBV), sedation (to prevent agitation, reduce muscular activity, and reduce the cerebral metabolic rate for oxygen, CMRO$_2$), osmotic diuresis (to extract water from cells down an osmolar gradient in areas with an intact BBB), and ventricular drainage (to reduce the volume of CSF).

AIRWAY AND BREATHING

Airway control and hyperventilation can be lifesaving in the patient with a severe head injury.[11] Control of the airway should be obtained in all patients in coma (i.e., GCS ≤ 8). This is most safely and expeditiously performed with endotracheal intubation. Provided that the patient is hemodynamically stable after intubation, paralysis with vecuronium (0.1 mg/kg) and sedation with morphine sulfate (0.1 mg/kg) are recommended. Paralysis and sedation decrease $CMRO_2$ and prevent the patient from breathing dysynchronously with the ventilator. Dysynchronous breathing causes the patient to "buck" the ventilator, increasing intrathoracic pressure and decreasing cerebral venous return. Sedation and neuromuscular paralysis are necessary to obtain a computed tomographic (CT) scan in the combative patient.[55] Vecuronium and morphine sulfate have a duration of action sufficient to complete a cranial CT but short enough to allow repetitive neurologic evaluation.

Initial ventilator settings should strive for adequate oxygenation and moderate hyperventilation. This can be achieved in most adults with an FIO_2 of 0.5, a tidal volume of 15 ml/kg, and a ventilator rate of 10 breaths per minute. The ventilator rate should be adjusted to maintain a P_{CO_2} of 25 to 30 mmHg using either arterial blood gas analysis or the end-tidal CO_2 concentration.[56] It is important to remember that a large tidal volume combined with a high ventilator rate will increase the mean intrathoracic pressure and decrease cerebral venous return, thus potentially increasing the CBV and ICP.[28] Furthermore, a decrease in systemic venous return as a result of increased intrathoracic pressure can decrease cardiac output and reduce the CPP. For similar reasons, positive end-expiratory pressure should not be used initially to treat hypoxia because it will also increase mean intrathoracic pressure. Rather, hypoxia should be treated by increasing oxygen concentration in the inspired gases.

The effectiveness of hyperventilation in producing vasoconstriction of the pial vessels has been well demonstrated.[57] The effect on vessel size and CBV is rapid but transient. Muizelaar and colleagues[57] have demonstrated that the effects of hyperventilation to 25 mmHg are diminished by 4 h and totally absent by 20 h. This is probably due to a compensatory normalization of the pH of the CSF induced by a reduction in secretion of bicarbonate ion by the choroid plexus. Any transient increases in P_{CO_2} after this compensation will cause a relative increase in the concentration of hydrogen ions, thereby causing vasodilation and an increase in the ICP. These investigators have recently demonstrated, in a controlled, randomized clinical study, that prophylactic chronic hyperventilation was deleterious in a subset of head-injured patients.[58] Ward et al.[58] found that patients maintained at a P_{CO_2} of 24 ± 2 mmHg had a significantly worse outcome than did patients maintained at a P_{CO_2} of 35 ± 2 mmHg. In the acute phases of care, hyperventilation should be used in all patients suspected of having a severe head injury and intracranial hypertension, but its *continued* use should be reserved for those patients with a *demonstrated* increase in ICP. Current data suggest that hyperventilation is not effective prophylaxis against intracranial hypertension. It does, however, remain a valuable technique for acutely reducing intracranial pressure.

CIRCULATION

Maintenance or restoration of the CPP is of paramount importance in the head-injured patient who is hypovolemic. Restitution of intravascular volume is achieved with asanguinous solutions followed by blood products if the deficit is persistent and physiologically significant.[59] There is controversy regarding the constituents of the optimal asanguinous fluid for the patient with a head injury.[10]

ASANGUINOUS FLUIDS: CRYSTALLOIDS

Fluid and salt restriction have been advocated to control ICP in an attempt to reduce vasogenic edema formation in areas of BBB disruption.[60,61] Since edema formation is driven by the capillary hydrostatic pressure acting at the site of injury,[62] it is logical to minimize the hydrostatic gradient between the capillary and cerebral tissue whenever possible. Fluid restriction or active diuresis can lower the capillary hydrostatic pressure and, theoretically, reduce edema formation.

Despite the theoretical advantages of fluid restriction, there have been no controlled studies which demonstrate its benefit. In fact, several studies have shown that no relationship exists between fluid balance and ICP or cerebral water content.[63–67] Morse and associates[66] specifically examined this question by comparing the effects of fluid restriction with those of *over*hydration in animals with brain injury. Control animals received maintenance fluid, while fluid-restricted animals received 66 percent of the maintenance volume and overhydrated animals received 133 percent of the maintenance volume. There was no difference in cerebral water content between the groups despite the fact that the overhydrated group had a 13 percent gain in body weight. Unfortunately, Morse and colleagues did not measure MAP or CVP to determine if the overhydrated animals were truly hypervolemic in the intravascular space.

It is often not possible to restrict fluids in patients sustaining head injury in association with other injuries, especially if they are hypotensive[68] or require operative therapy. Asanguinous fluid and blood are necessary, often in volumes that exceed the amount of blood loss.[59,68] In fact, restricting fluids in hypovolemic patients could lead to hypotension and decreased perfusion to vulnerable areas of injured brain.

The apparent controversy regarding whether or not to restrict fluid in the head-injured patient can be rectified by understanding that the *volume of fluid* administered to a patient is not a surrogate for the capillary hydrostatic pressure in the brain. On the other hand, MAP, CVP, or pulmonary capillary wedge pressure (PCWP) may be more appropriate parameters. It is important to remember that resuscitation should be driven by *physiologic endpoints* which reflect the adequacy of perfusion, rather than by arbitrary estimates of hydration. Since the capacity to measure CBF at the bedside in the head-injured patient is limited, it is appropriate to use indicators of perfusion, such as MAP, cardiac output, base deficit,[68] or jugular venous oxygen saturation.[69] The physician treating a hypotensive patient with a severe head injury must rapidly restore perfusion, avoid excessive elevations in the capillary hydrostatic pressure, and control ICP in order to prevent secondary injury. Management of hypotension in the head-injured patient has conventionally been achieved by the infusion of a balanced salt solution. Ringer's lactate (RL, Table 12–2), a slightly hypotonic solution, has been recommended for replacement of volume deficits until blood is available.[70] After stabilization of volume deficits, active diuresis and restriction of fluid and salt are advocated in patients with elevated ICP.[17,61,71] Hypotonic fluid (0.45% saline, ½NS, Table 12–1) has been recommended to provide maintenance fluid and solute, to keep intravenous lines open, and to administer medications.[17,61,71] Such therapy is directed at restricting salt administration to prevent retention of water which might contribute to edema formation or to cerebral swelling.[17]

TABLE 12–2. Asanguinous Crystalloid Fluids: Compositional Differences

Fluid	%Na	Na[a]	K[a]	Cl[a]	Ca[a]	Lactate[a]	Osmol[b]	COP[c]
RL[d]	0.7	130	4	109	3	28	274	0
1/2 NS[e]	0.45	77	0	77	0	0	154	0
HSL[f]	1.6	250	4	180	3	77	514	0
NS	0.9	154	0	154	0	0	308	0
HS[g]	7.5	1200	0	1200	0	0	2400	0

[a]mEq/liter
[b]Osmol: mosmol/liter
[c]COP: colloid osmotic pressure (mmHg)
[d]RL: Ringer's lactate
[e]NS: normal saline
[f]HSL: hypertonic sodium lactate
[g]HS: hypertonic saline

There have been no studies, however, that have documented that salt restriction either decreases vasogenic edema formation or reduces ICP.[10] On the contrary, Bakay and coworkers[60] showed that administration of a slightly hypertonic salt solution (0.9%) lowered the CSF pressure by 30 to 50 percent in patients in chronic coma, while a hypotonic salt solution (½NS) produced no change. The administration of fluid without ionizing solute (dextrose in water) resulted in a 14 to 100 percent *increase* in the CSF pressure. Furthermore, it does not appear that either the amount of sodium administered or the sodium balance during the first 72 h of hospitalization has any meaningful relationship to ICP in patients with severe head injury.[67]

Hypertonic salt solution would seem to be ideal for the treatment of head-injured hypovolemic patients. It restores blood pressure and cardiac output with significantly less volume and at a lower capillary hydrostatic pressure than does Ringer's lactate.[72–75] Hypertonic fluids achieve this by having a positive inotropic effect[76–80] and by extracting water from the intracellular space to restore intravascular losses.[81,82] It also appears that hypertonic fluids may act to lower vascular resistance and improve blood flow to the brain, kidney, and gut.[83–86] Whether hypertonicity induces active vasodilation or simply increases the size of the capillary lumen by reducing the volume of endothelial cells is, at this time, unknown. Mazzoni and coworkers[87] have emphasized the importance of the latter mechanism (i.e., reduction of endothelial cell volume resulting in a decrease in hydraulic resistance) in improving blood flow after resuscitation from hypovolemic shock. Using intravital microscopy of a skeletal muscle bed, they observed a 20 percent reduction in capillary lumenal diameter after shock (Fig. 12–3). Resuscitation with Ringer's lactate caused only a transient increase in flow and no change in the lumenal diameter. Resuscitation with a hypertonic solution resulted in a persistent increase in flow with return of the lumenal diameter to the control value.

The use of *very hypertonic* fluids (1.8 to 7.5%) to treat laboratory models of head injury, with and without hypovolemic shock, has resulted in significantly lower ICP, improved CBF, and a significantly lower cerebral water content than treatment with either hypotonic or isotonic fluids.[64,88–94] Gunnar and cowork-

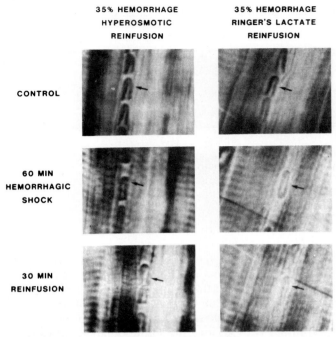

FIG. 12–3. Comparative photograph sequence during shock and resuscitation of a muscle capillary from an animal treated with Ringer's lactate (RL) and from one treated with hyperosmotic 7.5% hypertonic saline and dextran (HSD). The arrows point to the same location in each respective capillary. HSD completely restored the lumenal diameter narrowed during shock, whereas RL had no effect. (Reprinted from Mazzoni et al.[87] with permission.)

ers,[88] using a canine model of hemorrhagic shock combined with an epidural balloon to simulate an intracranial injury, compared 0.9% saline (NS, Table 12–1), 3% hypertonic saline, and 10% dextran. After resuscitation, the ICP increased rapidly in the normal saline and dextran groups to 46 and 45 mmHg, respectively, but decreased to levels lower than baseline in the group resuscitated with 3% hypertonic saline. Ducey and colleagues[89] compared 0.9% saline, 6% saline, and hydroxyethyl starch in a porcine model of shock and head injury (epidural balloon). Hypertonic resuscitation resulted in a significantly lower ICP and a significantly lower cerebral elastance (the reciprocal of compliance) compared with the other fluids. Wisner et al,[64] using an ovine model of cryogenic injury and hemorrhagic shock, compared Ringer's lactate with 7.5% hypertonic saline (HS, Table 12–1). Ringer's lactate and the 7.5% hypertonic saline equally restored hemodynamic parameters, but the Ringer's lactate group required significantly more fluid (48 ± 17 ml/kg) than the hypertonic group (9 ± 4 ml/kg) to achieve hemodynamic stability ($p < 0.0002$). The ICP rose in all Ringer's lactate animals and *decreased* in all hypertonic animals. The mean ICP at the conclusion of the study (2 h after insult) was significantly greater in the Ringer's lactate group ($p < 0.002$). The experiments cited utilized relatively short periods of study, usually less than 6 h, which may limit their applicability to the clinical situation. Observations of ICP during the first 6 h after insult may be irrelevant, since major increases in ICP after injury, shock, and resuscitation do not occur until 18 and 24 h.[95]

We have made similar observations in animals exposed to shock alone,[72] animals exposed to shock and a focal cryogenic brain injury,[96] and animals exposed to a focal cryogenic brain injury without shock.[94] We used a porcine model and study paradigm that allowed for 24 h of observation after the insult. We selected a porcine model because the neurohumoral and cardiovascular responses of swine to hemorrhage are similar to those of humans and because swine have a relatively large brain that facilitates study.[97] To determine the safety and efficacy of hypertonic resuscitation of hypovolemic shock in terms of its effects on systemic parameters, in anticipation of future clinical trials with trauma patients, we studied awake animals hemorrhaged 40 percent of their blood volume and resuscitated with either Ringer's lactate or hypertonic sodium lactate[72] (HSL, Table 12–1). The animals were studied hourly for 24 h and then daily for 3 days. Resuscitation with Ringer's lactate required significantly more fluid and produced a significantly greater rise in ICP than hypertonic sodium lactate. Hypertonic sodium lactate produced significant increases in serum sodium level and osmolality which resolved within 48 h. Hypernatremia and hyperosmolality were not associated with either cerebral dysfunction (by physical examination and EEG analysis) or renal dysfunction. Increases in serum sodium level and osmolality as a result of hypertonic resuscitation resolved spontaneously by increased renal sodium clearance, free water intake, and a negative free water clearance. There was no late rise in ICP, suggesting that late onset of edema does not occur after resuscitation with hypertonic solution.

To determine the effects of hypertonic resuscitation on cerebral perfusion in a model of hypovolemic shock without brain injury, we studied anesthetized swine for 24 h after hemorrhagic shock and resuscitation with either hypertonic sodium lactate or Ringer's lactate.[9] Both fluids restored MAP to baseline, the Ringer's lactate group requiring significantly more fluid ($p < 0.01$). When compared with Ringer's lactate, hypertonic sodium lactate significantly increased CBF and cerebral oxygen delivery (cO_2del) for the 24 h after shock ($p < 0.05$) (Fig. 12–4). ICP and cerebral water content were significantly lower in the hypertonic sodium lactate group ($p < 0.05$). We attributed these effects to hypertonic dehydration of the brain parenchyma, resulting in a decrease in ICP, and to dehydration of the cerebrovascular endothelium, causing a decrease in vascular resistance and improved CBF. These data suggest that by decreasing ICP and increasing CBF, hypertonic resuscitation might be useful in decreasing secondary brain injury. To determine the early and late effects of hypertonic resuscitation on the injured brain after shock, we used a porcine model of focal cryogenic injury and hemorrhagic shock and compared Ringer's lactate, 7.5% hypertonic saline with 6% dextran (HSD), and hypertonic sodium lactate.[96] Shock and injury significantly reduced CBF to the penumbra (the halo area surrounding the injured brain) in all experimental animals. Hypertonic resuscitation resulted in an improved CBF and a lower ICP than Ringer's lactate. It

CEREBRAL BLOOD FLOW

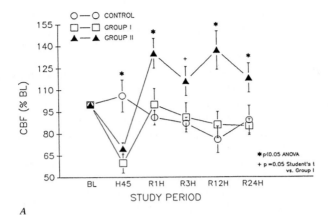

A

CEREBRAL OXYGEN DELIVERY

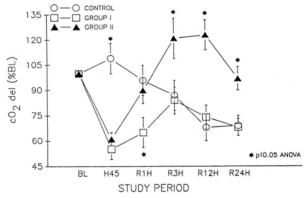

B

FIG. 12–4. *A.* Cerebral blood flow during shock and resuscitation in a porcine model without a head injury. Group I animals were resuscitated with RL, and Group II animals were resuscitated with HSL. Hemorrhage significantly reduced CBF in both groups. HSL resuscitation resulted in a significantly greater CBF compared with RL throughout the resuscitation period. *B.* Cerebral oxygen delivery during the study. Hemorrhage significantly reduced the cerebral oxygen delivery in both experimental groups compared with controls. HSL resuscitation (group II) restored cerebral oxygen delivery to values no different than controls by 1 h. In contrast, cerebral oxygen delivery in group I (RL) animals remained significantly below control and group II at 1 h. By 3 h, and for the remainder of the study, cerebral oxygen delivery in group II remained significantly greater than in group I and controls. Abbreviations: BL, baseline; H45, at the end of hemorrhage; R1H, R3H, R12H, and R24H represent 1, 3, 12, and 24 h after the start of resuscitation. (Reprinted from Schmoker et al.[9] with permission.)

appeared that the early benefits of lowered ICP and improved CBF derived from the bolus of hypertonic saline with dextran were abrogated by further resuscitation with Ringer's lactate. Continued resuscitation with hypertonic sodium lactate, however, prolonged the period of improved CBF and low ICP (Fig. 12–5). At 24 h, CBF had deteriorated to the penumbra in all animals and to the uninjured cortex in animals receiving Ringer's lactate. These data suggest that hypertonic resuscitation of hemorrhagic shock and brain injury, by maintaining CBF without elevating the ICP, could effectively prevent secondary brain injury when focal contusion and shock occur together.

To investigate the role of intravenous fluid tonicity in determining ICP and CBF after isolated brain injury without shock, we compared maintenance infusions of Ringer's lactate and hypertonic sodium lactate in a porcine model of focal cryogenic injury alone studied for approximately 30 h after injury.[94] The cryogenic injury produced a significant increase in ICP and a significant decrease in CBF to the penumbra, as we had previously observed. Maintenance infusion of hypertonic sodium lactate resulted in a significantly lower ICP and higher CBF than Ringer's lactate (Fig. 12–6). Cortical water content in the area of the lesion was similar in both groups, but cortical water content in the uninjured hemisphere was significantly lower in the hypertonic sodium lactate group. As in all of our previous studies, we measured lesion volume (all animals had been injected with Evan's blue dye to ascertain areas of BBB disruption). While lesion volumes were not significantly different between groups, the area of Evan's blue

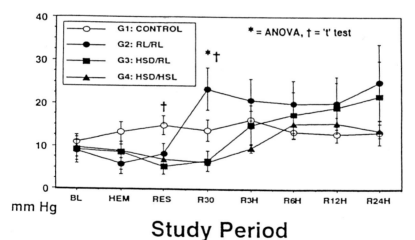

Study Period

FIG. 12–5. Intracranial pressure after shock, head injury, and resuscitation in a porcine model. This study compared the use of bolus HSD followed by RL (group 3) with either bolus HSD followed by HSL (group 4) or RL alone (group 2). Resuscitation with RL alone increased the ICP significantly. A small bolus infusion of HSD did not increase the ICP, but continued resuscitation with RL increased the ICP. Resuscitation with HSD followed by HSL increased the ICP slightly, but the increase was not significant and was no greater than in uninjured controls. Abbreviations: BL, baseline; HEM, immediately after hemorrhage; RES, immediately after the bolus infusion; R30, 30 min after RES; R3H, R6H, R12H, and R24H, 3, 6, 12, and 24 h after HEM. (Reprinted from Walsh et al.[96] with permission.)

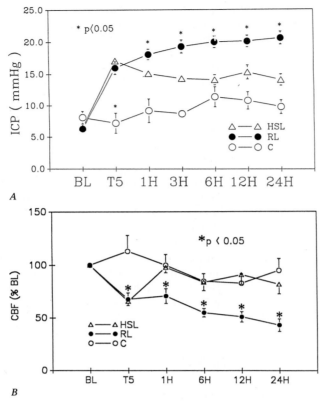

FIG. 12–6. *A.* Intracranial pressure following head injury in a porcine model. The ICP increased in the experimental animals after injury and continued to increase in the group receiving RL. ICP decreased in the group receiving HSL, resulting in a significant difference between the groups at 6, 12, and 24 h postinjury. *B.* Cerebral blood flow during the study. CBF was reduced in both experimental groups immediately after injury and continued to deteriorate in the RL group. Infusion of HSL significantly increased the CBF to contol levels. Abbreviations: BL, baseline; T5, 5 minutes after injury; R1H, R6H, R12H, and R24H, 1, 3, 12, and 24 h after the start of resuscitation. (Reprinted from Shackford et al.[94] with permission.)

staining was always larger in the animals resuscitated with or maintained on hypertonic sodium lactate. Similar observations had been made by others in animals receiving hypertonic solutions,[88,98] leading them to suggest that hypertonic solutions were *increasing* the size of the lesion. Rather, it is our belief that the area of staining was increased because movement of edema fluid (and Evan's blue dye) away from the injury was being facilitated by the hypertonic fluid. Edema formation, as previously stated, is dependent on the creation of a hydrostatic gradient; the same should be true of edema resolution. That is, since hypertonic fluids extract water from cells and decrease ICP, they logically reduce the intracellular volume. Reduction of the intracellular volume of those cells surrounding the lesion should decrease the resistance to bulk flow of edema fluid. The role of cellular volume in edema spread has been demonstrated by Reulan and coworkers,[62] who induced intracellular edema in the brain with hexachlorophene. They found that extracellular edema formation from an area of disruption of the BBB was impeded when intracellular edema was present. If intracellular swelling impedes edema movement, cell shrinkage may facilitate it. We suggest that cerebral dehydration induced by hypertonic resuscitation decreases resistance to bulk flow and thus facilitates edema resolution. Hypotonic fluids, which increase cellular volume, should have the opposite effect. We therefore attribute the observed increase in Evan's blue staining to the more expeditious movement of edema fluid through the white matter toward the ventricle. Rapid resolution of edema may represent another mechanism by which ICP is controlled or reduced with hypertonic resuscitation.

In summary, the mechanism proposed for the reduction of ICP by hypertonic fluids is the extraction of intracellular water from uninjured cerebral tissue down an osmolar gradient. The extraction of water from the cerebrovascular endothelium and from erythrocytes is the probable mechanism for improvement of CBF. The reduction in intracellular volume also may aid in edema resolution. Concerns that mild hypertonicity is injurious to the brain or that return of the osmolarity to the normal range would result in an increase in intracellular volume and a late increase in ICP appear unwarranted. These laboratory data suggest that hypertonic resuscitation, by improving intracranial compliance and CBF, may reduce secondary brain injury after trauma and hemorrhage.

While hypertonic resuscitation is common in the treatment of patients with burn injury,[99,100] there have been only four published trials of hypertonic resuscitation in trauma patients with and without head injury.[101-104] Unfortunately, all these trials evaluated a single bolus of 250 ml 7.5% hypertonic saline in 6% dextran (HSD), followed by resuscitation with conventionally used crystalloid solutions. Therefore, these studies were not a true evaluation of hypertonic resuscitation, since serum osmolarity and serum sodium level were normalized very shortly after admission to the hospital. All the studies have shown, however, that administration of hypertonic saline to severely injured trauma patients is safe and at least as effective in initial resuscitation as conventional crystalloid. In each of the studies, the bolus of hypertonic saline with dextran resulted in a greater increase in blood pressure than did an equivalent volume of isotonic crystalloid. The patients treated with hypertonic saline with dextran tended to require less blood and fluid than did the Ringer's lactate patients. Furthermore, in the largest study to date, there were trends indicating improved survival and fewer complications in patients receiving hypertonic saline with dextran.[101] Holcroft and colleagues,[103] in their initial study of 20 patients, observed significantly better survival in the hypertonic saline with dextran group ($p < 0.05$). Holcroft and coworkers have now expanded their experience to 166 patients.[105] While overall survival was similar in both the Ringer's lactate and hypertonic saline with dextran groups in this expanded study, survival after severe head injury was greater in patients treated with hypertonic saline with dextran (32 percent) than in patients treated with Ringer's lactate (16 percent) and approached statistical significance ($p = 0.07$).

Based on solid laboratory data and an early clinical experience, it appears that the use of hypertonic fluid for the resuscitation of head-injured patients is justified. The early experience with hypertonic saline with dextran followed by

Ringer's lactate may not be a valid evaluation of hypertonic resuscitation, since the patients eventually received large volumes of solute-free water in the Ringer's lactate. Rather, the use of hypertonic saline with dextran as a bolus injection followed by continued hypertonic resuscitation, compared to Ringer's lactate resuscitation, would seem to be a more reasonable paradigm to evaluate hypertonic resuscitation. Additional investigation of hypertonic resuscitation is required to determine the levels of serum sodium and osmolarity that are safely tolerated in this patient group.

ASANGUINOUS FLUIDS: COLLOIDS

Colloid solutions contain large-molecular-weight solutes ($>$60,000 Da) that generally exceed the pore size of most capillaries and are retained, at least temporarily, in the vascular compartment. The administration of a colloid solution will increase the colloid osmotic pressure and, according to Starling's hypothesis, should reduce the transcapillary fluid flux at a given hydrostatic pressure, provided there is no increase in capillary permeability. Colloid solutions have been shown to be very effective in the resuscitation of hypovolemic shock, adequately restoring perfusion with a smaller volume of fluid than is necessary with isotonic salt solution. Studies comparing colloids and electrolyte solutions have focused primarily on the lung,[106] where edema formation can be detrimental to function.

A few studies have examined the effects of colloid administration on the injured brain. Clasen and associates[107] compared hypertonic glucose (50%, 50 ml) with albumin (25%, 50 ml) in normovolemic dogs with a cryogenic brain injury. The authors postulated that an oncotic gradient might reduce cerebral water content and lower ICP. Treatment with albumin lowered the cisternal pressure, but not significantly, whereas hypertonic glucose therapy resulted in a significant drop in the ICP. Postmortem cerebral water content was not affected by either treatment. The authors concluded that the solutions decreased ICP by a mechanism other than interstitial dehydration. One has to wonder, however, if the small dosages of albumin and glucose were sufficient to establish oncotic or osmotic gradients capable of dehydration. Albright and Phillips[108] compared 25% albumin (1 g/kg) with an electrolyte solution in normovolemic dogs with a cryogenic lesion, also postulating that the oncotic gradient produced by the infusion would result in the withdrawal of cerebral interstitial water and lower the ICP. They found no difference between study groups in the cerebral water content in either the injured hemisphere or the contralateral hemisphere and concluded that the dosage of albumin was insufficient to produce the desired oncotic effect. In a subsequent investigation Albright and colleagues[80] studied three groups of normovolemic dogs subjected to a cryogenic lesion. A control group was given a crystalloid solution, and experimental groups received either 12% hydroxyethyl starch (a synthetic colloid) or 24% hydroxyethyl starch and furosemide. At the end of the 6-h study period, the dogs receiving starch had a significantly higher colloid osmotic pressure (COP) and significantly lower ICP than the group receiving crystalloid ($p < 0.05$). Cerebral water content in the area of the lesion was significantly lower in the dogs receiving hydroxyethyl starch than in those receiving crystalloid. In the group treated with 24% hydroxyethyl starch and furosemide, the water content of the contralateral uninjured hemisphere also was significantly lower than control ($p < 0.05$). In another study, Albright and coworkers[109] compared five groups of normovolemic dogs with a cryogenic lesion treated with either crystalloid (control), mannitol (20%, 1.5 g/kg), furosemide, albumin (25%, 2 g/kg), or albumin and furosemide. Albumin alone failed to decrease the mean ICP compared with control, whereas albumin and furosemide did lower the mean ICP significantly ($p < 0.05$). The water content in the lesioned area of the albumin-treated dogs was significantly lower than in control animals ($p < 0.05$). The water content of the uninjured cortex in the experimental groups was lower than control, but the difference was not statistically significant. The authors point out, however, that small differences in cerebral water content can result in significant volume displacement within the cranium and could have been responsible for the observed difference in ICP. They conclude from this and their previous studies that colloid therapy, especially when combined with furosemide, is effective in lowering ICP through normovolemic dehydration of the lesioned area and the uninjured brain.

Poole and associates[110] compared crystalloid with 6% hydroxyethyl starch in dogs subjected to hemorrhage and an inflated epidural balloon. After resuscitation, the ICP was significantly higher in the crystalloid group but was not clinically elevated ($p < 0.05$). CBF was not restored to baseline level in either group, suggesting inadequate volume expansion.

Zornow and colleagues[111] induced normovolemic hemodilution with either crystalloid or colloid (hydroxyethyl starch) in rabbits without brain injury and studied ICP and cerebral water content. There were no significant differences between the groups for either variable despite a significantly reduced COP in the crystalloid group. The authors concluded that the pivotal factor in water movement across the BBB was independent of the COP. Wisner and coworkers,[64] using an ovine model of combined trauma (crush injury of the leg) and hemorrhagic shock, compared the effects of colloid (4% albumin) and crystalloid resuscitation in groups of animals with and without a cryogenic brain injury. In the animals without brain injury, the crystalloid group required significantly more fluid to achieve resuscitation than did the colloid group ($p < 0.01$). ICP increased with resuscitation in both groups but was not significantly different from baseline in either group, nor was there any difference between the groups in cerebral water content. Similar results were obtained when the cryogenic brain injury was added to traumatic hemorrhagic shock: ICP rose with resuscitation in both groups, but it was not significantly different than baseline values and there was no difference between the groups in cerebral water content in either the area of the lesion or the uninjured brain tissue. The authors concluded that maintaining the COP had no beneficial effect on ICP or water content. Further, they believe that their data demonstrate that the large volume of crystalloid necessary to restore baseline hemodynamic function does not adversely affect either the ICP or the cerebral water content. The volume of hemorrhage in this study was relatively small (approximately 14 ml/kg, or 20 percent of the blood volume), and the results might have been different had the shock been more severe. The duration of study was only 2 h after completion of shock, and the delayed effects of resuscitation could not be evaluated. Nevertheless, this well-controlled study does suggest that colloid resuscitation offers no advantage over isotonic crystalloid in the resuscitation of brain injury with or without hemorrhage.

Warner and Boehland[112] studied the effects of iso-osmolal 6% starch and crystalloid in a murine model of hemorrhage and ischemia at intervals up to 24 h. Edema was noted in animals sacrificed within 1.5 h of injury, independent of the type of fluid used. At 24 h, there was no difference between the groups in cerebral water content. They concluded that the magnitude of edema was independent of the fluid used, provided osmolality was constant. Based on their data, it seems unlikely that COP plays a substantial role in early edema formation.

Tranmer and colleagues[113] also evaluated colloid therapy in a model of cryogenic injury without hemorrhage. Animals received excessive amounts of fluid (up to 30 ml/kg/h, equivalent to 2100 ml/h in a 70-kg person). Although no statistical analysis was performed to compare the groups,[114] the greatest increases in ICP following fluid infusion occurred in the normal saline and D_5W groups. In addition, a deterioration in the power ratio index of the EEG was noted in the normal saline group. Unfortunately, the authors did not measure either COP or osmolarity, and it is difficult to determine the significance of the observed EEG changes.

Many of the previous studies have been flawed because important variables were either not controlled (i.e., osmolarity of the colloid solutions) or not measured (i.e., COP) or agents known to reduce ICP were used in conjunction with colloid therapy (i.e., diuretics). To clarify the relative importance of COP and osmolarity, Kaieda and associates,[115] in a well-controlled experiment, infused fluids of varying oncotic and osmotic pressures in a model of focal cryogenic brain injury in which the animals had undergone plasmapheresis; experimental fluids were given to maintain the MAP and the CVP. Animals receiving hypo-osmolar fluids, regardless of the oncotic pressure of the fluid, had significant increases in ICP and cerebral water content in the uninjured cortex. The COP had no effect on either the ICP or the cerebral water content by regression analysis. On the other hand, there was a significant inverse relationship between the osmolarity of the fluid and the water content of the uninjured brain. Similar results were obtained by Zornow and coworkers[116] in a model of cryogenic brain injury and isovolemic hemodilution. Despite a 53 percent reduction in COP and a significantly increased fluid requirement to maintain hemodynamic stability, animals receiving normal saline had a similar ICP and a similar cerebral water content to animals receiving 5% albumin or 6% hetastarch.

In summary, colloids, while effective in restoring hemodynamic parameters with significantly less fluid than crystalloid, do not decrease either ICP or cerebral water content. This is not surprising given that the BBB, with a pore size of 8 Å, is not permeable to sodium but is permeable to water. The possibility therefore exists for large osmotic gradients with significant absorptive power (a 1-mosmol/kg gradient is equivalent to a 19-mmHg hydrostatic gradient). Thus osmotic (not oncotic) forces are the major factors determining water movement in the brain. Such is not the case in the peripheral muscle capillary (pore size 19 Å), which is freely permeable to sodium and to water but not to large protein moieties. Thus a large oncotic gradient exists between the intravascular and the extravascular spaces and is the determining factor in water movement between those spaces.

The lack of consistency in reducing either ICP or cerebral water content, combined with the increased cost,[117] a small risk of anaphylaxis,[118] and the potential for increased bleeding,[119] limits the usefulness of colloids as a primary choice in the resuscitation of head injury.

INITIAL DIAGNOSTIC MEASURES

COMPUTED TOMOGRAPHY (CT)

Following complete evaluation of the patient in the emergency room, which includes determination of the Glasgow coma score (GCS),[12] it is essential to obtain a CT scan for any patient with a GCS ≤ 8. Patients with a GCS score of 9 to 13 also should be scanned,[120,121] although this policy has yet to be validated prospectively. Controversy exists about the need for CT scanning of patients with GCS scores of 14 to 15.[122–124] A recent retrospective multicenter study of 2766 patients demonstrated that 22 percent of patients with a GCS of 13 to 15 had a positive CT scan (i.e., indicative of injury to the brain).[120] Problems of CT availability and cost preclude us from suggesting that all patients with a history of head injury require CT scanning.

SKULL X-RAYS

The routine use of skull x-rays in patients with severe head injury has decreased with the widespread use of CT scanners. The skull x-ray is useful for detecting skull fractures, which are often indicators of significant intracranial pathology. In a recently completed study of patients with minor head injury, the presence of skull fracture increased the likelihood of a significant intracranial lesion by a factor of 3.[120] Macpherson et al.[125] noted that 71 percent of patients with skull fractures had concomitant cerebral contusions or hematomas, while only 46 percent of patients without skull fracture demonstrated contusion or hematoma. It is, however, rare that a skull x-ray will be of clinical importance to the neurosurgeon. Since CT is also very sensitive in the detection of skull fractures, we rarely obtain skull x-rays in patients with severe head injuries. In patients with moderate head injuries (GCS 9 to 12), CT scans are indicated and, therefore, preclude the need for a skull x-ray. In patients with minor head injuries (as defined by a GCS of 14 to 15), no neurologic deficit, normal mental status examination, but with historical evidence of concussion, skull x-rays are often obtained. Dacey et al.[126] demonstrated that 11.1 percent of this group will demonstrate a fracture and therefore have a much greater likelihood of requiring neurosurgical intervention. Patients without evidence of concussion who are asymptomatic and without scalp lacerations are not recommended for x-ray. The general recommendations regarding skull x-rays if CT is not available are summarized in Table 12–3.

MAGNETIC RESONANCE IMAGING (MRI)

MRI has changed many aspects of neuroradiology. Although technically very difficult in the acute stages of head injury, MRI provides valuable information about subcortical structures and the brainstem. As with CT scanning, sedation

TABLE 12–3. Indications for Skull Radiographic Examination When CT Scanning Is Unavailable

Loss of consciousness or amnesia
Neurologic symptoms or signs
Cerebrospinal fluid or blood from the ears or nose
Suspected penetrating injury
Suspected facial fracture

is often required. We have found the MRI to be helpful when the findings on CT scan fail to account for the patient's neurologic status. Gentry et al.[127] compared the diagnostic efficacy of CT with that of MRI, finding that both were highly sensitive in detecting hemorrhagic lesions. MRI scans, however, were much more sensitive in defining nonhemorrhagic regions (ischemia) and for evaluation of the brainstem. Only subarachnoid blood was more frequently detected by CT than by MRI.

MONITORING

HEMODYNAMIC VARIABLES

Patients with head injury severe enough to produce coma (i.e., GCS $\leq$ 8) should have an arterial line and a central venous line placed. The arterial line will allow continuous monitoring of blood pressure and derivation of the CPP. Arterial access also will allow repetitive sampling of arterial blood gases to guide ventilator adjustments—especially if transcutaneous oximetry and end-tidal CO_2 monitoring are unavailable. A central line will allow monitoring of central venous pressure to modulate the volume of fluid infusion and the efficacy of diuresis. In older patients and those who have required large volumes of asanguinous fluid and blood for resuscitation, we advocate the use of a pulmonary artery catheter. This will allow the clinician to measure filling pressures and cardiac output and will provide access to mixed venous blood in order to calculate systemic oxygen delivery and utilization. Such calculations allow a more careful titration of fluid to meet metabolic demand.

INTRACRANIAL PRESSURE

The technology for ICP monitoring was first described over 30 years ago, with the last decade having witnessed refinement of indications and methods for treatment.[128,129] Insertion of an ICP monitoring device is considered routine in most institutions for patients with a GCS of 8 or less. Monitoring the ICP in this group of patients is especially important, since many standard treatment protocols advocate intubation and either sedation or paralysis, severely limiting the clinical neurologic examination of the patient. The incidence of elevated ICP in this cohort is approximately 60 percent.[130] The use of ICP monitoring for patients with a GCS of 9 to 12 (i.e., moderate head injury) is still debated. We generally do not monitor patients who are able to follow simple commands. This decision presupposes the ability to carefully and frequently monitor the patient's neurologic condition. Patients in the moderate head injury group who require general anesthesia are often monitored because the anesthetic prohibits serial neurologic evaluation over a prolonged period of time. It is rarely necessary to monitor patients with mild head injuries (GCS 13 to 15). Finally, we recommend monitoring all patients who have undergone a neurosurgical procedure for trauma, except those with epidural hematomas who were able to follow commands prior to surgery.

CEREBRAL BLOOD FLOW (CBF) AND METABOLISM

Basing treatment decisions solely on the results of ICP measurements may not prevent secondary injury, since the ICP does not necessarily reflect changes in blood flow or oxygen requirement. We currently lack an accessible, repeatable, and accurate modality to measure CBF and $CMRO_2$, although the technology may soon be available to routinely assess these parameters.

Several methods for measuring CBF are available for intermittent recordings, only a few of which are applicable to the ICU setting. Intravenous, intraarterial, and inhalation xenon-133 are frequently used because they allow measurement of regional flow. Recent reports using thermal diffusion technology or laser Doppler are promising but have yet to be carefully validated.[131,132] All these techniques primarily measure cortical flow. A modification of the xenon-133 technique, which employs a stable xenon molecule and CT detection, is capable of determining flow to individual cerebral lobes, basal ganglia, and brainstem.[133] Single photon emission computed tomography (SPECT) also generates an image of regional CBF and is more sensitive than CT in detecting regional areas of ischemia or hyperemia. One of the most useful methods for assessing cerebral hemodynamics and metabolism is positron emission tomography (PET) scanning. This study is generally limited to nonacute situations but measures regional CBF, regional CBV, permeability of cerebral vessels, and regional $CMRO_2$ sequentially, serially, and simultaneously.[134]

Transcranial Doppler ultrasonography is able to detect direction and flow velocity of the major cerebral vessels in the majority of patients.[131] Normally, the end-diastolic flow velocity is 50 percent of the systolic peak value. As ICP increases, the diastolic flow velocity decreases and the systolic peak increases, resulting in an increased pulsatility amplitude. When ICP rises to diastolic pressures, flow ceases. Further elevation of ICP to the level of the MAP results in reversal of flow direction. Doppler ultrasonography is also able to provide useful information about vasospasm. Although the incidence of vasospasm in head injury is unknown, it has been increasingly recognized and may contribute to secondary injury. Few would argue with the potential need for monitoring CBF in severely head-injured patients. Many investigators, however, feel that cerebral metabolism, which normally is coupled to CBF, is a more relevant measure of brain function than either ICP or CBF. In a recent clinical study, the $CMRO_2$ was found to be second only to age as the most important predictor of outcome.[39]

Since CBF and metabolism may be uncoupled during the acute phase of head injury, it would theoretically be of clinical importance to relate these two parameters in an effort to determine treatment and predict outcome. The placement of a catheter in the jugular bulb provides the ability to determine cerebral venous oxygen saturation, which then permits the calculation of cerebral arterial-venous oxygen difference $(a\text{-}vD_{O_2})$.[69] $a\text{-}vD_{O_2}$ is a reflection of the relative adequacy of CBF to meet the metabolic needs of the brain; an increase in the $a\text{-}vD_{O_2}$ represents inadequate CBF to meet cerebral metabolic demand. Cruz et al.[69] recently noted an increase in the $a\text{-}vD_{O_2}$ in nearly half of a group of severely head injured patients. During this period of desaturation, patients developed a mean decrement of GCS from 6.7 to 3.8.

The recent report by Bouma et al.[135] underscores the importance of CBF and $a\text{-}vD_{O_2}$ measurements. These investigators demonstrated early transient ischemia in 186 head-injured patients. If this ischemia is due to vasospasm, the commonly employed technique of hyperventilation may actually be detrimental, since further reduction in vessel caliber would only exacerbate preexisting ischemia. Preferably, one could speculate that artificial elevation of systemic pressure might alleviate the ischemic condition, as has been suggested by Rosner et al.[136]

Intracerebral microdialysis has, until recently, been a laboratory technique which extracts and analyzes extracellular fluid from the brain parenchyma. The dialysate can be analyzed for electrolytes, lactate, pyruvate, purines, and neurotransmitter amino acids such as glutamate, aspartate, and taurine. Persson et al.[137] have recently used this technique in three patients with head injury. The dialysate catheters were attached to ICP monitors and left in place for 2 to 8 days. Although no conclusions can be drawn from such a small series, all three head injury patients demonstrated a consistent elevation of lactate, hypoxanthine, and lactate/pyruvate ratio, suggesting a profound disturbance of energy metabolism in the cerebral cortex. A single patient with a severe head injury and shock was studied for 65 h. Elevations of the lactate/pyruvate ratio and hypoxanthine concentration correlated with episodes of seizures, hemodynamic instability, and fluid and electrolyte disturbances. The use of this technique offers tremendous potential in furthering our understanding of local metabolic events after head injury.

ADJUVANT THERAPEUTIC AGENTS FOR TREATMENT

MANNITOL

Hyperosmolar solutions containing nonionizing solutes such as urea or mannitol have been shown to decrease ICP and cerebral water content in the normal brain. Because these are low-molecular-weight substances which are filtered but not reabsorbed by the kidney, they induce an osmotic diuresis.[138,139] The capacity of hyperosmolar nonionizing solutes to reduce ICP and cerebral water content has long been attributed to this diuretic property. Reed and Woodbury,[140] performing studies of urea in nephrectomized rats, demonstrated that these changes were independent of a forced diuresis. The decrease in ICP occurred rapidly (within 20 to 30 min) and returned to baseline within 2 h owing to compensatory increases in the volumes of the other intracranial contents. The decrease in cerebral water content occurred within 1 h and returned to normal by 8 h as urea crossed the BBB and entered cells. Kassell and associates[141] demonstrated a transient increase in CBF associated with mannitol administration in the normal brain and postulated that the beneficial effects of hyperosmolar therapy were due to a reduction in endothelial and perivascular cell volume, reduced blood viscosity, and an increase in cardiac output. Muizelaar and colleagues,[142] using a cranial "window" technique to observe pial arterioles directly, demonstrated a reduction in pial arteriolar diameter associated with a reduction in blood viscosity and a decrease in ICP. They postulated that reduced viscosity improves flow (by Poiseuille's law), which increases oxygen delivery and improves the removal of cerebral metabolites that are thought to reduce cerebral vascular tone. They suggested that the improved flow caused pial vasoconstriction that led to a reduction in cerebral blood volume and ICP. Whatever the mechanism of the rapid decrease in ICP, it has been shown by Nath and Galbraith[143] that even low-dose mannitol (0.28 g/kg) decreases the water content of the white matter, suggesting that dehydration plays some role in the reduction of ICP by hyperosmolar solutions in the normal brain.

Mannitol and urea also have been shown to consistently decrease ICP and cerebral water content in the presence of a brain injury. Mannitol appears to have a variable effect on CBF in brain injury, causing an increase when autoregulation is lost and no change when autoregulation is intact. Bruce and colleagues[34] found that mannitol decreased the ICP in 11 of 13 patients, increased the CBF in 12 of 13, and increased the $CMRO_2$ in 10 of 13. They found that the increase in CBF appeared to be independent of the effects on ICP. Further, mannitol was equally effective in patients with and without a mass lesion. Similar results were obtained by Mendelow and colleagues.[36] The magnitude of the decrease in ICP appears to be affected by two factors: the ICP itself (higher pressures tend to have greater decreases) and the dose of mannitol.[144] Marshall and coworkers[145] suggest that doses as low as 0.25 g/kg are effective in lowering the ICP, but the larger doses (1.0 g/kg) are associated with a more persistent reduction.

Most of the studies involving mannitol have been performed in hemodynamically stable patients with supposedly normal blood volumes. Until recently, mannitol has not been advocated for reduction of ICP in hypovolemic subjects because it can cause or exaggerate hypotension. Cote and associates[146] have suggested that the hypotension due to mannitol infusion is a result of vasodilation in skeletal muscle and is proportionate to the dose and rate of administration. Even with maximal doses and rapid administration, the hypotension is transient and self-limited, with blood pressure returning to normal in 85 to 115 s. Brown and coworkers[147] observed an increase in MAP, CPP, and CBF when animals with a penetrating brain injury were given mannitol. They attributed the improved hemodynamics to a positive inotropic effect and to decreased blood viscosity, suggesting that mannitol could be used early as a resuscitative therapy.

The consistent reduction in ICP and, in some studies, improved CBF rekindled interest in mannitol for the treatment of hypovolemic shock associated with a head injury. Israel and associates[7] compared 25% mannitol with normal saline in dogs that were hemorrhaged 25 ml/kg (approximately 35 percent of blood volume). The dogs also were subjected to a brain injury by the inflation of an epidural balloon that created a mass effect and intracranial hypertension. Both solutions restored MAP, and no hypotension was observed after mannitol infusion. In the dogs resuscitated with mannitol, the ICP was significantly lower, and left ventricular stroke work index, cardiac index, CPP, and urine output were significantly higher than in dogs resuscitated with normal saline ($p < 0.01$).

Based on these studies, it would appear that mannitol may be useful in maintaining CPP and decreasing ICP after head injury. The work of Israel and colleagues[7] suggests that it also may be useful in head injury associated with hypovolemic shock, but this will require further study.

CORTICOSTEROIDS

The efficacy of corticosteroid administration has been a topic of debate among neurosurgeons for nearly two decades. While experimental work using various models of head injury have demonstrated benefits from the administration of steroid compounds, several double-blind, prospective, controlled trials instituted in the 1970s failed to demonstrate any advantage in outcome to patients treated with glucocorticoids.[148–150] It was then suggested that a subset of patients with intracranial hypertension might benefit from the administration of high-dose steroids. Dearden and colleagues,[151] however, demonstrated no advantage in the control of intracranial hypertension using high-dose dexamethasone therapy and no benefit in final outcome for treated patients.

The incidence of side effects related to steroid administration has been investigated in numerous studies.[4–6] It is now reasonably established that steroids do not increase the incidence of gastrointestinal bleeding, nor do they increase the frequency of infection in head-injured patients.[40,148,149,152] Hyperglycemia is common in most patients on steroids, although rarely significant. Deutschman et al.[153] demonstrated that steroids prolong the abnormal catabolic response of head injury and suggested that the use of this class of drug in severe head injury is inappropriate.[153] Recent data demonstrating beneficial effects of high-dose glucocorticoids in spinal cord injury[154] and their known ability to scavenge toxic oxygen radicals may renew interest in their use in head injury.

CALCIUM CHANNEL BLOCKERS

Since ischemic secondary brain injury could be due to vasospasm, it is logical that calcium channel blockers might prove efficacious in improving the outcome of patients with severe head injury. Initial anecdotal clinical reports suggested a potential benefit, but subsequent larger series and a recently completed multicenter European trial have failed to substantiate improved outcome.[155–157] Compton and coworkers[156] did show a reduction in Doppler flow velocity by nicardipine in vessel segments with initially elevated flow velocities. Because flow was not elevated in the ipsilateral carotid, the authors speculated that spasm was present in the cranial vessels with increased velocity and that the spasm was relieved by calcium channel blockade. The use of these agents in head injury must be considered to be experimental at this point, since their use is not without risk. Hollerhage et al.[158] have demonstrated a loss of normal pressure autoregulation with the use of calcium channel blockers in rats. They also demonstrated extravascular extravasation of Evan's blue dye from cerebral vessels, suggesting that calcium channel blockers induce BBB dysfunction associated with the loss of pressure autoregulation. The clinical use of calcium channel blockers also has been associated with a decrease in MAP, which could have deleterious effects on CPP.

ANTICONVULSANTS

The risk of seizures after head injury is related to multiple factors, including age, the presence of an intracranial hematoma, and dural penetration. Decisions regarding the use of anticonvulsants have often been empiric despite a wealth of clinical information.

Neurosurgeons have classically divided seizures related to head trauma into *early*, defined as epileptic events occurring within the first week or two, and *late*. Patients with early seizures are at an increased risk for delayed epilepsy, although the risk is relatively low. In the study by Jennett and coworkers,[159] absence of risk factors such as intracranial hematoma, depressed skull fracture, and early seizure resulted in a risk of late seizures of no more than 1 percent. In a population-based study, Annegers et al.[160] reported that early posttraumatic seizures occurred in about 1.9 percent of civilian head injuries. In a randomized, double-blind study of phenytoin for the prevention of seizures, investigators at the Harborview Medical Center enrolled 586 patients with a GCS ≤ 10 and an abnormal CT scan.[161] Of the 404 patients who met all criteria and successfully completed the study, 33 developed a seizure during the first week (8.1 percent). The phenytoin group had a cumulative seizure rate of 3.6 percent compared with the placebo group, which had a rate of 14.2 percent. The data from this highly selected group may not be indicative of the general population of head injuries, but they do suggest a significant risk of early seizures for patients with serious head injuries. Based on the work of Jennette et al.[159] and the Harborview experience,[161] it seems prudent to begin anticonvulsants during the early phase of treatment in patients with penetrating injuries, intracranial hematomas, and compound depressed skull fractures.

Young et al.[162] examined the incidence of late seizures in 179 head-injured patients treated with phenytoin or placebo over an 18-month period. At the conclusion of this study, seizures had occurred in 12.9 percent of the treated patients and in 10.8 percent of the control group, suggesting no significant benefit for phenytoin in preventing late seizures.

Based on a review of multiple studies, it seems clear that there is a prophylactic role for phenytoin during at least the first week following a severe head injury. There is, however, no effect on seizure occurrence or frequency after the first week. At present, we have no proven way to prevent delayed posttraumatic seizures. While most studies have concentrated on the use of phenytoin in the setting of head injury, the use of other anticonvulsants is now the focus of further clinical studies.

FUROSEMIDE

Furosemide has been shown to decrease the ICP of patients undergoing elective craniotomy.[163] The lowered ICP is a result of the diuresis, decreased CSF production, and a lower CVP.[65,164] Because of its success in lowering ICP in elective craniotomy patients, furosemide has been advocated for the treatment of intracranial hypertension in trauma patients. Cottrell and Marlin[165] found that furosemide dramatically decreased the ICP after head injury. Because it crosses the BBB, these authors suggested that furosemide may act at the astrocyte membrane to limit uptake of chloride and sodium ions and thus may limit brain edema.

Loop diuretics seem to produce a synergistic action on ICP when combined with mannitol.[65,163,164,166] Pollay and colleagues[164] attribute the synergy to the diuretic effects of both agents, which act by differing mechanisms. The osmotic diuresis produced by mannitol will create a solute drag in the proximal tubule. Furosemide, acting in the ascending limb of Henle, will block reabsorption of much of the solute, resulting in a greater diuresis. Not only does the combination reduce ICP to a greater degree, but it also results in a more persistent reduction. Schettini and associates[166] have cautioned that the combination will produce significant losses of sodium and potassium, which could result in symptomatic hyponatremia. They observed severe postoperative lethargy in some of their patients which was reversed with administration of sodium chloride.

When compared with mannitol alone, furosemide alone produces less change in ICP and has a shorter duration of action.[65,164] Moreover, mannitol achieves its maximal effect on ICP in less than 15 min, while the maximal ICP effect with furosemide requires approximately 60 min.[65] Furosemide, on the other hand, has less of an effect on serum osmolarity.[164] Administration of furosemide would therefore seem appropriate for those patients with hyperosmolarity (due to a prior osmotic diuresis) who require further treatment for intracranial hypertension.

SODIUM BICARBONATE

An uncompensated systemic metabolic acidosis frequently accompanies hypovolemic shock.[167,168] A significant acidosis can depress cardiac function and should therefore be treated. Acidemia, on the other hand, shifts the oxyhemoglobin dissociation curve to the right and thereby favors oxygen unloading in peripheral capillary beds. In terms of oxygen delivery, therefore, not all acidosis is disadvantageous.

We advocate treating moderately severe acidosis (pH < 7.20) with sodium bicarbonate using the base deficit as a rough approximation of the extracellular bicarbonate deficit.[167,168] We recommend replacing only 50 percent of the calculated deficit (see Table 12–4 for an example) with any single infusion to lessen the chances of producing a significant alkalosis. It is important to remember that the lactate in Ringer's lactate will be metabolized to bicarbonate when flow has been reestablished to the liver.[167] This has the potential of leading to a significant "rebound" alkalosis in those patients receiving large volumes of Ringer's lactate. If respiratory reserve is limited or ventilation is not well controlled, the metabolism of bicarbonate can result in an increase in the P_{CO_2}, which will increase the CBV and ICP. Therefore, it is important to monitor arterial blood gases closely during and after resuscitation, especially if sodium bicarbonate is used.

THAM

Multiple clinical studies of head injury have demonstrated elevated levels of lactate in the CSF.[169-171] It is assumed that these elevated levels produce brain

TABLE 12–4. Sodium Bicarbonate Treatment Using the Base Deficit

Problem: A 25-year-old male weighing approximately 70 kg presents with hypotension. An arterial blood gas reveals an arterial pH of 7.15 with a base deficit of − 10. Since this approximates a bicarbonate deficit of approximately 10 mEq/liter of extracellular fluid (ECF), we can calculate the total deficit as follows:

Body weight: 70 kg

ECF: 25% of body weight in kg = 17.5 liters

Total bicarbonate deficit = base deficit × ECF volume
= 10 mEq/liter × 17.5 liters
= 175 mEq

Solution: Replace 50 percent of the total deficit (to avoid alkalosis). Since the calculated deficit is 175 mEq, 85.5 mEq are indicated. Since an ampule of bicarbonate contains 50 mEq, give 1.75 ampules, continue the resuscitation, and repeat the blood gas analysis after treatment.

---

tissue acidosis, which further potentiates cellular injury and impairs reestablishment of cellular ionic homeostasis. Buffering agents such as *tris*-hydroxymethyl-aminomethane (THAM) have been proposed as a method to reduce cerebral acidosis.

THAM is a systemic and intracellular alkalinizing agent that has been used clinically and studied extensively in the laboratory.[172–175] Since 30 percent of THAM is in the nonionized form, it can easily cross plasma membranes and enter the intracellular space. Sodium bicarbonate is not effective in raising cerebral intracellular pH because of its inability to cross the BBB. Yoshida and Marmarou[175] studied the effect of immediate treatment with THAM after a percussion injury in cats.[175] Animals were randomized into three treatment groups: THAM alone, hyperventilation alone, and THAM and hyperventilation. The THAM-treated animals demonstrated a marked reduction in lactate production, a direct metabolic effect not previously reported, as well as a reduction in cerebral edema. Chronically hyperventilated animals had the highest lactate levels of any group. Moreover, intracellular pH, as assessed by MR spectroscopy, was increased by THAM and remained at nearly normal levels for the duration of the study. In a randomized clinical trial of THAM, Rosner et al.[172] demonstrated a lowering of CSF lactate levels and improvement in ICP. A preliminary clinical report by Ward et al.[58] comparing hyperventilation alone with hyperventilation and THAM found no difference in neurologic outcome between the groups at 3 and 6 months following head injury. The direct treatment of cerebral acidosis with THAM will require further evaluation in both the laboratory and clinical setting before it can be recommended for general clinical use.

BARBITURATES

Intracranial hypertension resistant to standard therapeutic modalities is one of the leading causes of death in the head-injured population. Following Shapiro's report[176] that thiopental reduced ICP in patients undergoing induction of anesthesia, several investigators began studying the use of barbiturates for the treatment of resistant intracranial hypertension. Despite the methodologic shortcomings of some of these studies, it appears that barbiturates do play a role in reducing intracranial hypertension and improving the nearly uniform mortality associated with uncontrolled intracranial hypertension.

Rockoff et al.[177] first reported their experience with high-dose barbiturate in treating 45 patients with severe head injuries. Twenty-nine patients responded favorably with a significantly better outcome than would have been expected without successful treatment. In 1979, Marshall et al.[178] analyzed a consecutive series of 100 patients, 25 of whom were resistant to standard therapeutic modalities for the treatment of intracranial hypertension. ICP normalized in 13 patients and was improved in 6 patients. All the patients failing to respond to barbiturates died, while 10 of the 19 responders made a good recovery. In the five-center study by Eisenberg et al.[179] 75 patients with intracranial hypertension were randomized into two treatment groups: conventional therapy or conventional therapy plus pentobarbital. These authors concluded that barbiturate therapy is effective in the management of elevated ICP refractory to standard therapy. Ward et al.[180] studied the use of pentobarbital as a prophylactic agent in a prospective trial with 53 head-injured patients. The mortality rate and ICP characteristics were similar between the barbiturate-treated group and the conventional plus barbiturate group, leading these authors to conclude that the prophylactic use of pentobarbital affords no advantage.

A variety of dosage schedules have been offered, ranging from 3 to 10 mg/kg given over 0.5 to 3 h. This is followed by a maintenance infusion of 0.5 to 3.0 mg/kg/h to maintain a therapeutic concentration ranging from 2.5 to 4.0 mg/dl. Physiologic monitoring using continuous EEG recordings to achieve "burst suppression" may be advantageous. At these levels, the patient will be comatose, lacking voluntary respiration and requiring mechanical ventilation. Barbiturate-induced coma requires extensive monitoring and vigilance by the attending and nursing staff. Hemodynamic monitoring is invaluable because barbiturates depress the cardiovascular system. Inotropic agents and intravenous therapy may be required to support the blood pressure and systemic oxygen delivery. Barbiturates also suppress coughing and ciliary action within the tracheobronchial tree, making pneumonia an almost uniform complication in patients receiving barbiturate therapy.

The routine use of high-dose barbiturates cannot be recommended. There is, however, a subset of patients who are resistant to conventional means of controlling intracranial hypertension and will respond to this medication. As yet, it is not known how to identify this group of patients prior to the failure of standard means of therapy.

NALOXONE

Narcotic antagonists have been shown to reduce the hypotension associated with various experimental shock models and to improve the neurologic recovery in models of compressive spinal cord trauma.[181] These data suggest that endogenous opiate mechanisms may be involved in the depressed cardiovascular function observed after these insults.[182] Because hypotension has been observed following experimental percussion head injury, endogenous opiates also have been implicated as contributing to ischemic secondary injury of the brain. Naloxone (10 mg/kg) has been shown to reverse the hypotensive effects of high-grade (3.9 atm) brain percussion injury in the cat.[183] The improved blood pressure, however, was associated with a significantly higher ICP than was observed in saline-treated controls, leading the authors to hypothesize that the increased blood pressure resulted in increased CBV secondary to a higher CBF. The significant increase in EEG amplitude associated with the improved CPP was consistent with this hypothesis. Surprisingly little has been done since these initially promising studies, and as yet there are no clinical data to support the use of narcotic antagonists in head-injured patients. Their use remains an area of potentially fruitful research.[182]

DIMETHYL SULFOXIDE (DMSO)

Dimethyl sulfoxide (DMSO) is a dipolar, aprotic, hygroscopic solvent that is capable of replacing the water molecule in the membranes of different cell lines. Although much of the clinical information is anecdotal, the drug has profound and rapid effects on ICP. To date, no series has accumulated an adequate number of patients to be statistically analyzed.[184–186] Marshall and coworkers[184] studied six patients unresponsive to conventional therapy and found that DMSO produced a rapid reduction in ICP (within 3 to 18 min), suggesting a direct role on the cerebral vasculature. The precise mechanism of the ability of DMSO to acutely lower ICP remains unknown. DMSO may facilitate the transport of oxygen molecules to hypoxic or ischemic areas of the brain and may limit the formation of superoxide radicals.[187]

Because the drug is capable of leaching polyvinyl chloride from plastic tubing within minutes, DMSO infusion requires the use of a special plastic-coated tubing and glass storage bottles. Additionally, marked hypernatremia occurs in the majority of patients. A variety of studies have indicated that there is a potential of severe hemolysis and hemoglobinuria,[188] and Broadwell noted that DMSO is capable of opening the BBB.[189]

The role of DMSO in the treatment of patients with serious head injuries remains entirely experimental. The results of a controlled, randomized study will be required prior to the universal acceptance of the drug in the management of intracranial hypertension.

OXYGEN RADICAL SCAVENGERS

Because oxygen free radicals can cause lipid peroxidation and increase capillary permeability resulting in edema formation,[190] it was logical to implicate them in the pathophysiology of secondary brain injury.[191] As Hall[192] points out, of all the organs in which oxygen free radicals can contribute to injury, the central nervous system provides an extremely supportive environment for radical generation and lipid peroxidation. The brain and spinal cord contain large amounts of polyunsaturated fatty acids which are the primary targets of free radical reactions.

There is now a considerable body of biochemical and pharmacologic data which suggests that oxygen free radicals increase vascular permeability and edema formation associated with experimental models of brain injury.[169,193–196] Oxygen free radical generation and lipid peroxidation are associated with both percussion and cryogenic injury.[193,196] Furthermore, cyclooxygenase inhibition and the use of free radical scavengers have been associated with a reduction in lesion volume, amount of edema, and degree of BBB permeability associated with these models.[195,196] Most of the benefit, however, has been associated with models using a pretreatment regimen. Bochicchio and colleagues[197] have provided some clinical data to support the role of lipoperoxidation in brain injury. They found a significant increase (compared with healthy controls) in the concentration of the products of polyunsaturated fatty acid peroxidation in the serum of 10 patients within 2 h of a diffuse axonal injury. These elevations were persistent for up to 5 days.

Clinical trials of free radical scavengers are ongoing, and the results are awaited with interest. Early analysis of the data suggests that polyethylene glycol–conjugated superoxide dismutase significantly improved 3-month survival when given within 4 h of injury to patients with severe head injury (Paul Muizelaar, personal communication). Since both mannitol and glucocorticoids are known to be free radical scavengers[192] and have long been used in the management of head-injured patients, it is interesting to speculate that their efficacy may have been due to their effects in limiting the toxic effects of oxygen.

GLUTAMATE

Using microdialysis probes, it has been demonstrated that the concentrations of two amino acid neurotransmitters, glutamate and aspartate, are markedly increased when CBF falls to critical levels.[198,199] The release of glutamate activates several receptors, the most important of which is the N-methyl-D-asparate (NMDA) receptor. This results in sodium and calcium influx. Elevation of intracellular sodium results in cell swelling and, ultimately, physical disruption of membranes, while elevated intracellular calcium damages organelle membranes and may play a major role in cell death.[200] Further support for this hypothesis comes from studies in which the toxic effects of these excitatory amino acids have been reduced by treatment with specific antagonists.[201-203] Specific glutamate antagonists offer the potential for ameliorating the secondary neuronal damage seen in patients with cerebral injuries and hypotension.

SUMMARY

Head injury remains the leading cause of traumatic death. Much of the associated morbidity and mortality is due to secondary ischemic injury, which may be preventable or reversible with aggressive resuscitation and early treatment. Experimental and clinical data demonstrate that hypotension has a significant adverse impact on the outcome of head-injured patients. Resuscitation of the head-injured patient should be guided by restoration of blood pressure, restitution of the blood volume, and control of ICP. Intense investigation is currently underway not only to develop new treatments but also to develop methodologies for measuring CBF and metabolism at the bedside.

REFERENCES

1. Shackford SR, Mackersie RC, Davis JW, et al: Epidemiology and pathology of traumatic deaths occurring at a level I trauma center in a brain injury. *J Trauma* 29:1392, 1989.
2. Sosin DM, Sacks JJ, Smith SM: Head injury–associated deaths in the United States from 1979 to 1986. *JAMA* 262:2251, 1989.
3. Adams JH, Graham DI, Scott G, et al: Brain damage in fatal non-missile head injury. *J Clin Pathol* 33:1132, 1980.
4. Graham DI, Adams JH, Doyle D: Ischaemic brain damage in fatal non-missile head injuries. *J Neurosci* 39:213, 1978.
5. Graham DI, Ford I, Adams JH, et al: Ischemic brain injury is still common in fatal non-missile head injuries. *J Neurol Neurosurg Psychiatry* 52:346, 1989.
6. Miller JD, Sweet RC, Narayan R, Becker DP: Early insults to the injured brain. *JAMA* 240:439, 1978.
7. Chestnut RM, Marshall LS, Klauber M: The role of secondary brain injury in determining outcome from severe head injury. *JAMA* (submitted).
8. Wald S, Fenwick J, Shackford SR: The effect of secondary insults on mortality and longterm disability of severe head injury in a rural region without a trauma system (abstract). *J Trauma* 31:1038, 1991.
9. Schmoker JD, Zhuang J, Shackford SR: Hypertonic fluid resuscitation improves cerebral oxygen delivery and reduces intracranial pressure after hemorrhagic shock. *J Trauma* 31:1607, 1991.
10. Shackford SR: Fluid resuscitation in head injury. *Intensive Care Med* 5:59, 1990.
11. Shackford SR, Baxt WG, Hoyt DB, et al: Impact of a trauma system on outcome of severely injured patients. *Arch Surg* 122:523, 1987.
12. Jennett B, Bond M: Assessment of outcome after severe brain damage: A practical scale. *Lancet* 1:480, 1975.
13. Eisenberg HM, Cayard C, Papanicolaou A, et al: The effects of three potentially preventable complications on outcome after severe closed head injury. In *Intracranial Pressure V.* Berlin, Springer-Verlag, 1983, pp 549–553.
14. Miller JD, Becker DP, Ward JH, et al: Significance of intracranial hypertension in severe head injury. *J Neurosurg* 47:503, 1977.
15. Miller JD, Butterworth JF, Gudeman SK, et al: Further experience in the management of severe head injury. *J Neurosurg* 54:289, 1981.
16. Becker DP, Miller JD, Ward JD, et al: The outcome from severe head injury with early diagnosis and intensive management. *J Neurosurg* 47:491, 1977.
17. Pacult A, Gudeman SK: Medical management of head injuries. In DP Becher, SK Gudeman (eds): *Textbook of Head Injury.* Philadelphia, Saunders, 1989, pp 192–220.
18. Civetta JM: A new look at the Starling equation. *Crit Care Med* 7:84, 1979.
19. Staverman AJ: Non-equilibrium thermodynamics of membrane processes. *Trans Faraday Soc* 48:176, 1952.
20. Zarins CK, Rice CL, Peters RM, Virgilio RW: Lymph and pulmonary response to isobaric reduction in plasma oncotic pressure in baboons. *Circ Res* 43:925, 1978.
21. Fenstermacher JD: Volume regulation of the central nervous system. In NC Staub, AE Taylor (eds): *Edema.* New York, Raven Press, 1984, pp 383–404.
22. Fenstermacher JD, Johnson JA: Filtration and reflection coefficients of rabbit blood-brain barrier. *Am J Physiol* 211:341, 1966.
23. Siesjo BK: Cerebral circulation and metabolism. *J Neurosurg* 60:883, 1984.
24. Heistad DD, Kontos HA: Cerebral circulation. In JT Shepard, FM Abboud (eds): *Handbook of Physiology: The cardiovascular system,* vol 3. Baltimore, Williams & Wilkins, 1983, pp 137–182.

25. Prough DS, Rogers AT: Physiology and pharmacology of cerebral blood flow and metabolism. *Crit Care Clin* 5:713, 1989.

26. Kontos HA: Regulation of the cerebral circulation. *Annu Rev Physiol* 43:397, 1981.

27. Wei EP, Dietrich WD, Povlishock JT, et al: Functional, morphological, and metabolic abnormalities of the cerebral microcirculation after concussive brain injury in cats. *Circ Res* 46:37, 1980.

28. Wagner EM, Traystman RJ: Cerebral venous outflow and arterial microsphere flow with elevated venous pressure. *Am J Physiol* 244:H505, 1983.

29. Reivich M: Arterial Pco_2 and cerebral hemodynamics. *Am J Physiol* 206:25, 1965.

30. Greenberg JH, Alavi A, Reivich M, et al: Local cerebral blood volume response to carbon dioxide in man. *Circ Res* 43:324, 1978.

31. Brown MM, Marshall J: Effect of plasma exchange on blood viscosity and cerebral blood flow. *Br Med J* 284:1733, 1982.

32. Brown MM, Wade JP, Marshall J: Fundamental importance of arterial oxygen content in the regulation of cerebral blood flow in man. *Brain* 108:81, 1985.

33. Brown MM, Marshall J: Regulation of cerebral blood flow in response to changes in blood viscosity. *Lancet* 1:604, 1985.

34. Bruce DA, Langfitt TW, Miller JD, et al: Regional cerebral blood flow, intracranial pressure, and brain metabolism in comatose patients. *J Neurosurg* 38:131, 1973.

35. Marion DW, Darby J, Yonas H: Acute regional cerebral blood flow changes caused by severe head injuries. *J Neurosurg* 74(3):407, 1991.

36. Mendelow AD, Teasdale GM, Russell T, et al: Effect of mannitol on cerebral blood flow and cerebral perfusion pressure in human head injury. *J Neurosurg* 63:43, 1985.

37. Muizelaar JP, Marmarou A, DeSalles AA, et al: Cerebral blood flow and metabolism in severely head-injured children: I. Relationship with GCS score, outcome, ICP, and PVI. *J Neurosurg* 71:63, 1989.

38. Obrist WD, Langfitt TW, Jaggi JL: Cerebral blood flow and metabolism in comatose patients with acute head injury: Relationship to intracranial hypertension. *J Neurosurg* 61:241, 1984.

39. Jaggi JL, Obrist WD, Gennarelli TA, Langfitt TW: Relationship of early cerebral blood flow and metabolism to outcome in acute head injury. *J Neurosurg* 72:176, 1990.

40. Overgaard J, Mosdal C, Tweed WA: Cerebral circulation after head injury: 3. Does reduced regional cerebral blood flow determine recovery of brain function after blunt head injury? *J Neurosurg* 55:63, 1981.

41. Marshall LF, Welsh F, Durity F: Experimental cerebral oligemia and ischemia produced by intracranial hypertension: 3. Brain energy metabolism. *J Neurosurg* 43:323, 1975.

42. DeSalles AA, Muizelaar JP, Young HF: Hyperglycemia, cerebrospinal fluid lactic acidosis, and cerebral blood flow in severely head-injured patients. *Neurosurgery* 21:45, 1987.

43. DeWitt DS, Jenkins LW, Lutz H: Regional cerebral blood flow following fluid percussion injury. *J Cereb Blood Flow Metab* 1(suppl):S579, 1981.

44. McIntosh TK, Vink R, Noble L, et al: Traumatic brain injury in the rat: Characterization of a lateral fluid-percussion model. *Neuroscience* 28:233, 1989.

45. DeWitt DS, Jenkins LW, Wei EP, et al: Effects of fluid-percussion brain injury on regional cerebral blood flow and pial arteriolar diameter. *J Neurosurg* 64:787, 1986.

46. Yuan XQ, Prough DS, Smith T, Dewitt DS: The effects of traumatic brain injury on regional cerebral blood flow in rats. *J Neurotrauma* 5:289, 1988.

47. Pfenninger EG, Reith A, Breitig D, et al: Early changes of intracranial pressure, perfusion pressure, and blood flow after acute head injury: I. An experimental study of the underlying pathophysiology. *J Neurosurg* 70:774, 1989.

48. Jenkins LW, Moszynski K, Lyeth BG, et al: Increased vulnerability of the mildly traumatized rat brain to cerebral ischemia: The use of controlled secondary ischemia as a research

tool to identify common or different mechanisms contributing to mechanical and ischemic brain injury. *Brain Res* 477:211, 1989.

49. Bakay R, Wood JH: Pathophysiology of cerebrospinal fluid in trauma. In DP Becker, J Povlishock (eds): *Central Nervous System Trauma Status Report*. Bethesda, MD, NINCDS, NIH 1985, pp 89–122.

50. Sood SC, Gulati SC, Kumar M, Kak VK: Cerebral metabolism following brain injury: II. Lactic acid changes. *Acta Neurochir* 53:47, 1980.

51. Ishige N, Pitts LH, Berry I, et al: The effects of hypovolemic hypotension on high-energy phosphate metabolism of traumatized brain in rats. *J Neurosurg* 68:129, 1988.

52. Rango M, Lenkinski RE, Alves WM: Brain pH in head injury: An image-guided P magnetic resonance spectroscopy study. *Ann Neurol* 28:661, 1990.

53. Schmoker J, Zhuang J, Shackford SR: Hemorrhagic hypotension after brain injury causes an early and sustained oxygen delivery despite normalization of systemic oxygen delivery (abstract). *J Trauma* 31:1038, 1991.

54. Bouma GJ, Muizelaar JP: Relationship between cardiac output and cerebral blood flow in patients with intact and with impaired autoregulation. *J Neurosurg* 73:368, 1990.

55. Redan JA, Livingston DH, Tortella BJ, Rush BF Jr: The value of intubating and paralyzing patients with suspected head injury in the emergency department. *J Trauma* 31(3):371, 1991.

56. Mackersie RC, Karagianes TG: Use of end-tidal carbon dioxide tension for monitoring induced hypocapnia in head-injured patients. *Crit Care Med* 18:764, 1990.

57. Muizelaar JP, van der Poel HG, Li ZC, et al: Pial arteriolar vessel diameter and CO_2 reactivity during prolonged hyperventilation in the rabbit. *J Neurosurg* 69:923, 1988.

58. Ward JD, Choi S, Marmarou A: Effect of prophylactic hyperventilation on outcome in patients with severe head injury. In JT Hoff, AL Betz (eds): *Intracranial Pressure VII*. Berlin, Springer-Verlag, 1989, p 630.

59. Shackford SR: Fluid resuscitation of the trauma victim. In SR Shackford, A Perel (eds): *Problems in Critical Care*, vol 1. Philadelphia, Lippincott, 1987, pp 576–587.

60. Bakay L, Crawford JD, White JC: The effects of intravenous fluids on cerebrospinal fluid pressure. *Surg Gynecol Obstet* 99:48, 1954.

61. Shenkin HA, Gutterman P: The analysis of body water compartments in postoperative craniotomy patients. *J Neurosurg* 31:400, 1964.

62. Reulen HJ: Vasogenic brain oedema: New aspects in its formulation, resolution and therapy. *Br J Anaesth* 48:741, 1976.

63. Walsh J, Zhuang J, Shackford SR: Fluid resuscitation of focal brain injury and shock (abstract). *Surg Forum* 41:56, 1990.

64. Wisner D, Busche F, Sturm J, et al: Traumatic shock and head injury: Effects of fluid resuscitation on the brain. *J Surg Res* 46:49, 1989.

65. Wilkinson HA, Rosenfeld SR: Furosemide and mannitol in the treatment of acute experimental intracranial hypertension. *Neurosurgery* 12:405, 1983.

66. Morse ML, Milstein JM, Haas JE, Taylor E: Effect of hydration on experimentally induced cerebral edema. *Crit Care Med* 13:563, 1985.

67. Schmoker JW, Shackford SR, Wald SL, Pietropaoli JA: An analysis of the relationship between fluid and sodium administration and intracranial pressure after head injury. *J Trauma* 33:476, 1992.

68. Davis JW, Shackford SR, Mackersie RC, Hoyt DB: Base deficit as a guide to volume resuscitation. *J Trauma* 28:1464, 1988.

69. Cruz J: Continuous versus serial global cerebral hemometabolic monitoring: Applications in acute brain trauma. *Acta Neurochir Suppl (Wein)* 42:35, 1988.

70. Ali J, Aprahamian C, Brown R, et al: *Advanced Trauma Life Support Program*. Chicago, American College of Surgeons, 1989, pp 1–706.

71. Shenkin HA, Bezier HS, Bouzarth WF: Restricted fluid intake: Rational management of the neurosurgical patient. *J Neurosurg* 45:432, 1976.

72. Shackford SR, Norton CH, Todd MM: Renal, cerebral, and pulmonary effects of hypertonic resuscitation in a porcine model of hemorrhagic shock. *Surgery* 104:553, 1988.

73. Velasco IT, Pontieri V, Rochae-Silva M Jr, Lopes OU: Hyperosmotic NaCl and severe hemorrhagic shock. *Am J Physiol* 239:H664, 1980.

74. Nakayama S, Sibley L, Gunther RA, et al: Small-volume resuscitation with hypertonic saline (2,400 mOsm/liter) during hemorrhagic shock. *Circ Shock* 13:149, 1984.

75. Shackford SR, Fortlage DA, Peters RM, et al: Serum osmolar and electrolyte changes associated with large infusions of hypertonic sodium lactate for intravascular volume expansion of patients undergoing aortic reconstruction. *Surg Gynecol Obstet* 164:127, 1987.

76. Kreimeier U, Brueckner UB, Schmidt J, Messmer K: Instantaneous restoration of regional organ blood flow after severe hemorrhage: Effect of small-volume resuscitation with hypertonic-hyperoncotic solutions. *J Surg Res* 49:493, 1990.

77. Wildenthal K, Skelton CL, Coleman HN: Cardiac muscle mechanics in hyperosmotic solutions. *Am J Physiol* 217:302, 1969.

78. Rowe GG, McKenna DH, Corliss RJ, Sialer S: Hemodynamic effects of hypertonic sodium chloride. *J Appl Physiol* 32:182, 1972.

79. Kien ND, Kramer GC, White DA: Direct cardiac effect of hypertonic saline in anesthetized dogs. *Anesth Analg* 68:S147, 1989.

80. Kien ND, Reitan JA, White DA, et al: Cardiac contractility and blood flow distribution following resuscitation with 7.5% hypertonic saline in anesthetized dogs. *Circ Shock* 35:109, 1991.

81. Mazzoni MC, Arfors BK, Intaglietta M: Dynamic fluid redistribution in hyperosmotic resuscitation of hypovolemic hemorrhage. *Am J Physiol* 139:H629, 1988.

82. Mazzoni MC, Lundgren E, Arfors KE, Intaglietta M: Volume changes of an endothelial cell monolayer on exposure to anisotonic media. *J Cell Physiol* 140:272, 1989.

83. Wahl M, Kuschinsky W, Bosse O, et al: Dependency of pial arterial and arteriolar diameter on perivascular osmolarity in the cat: A microapplication study. *Circ Res* 32:162, 1973.

84. Maningas PA: Resuscitation with 7.5% NaCl in 6% dextran-70 during hemorrhagic shock in swine: Effects on organ blood flow. *Crit Care Med* 15:1121, 1987.

85. Gazitùa S, Scott JB, Swindall B, et al: Resistance responses to local changes in plasma osmolality in three vascular beds. *Am J Physiol* 220:384, 1971.

86. Silva MR, Negraes GA, Soares AM, et al: Hypertonic resuscitation from severe hemorrhagic shock: Patterns of regional circulation. *Circ Shock* 19:165, 1986.

87. Mazzoni MC, Borgstrom P, Intaglietta M, Arfors KE: Capillary narrowing in hemorrhagic shock is rectified by hyperosmotic saline-dextran reinfusion. *Circ Shock* 31:407, 1990.

88. Gunnar W, Jonasson O, Merlotti G, et al: Head injury and hemorrhagic shock: Studies of the blood brain barrier and intracranial pressure after resuscitation with normal saline solution, 3% saline solution, and dextran-40. *Surgery* 103:398, 1988.

89. Ducey JP, Mozingo DW, Lamiell JM, et al: A comparison of the cerebral and cardiovascular effects of complete resuscitation with isotonic and hypertonic saline, hetastarch, and whole blood following hemorrhage. *J Trauma* 29:1510, 1989.

90. Todd MM, Tommasino C, Moore S: Cerebral effects of isovolemic hemodilution with a hypertonic saline solution. *J Neurosurg* 63:944, 1985.

91. Wisner DH, Schuster L, Quinn C: Hypertonic saline resuscitation of head injury: Effects on cerebral water content. *J Trauma* 30:75, 1990.

92. Prough DS, Johnson JC, Poole GV Jr, et al: Effects on intracranial pressure of resuscitation from hemorrhagic shock with hypertonic saline versus lactated Ringer's solution. *Crit Care Med* 13:407, 1985.

93. Prough DS, Johnson JC, Stump DA, et al: Effects of hypertonic saline versus lactated Ring-

er's solution on cerebral oxygen transport during resuscitation from hemorrhagic shock. *J Neurosurg* 64:627, 1986.

94. Shackford SR, Zhuang J, Schmoker J: Intravenous fluid tonicity: Effect on intracranial pressure, cerebral blood flow, and cerebral oxygen delivery in focal brain injury. *J Neurosurg* 76:91, 1992.

95. Pitts LH, Kaktis JV, Juster R, Heilbron D: ICP and outcome in patients with severe head injury. In K Shulman, A Marmarou, JD Miller, et al (eds): *Intracranial Pressure IV.* Berlin, Springer-Verlag, 1980, pp. 5–9.

96. Walsh JC, Zhuang J, Shackford SR: A comparison of hypertonic to isotonic fluid in the resuscitation of brain injury and hemorrhage shock. *J Surg Res* 50:284, 1991.

97. Bustad LK, Horstman VG, Swindle MM, et al: *Swing in Biomedical Research.* New York, Plenum Press, 1986, pp 1–698.

98. Waters DC, Hoff JT, Black KL: Effect of parenteral nutrition on cold-induced vasogenic edema in cats. *J Neurosurg* 64:460, 1986.

99. Monafo WW, Halverson JD, Schectman K: The role of concentrated sodium solutions in the resuscitation of patients with severe burns. *Surgery* 95:129, 1984.

100. Bowser-Wallace BH, Cone JB, Caldwell FT Jr: Hypertonic lactated saline resuscitation of severely burned patients over 60 years of age. *J Trauma* 25:22, 1985.

101. Mattox KL, Maningas PA, Moore EE, et al: Prehospital hypertonic saline/dextran infusion for post-traumatic hypotension: The U.S.A. Multicenter Trial. *Ann Surg* 213:482, 1991.

102. Maningas PA, Mattox KL, Pepe PE, et al: Hypertonic saline-dextran solutions for the pre-hospital management of traumatic hypotension. *Am J Surg* 157:528, 1989.

103. Holcroft JW, Vassar MJ, Turner JE, et al: 3% NaCl and 7.5% NaCl/dextran 10 in the resuscitation of severely injured patients. *Ann Surg* 206:279, 1987.

104. Vassar MJ, Perry CA, Holcroft JW: Analysis of potential risks associated with 7.5% NaCl/dextran for resuscitation of trauma patients undergoing helicopter transport. *Arch Surg* 126(1):43, 1991.

105. Teasdale G, Galbraith S, Murray L, et al: Management of traumatic intracranial haematoma. *Br Med J* 285:1695, 1982.

106. Virgilio RW, Metildi LA, Peters RM, Shackford SR: Crystalloid vs colloid volume resuscitation of patients with severe pulmonary insufficiency. *Surg Forum* 30:166, 1979.

107. Clasen RA, Prouty RR, Bingham WG, et al: Treatment of experimental cerebral edema with intravenous hypertonic glucose, albumin, and dextran. *Surg Gynecol Obstet* 104:591, 1957.

108. Albright AL, Phillips JW: Oncotic therapy of experimental cerebral oedema. *Acta Neurochir (Wien)* 60:257, 1982.

109. Albright AL, Latchaw RE, Robinson AG: Intracranial and systemic effects of osmotic and oncotic therapy in experimental cerebral edema. *J Neurosurg* 60:481, 1984.

110. Poole GV, Prough DS, Johnson JC, et al: Effects of resuscitation from hemorrhagic shock on cerebral hemodynamics in the presence of an intracranial mass. *J Trauma* 27:18, 1987.

111. Shackford SR, Mackersie RC, Hollingsworth-Fridlund P: The evolution, design, results, and cost of a successful trauma system. In AR Moossa (ed): *Problems in General Surgery.* Philadelphia, Lippincott, 1989, pp 32–45.

112. Warner DS, Boehland LA: Effects of iso-osmolal intravenous fluid therapy on post-ischemic brain water content in the rat. *Anesthesiology* 68:86, 1988.

113. Tranmer BI, Iacobacci RI, Kindt GW: Effects of crystalloid and colloid infusions on intracranial pressure and computerized electroencephalographic data in dogs with vasogenic brain edema. *Neurosurgery* 25:173, 1989.

114. Todd MM, Tommasino C, Moore S, et al: The effect of hypertonic saline on intracranial pressure, cerebral blood flow and brain water content (abstract). *Anesthesiology* 61:3A, 1984.

115. Kaieda R, Todd MM, Cook LN, Warner DS: Acute effects of changing plasma osmolality

and colloid oncotic pressure on the formation of brain edema after cryogenic injury. *Neurosurgery* 24:671, 1989.

116. Zornow MH, Scheller MS, Todd MM, Moore SS: Acute cerebral effects of isotonic crystalloid and colloid solutions following cryogenic brain injury in the rabbit. *Anesthesiology* 69:180, 1988.

117. Metildi LA, Shackford SR, Virgilio RW, Peters RM: Crystalloid versus colloid in fluid resuscitation of patients with severe pulmonary insufficiency. *Surg Gynecol Obstet* 158:207, 1984.

118. Ring JL, Messmer RJ: Incidence and severity of anaphylactoid reactions to colloid volume substitute. *Lancet* 1:466, 1977.

119. Johnson SD, Lucas CE, Gerrick SJ, et al: Altered coagulation after albumin supplements for treatment of oligemic shock. *Arch Surg* 114:379, 1979.

120. Shackford SR, Wald SL, Hoyt DB, et al: The utility of CT scanning in patients with minor head injury. *J Trauma* 33:385, 1992.

121. Task Force of the Committee on Trauma of the American College of Surgeons: *Resources for Optimal Care of the Injured Patient.* Chicago, American College of Surgeons, 1990, pp 1–79.

122. Mohanty SK, Thompson W, Rakower S: Are CT scans for head injury patients always necessary? *J Trauma* 31:804, 1991.

123. Livingston DH, Loder PA, Koziol J, Hunt CD: The use of CT scanning to triage patients requiring admission following minimal head injury. *J Trauma* 31:483, 1991.

124. Stein SC, Ross SE: The value of computed tomographic scans in patients with low-risk head injuries. *J Neurosurg* 26:638, 1990.

125. Macpherson CM, Macpherson P, Jennett B: CT evidence of intracranial contusion and haematoma in relation to the presence, site and type of skull fracture. *Clin Radiol* 42:321, 1990.

126. Dacey RG Jr, Alves WM, Rimel RW, et al: Neurosurgical complications after apparently minor head injury: Assessment of risk in a series of 610 patients. *J Neurosurg* 65:203, 1986.

127. Gentry LR, Godersky JC, Thompson B, Dunn VO: Prospective comparative study of intermediate-field MR and CT in the evaluation of closed head trauma. *AJR* 150:673, 1988.

128. Lundberg N: Continuous recording and control of ventricular fluid pressure in neurosurgical practice. *Acta Psychiatry Neurol Scand* 36:1, 1960.

129. Narayan RK, Kishore PR, Becker DP, et al: Intracranial pressure: To monitor or not to monitor? A review of our experience with severe head injury. *J Neurosurg* 56:650, 1982.

130. Narayan RK, Kishore PR, Becker DP, et al: Intracranial pressure: To monitor or not to monitor? A review of our experience with severe head injury. *J Neurosurg* 56:650, 1982.

131. Hassler W, Steinmetz H, Gawlowski J: Transcranial Doppler ultrasonography in raised intracranial pressure and in intracranial circulatory arrest. *J Neurosurg* 68:745, 1988.

132. Haberl RL, Heizer ML, Marmarou A, Ellis EF: Laser-Doppler assessment of brain microcirculation: Effect of systematic alterations. *Am J Physiol* 256:H1247, 1989.

133. Gur D, Good WF, Wolfson SK Jr: In vivo mapping of local cerebral blood flow by xenon-enhanced computed tomography. *Science* 215:1267, 1982.

134. Tenjin H, Ueda S, Mizukawa N, et al: Positron emission tomographic studies on cerebral hemodynamics in patients with cerebral contusion. *Neurosurgery* 26:971, 1990.

135. Bouma GJ, Muizelaar JP, Choi SC: Cerebral circulation and metabolism after severe traumatic brain injury: The elusive role of ischemia. *J Neurosurg* 75:685, 1991.

136. Rosner MJ, Daughton S: Cerebral perfusion pressure management in head injury. *J Trauma* 30:933, 1990.

137. Persson L, Hillered L: Chemical monitoring of neurosurgical intensive care patients using intracerebral microdialysis. *J Neurosurg* 76:72, 1992.

138. Stahl WM: Effect of mannitol on the kidney—Changes in intrarenal hemodynamics. *N Engl J Med* 272:381, 1965.

139. Gennari FJ, Kassirer JP: Osmotic diuresis. *N Engl J Med* 291:714, 1974.

140. Reed DJ, Woodbury DM: Effect of hypertonic urea on cerebrospinal fluid pressure and brain volume. *J Physiol* 164:252, 1962.

141. Kassell NF, Baumann KW, Hitchon PW, et al: The effects of high dose mannitol on cerebral blood flow in dogs with normal intracranial pressure. *Stroke* 13:59, 1982.

142. Muizelaar JP, Wei EP, Kontos HA, Becker DP: Mannitol causes compensatory cerebral vasoconstriction and vasodilation in response to blood viscosity changes. *J Neurosurg* 59:822, 1983.

143. Nath F, Galbraith S: The effect of mannitol on cerebral white matter water content. *J Neurosurg* 65:41, 1986.

144. McGraw CP, Howard G: Effect of mannitol on increased intracranial pressure. *Neurosurgery* 13:269, 1983.

145. Marshall LF, Smith RW, Rauscher LA, Shapiro HM: Mannitol dose requirements in brain-injured patients. *J Neurosurg* 48:169, 1978.

146. Cote CJ, Greenhow DE, Marshall BE: The hypotensive response to rapid intravenous administration of hypertonic solutions in man and in the rabbit. *Anesthesiology* 50:30, 1979.

147. Brown FD, Johns L, Jafar JJ, et al: Detailed monitoring of the effects of mannitol following experimental head injury. *J Neurosurg* 50:423, 1979.

148. Braakman R, Schouten JH, Blaauw-van Dishoeck M, Minderhoud JM: Megadose steroids in severe head injury: Results of a prospective double-blind clinical trial. *J Neurosurg* 58:326, 1983.

149. Cooper PR, Moody S, Clark WK, et al: Dexamethasone and severe head injury: A prospective double-blind study. *J Neurosurg* 51:307, 1979.

150. Saul TG, Ducker TB, Salcman M, Carro E: Steroids in severe head injury: A prospective randomized clinical trial. *J Neurosurg* 54:596, 1981.

151. Dearden NM, Gibson JS, McDowall DG, et al: Effect of high-dose dexamethasone on outcome from severe head injury. *J Neurosurg* 64:81, 1986.

152. Marshall LF, King J, Langfitt TW: The complications of high-dose corticosteroid therapy in neurosurgical patients: A prospective study. *Ann Neurol* 1:201, 1977.

153. Deutschman CS, Konstantinides FN, Raup S, Cerra FB: Physiological and metabolic response to isolated closed-head injury: 2. Effects of steroids on metabolism. Potentiation of protein wasting and abnormalities of substrate utilization. *J Neurosurg* 66:388, 1987.

154. Bracker MB, Shepard MJ, Collins WF Jr, et al: Methylprednisolone or naloxone treatment after acute spinal cord injury: One year follow-up data. Results of the second National Acute Spinal Cord Injury Study. *J Neurosurg* 76:23, 1992.

155. Kostron H, Twerdy K, Stampfl G, et al: Treatment of the traumatic cerebral vasospasm with the calcium channel blocker nimodipine: A preliminary report. *Neurosurg Res* 6:29, 1984.

156. Compton JS, Lee T, Jones NR, et al: A double-blind placebo-controlled trial of the calcium entry blocking drug, nicardipine, in the treatment of vasospasm following severe head injury. *Br J Neurosurg* 4:9, 1990.

157. Bailey I, Bell A, Gray J, et al: A trial of the effect of nimodipine on outcome after head injury. *Acta Neurochir* 110:97, 1991.

158. Höllerhage HG, Gabb MR, Zumkeller M, Walter GF: The influence of nimodipine on cerebral blood flow autoregulation and blood-brain barrier. *J Neurosurg* 69:919, 1988.

159. Jennett B: *Epilepsy after Nonmissile Injuries,* 2d ed. Chicago, Year Book Medical Publishers, 1975.

160. Annegers JF, Grabow JD, Groover RV: Seizures after head injury: A population study. *Neurology* 30:683, 1980.

161. Temkin NR, Dikmen SS, Wilensky AJ, et al: A randomized double-blind study of phenytoin for the prevention of post-traumatic seizures. *N Engl J Med* 323:497, 1990.

162. Young B, Rapp RP, Norton JA, et al: Failure of prophylactically administered phenytoin to prevent late posttraumatic seizures. *J Neurosurg* 58:236, 1983.

163. Cottrell JE, Robustelli A, Post K, et al: Furosemide- and mannitol-induced changes in intracranial pressure and serum osmolality and electrolytes. *Anesthesiology* 47:28, 1977.

164. Pollay M, Fullenwider C, Roberts PA, Stevens FA: Effect of mannitol and furosemide on blood-brain osmotic gradient and intracranial pressure. *J Neurosurg* 59:945, 1983.

165. Cottrell JE, Marlin AE: Furosemide and human head injury. *J Trauma* 21:805, 1981.

166. Schettini A, Stahurski B, Young HF: Osmotic and osmotic-loop diuresis in brain surgery: Effects on plasma and CSF electrolytes and ion excretion. *J Neurosurg* 56:679, 1982.

167. Roberts JP, Shackford SR, Peters RM: Metabolism of D-lactate in patients receiving hypertonic sodium lactate solution. *Surg Gynecol Obstet* 168:429, 1989.

168. Davis JW, Shackford SR, Holbrook TL: Base deficit as a sensitive indicator of compensated shock and tissue oxygen utilization. *Surg Gynecol Obstet* 173:473, 1991.

169. DeSalles AA, Kontos HA, Becker DP, et al: Prognostic significance of ventricular CSF lactate acidosis in severe head injury. *J Neurosurg* 65:615, 1986.

170. Gordon E: Some correlations between the clinical outcome and the acid-base status of blood and cerebrospinal fluid in patients with traumatic brain injury. *Acta Anaesthesiol Scand* 15:209, 1971.

171. Enevoldsen EM, Jensen FT: Cerebrospinal fluid lactate and pH in patients with acute severe head injury. *Clin Neurol Neurosurg* 80:213, 1977.

172. Rosner MJ, Elias KG, Coley I: Prospective, randomized trial of THAM therapy in severe brain injury: Preliminary results. In JT Hoff, AL Betz (eds): *Intracranial Pressure VII.* Berlin, Springer-Verlag, 1989, p. 611.

173. Becker DP: Brain acidosis in head injury: A clinical trial. In DP Becker, JT Povlishock (eds): *Central Nervous System Trauma Status Report.* Richmond, Byre Press, 1985, p 229.

174. Gaab MR, Seegers K, Goetz C: THAM (trimethamine, "trisbuffer"): Effective therapy of traumatic brain swelling? In JT Hoff, AL Betz (eds): *Intracranial Pressure VII.* Berlin, Springer-Verlag, 1989, p 616.

175. Yoshida K, Marmarou A: Effects of tromethamine and hyperventilation on brain injury in the cat. *J Neurosurg* 74:87, 1991.

176. Shapiro HM, Galindo A, Wyte SR, Harris AB: Rapid intraoperative reduction of intracranial pressure with the open tone. *Br J Anaesth* 45:1057, 1973.

177. Rockoff MA, Marshall LF, Shapiro HM: High-dose barbiturate therapy in humans: A clinical review of 60 patients. *Ann Neurol* 6:194, 1979.

178. Marshall LF, Smith RW, Shapiro HM: The outcome with aggressive treatment in severe head injuries: II. Acute and chronic barbiturate administration in the management of head injury. *J Neurosurg* 50:26, 1979.

179. Eisenberg HM, Frankowski RF, Contant CF, et al: High-dose barbiturate control of elevated intracranial pressure in patients with severe head injury. *J Neurosurg* 69:15, 1988.

180. Ward JD, Becker DP, Miller JD, et al: Failure of prophylactic barbiturate coma in the treatment of severe head injury. *J Neurosurg* 62:383, 1985.

181. Faden AI: Opiate antagonists and thyrotropin-releasing hormone: II. Potential role in the treatment of central nervous system injury. *JAMA* 252:1452, 1984.

182. Gillman MA, Lichtigfeld FJ: The opiate system in traumatic brain death (letter). *Lancet* 2:156, 1981.

183. Hayes RL, Galinat BJ, Kulkarne P, Becker DP: Effects of naloxone on systemic and cerebral responses to experimental concussive brain injury in cats. *J Neurosurg* 58:720, 1983.

184. Marshall LF, Camp PE, Bowers SA: Dimethyl sulfoxide for the treatment of intracranial hypertension: a preliminary trial. *Neurosurgery* 14:659, 1984.

185. Karaca M, Bilgin UY, Akar M, de la Torre JC: Dimethyl sulphoxide lowers ICP after closed head trauma. *Eur J Clin Pharmacol* 40:113, 1991.

186. Waller F, Tanabe C, Paxton H: Treatment of elevated intracranial pressure with dimethyl sulfoxide. *Ann NY Acad Sci* 411:286, 1983.

187. de la Torre JC: Role of dimethyl sulfoxide in prostaglandin-thromboxane and platelet systems after cerebral ischemia. *Ann NY Acad Sci* 411:293, 1983.

188. Egorin MJ, Kaplan RS, Salcman M, et al: Cyclophosphamide plasma and cerebrospinal fluid kinetics with and without dimethyl sulfoxide. *Clin Pharmacol Ther* 32:122, 1982.

189. Broadwell RD, Salcman M, Kaplan RS: Morphologic effect of dimethyl sulfoxide on the blood-brain barrier. *Science* 217:164, 1982.

190. McCord JM: Oxygen-derived free radicals in postischemic tissue injury. *N Engl J Med* 312:159, 1985.

191. Ikeda Y, Long DM: The molecular basis of brain injury and brain edema: The role of oxygen free radicals. *Neurosurgery* 27:1, 1990.

192. Hall ED: Free radicals and CNS injury. *Neurol Crit Care* 5:793, 1989.

193. Ando Y, Inoue M, Hirota M, et al: Effect of a superoxide dismutase derivative on cold-induced brain edema. *Brain Res* 477:286, 1989.

194. Wei EP, Kontas HA, Dietrich WD, et al: Inhibition by free radical scavengers and by cyclo-oxygenase inhibitors of pial arteriolar abnormalities from concussive brain injury in cats. *Circ Res* 48:95, 1981.

195. Chan PH, Longar S, Fishman RA: Protective effects of liposome-entrapped superoxide dismutase on posttraumatic brain edema. *Ann Neurol* 21:540, 1987.

196. Chan PH, Yang GY, Chen SF, et al: Cold-induced brain edema and infarction are reduced in transgenic mice overexpressing CuZn-superoxide dismutase. *Ann Neurol* 29:482, 1991.

197. Bochicchio M, Latronico N, Zani DG, et al: Free radical-induced lipoperoxidation and severe head injury: A clinical study. *Intensive Care Med* 16:444, 1990.

198. Shimada N, Graf R, Rosner G, et al: Ischemic flow threshold for extracellular glutamate increase in cat cortex. *J Cereb Blood Flow Metab* 9:603, 1989.

199. Faden AI, Demediuk P, Panter SS, Vink R: The role of excitatory amino acids and NMDA receptors in traumatic brain injury. *Science* 244:798, 1989.

200. Becker DP, Katayama Y, Tamura T, et al: Excitotoxic ion fluxes and neuronal dysfunction following traumatic brain injury. *J Cereb Blood Flow Metab* 9:302, 1989.

201. Bullock R, McCulloch J, Graham DI, et al: Focal ischemic damage is reduced by D-CPP-ene studies in two animal models. *Stroke* 21:32, 1990.

202. Ozyurt E, Graham DI, Woodruff GN, McCulloch J: Protective effect of the glutamate antagonist, MK-801 in focal cerebral ischemia in the cat. *J Cereb Blood Flow Metab* 8:138, 1988.

203. Park CK, Nehls DG, Graham DI, et al: Focal cerebral ischaemia in the cat: Treatment with the glutamate antagonist MK-801 after induction of ischaemia. *J Cereb Blood Flow Metab* 8:757, 1988.

13

PEDIATRIC RESUSCITATION

Thomas M. Biancaniello

The need for resuscitation in the pediatric patient most commonly occurs in the first moments after birth, during the transition from fetal to newborn life. The most important causes of these difficulties are prematurity and obstetrical complications. Thereafter, in the developed parts of the world, injury is the leading cause of cardiovascular collapse, respiratory failure, and death. Other significant causes of these events include infection (sepsis, meningitis, epiglottitis, croup, pneumonia), dehydration, asthma, foreign body aspiration, toxic ingestions, and sudden infant death syndrome. Primary cardiac events may occur in childhood as a result of congenital cardiac defects, myocardial disease, dysrhythmias, and as complications following cardiac surgery, but these events are much less common than in adults.

While this chapter addresses aspects of resuscitation, the most important approach is prevention and anticipation. While this approach pertains to all health problems, it is especially true in children. A widely held misconception is that children are more resistant and recovery is more likely from cardiovascular collapse. This could not be further from the truth. In a study by Eisenberg and colleagues,[1] 31 percent of adults who experienced out-of-hospital cardiac arrest survived to be discharged from the hospital. Others, however, have found the results to be less encouraging in adults not initially resuscitated successfully.[2] In contrast, the outlook for children is dismal for both in-hospital and out-of-hospital arrests. Gillis and colleagues[3] evaluated the outcome of 42 inpatient arrests in children and found only a 17 percent overall survival in respiratory arrest alone and only 9 percent survival following full cardiac arrest. They also found that no patient survived if resuscitation was not successful within 15 minutes. Torphy et al.[4] reviewed the outcome following resuscitation of 183 children treated over a 5-year period. Only 3.3 percent in whom resuscitation was started at the scene and only 5.5 percent in whom resuscitation was performed in the emergency department survived. Five of the eight survivors from the combined groups had good neurologic recovery; this outcome was clearly related to prompt initiation of resuscitation and rapid clinical response. The findings of these studies demonstrate that the myth of children being more resistant than adults to these catastrophic events is false and that even a witnessed arrest in the best of circumstances has a poorer prognosis than the out-of-hospital adult collapse. Clearly, the course to take to reduce the morbidity and mortality for infants and children is better prenatal care, better training and preparation for resuscitation of newborns, programs to educate the population to reduce injury risks for infants and children, and good preventative health care and immunization programs.

While other chapters in this book address the basics of the physiology and pathophysiology of shock, only a brief review of these principles as they pertain to pediatrics will be presented. Since children are not merely "small adults," this review will concentrate on how infants and children differ from adults and how these differences influence the approach to management. Finally, some special conditions which are either unique to children or have unique aspects involved in their treatment will be presented in greater detail.

CARDIOPULMONARY RESUSCITATION (CPR) IN INFANTS AND CHILDREN

The *A,B,C approach* to basic life support (CPR) in infants and children is similar to that in adults: (1) *A*irway—assess for patency and attain proper positioning of the head; (2) *B*reathing—evaluate whether air is being exchanged by listening and watching for chest excursion and, if absent, begin ventilation; (3) *C*irculation—evaluate for effectiveness by assessing pulses and perfusion and, if inadequate, begin chest compressions.

To adequately assess the pediatric patient, one must be cognizant of the normal vital signs and differing requirements for resuscitation. Respiratory rates in children are faster than in adults. Infants may breathe at 20 to 40; children, about 20; and adolescents, 12 to 20 breaths per minute. Therefore, what would be considered tachypnea in an adult might be normal for an infant. Similarly, heart rates vary by age and size; infants have a mean heart rate of about 125 beats per minute (range 70 to 160); children at 4 years, a rate of 100 beats per minute (range 80 to 120); adolescents, a rate of 75 beats per minute (50 to 90). What is tachycardia in an adult may therefore be normal in an infant or child. Conversely, blood pressures increase with age. A systolic pressure of 65 mmHg is acceptable in an infant, 80 mmHg in children 2 to 8 years old, and 90 mmHg after 10 years of age. Therefore, what might be considered hypotension in an adult could be perfectly acceptable in a child. In addition to being familiar with the concept of norms for age, anticipation and prevention are critical. One must recognize that situations do not remain static, and therefore, serial assessment and attention to trends or changes may be the first harbinger of disaster. For example, an infant with a ventilation problem who develops bradycardia is headed for serious trouble, while one with tachycardia is still compensating. It is also important to keep in mind that blood pressure is maintained by vasoconstriction in compensated shock states and that adequacy of circulation is better determined by assessing perfusion. Capillary refill should occur within 2 s.

A joint committee of the American Heart Association and the American Academy of Pediatrics established recommendations for CPR and Pediatric Advanced Life Support (PALS), the details of which appear in a textbook edited by Chameides.[5] Here, only important differences between the resuscitation of adults and children will be pointed out and summaries of these pediatric recommendations presented. Those wishing the complete descriptions should consult this source.

If breathing is deemed inadequate, artificial ventilation should be started in infants and children with two initial breaths. Ventilation is continued in infants at 20 breaths per minute and at 15 breaths per minute in children. If, in addition, pulses are deemed absent or the heart rate is below 60 beats per minute in an infant with inadequate perfusion, chest compressions should be started with a ratio of five compressions to each respiration (5:1).

AIRWAY: IMPORTANT CONSIDERATIONS

The most common cause of complete cardiovascular collapse in children is respiratory compromise. Therefore, a search for airway pathology should be integrated into the initial approach to resuscitation, since prompt recognition and treatment of these causes can halt the cascade before full arrest.

The pediatric airway differs from the adult both quantitatively and qualitatively. Since resistance in the airway to laminar flow is inversely proportional to the radius of the airway raised to the fourth power, resistance rises dramatically in the anatomically smaller child's airway. Furthermore, disease states such as laryngotracheitis (croup), in which the edema further reduces the radius of the airway, can profoundly alter the resistance to airflow and markedly increase the work of breathing. Consequently, in order to achieve adequate ventilatory volumes in small infants or sick children, it is often necessary to generate higher airway pressures. These higher pressures increase the risk of complications of barotrauma, such as pneumothorax. Qualitatively, since the larynx is more cephalad and the vocal cords shorter and more concave, the skills required for endotracheal intubation are different. The narrowest part of the trachea in children under 8 years of age is just below the cords at the cricoid cartilage. Therefore, the tube size is not determined by the cord size, as it is in adults. A useful rule in determining the size of the endotracheal tube required is that the internal diameter of the tube in millimeters is 4 plus $\frac{1}{4}$ of the child's age in years.[6] Tube size for premature infants is 2.5 mm, and in the first year of life it is 3 to 4 mm. Since the narrow cricoid area of the trachea tends to afford some natural protection against aspiration, cuffed endotracheal tubes are generally not used or necessary in the child younger than 8 years old. Learning to intubate infants and children requires formal instruction and practice.

A critical decision in pediatric resuscitation relates to intubation. Since intubation is traumatic, often initiates vagal reflexes that slow the heart rate and lower blood pressure, tends to interrupt CPR, and halts air exchange during the procedure, the risks and benefits must be weighed and the timing correct. Given the factors discussed above, the individual performing the procedure in the pediatric patient must be specially trained. *If a patient cannot be intubated expedi-*

tiously and with minimal trauma, it is far better to bag-mask ventilate than to further worsen or reverse any improvement that has been achieved in the patient's condition by imposing the stress of a poorly performed or failed intubation. Adequate ventilation can be attained in most patients by the bag-mask technique and maintained for prolonged periods if necessary.

To bag-mask ventilate infants and children successfully, one must understand additional important considerations in providing ventilation for children. First, positioning the child to establish a straight pathway from the oropharynx to the trachea is important. The head and neck should be in the head-tilt ("sniffing") position (Fig. 13–1). Since the neck is more flexible in infants and children, it is possible to overextend the airway in the opposite direction. In an infant, a rolled diaper or blanket may be positioned under the neck and shoulders to support this position. If there is suspected cervical injury, hyperextension of the neck is to be avoided. The airway is then positioned with a jaw-thrust maneuver (Fig. 13–2) while the neck is immobilized. Second, a mask of the appropriate size must be used. The mask should cover the mouth and nose, but not the eyes. A tight seal between mask and face must be accomplished in the head-tilt position, taking care not to compress the soft airway in children. Third, the child should be ventilated with the correct size self-inflating bag. Self-inflating bags are preferred because they do not require that a source of oxygen be available. The correct bag size can be estimated using a tidal volume of 10 to 15 ml/kg. Many of these bags are equipped with pop-off valves to reduce the risk of barotrauma. It may be necessary to occlude this valve in the resuscitation situation in which more than 40 cmH_2O is required to establish initial ventilation. The required pressure is that which creates good chest excursion. The appropriate rate for infants is 20 breaths per minute and for children 15 breaths per minute.

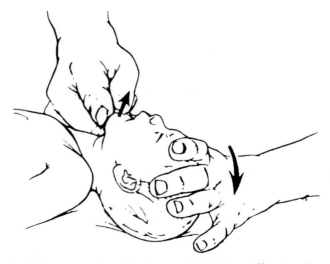

FIG. 13–1. Position of the head and neck. "Sniffing" position necessary to establish good ventilation. (*Textbook of Pediatric Advanced Life Support,* 1988, 1990. Copyright American Heart Association. Reproduced with permission.)

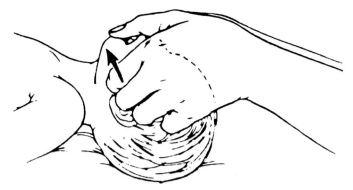

FIG. 13–2. Jaw-thrust maneuver. With elbows resting on a firm surface if possible, fingers are placed under each side of the lower jaw at its angle and the jaw lifted upward. (*Textbook of Pediatric Advanced Life Support,* 1988, 1990. Copyright American Heart Association. Reproduced with permission.)

Two other considerations regarding airway management in children should be mentioned. Children will generally assume the position that allows them to maintain a patent airway if they can. Therefore, in conscious children who are breathing on their own, one must allow them to keep the position they assume. *Do not force a child to lie down.* Second, there has never been a report of toxicity from supplemental oxygen administered during resuscitation. Therefore, *oxygen should be administered in all children who require resuscitation or manifest symptoms of an obstructed airway.*

Finally, in infants with respiratory depression from narcotics given during labor or in infants and children who receive accidental or self-administered narcotic overdose, naloxone hydrochloride may be lifesaving. Given at 0.1 mg/kg, it may be repeated every 2 to 3 minutes due to its short half-life and lack of respiratory depressive effects. The maximum total dose is 2.0 mg.

CAUSES OF VENTILATORY FAILURE

Common causes of respiratory distress in infants and children include croup, asthma, foreign body aspiration, bronchiolitis, epiglottitis, burns, smoke inhalation, near-drowning, pneumonia, pneumothorax, and flail chest. Foreign body aspiration and epiglottitis, although not unique to the pediatric population, are especially common. Most important, early recognition and treatment of these two conditions can result in a good outcome.

Foreign body aspiration most commonly occurs in the preschool child and becomes a threat as soon as infants at about 4 months begin to grab objects and bring them to their mouths. Children may aspirate food (especially peanuts and hard candies), toys or parts of toys, or anything small enough to fit into their mouths. Foreign body aspiration should be suspected in this age group in any child who suddenly develops stridor or cannot breathe.

The procedures to be followed depend on the clinical state and the age of the child.[5,7] If a child is able to breathe and cough effectively, then it is best to provide supportive care and avoid agitating the child. Leave the child in the position of comfort he or she has assumed, and provide oxygen if available. The child should be moved to an area or facility where bronchoscopy and laryngoscopy are available. During this period, the child should be observed carefully to see if he or she coughs up any objects, since the coughing may persist after the object has been expelled. One should not gain a false sense of security if a single object is found, since there may be more than one object involved. If either the child is unable to breathe or the child's cough and breathing become ineffective, active intervention is required. In the infant less than 1 year old, back blows and chest thrusts are preferred to abdominal thrusts to expel foreign bodies, since abdominal thrusts may cause intraabdominal injury. The infant is placed with the head down in the prone position over the rescuer's arm with the hand holding the jaw. Four back blows are administered between the shoulder blades. If the object is not expelled, then the infant is turned over and placed in the supine position on the rescuer's thigh with the head lower than the trunk. Four chest compressions are then performed in the same location as compressions for CPR. In the child more than 1 year old, the Heimlich maneuver[8] is recommended: Subdiaphragmatic thrusts are performed sequentially until the object is expelled or 10 thrusts have been completed. Standard rescue breathing techniques should be used if, after completion of the preceding, the infant or child does not resume spontaneous respirations.

Epiglottitis is an acute, life-threatening bacterial infection of the epiglottis most common in children 2 to 6 years old. Edema of the epiglottis and associated structures, usually resulting from *Haemophilis influenzae* infection (occasionally by staphylococcal or streptococcal infection), causes these laryngeal structures to be sucked into the airway on inspiration. This results in a characteristic presentation that may include fever (often high), stridor, drooling, difficulty swallowing, hoarse cough, respiratory distress, anxiety, toxicity, and the "tripod" position of comfort for the child. In this position, the child sits forward with neck extended, chin forward, and hands on the examination table. A lateral neck radiograph showing a swollen epiglottis ("thumb print" sign) is helpful in making the diagnosis. However, radiographic examination should only be attempted when a physician accompanies the child to a radiology suite that is in close proximity to the treatment area. The patient should remain in the upright position (position of comfort) at all times.

Nothing should be done to agitate the child. Parents should be allowed to stay with the child while the child is closely observed in a nonthreatening manner. Supplemental oxygen may be administered while preparations are made to bring the child to the operating room. There, an experienced anesthesiologist and surgeon can secure the airway, visualize the epiglottis, and obtain swabbings for culture. Parents should accompany the child to the operating room, where often they remain until sedation is administered. Emergency tracheostomy may be necessary if the airway becomes occluded and intubation fails.

Nowhere in medicine is the "first do no harm" rule more important. The "don'ts" of epiglottitis are potentially lifesaving. *Don't* attempt to look into the pharynx unless ready to immediately secure the airway. *Don't* do routine blood work. *Don't* allow unnecessary personnel to gather around. Generally, with successful airway management and antibiotic therapy, the edema will subside significantly within 2 to 3 days, allowing extubation.

CARDIAC ARREST

CHEST COMPRESSIONS

If preventive measures fail, or if the cascade to cardiac arrest is not halted by the reestablishment of ventilation, or if cardiac arrest is the manner of presentation, then chest compressions must be initiated. The rate and manner in which chest compressions are performed in infants and children are influenced by size and age. The ratio of 5:1 (compressions to ventilations) is recommended. To meet physiologic needs, 100 compressions and 20 breaths per minute in the infant and 75 compressions and 15 breaths per minute in children are required. A firm surface or support behind the back is necessary to ensure that compressions will generate flow. The depth of compression necessary is reduced in the smaller infant and child. Anatomic differences in the infant, as compared with the older child and adult, require a different location for compressions. Orlowski[9] showed by chest radiograph that the heart is located under the lower third of the sternum in infants and young children. In this study, the author found in 10 monitored patients in the pediatric intensive care unit that better systolic and mean arterial pressures were attained by compressions performed 1.5 to 2.0 cm above the xyphoid than by midsternal compressions, with each patient serving as his or her own control. For infants,[5,7] the sternum is compressed ½ to 1 inch using two or three fingers 100 times per minute at a point one finger breadth below an imaginary line between the nipples. Care should be taken not to compress the xyphoid. In a small infant, an additional modification may improve the technique, especially for rescuers with larger hands. Both thumbs are placed side by side (Fig. 13–3) or superimposed (Fig. 13–3, *inset*) on this portion of the sternum, and the fingers encircle the chest. This helps produce smoother compressions with less trauma and better control. In the young child,[5,7] compressions are made with the long axis of the heel of one hand parallel to the long axis of the sternum, with the inferior portion of the heel one finger breadth up from the inferior end of the sternum. Compression is 1 to 1½ inches at 80 to 100 times per minute. In the larger child (about 8 years and older), compression is performed with one or two hands 1½ to 2 inches at 80 to 100 times per minute as it is in an adult.

PHARMACOLOGIC TREATMENT OF ASYSTOLE

If effective cardiac action and perfusion are not rapidly restored, then pharmacologic measures are instituted. Doses recommended in this section follow PALS guidelines.[5] Those experienced in the critical care of infants and children have long recognized that, unlike adults, most children die in asystole. This experience was confirmed in the two studies previously cited,[2,3] where 91 percent of the cardiac arrests were asystole or bradydysrhythmias. Therefore, there is no

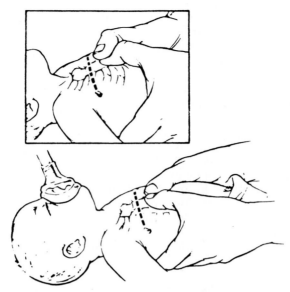

FIG. 13–3. Encirclement technique for chest compressions in neonates and small infants. Inset shows overlapping of thumbs (see text). (*Textbook of Pediatric Advanced Life Support,* 1988, 1990. Copyright American Heart Association. Reproduced with permission.)

role for defibrillation in unmonitored pediatric arrests. In order to determine the underlying cardiac rhythm, CPR should be interrupted briefly to enable cardiac rhythm determination from the monitor, rhythm strip, or electrocardiogram.

Epinephrine is the main pharmacologic agent for the treatment of asystole or bradycardia with ineffective circulation. Epinephrine not only stimulates cardiac contractility and rhythm but also improves myocardial and cerebral perfusion.[10,11] Epinephrine reverses arterial collapse during CPR, resulting in increased cerebral perfusion pressure and blood flow. Improved perfusion in the brain and myocardium has been demonstrated with radiolabeled microspheres. Oxygen uptake in these vital organs is also improved by epinephrine's selective vasoconstrictive effect on other vascular beds, thus preventing runoff during CPR.

The currently recommended dose of epinephrine for resuscitation is 0.01 mg/kg or 0.1 ml/kg of a 1:10,000 solution given by intravenous, endotracheal, or intraosseous route. Because of its short duration of action, it can be repeated at 5-minute intervals. Its positive effects include increased cardiac rate, automaticity, and contractility and increased vascular resistance resulting in increased blood pressure and favorable redistribution of blood flow to vital organs. The detrimental effects of epinephrine in this situation relate to increased myocardial oxygen consumption at a time when the oxygen supply to the myocardium is compromised.

Recently, higher doses of epinephrine have been suggested to improve outcome. Goetting and Paradis[12] compared the outcome prospectively of 20 consecutive patients who received high-dose epinephrine (HDE) with similar recent historic controls. They administered epinephrine at 0.2 mg/kg (20 times current recommendation) to children not responding to two standard doses. They found that 14 (70 percent) of the HDE-treated patients had return of spontaneous circulation within 5 minutes, whereas none of the controls demonstrated response ($p < 0.001$). Although all HDE-treated patients had sinus tachycardia for 15 minutes and mild to moderate hypertension, none developed life-threatening dysrhythmias or severe hypertension. Eight (40 percent) of the HDE-treated group survived to discharge, six neurologically intact. This compares favorably with the 5.5 percent survival rate described earlier in this chapter for patients suffering in-hospital arrest. However, two recently published prospectively randomized, large-scale studies in adults have failed to demonstrate improved outcome using HDE.[12a,12b]

Sodium bicarbonate ($NaHCO_3$) 1.0 mEq/kg may be required for the treatment of metabolic acidosis. Anaerobic metabolism from hypoxia and poor perfusion result in lactic acid production. Hypoventilation and resultant hypercapnia may cause concurrent respiratory acidosis. If the arrest does not respond to CPR, epinephrine, and hyperventilation and acidosis is severe, then $NaHCO_3$ should be infused intravenously or by intraosseous route. Additional doses should be guided by blood gas determinations. Treatment of the acidosis at this time is necessary because catecholamines such as epinephrine are not effective in an environment that is too acidotic (or alkalotic). The standard preparation of $NaHCO_3$ (8.4%) is hyperosmolar and may cause central nervous system hemorrhage in infants. A preparation with 0.5 mEq/ml (or the standard solution diluted with sterile water 1:1) is infused at double the volume to give the equivalent dose in infants weighing less than 5 kg (about 3 months of age).

It is preferable to treat acidosis with hyperventilation because of the negative consequences associated with the administration of $NaHCO_3$. Paradoxical cerebral intracellular acidosis can occur as the resultant carbon dioxide (CO_2) produced by $NaHCO_3$ more readily crosses the blood-brain barrier than the bicarbonate ion. Although the potential adverse effects on the central nervous system are speculative, they require consideration in the decision process. This increased CO_2 production also requires adequate ventilation to prevent its accumulation in the body. Other harmful consequences include excess water and sodium load (for each milliequivalent of bicarbonate administered, 1.0 mEq of sodium is given), decreased oxygen delivery due to left shift of the oxyhemoglobin disassociation curve, decreased ionized calcium due to enhanced protein binding, and decreased serum potassium as it shifts intracellularly.[5] Because $NaHCO_3$ is hyperosmolar, it would damage the respiratory mucous membranes, and therefore it cannot be administered by endotracheal instillation. Finally, since catecholamines are inactivated in alkaline solutions and calcium precipitates with $NaHCO_3$, these agents should not be administered with $NaHCO_3$ or without a flush between them through the same line.

Most bradycardia in infants and children is due to hypoventilation. If adequate ventilation is restored, heart rate will improve. However, if CPR, hyperventilation, and epinephrine do not improve heart rate and perfusion is poor, then 0.02 mg/kg of atropine is given at 5-minute intervals. Atropine is given via vein, intratracheal, or intraosseous routes. The maximum dose is 1.0 mg for a child and 2.0 mg for an adolescent. Since low doses may cause a paradoxical bradycardia, the minimum dose should be 0.1 mg. Atropine also may be administered to patients with atrioventricular block (since it enhances conduction through the atrioventricular node).

While complete heart block is best treated by temporary artificial pacing, isoproterenol may temporize the situation by enhancing conduction or increasing the rate of the escape rhythm. This pure beta-adrenergic agent increases heart rate, conduction velocity, and contractility while causing peripheral vasodilation. The infusion should be started at 0.1 μg/kg/min and increased until either the desired effect or significant side effects are encountered or the maximum dose of 1.0 μg/kg/min is reached.

During periods of stress, infants and small children may rapidly deplete glycogen stores, resulting in hypoglycemia. Not only is glucose availability important during the increased demands of the heart during resuscitation, but it is necessary to maintain central nervous system integrity. If an infant is allowed to remain hypoglycemic during resuscitation, severe neurologic impairment is likely. Dextrostix should be monitored in all critically ill infants. Glucose should be administered intravenously at 0.5 to 1.0 g/kg using $D_{25}W$, which is 2 to 4 ml/kg in the child. In infants (especially neonates), it is preferable to use $D_{10}W$ (5 to 10 ml/kg) to avoid possible side effects from the more hyperosmolar solution.

The use of calcium in resuscitation is controversial. While calcium may improve contractility transiently, it has been implicated in causing increased cell death. This negative effect may preclude its use for whatever short-term improvement may be gained. The only currently accepted indications for the use of calcium include treatment to reverse calcium channel blocker–induced hypotension and bradycardia and treatment of hyperkalemia, hypermagnesemia, and true hypocalcemia. A dose of 0.2 to 0.25 ml/kg of a 10% calcium chloride solution will provide 5 to 7 mg/kg ionized calcium. Heart rate should be monitored carefully during administration, since bradycardia may occur. Caution is also advised in its use in patients receiving digitalis, since calcium may potentiate digitalis-induced dysrhythmias.

TREATMENT OF VENTRICULAR DYSRHYTHMIAS

Ventricular dysrhythmias in infants and children are not common. They may, however, occur in the arrest situation. Patients at risk for ventricular dysrhythmias include those with congenital cardiac defects, congestive heart failure, or electrolyte imbalances. Postoperative cardiac surgery patients, patients on cardiac medications or tricyclic antidepressants, electric shock victims, and near-drowning victims are also at risk. However, ventricular dysrhythmias are not unique to these situations and may be seen in any patient experiencing hypoxic arrest.

Ventricular fibrillation requires immediate electrical defibrillation using direct current. The current administered to infants and children is 2 J/kg. If unsuccessful, the current is doubled.[13] Effective and safe delivery of electrical energy requires a calm, thoughtful approach with attention to detail. The largest paddle size that will allow good skin contact and separation of the paddles should be chosen. An electrode gel or cream is necessary to ensure good conductivity and to help avoid skin burns. Firm pressure should be applied to the paddles while administering current. Paddle position during CPR is at the second rib to the right of the sternum and at the midclavicular line to the left of the sternum at the level of the xyphoid. CPR should be continued until one is ready to administer the current. It is imperative that the operator of the defibrillator delineate the steps in a clear command voice, checking and announcing that there is no contact between rescue personnel (including the operator) and the patient, bed, or equipment attached to the patient. The rhythm should be rechecked to be sure that it is still ventricular fibrillation prior to shocking the patient. Immediately after the shock has been delivered, the rhythm should be ascertained and CPR continued.

The key pharmacologic agent in the treatment of ventricular dysrhythmias is lidocaine. A bolus of 1.0 mg/kg lidocaine is administered via the intravenous or intraosseous route. This should be followed by an infusion of 20 to 50 μg/kg/min to suppress ventricular ectopy and prevent recurrence. Whether lidocaine is used to treat a ventricular tachyarrhythmia following defibrillation or one that has occurred spontaneously, it is necessary to give a second bolus of 1.0 mg/kg in 10 to 20 minutes, even as the continuous infusion is being started. Due to the short half-life of lidocaine, failure to administer the additional bolus may allow the blood level to become subtherapeutic before the continuous infusion can attain a therapeutic level.

Bretylium use in children is problematic. There are no studies of its effectiveness in children or data to support 5 mg/kg as the recommended dose.

ADVANCED SUPPORT

Shock, simply defined, is the inability of the cardiovascular system to meet the metabolic demands of the body. Following initial resuscitation, or in infants and children heading down the cascade to cardiac arrest, it is necessary to maintain a cardiac output that will prevent or reverse shock. Note that hypotension is not included in this definition. Shock usually begins in a compensated state with the vascular system maintaining blood pressure despite inadequate cardiac output. Therapy is much more likely to reverse shock if it is recognized at this early, compensated stage. Therefore, to stay ahead of the cascade, it is imperative to recognize signs of compensated shock before hypotension occurs. Vasoconstriction results in grayish, cold, clammy skin with delayed capillary refill (>2 s) and decreased renal blood flow with resultant low urine output (<0.8 to 1.0 ml/kg/h). The heart compensates by increasing rate to improve output, so tachycardia or a trend toward increasing heart rate is observed. Inadequate tissue perfusion with hypoxia drives ventilation, leading to tachypnea. To understand the prevention and treatment of shock, it must be recognized that four principal components determine cardiac output and effective circulation. One must be prepared to treat one or all of these components to attain maximal results. Schematically, this system can be represented as follows:

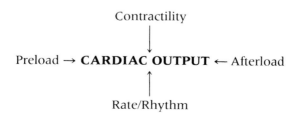

PRELOAD

Adequate preload is necessary to maintain effective circulation. After respiratory failure, the next most important cause of cardiovascular collapse in infants and children is hypovolemia. Hypovolemia may be absolute, as a consequence of inadequate circulating volume, or relative to an increased vascular capacitance. Absolute hypovolemia can result from hemorrhage (trauma, accidents of birth), plasma leakage (sepsis, crush injury, burns, toxins), and dehydration (vomiting, diarrhea, diabetic ketoacidosis, heat stroke, anorexia, cystic fibrosis, adrenogenital syndromes, diabetes insipidus, anaphylaxis). Relative hypovolemia leads to states that increase capacitance, requiring increased circulating volume. This condition can result from sepsis (vasodilatation, cell injury), central nervous system injury (vasodilation, loss of vascular control), anaphylaxis (vasodilation), toxins, or drugs. Note that the etiology may lead to combined absolute and relative hypovolemia. This may occur in sepsis and anaphylaxis, with capillary leakage contributing to absolute hypovolemia and vasodilation contributing to the relative component.

Treatment principles include obtaining a good history and physical examination. The goals are to ascertain the etiology and address the specific problems resulting from that condition, to restore circulating fluid volume as rapidly as possible, and to provide fluids to compensate for ongoing losses and maintenance requirements. While the most important initial step is to rapidly restore circulating fluid volume, one must not lose sight of the importance of diagnosis. For example, if sepsis is not recognized as the underlying cause, although circulating volume may be initially restored, the infection will lead to irreversible shock if untreated.

The initial treatment and first priority are to restore circulating fluid volume. Colloid solutions may be employed because they tend to stay in the vascular space longer than crystalloid and because smaller volumes are required to expand the circulating volume. Albumin may be administered as rapidly as needed, at 0.5 to 1.0 g/kg, which is 10 to 20 ml/kg of 5% albumin or 2 to 4 ml/kg of 25% albumin. The disadvantages of colloid solutions include the possibility of allergic reaction (rare), high sodium load (130 to 160 mEq/liter), and expense. Alternatively, fresh frozen plasma given at 10 to 20 ml/kg can be used to expand circulating volume and has the added advantage of supplying clotting factors that may be depleted. The disadvantages include that it must be thawed and is a blood product. Crystalloid solutions such as normal saline and Ringer's lactate are usually more readily available for immediate administration and are infused at 20 ml/kg. The disadvantage is that only about 25 percent of the infused solution remains in the vascular space. Additional fluid pushes are given until there is evidence that circulating volume has been restored, as judged by improved heart rate and blood pressure, brisk capillary refill, urine output of at least 1.0 ml/kg/h, or normalized central venous pressure. The most common error is undertreatment. Although it is preferable to replace blood loss with blood, it is worse for the patient to be hypovolemic and anemic than to be just anemic; therefore, restoration of circulating volume is accomplished while waiting for blood to be readied.

Known or estimated ongoing losses should be quantified, if possible, and replaced milliliter for milliliter with the appropriate fluids. Several methods have been advocated for common dehydration states. Basically, all accomplish replacement of ongoing losses and maintenance fluids. General pediatric textbooks should be consulted for details. Finally, ultimate outcome is critically dependent on treatment of the underlying condition with the appropriate therapy.

Cardiac tamponade deserves special mention in the pediatric patient. Although it is generally associated with thoracic trauma and heart surgery, bacterial infections in childhood may cause purulent pericarditis resulting in tamponade. The typical presentation is that of an infant or child who appears to be making satisfactory progress with treatment for sepsis or pneumonia but who then suddenly begins to look toxic. Tachypnea, dyspnea, and tachycardia develop. On examination, there may be pulsus paradoxus, hepatomegaly, and distant or muffled heart sounds. Jugular venous distension is not easily detected in babies who have short necks and a lot of subcutaneous tissue. The diagnosis is confirmed by echocardiography. Since elevated pericardial pressure interferes with the filling of the heart, volume infusion can provide adequate preload to improve output while preparing for an emergency pericardiocentesis. The method I prefer[14] is to use a 16-gauge angiocatheter from the left subxyphoid approach and relieve the pressure by draining fluid from the pericardial space. After the hemodynamics are improved, a Teflon-coated floppy-tipped guidewire is advanced into the pericardial space. The angiocatheter is removed, and after dilating the entry site, a pigtail catheter is advanced and left in the pericardium to continue to drain the purulent fluid. If successful, surgical drainage, which was often required in the past, may not be necessary.

Excess fluid can increase end-diastolic pressure in the heart, stretching the muscle and thus causing the heart to function on the downward or flattened portion of the Starling curve. The result is congestive heart failure. This problem may be caused by injudicious fluid administration or renal failure. Conversely, if congestive heart failure is present, decreased renal blood flow will result in decreased urine output, resulting in increased preload and worsening heart failure. The most common cause of congestive heart failure in infants and children is a congenital cardiac defect with right, left, or biventricular failure. Regardless of type, the initial therapy is to decrease preload by diuresis and fluid restriction. Furosemide given intravenously at 0.5 to 1.0 mg/kg slowly is the initial drug of choice. If the patient is unresponsive, double or triple the dose may be given. If there is renal failure, either as a cause or result of congestive heart failure, then renal dialysis may be necessary to remedy the situation.

CONTRACTILITY AND AFTERLOAD

Historically, treatment of shock was aimed at increasing contractility and blood pressure, and afterload was not of paramount consideration. However, it came to be understood that this therapeutic rationale often resulted in the state of compensated shock and that if improved perfusion of vital organs was not attained, the patient would die. Because the available pharmacologic modalities that treat contractility also affect afterload, one must be cognizant of the effects of one on the other.

Epinephrine is a powerful alpha- and beta-adrenergic agonist that is useful in the treatment of profound shock, especially if blood pressure has not responded to other adrenergic agents. Infused at 0.1 to 2.0 μg/kg/min, it will improve contractility, rate, automaticity, and blood pressure. The dose determines its effects. At lower doses, its beta properties will result in vasodilation. At doses greater than 0.5 μg/kg/min, it is principally an alpha agonist. The resultant vasoconstriction may cause significant ischemia to the mesentery, renal vascular bed, and skin.

Dopamine, because its behavior is determined by dose, is best considered as three drugs in one. At doses less than 5.0 μg/kg/min, dopamine stimulates receptors (dopaminergic) that dilate the renal vascular bed, and thus it can be used to improve compromised renal blood flow. At doses about 5 to 10 μg/kg/min, it has both alpha- and beta-adrenergic properties, improving contractility and cardiac output and increasing blood pressure. At doses exceeding 10 μg/kg/min, it is principally alpha-adrenergic, inducing increased vasoconstriction.

Dobutamine is a relatively selective beta-adrenergic agent. Infused at 2.5 to 20 μg/kg/min, it increases cardiac contractility and output. Combining dobutamine and dopamine allows one to manipulate contractility and afterload to obtain an optimal cardiovascular state. If one infuses dopamine at a low dose (<5.0 μg/kg/min) to maintain renal blood flow through its dopaminergic stimulation, one can infuse dobutamine concurrently at doses chosen to maximize cardiac output and contractility with minimal vasoconstrictive effects. The net effect should be to improve cardiac output and contractility, renal blood flow, and perfusion of vital organs.

Nitroprusside is a vasodilator that has been useful in reducing afterload in infants and children. Infusion is begun at 0.5 μg/kg/min and is titrated to its desired effect (up to 10 μg/kg/min). Because nitroprusside may cause hypotension, preload must be adequate. It may be desirable to monitor central venous and/or pulmonary capillary wedge pressure as well as arterial pressure during infusion. Nitroprusside decreases systemic and pulmonary vascular resistance, resulting in a lower workload for the heart and thus producing an increase in cardiac output and improved vital organ perfusion. It is often combined with dopamine or other adrenergic agents when used to maximize cardiac output. Once nitroprusside infusion is begun, it is increased every 5 minutes by 0.5 μg/kg/min until a fall in arterial blood pressure is noted. The infusion rate is immediately reduced by 0.5 to 1.0 μg/kg/min, which should result in maximum forward flow and perfusion. If practical, this can be monitored by measuring cardiac output as well. Severe, sudden hypotension may be a serious consequence, but since nitroprusside is short-acting, prompt recognition and termination or reduction of the infusion may restore blood pressure. If necessary, volume infusion and increased inotropic support can be utilized to help reverse the hypotension. Cyanide is produced by the metabolism of nitroprusside. To avoid toxicity, especially in infants, thiocyanate levels are monitored after 48 h.

Although these vasoactive drugs are lifesaving in the resuscitation situation, their potent effects necessitate a discussion of some practical and safety considerations for safe and effective use. Proper dosages and rates of administration should be carefully calculated and double-checked. The formula to convert μg/kg/min to ml/h is as follows:

$$\text{ml/h} = \frac{\text{kg wt} \times \text{μg/kg/min} \times 60\ \text{min/h}}{\text{μg/ml in the solution}}$$

These drugs, especially those with alpha-adrenergic properties, should be infused in the largest vein that can be cannulated (central is preferable) because extravasation may lead to necrosis. If there is doubt about the integrity of the infusion site, the site should be changed immediately. These drugs should be given by infusion pumps to ensure accurate, stable rates of administration. Rates and concentrations should be checked carefully. It is recommended that solutions be formulated in uniform concentrations for each drug to minimize the chance of error. If the solution compositions and rates are familiar to all personnel, then personnel are more likely to note errors in administration. Patients should be monitored carefully and, most important, *observed* carefully.

RATE/RHYTHM

When stressed, most patients optimize cardiac output by increasing heart rate to about 20 to 25 percent above mean rate for age, and manipulation is not necessary. However, certain pathologic states, such as heart block or tachydysrhythmias or the presence of toxins or drugs, may cause the rate to be too slow or too fast. In these situations, cardiac output may be compromised.

As mentioned earlier, atropine and isoproterenol may be useful in temporizing patients who are compromised by complete heart block. These agents increase the escape rhythm if the inherent escape rhythm is not fast enough. Insertion of temporary transvenous or epicardial pacemakers in this situation is lifesaving. Pacemaker insertion should be accomplished as soon as possible to enable control of the rate. The transvenous route has an advantage because it allows dual-chamber pacing so that sequential atrioventricular activity can be restored. The loss of sequential activity in complete heart block reduces cardiac output by 25 percent independent of rate effect. If pacing is needed beyond the early resuscitation period, dual-chamber pacing can help by restoring the atrial contribution to cardiac output in the management of low-output states.

Tachydysrhythmias, atrial as well as ventricular, may be acutely life-threatening in infants and children. Supraventricular tachycardia may cause congestive heart failure and death in newborns. Prompt recognition and treatment are imperative. In fact, the most common cause of hydrops fetalis and congestive heart failure in the first days of life is supraventricular tachycardia. Newborn infants do not tolerate rapid heart rates. Regardless of whether the rhythm is deemed supraventricular or ventricular in origin, the presence of hemodynamic compromise is an indication for immediate synchronous electrical cardioversion. Using the paddle technique described earlier for defibrillation, a *synchronized* shock is administered at 0.5 to 1.0 J/kg. Care must be taken to be sure that the defibrillation unit is in the synchronized mode and that the monitor shows synchronization with the patient's rhythm, because a randomly administered electric current may result in a more disorganized and dangerous rhythm than the one being treated. If unsuccessful, double the current and repeat. If still unsuccessful, additional treatment depends on whether the rhythm is thought to be ventricular or atrial in nature. For wide QRS tachycardia or suspected ventricular tachycardia, synchronized cardioversion after administration of a 1.0-mg/kg lidocaine bolus is repeated at 2.0 J/kg. Another condition that can be confused with ventricular tachycardia in infants with wide QRS complexes is hyperkalemia, which may be suspected in babies with sepsis or renal failure. The heart rate is usually slower in hyperkalemia than in ventricular tachycardia. The treatment is to lower the potassium; antidysrhythmia therapy is not indicated and will not change this pattern.

For narrow QRS tachycardia, digoxin administration may be necessary if initial conversion is unsuccessful or if a sinus rhythm cannot be maintained after cardioversion. The administration and dosing of digoxin to infants and children should be done under the supervision of a pediatric cardiologist.

Supraventricular dysrhythmias not associated with hemodynamic compromise may be treated initially with vagal maneuvers such as carotid massage, Valsalva maneuver, or a large ice bag over the face (diving reflex). Subsequent pharmacologic therapy is tailored to the patient's condition and age. Verapamil can be given intravenously at 0.1 to 0.2 mg/kg over 2 to 3 minutes (maximum 5.0 mg) or 5 to 10 mg in an adolescent. Verapamil should not be used in infants because fatalities from its use have been reported.[15] When verapamil is used, a secure intravenous line should be available to infuse volume, calcium, and, if severe hypotension or bradycardia occur, inotropic agents. Digoxin remains a very effective drug for supraventricular tachycardia both for immediate and long-term treatment. Digoxin therapy requires supervision by a pediatric cardiologist. Propanolol given by slow intravenous infusion at 0.01 to 0.1 mg/kg (maximum 1.0 mg) may be used. Propanolol is contraindicated in patients with asthma, and one should be prepared to administer volume and inotropic agents if severe hypotension and bradycardia occur. Finally, adenosine has been used recently to treat supraventricular tachycardia in infants and children.[17] It is given by rapid intravenous bolus at 0.1 to 0.3 mg/kg because its half-life is less than 10 s. Transient flushing, irritability, dyspnea, and bradycardia may occur.

OBTAINING VASCULAR ACCESS

Obtaining vascular access during an arrest or in a patient in shock may be difficult due to vascular collapse. If one considers the additional problems in pediatrics of small size and the infant with significant subcutaneous tissue, vascular access may be a real dilemma. The standard peripheral and central venous sites of subclavian, internal jugular, and femoral veins may be used. The femoral vein is generally recommended as the preferred central site because there is no danger of causing pneumothorax and its use does not interfere with CPR. The latter is of real practical significance because in the small child there simply may not be room available to do chest compressions, ventilations, and also prepare the chest or neck for venipuncture. Details of cannulation of these sites are available in the textbook edited by Chameides.[5] In addition, during the initial phase, the trachea may be used to give epinephrine, atropine, and lidocaine. However, there still must be vascular access to infuse other medications (e.g., $NaHCO_3$), give volume, and administer adrenergic drips.

In children under 3 years of age, infusion via the intraosseous space is safe and effective. The area one finger breadth below the tibial tuberosity is antiseptically prepared (Fig. 13–4). A 16- or 18-gauge needle with stylet or a bone marrow needle is advanced into the periosteum, perpendicular to the skin and away from the epiphyseal plate. When the marrow is penetrated, a sudden de-

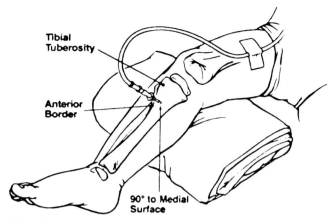

FIG. 13–4. Intraosseous cannulation technique. See text. (*Textbook of Pediatric Advanced Life Support,* 1988, 1990. Copyright American Heart Association. Reproduced with permission.)

crease in resistance is felt. The stylet is removed, and marrow is aspirated with a saline-filled syringe. Saline is then infused to clear clot and confirm position in the marrow before other medications or solutions are given.[18] This procedure may be accomplished in about the same time as a standard venipuncture.

NEONATAL RESUSCITATION

A complete discussion of the resuscitation of newborns is beyond the scope of this chapter but can be found in the *Textbook of Neonatal Resuscitation.*[19] The principles of neonatal resuscitation are similar to those described earlier. Several important points will be highlighted here.

Heat loss is a significant problem for the newborn because of the large surface area to weight ratio. Cold stress increases metabolic demand and delays resolution of acidosis. One of the priorities in management after the infant emerges from the birth canal is to dry off the skin as quickly as possible to reduce heat loss from evaporation. One must be cognizant that even if the newborn is in an overhead warmer, he or she will continue to lose heat to the cooler room air by convection and to the walls of the room by radiation. Therefore, as soon as possible, the child should be transferred to a heated isolette.

In newborn resuscitation, restoring adequate ventilation is often all that is required. The mouth is suctioned first to prevent aspiration, followed by suctioning of the nose. Since deep suctioning may induce a vagal response, heart rate should be watched and suction limited to less than 10 s. One should keep in mind that infants are obligate nose breathers at birth and must learn to breathe from the mouth; therefore, nasal passages must not be occluded. Rescue breathing in infants requires that the seal include the nose within the mask or mouth to prevent the possible escape of air. Meconium aspiration is a deadly condition that may be treated by vigorous airway management. If meconium is present, the airway should be suctioned as soon as the head is delivered and, if possible, before the baby's first breath. Intubation and suctioning may be required to remove as much meconium from the airway as possible. One should avoid positive-pressure breathing until meconium is removed, since it may drive the meconium into the lungs.

Infants with severe congenital cardiac defects may deteriorate and die quickly as the ductus arteriosus closes. There are two classes of congenital lesions in which infants may be "ductal dependent": cyanotic lesions and left ventricular outflow obstructive lesions. Prompt recognition and treatment of these infants with prostaglandin E_1 (PGE_1) may be lifesaving and palliative until further treatment or transfer to an appropriate facility can be accomplished. Infants with severe cyanotic lesions from right to left shunts within the heart can develop severe hypoxia, resulting in metabolic acidosis. Cyanosis can result either from lesions such as transposition of the great arteries, where there is inadequate mixing within the heart to provide enough oxygen to the systemic circulation, or from lesions such as pulmonary valve atresia, where pulmonary blood flow does not come from the heart directly. Infants with such lesions are recognized by their deep cyanotic appearance which fails to improve with the administration of oxygen. If the arterial P_{O_2} fails to increase to above 150 mmHg after the administration of 100% oxygen for 10 minutes, then a critical cyanotic heart lesion is likely. Administration of PGE_1 at 0.05 to 0.1 μg/kg/min may improve the oxygenation and acidosis. Lesions that obstruct left ventricular or systemic output, such as critical aortic stenosis or coarctation of the aorta, may cause life-threatening congestive heart failure. A patent ductus can provide adequate systemic blood flow by shunting from the pulmonary circulation, which is usually a high-pressure circulation in these newborns, into the aorta, thus providing flow to critical organs. Natural closure of the ductus may cause shock. PGE_1 at the preceding dose with inotropic support may be lifesaving. PGE_1 should be administered in consultation with the pediatric cardiologist who is to care for the infant, since its side effects or misuse also may be life-threatening. PGE_1 is a potent vasodilator that may cause hypotension. Serious side effects include apnea, bradycardia, and seizures.

Vascular access can be attained through the umbilical cord. There are usually three vessels within the cord, with the vein being the largest and having a thin wall. Umbilical tape is tied around the base of the cord, and the cord is cut about 1.0 cm above the tape. An umbilical catheter is passed until easy blood return is obtained; then medications can be administered. The catheter should not be advanced too far, since it may lodge in the liver, where vasoactive drugs may cause necrosis.

PEDIATRIC TRAUMA

Preceding sections in this chapter have dealt with volume resuscitation, management of shock, and airway management in children. Other chapters in this book discuss head injury, neurogenic shock, and burn resuscitation. These principles are applied to the resuscitation of childhood trauma victims in conjunction with specific specialty treatment.

MANAGEMENT STRATEGY

A pediatric code team or resuscitation team should be organized in all facilities that treat infants and children. The team should include a pediatrician (preferably a pediatric intensivist), a surgeon, an anesthesiologist, experienced pediatric nurses, and a respiratory therapist. Ideally, all the members of the team should be pediatric subspecialists or intensive care unit personnel. Resuscitation in the delivery room requires a team with a pediatrician, nurse practitioner, anesthesiologist, and neonatal nurse. Ideally, mock arrests and resuscitation exercises should be conducted on a regular basis to keep personnel current on infant and pediatric resuscitation. Preparation is important to ensure that the appropriate supplies, equipment, and drugs are available for pediatric needs.

It is also helpful to have available and accessible data sheets or cards that present the information needed to assess and treat infants and children of various sizes and ages. Hospital computer systems may be programmed to print out the correct endotracheal tube size, resuscitation doses, and infusion doses and concentrations required if the age and estimated size of the child are entered. Tables 13–1 to 13–5 relate the data presented in this chapter and may be used to construct data sheets or prepare computer programs.

TABLE 13–1. Useful Normal Parameters for Children

Age	Respiratory Rate	Heart Rate	Lower Limit, Systolic BP	Compressions/Ventilations per Minute of CPR and Depth
Infants	20–40	70–160	~65	100/20, ½ to 1 inches
Children	~20	80–120	~80	75/15, 1 to 1½ inches
Adolescents	12–20	50–90	~90	75/15, 1½ to 2 inches

TABLE 13–2. Useful Formulas for Pediatrics

Endotracheal tube internal diameter (mm) $= 4 + \frac{1}{4}$ age (in years)
Tidal volume $= 10\text{--}15$ ml/kg
Defibrillation $= 2$ J/kg—double if unsuccessful
Synchronized cardioversion $= 0.5$ to 1.0 J/kg—double prn
Minimum urine output $= 1.0$ ml/kg/h; capillary refill <2 s
$$\text{Infusion (ml/h)} = \frac{\text{kg body wt} \times \mu\text{g/kg/min} \times 60 \text{ min/h}}{\mu\text{g/ml solution concentration}}$$

TABLE 13–3. "Arrest" Medications and Advanced Support

Drug	Dose for Arrest	Infusion Rate
Epinephrine	0.1 ml/kg 1:10,000 sol = 0.01 mg/kg q5min	0.1–2.0 µg/kg/min
NaHCO₃	1.0 mEq/kg	
Atropine	0.02 mg/kg, min. 0.1, max. 2.0 mg	
Isproterenol		0.1–1.0 µg/kg/min, increase q2–3min
Naloxone HCl	0.1 mg/kg q2–3min, max. 2.0 mg	
Glucose	0.5–1.0 g/kg	2–4 ml/kg D₂₅W 5–10 ml/kg D₁₀W infants
Lidocaine	1.0 mg/kg bolus, repeat in 10 to 20 min	20–50 µg/kg/min
Dopamine		1–4 µg/kg/min renal 5–10 µg/kg/min alpha/beta 10–20 µg/kg/min alpha
Dobutamine		2.5–20 µg/kg/min
Nitroprusside		0.5–10.0 µg/kg/min
PGE₁		0.05–0.1 µg/kg/min

TABLE 13–4. Volume Expanders

Agent	Infusion Rate
Albumin	0.5–1.0 g/kg q10–20min prn
5%	10–20 ml/kg
25%	2–4 ml/kg
Fresh frozen plasma	10–20 ml/kg q10–20min prn
NS/Ringer's lactate	20 ml/kg q10–20min prn

TABLE 13–5. Antidysrhythmia Drug Dosages

Drug	Dosage
Lidocaine	1.0 mg/kg bolus; repeat in 10 to 20 min
Verapamil	0.1–0.2 mg/kg 2 to 3 min; max. 5–10 mg
Propanolol	0.01–0.1 mg/kg slow; max. 1.0 mg
Adenosine	0.1–0.3 mg/kg rapid bolus
Bretylium	5 mg/kg

REFERENCES

1. Eisenberg M, Bergner L, Halstrom A: Paramedic programs and out-of-hospital cardiac arrest: I. Factors associated with successful resuscitation. *Am J Public Health* 69:30, 1979.

2. Gray WA, Capone RJ, Most AS: Unsuccessful emergency medical resuscitation: Are continued efforts in the emergency department justified? *N Engl J Med* 325:1393, 1991.

3. Gillis J, Dickson D, Rieder M, et al: Results of inpatient pediatric resuscitation. *Crit Care Med* 14:469, 1986.

4. Torphy DE, Minter MG, Thompson BM: Cardiopulmonary arrest and resuscitation of children. *Am J Dis Child* 138:1099, 1984.

5. Chameides L (ed): *Textbook of Pediatric Advanced Life Support.* Dallas, American Heart Association, 1988, 1990.

6. Jaffe DJ, Wesson D: Emergency management of blunt trauma in children. *N Engl J Med* 324:1477, 1991.

7. Silverman BK (ed): *Advanced Pediatric Life Support.* Elk Grove Village/Dallas, American Academy of Pediatrics/American College of Emergency Physicians, 1989.

8. Heimlich HJ: A life-saving maneuver to prevent food choking. *JAMA* 234:398, 1975.

9. Orlowski JP: Optimum position for external cardiac compressions in infants and young children. *Ann Emerg Med* 15:667, 1986.

10. Michael JR, Guerci AD, Koehler RC, et al: Mechanisms by which epinephrine augments cerebral and myocardial perfusion during cardiopulmonary resuscitation in dogs. *Circulation* 69(4):822, 1984.

11. Schleien CL, Dean JM, Koehler RC, et al: Effect of epinephrine on cerebral and myocardial perfusion in an infant animal preparation of cardiopulmonary resuscitation. *Circulation* 73(4):809, 1986.

12. Goetting MG, Paradis NA: High-dose epinephrine improves outcome from pediatric cardiac arrest. *Ann Emerg Med* 20(1):22, 1991.

12a. Brown CG, Martin DR, Pede PE, et al and the Multicenter High Dose Epinephrine Study Group: A comparison of standard dose and high dose epinephrine in cardiac arrest outside the hospital. *New Engl J Med* 327:1051, 1992.

12b. Stiell IG, Hebert PC, Weizman BN, et al: High-dose epinephrine in adult cardiac arrest. *N Engl J Med* 327:1045, 1992.

13. Chameides L, Brown G, Raye JR, et al: Guidelines for defibrillation in infants and children. *Circulation* 56(3):502A, 1977.

14. Biancaniello TM, Anagnostopoulos CE, Bernstein HE, Proctor C: Purulent meningococcal pericarditis: Chronic percutaneous drainage with modified catheter aided by echocardiography. *Clin Cardiol* 8:542, 1985.

15. Radford D: Side effects of verapamil in infants. *Arch Dis Child* 58:465, 1983.

16. Epstein ML, Kiel EA, Victorica BE: Cardiac decompensation following verapamil therapy in infants with supraventricular tachycardia. *Pediatrics* 75:737, 1985.

17. Overholt ED, Rheuban KS, Gutgesell HP, et al: Usefulness of adenosine for arrhythmias in infants and children. *Am J Cardiol* 61:336, 1988.

18. Rosetti VA, Thompson BM, Miller J, et al: Intraosseous infusion: 'An alternative route of pediatric intravascular access. *Ann Emerg Med* 14:885, 1985.

19. Chameides L (ed): *Textbook of Neonatal Resuscitation.* Dallas, American Heart Association, 1987, 1990.

14

ANAPHYLAXIS

Kathy R. Sonenthal
Roy Patterson

CLINICAL SYNDROME

HISTORY AND DEFINITIONS

Anaphylaxis is a severe systemic form of immediate hypersensitivity. It results from the sudden release into the circulatory system of mediators derived from mast cells and/or basophils. Urticaria, asthma, airway edema, vascular collapse, diarrhea, and abdominal pain are common clinical signs. In severe cases, anaphylaxis can cause death.

This chapter reviews the historical background of anaphylaxis, its epidemiology and etiology, as well as the mechanisms and mediators of the reaction. In addition, this chapter examines the clinical manifestations, diagnosis, treatment, and various methods of prophylaxis of this syndrome.

Retrospectively, the initial report of anaphylaxis may have been recorded in 2640 B.C. in hieroglyphics describing the sudden death of an Egyptian pharoah after a wasp sting.[1] The term *anaphylaxis* was coined in 1902 by Portier and Richet,[2] who used it to denote a paradoxical effect that occurred when they were using a specific immunization protocol. They had attempted to induce tolerance or resistance in dogs to a toxin derived from the sea anemone by repeatedly injecting large, but sublethal, doses of toxin into the dogs. Weeks later, when they injected a much smaller dose of the toxin into the dogs, the animals died almost immediately. Instead of the protective or prophylactic effect they had anticipated, they believed that these dogs had an increased sensitivity to the toxin. This increased sensitivity was referred to as *anaphylaxis*, based on the Greek words *ana*, meaning "without," and *phylaxis*, meaning "protection."

Since 1902, anaphylaxis has been studied extensively. Early investigation led to the finding that anaphylactic sensitivity is acquired; that is, previous exposure and a delay before reexposure are required. Subsequent studies demonstrated that anaphylaxis could be induced by a wide array of foreign materials, including proteins and low-molecular-weight substances acting as haptens that bind to human proteins. Later, it was determined that anaphylactic reactions are the result of the production of antigen-specific immunoglobulin E (IgE) during the sensitization period. These IgE molecules fix to mast cells and basophils, sensitizing them so that a rapid release of their mediators, including histamine, occurs when an antigen bridges two IgE antibody molecules.

Various mechanisms result in anaphylaxis. Strictly speaking, the term *anaphylaxis* should only be used to describe the syndrome when it is mediated by IgE antibodies. The term *anaphylactoid* has been used to describe this syndrome when it is the result of non-IgE-mediated reactions. Some authors prefer the term *immediate generalized reaction* because it encompasses both IgE-mediated reactions and non-IgE-mediated reactions. In this chapter, for the sake of simplicity, *anaphylaxis* will be used to refer to both IgE-mediated and non-IgE-mediated reactions.

EPIDEMIOLOGY

Age, sex, and race are not factors in a person's predisposition to anaphylaxis.[3] The incidence of anaphylaxis caused by penicillin and insect stings is not increased in individuals with a personal or family history of atopy. However, once a person is sensitized to an antigen and has a positive skin test, that person has a greater incidence of anaphylaxis than the general population.

TABLE 14–1. IgE-Mediated Anaphylaxis

Mechanism	Agent	Examples
Against proteins	Venoms	Hymenoptera, fire ants
	Foods	Peanuts, milk, tree nuts, seafood
	Enzymes	Trypsin, L-asparaginase, chymopapain
	Human or animal proteins	Insulin, vasopressin, seminal proteins
	Allergen extracts	Ragweed, Bermuda grass, cotton seed
	Heterologous serum	Tetanus antitoxin, antilymphocyte globulin, bovine serum albumin
	Vaccines	Influenza, measles
	Others	Latex
Against polysaccharides		Dextran
		Iron dextran
Against protein-hapten conjugates	Antibiotics	Penicillins, cephalosporins, sulfonamides, tetracycline, streptomycin
	Vitamins	Thiamine
	Disinfectants	Ethylene oxide

Data on the overall incidence of anaphylaxis are vague and produce vastly different rates of incidence. One estimated rate of anaphylaxis from any cause is 0.4 cases per million individuals per year.[4] In another study involving a series of 11,526 medical inpatients, drug anaphylaxis was recorded in 8 patients (0.6 per 1000) with one fatality.[5] In this study, anaphylaxis was most common following infusions of protein-containing agents such as blood or its derivatives and was intermediate following the administration of parenteral penicillin derivatives. Other authors estimate that 3 percent of the population has a history of systemic reactions to insect venoms.[6] Finally, Kaliner[7] believes that the most common causes of anaphylactic reactions and death include penicillin reactions (400 to 800 deaths), Hymenoptera stings (100 or more deaths), and radiocontrast media reactions (250 to 1000 deaths).

True IgE-mediated anaphylaxis requires previous exposure to the antigen with synthesis of IgE antibodies. It usually occurs after the inciting allergen enters the body by injection, ingestion, or inhalation.

ETIOLOGY

The causes of anaphylaxis may be categorized based on the mechanism of mediator release from the mast cells and basophils. Specific causes for anaphylaxis are presented in Tables 14–1 and 14–2. These lists, though not exhaustive, are representative.

Systemic anaphylaxis may be IgE-mediated (Table 14–1). The exposure of a susceptible person to a foreign protein (either in its native state or as a hapten after covalent conjugation with a carrier protein) or polysaccharide results in the generation of IgE antibodies. Therapy with antibiotics, particularly penicillin and the other beta-lactam antibiotics, is the most frequent cause of anaphylaxis from drug treatment.[8] Foods are also a significant cause of IgE-mediated anaphylaxis.[9]

TABLE 14–2. Non-IgE-Mediated Anaphylactoid Reactions

Mechanism	Agent	Example
Complement-mediated	Human proteins	Gamma globulin, transfusion reaction with IgA deficiency, other blood products
	Dialysis	Contact of blood with cuprophane membranes
Direct activation of mast cells, basophils, or both	Hypertonic solutions, drugs	Radiocontrast medium, mannitol, opiates, tubocurarine, vancomycin, deferoxamine, pentamadine
Arachidonate-mediated*	Aspirin, and other nonsteroidal anti-inflammatory agents	Aspirin, indomethacin, mefenamic acid
Unknown mechanisms	Exercise	
	Exercise and food	
	Idiopathic anaphylaxis	

*Presumptive explanation.[11,12]

Many biologic agents, including human insulin and enzyme preparations, have been incriminated in systemic reactions. Venom from insects of the order Hymenoptera, including honeybees, hornets, wasps, yellow jackets, and fire ants, also contains proteins that are antigenic.[8]

Another type of reaction leading to anaphylactic symptoms occurs when immune complexes or other agents activate the complement cascade, resulting in the formation of anaphylotoxins (C3a and C5a) that can trigger the release of mediators from mast cells (Table 14–2). This mechanism can be seen in IgA-deficient patients who produce antibodies against IgA after a blood transfusion and then receive a subsequent blood transfusion containing IgA.[10] IgA-deficient patients also may have IgE against IgA, leading to IgE-mediated anaphylaxis. This mechanism also can be seen in patients undergoing dialysis in whom the cuprophane membrane of the dialyzer activates the complement cascade.

There are also certain agents that can stimulate the release of mediators from mast cells and basophils directly without the presence of IgE antibody or complement activation. The exact mechanism behind this process is not known. Examples of agents that cause direct activation include opiates, radiocontrast media, mannitol, and vancomycin.

In some individuals, aspirin and other nonsteroidal anti-inflammatory agents can provoke asthma and urticaria. It is hypothesized, though not proven, that these analgesics may precipitate asthma in sensitive patients by inhibiting cyclooxygenase and thus the production of prostaglandins in the respiratory tract.[11,12] Furthermore, other unknown mechanisms may lead to anaphylaxis in patients sensitive to aspirin. These may be a different group than those susceptible to aspirin-induced asthma.

There have been reports of several hundred patients who have anaphylaxis associated with exercise.[13,14] Although these patients do not experience anaphylaxis with every episode of exercise, there is a sufficient degree of recurrence and uniformity of symptoms to suggest that exercise-induced anaphylaxis is a distinct clinical entity. Moreover, there are some reports of individuals who appear to develop symptoms only when they exercise after ingesting a particular food. The exact mechanisms by which the anaphylaxis develops is not known.

Finally, *idiopathic anaphylaxis* is anaphylaxis of unknown etiology in which no identifiable precipitant or event is noted.[15,16] This diagnosis is considered only after repeated careful evaluations have failed to identify an inciting allergen or precipitating event. It is believed that the clinical manifestations of idiopathic anaphylaxis may be due to episodic systemic release of histamine and other vasoactive substances from mast cells, basophils, or both.[17]

MECHANISMS OF ANAPHYLAXIS

MECHANISMS OF MEDIATOR RELEASE

Anaphylactic reactions are IgE-mediated reactions. IgE-mediated reactions consist of sensitization to the antigen, reversible binding of the IgE molecule to mast cells and basophils, and cross-bridging of the IgE molecules to release mediators.[18] Sensitization to antigens occurs when the antigen is introduced into the body. This may be done through the skin; via the respiratory, gastrointestinal, or genitourinary tract; or intramuscularly or intravenously. The antigen, once in the body, stimulates the immune system to produce IgE antibodies. An IgE antibody consists of two light chains and two heavy chains (Fig. 14–1). The heavy chain is of the epsilon class to distinguish IgE from other types of immunoglobulins. The antibody then consists of the F_{ab} fragment (with two light chains and part of two heavy chains), which is able to recognize and bind antigen, and the F_c fragment (consisting of the remainder of the heavy chains), which can bind to mast cells and basophils.

Once the immune system is stimulated by antigen to produce IgE antibodies, the IgE antibody interacts with specific receptors for the F_c region on mast cells and basophils. Finally, when an antigen is reintroduced into an organism after the organism has been sensitized to the antigen, the antigen interacts with the IgE molecule. The antigen is recognized by the F_{ab} portion of the molecule. When an antigen binds two adjacent receptor-bound IgE molecules, cross-bridging occurs. This activates intracellular biochemical events within mast cells and basophils which culminate in the release of mediators from the cells.

Mast cells and basophils also can release their mediators by other mechanisms. The activation of the complement cascade, either via the classic or alternate pathway, leads to the generation of anaphylotoxins C3a and C5a. These compounds have direct effects on target organs and can cause mediator release. Lysosomal proteases, kinins, and lymphokines also can stimulate the release of mediators. Moreover, certain substances can elicit the release of mediators directly. Such substances include iodinated contrast materials and dextran. Opioids (e.g., morphine) can cause cutaneous mast cell degranulation through a naloxone-sensitive receptor.[19] In these situations, prior exposure to the inciting agent is not required.

When mast cells and basophils are activated, a biphasic response in the intracellular level of cyclic adenosine-3',5'-monophosphate (cAMP) occurs, as well as changes in the level of cyclic guanosine-3',5'-monophosphate (cGMP).[18] An

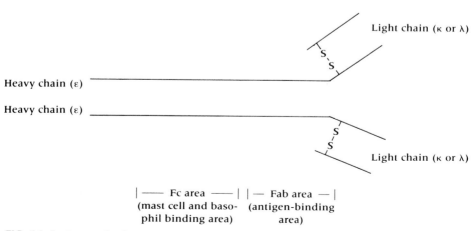

Heavy chain (ε)

Heavy chain (ε)

Light chain (κ or λ)

Light chain (κ or λ)

|—— Fc area ——| |— Fab area —|
(mast cell and baso- (antigen-binding
phil binding area)   area)

FIG. 14–1. IgE antibody.

initial rise in the level of cAMP is followed by a dramatic decline. The decline in the level of cAMP corresponds to the release of mediators into the extracellular environment. Intracellular calcium flux is also important in mediator release. A flow of calcium into the cells causes a decrease in cAMP. Magnesium and manganese concentrations also can affect mediator release. The steps leading to mediator release are quite complex and involve an active, energy-consuming process.

A knowledge of the mechanisms behind mediator release is important to an understanding of treatment rationale. Catecholamines with beta-adrenergic properties, such as epinephrine, can enhance cAMP production by stimulating adenylate cyclase. When the level of intracellular cAMP is maintained or raised, mediator release is inhibited.

MEDIATORS OF ANAPHYLAXIS

Two different cells, mast cells and basophils, participate in IgE-mediated generation and release of active mediators. Basophils are members of the polymorphonuclear leukocyte series formed in the bone marrow and comprise 0.2 to 1 percent of the nuclear cells in the peripheral blood.[20] These cells are normally only found in the blood or bone marrow. Basophils have a lobulated nucleus and large granules that stain with metachromatic dyes.

Mast cells also have high-affinity membrane receptors for IgE. Mast cells are found mainly in the skin and respiratory tract, as well as within the gastrointestinal mucosa. They are also found free in the bronchial lumen and in loose connective tissue, especially around blood vessels and nerves. They are present at a concentration of 1×10^6 per gram in lung and 10,000 per cubic millimeter in skin.[20] Mast cells have a rounded nucleus. Their granules stain more intensely with metachromatic dyes than those of basophils. Two types of human mast cells have been identified to date.[21] The first is the T mast cell, which contains tryptase but not chymase and predominates in the lung (particularly in the alveoli) and intestinal mucosa. The TC mast cells contain both chymase and tryptase and are found predominantly in the skin and the intestinal submucosa.

When the mast cells and basophils are activated, they release preformed granular mediators into the extracellular fluid. These activated cells also generate new mediators that together constitute the mediators of immediate hypersensitivity (Table 14–3). The preformed mediators include histamine, proteases, heparin, chondroitin sulfate, and chemotactic factors. The membrane-derived lipid mediators include prostaglandin D_2 (PGD_2); the leukotrienes C_4, D_4, and E_4 (LTC_4, LTD_4, and LTE_4), previously known as the slow-reacting substances of anaphylaxis (SRS-A); and platelet activating factor (PAF).

Histamine constitutes about 10 percent of the weight of mast cell granules.[22] The actions of histamine are mediated through three distinct receptors.[19] The H_1 receptor mediates most of the important histamine effects in allergic diseases. These include smooth-muscle contraction, pruritus, increased capillary permeability, prostaglandin generation, decreased atrioventricular node conduction time (which results in tachycardia), activation of vagal reflexes, and increased cGMP. The H_2 receptor mediates such effects as increased lower airway mucus secretion, gastric acid secretion, increased cAMP, esophageal contraction, inhi-

TABLE 14–3. Mediators of Immediate Hypersensitivity

Mediator	Source	Function
	Preformed Mediators	
Histamine	Basophils/mast cells	Vasodilation, vasopermeability, pruritus, bronchoconstriction
Proteases (tryptase, chymase, etc.)	Basophils/mast cells	Degradation of blood vessel basement membrane, generation of C3a
Heparin	Mast cells	Formation of complexes with protease and histamine
Chondroitin sulfates	Basophils predominantly	Formation of complexes with proteases and histamine
Eosinophil chemotactic factor of anaphylaxis	Mast cells	Attracts and deactivates eosinophils
Neutrophil chemotactic factor	Mast cells	Attracts and deactivates neutrophils
	Membrane-Derived Lipid Mediators	
Prostaglandin D_2	Mast cells	Vasopermeability, bronchoconstriction
Leukotrienes C_4, D_4, and E_4	Mast cells/basophils	Vasopermeability, bronchoconstriction
Platelet activating factor (PAF)	Mast cells	Aggregates platelets, vasopermeability, bronchoconstriction, chemotaxis

bition of basophil histamine release, induction of suppressor T cells, and inhibition of neutrophil chemotaxis and enzyme release. Several effects are mediated through combined H_1/H_2 receptor stimulation, including vasodilatation symptoms and tachycardia resulting indirectly via vasodilatation and catecholamine secretion. An H_3 receptor, believed to mediate negative feedback on histamine synthesis, also has been described.[19]

Intragranular proteases are released from mast cells and basophils upon activation. In some species these proteases make up almost 50 percent of the total mast cell protein.[22] These proteases are active at a neutral pH, at which they are strongly positively charged. Tryptase, a neutral protease, is known to be the dominant protein component of the secretory granules of mast cells; it is present only in very small amounts in basophils.[23] Another important protease is chymase. The possible actions of these proteases include degradation of the blood vessel basement membrane with resultant increased vascular permeability, digestion of connective tissue components allowing secondary inflammatory cells to flow into inflamed regions, and finally, degradation of debris and activation of growth factors promoting wound healing.

The proteoglycans serve to package the proteases within the granules. In mast cells, the proteoglycan is heparin sulfate, whereas in basophils, the proteoglycan is chondroitin sulfate. These molecules are very negatively charged, so they can bind the proteases, which are positively charged.

Chemotactic factors allow mast cells to recruit secondary inflammatory cells into the sites of immediate hypersensitivity reaction. Preformed cells include the eosinophil chemotactic factors of anaphylaxis (ECF-A) and neutrophil chemotactic factor (NCF). The lipid mediators are not made until after the mast cell has been activated. These mediators include arachidonic acid metabolites (Fig. 14–2) and the phospholipid-derivative platelet activating factor (PAF). The production of arachidonic acid via phospholipase A_2 from membrane phospholipids can be blocked by corticosteroids (Fig. 14–2). Prostaglandin D_2 (PGD_2) is synthesized only from mast cells via the cyclooxygenase pathway. PGD_2 causes increased vasodilation, vasopermeability, and can lead to bronchoconstriction. It does not lead to pruritus.

Leukotrienes C_4, D_4, and E_4 are produced in both mast cells and basophils. They are produced from arachidonic acid via the lipoxygenase pathway. These mediators cause erythema and wheal formation when injected under the skin. They also cause bronchospasm, with more effect on the small airways. Moreover, LTC_4, D_4, and E_4 are very potent stimulators of airway mucus secretion. Leukotriene B_4 (LTB_4), another leukotriene produced by the lipoxygenase pathway, is a potent chemotactic factor which may be important in anaphylaxis.

Platelet activating factor (PAF) is produced within mast cells, in addition to other cell lines, but not within basophils. PAF causes aggregation of platelets. It also causes vasodilation, vasopermeability, and bronchoconstriction. Moreover, it is a strong chemotactic agent for polymorphonuclear cells.

There are many secondary mediators of anaphylaxis (Table 14–4). These include the end products of several enzyme-dependent cascading reactions, such as the kinin, complement, coagulation, and fibrinolytic systems, as well as the products of circulating formed elements.[18]

When the complement system is activated either by the classic or the alternative pathway during anaphylaxis, C3a and C5a are produced. These are anaphylatoxins. They increase vascular permeability, cause smooth-muscle contraction, and enhance histamine release. The final complement product can cause further membrane damage and cell destruction.

After the primary mediators injure the vascular epithelium, exposed collagen in the basement membrane activates Hageman factor (factor XII). Activated Hageman factor triggers the intrinsic coagulation and fibrinolytic systems, resulting in intravascular coagulation that can lead to further vascular endothelium damage. Activated Hageman factor also can trigger the formation of

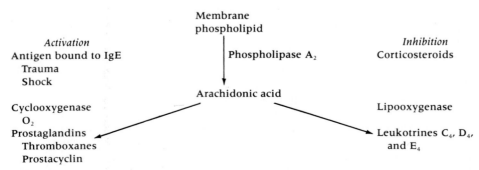

FIG. 14–2. Mediators derived from arachidonic acid metabolism.

TABLE 14–4. Secondary Mediators of Anaphylaxis

1. Activation of enzyme cascading reactions
   a. Complement system
   b. Kinin-kallikrein system
   c. Intrinsic coagulation pathways
   d. Fibrinolytic system
2. Products of white blood cells, platelets, and eosinophils
   a. Oxygen radicals
   b. Interleukins
   c. Vasoactive amines
   d. Phospholipase
   e. Fibrinolysin
   f. Collagenases
   g. Elastase

bradykinin, which is a powerful vasodilator that also increases vascular permeability.

White blood cells, platelets, and eosinophils elaborate additional mediators. These cells accumulate near areas of mast cell degranulation. A variety of enzymes and other substances are released by white blood cells. Among these, unstable oxygen radicals act as powerful mediators of tissue destruction.

CLINICAL MANIFESTATIONS OF ANAPHYLAXIS

SYMPTOMS

The clinical manifestations of anaphylaxis are variable. Anaphylaxis may present with relatively mild symptoms, or it may be rapidly fatal. Most reactions occur within 1 h of antigen exposure, but they can be variable, ranging from seconds to hours.[1] The variability depends on the dose of the inducing antigen, the route of administration, and the degree of the host immunologic sensitivity. There appears to be a correlation between the rapidity of onset of the symptoms and the severity of the reaction. Reactions occurring immediately following antigen exposure tend to be more severe. Occasionally, biphasic reactions occur in which symptoms recur several hours after the initial reaction.[24] Moreover, the reactions sometimes may be protracted over several hours.[24]

The most common features of anaphylaxis include urticaria, erythema, and angioedema. Diffuse erythema alone is the most common skin change. The urticarial lesions are well demarcated with raised, erythematous, serpiginous borders and dulled centers. These usually are highly pruritic. The urticarial lesions are evanescent. Angioedema involving the head, neck, and upper airways occurs in about 22 percent of patients.[25] Angioedema is a localized subcutaneous process that results in nonpitting edema of the deeper skin components. Although disfiguring, it may be asymptomatic or accompanied by a burning sensation. Angioedema can progress slowly during antigen-induced anaphylaxis.

TABLE 14–5. Clinical Manifestations of Anaphylaxis

Organ	Symptom
Skin	Erythema, urticaria, angioedema
Respiratory tract	Rhinorrhea, laryngeal edema, wheezing, bronchorrhea, asphyxiation
Cardiovascular system	Tachycardia, hypotension, shock, syncope, arrhythmias, diaphoresis
Gastrointestinal system	Abdominal cramps, nausea, vomiting, diarrhea
Genitourinary tract	Urinary incontinence, uterine contractions
Blood	Prolonged clotting, disseminated intravascular coagulation
Other	Pruritus, weakness, metallic taste in mouth, feeling of doom

Angioedema of the tongue, epiglottis, or larynx can result in upper airway obstruction with resultant stridor and possibly asphyxiation.

Aside from the upper airway obstruction due to angioedema, the rest of the respiratory tract is also a target for anaphylaxis. There is often associated congestion and pruritus of the mucous membranes of the eyes, nose, and mouth. Patients also may develop bronchospasm and bronchorrhea that can lead to severe hypoxemia, hypercarbia, and cardiovascular collapse.[26] Bronchospasm can result in cough, tachypnea, and wheezing which may not be heard if the bronchospasm is severe. Autopsy examination of patients who die of acute anaphylaxis often reveals bronchial obstruction and hyperinflation. On microscopic examination, these specimens exhibit peribronchial congestion, submucosal edema, eosinophilic infiltration, and luminal secretions in the bronchi.[27]

Cardiovascular collapse and hypotensive shock are major manifestations of anaphylaxis. The mechanisms causing these serious manifestations appear to be peripheral vasodilatation, increased vascular permeability, plasma extravasation, and intravascular volume depletion. Direct depression of the myocardium may appear in patients with previous cardiac disease. In a study of 205 patients who experienced anaphylactic shock during anesthesia with cardiovascular manifestations of the shock, patients with cardiac disease were more likely to have nonbenign arrhythmias and elevated filling pressures than healthy patients.[28] In this study, supraventricular tachycardia (SVT) was the most common arrhythmia. Four patients developed ventricular fibrillation following SVT which was associated with intravenous injections of epinephrine and halothane. Arrhythmias other than SVT are uncommon in the absence of cardiac disease. Other cardiovascular manifestations of anaphylaxis include dizziness, syncope, seizures, diaphoresis, and disorientation.

Other organ systems are also affected in anaphylaxis. The gastrointestinal tract is a frequent target organ. The symptoms here include abdominal cramping, nausea, vomiting, and diarrhea. Uterine contractions and urinary incontinence are some of the manifestations of anaphylaxis in the genitourinary tract. Anaphylaxis also can interfere with the coagulation system, sometimes resulting in prolonged clotting times and disseminated intravascular coagulation.

Finally, many patients with anaphylaxis develop nonspecific symptoms, including pruritus, weakness, a metallic taste in the mouth, and a feeling of impending doom (Table 14–5).

DIAGNOSIS

When a patient has urticaria, hypotension, and bronchospasm within minutes of exposure to an inciting agent, the diagnosis of anaphylaxis is obvious. However, when symptoms involve only one organ system, the differential diagnosis expands. Vasovagal reaction is probably the disorder most often confused with anaphylaxis.[7] In vasovagal reactions, hypotension is accompanied by bradycardia, which may be masked if the patient is treated with epinephrine.[29] Other disorders that involve the sudden loss of consciousness and may be confused with anaphylaxis include seizures, myocardial infarction, cardiac arrhythmias, pulmonary embolism, asphyxiation, cerebral vascular accident, and hypoglycemia.

If angioedema is the presenting condition, venous or lymphatic obstruction must be considered. Hereditary angioedema (HAE), a condition associated with low levels of active C1 inactivator, is also an important factor in the differential diagnosis. HAE is manifested by painless, nonpruritic angioedema, gastrointestinal cramps and bloating, recurrent attacks, and often a family history of similar attacks.

Another disease in the differential diagnosis of anaphylaxis is serum sickness.[7] Serum sickness is manifested by fever, macular papular and urticarial rashes, lymphadenopathy, arthralgia, and arthritis. Sometimes nephritis and neuritis are seen in serum sickness. Differing from anaphylaxis, serum sickness usually develops 1 to 2 weeks after exposure to the inciting antigen, and it may last for several weeks.

Acute respiratory distress, often seen in anaphylaxis, is also present in other diseases. These conditions include status asthmaticus, tension pneumothorax, epiglottitis, airway obstruction secondary to a foreign body, and pulmonary embolus.

Urticarial and flushing lesions are also seen in other disease states besides anaphylaxis. These disease states include mastocytosis, carcinoid syndrome, cold urticaria, pheochromocytoma, and idiopathic urticaria.

TREATMENT

The specific treatment of anaphylaxis is enhanced by early recognition that the patient is indeed having anaphylaxis, since rapid deterioration and even death may occur within a few minutes after the first symptoms. Regardless of the cause of the anaphylactic symptoms, certain common measures are useful and should influence the outcome. These measures include quick initial assessment of the extent and severity of the reaction, attempts to obtain a history of the reaction, halting administration of the offending agent (e.g., discontinuing intravenous medications), careful monitoring of the patient's vital signs, cardiac rhythm, and pulmonary status, and, once the patient's condition is stabilized, obtaining the patient's past medical history. This history should include his or her current condition and medication use.[1] Evaluation must be rapid. Prolonged evaluation should not replace early treatment with epinephrine followed by more extensive evaluation.

This section will first discuss the major drugs used in anaphylaxis and then review specific interventions.

DRUG THERAPY

The four major drugs used as treatment for acute anaphylaxis are epinephrine, oxygen, antihistamines, and corticosteroids (Table 14–6).

EPINEPHRINE

Epinephrine is the drug of first choice in the treatment of anaphylaxis.[1,30] This medication is important regardless of the presenting symptoms of anaphylaxis. Epinephrine has potent alpha, beta$_1$, and beta$_2$ properties that counteract the actions of the mediators. Epinephrine is an alpha agonist in that it increases blood pressure and reverses peripheral vasodilation. This vasoconstrictor activity helps to reverse systemic hypotension and also may decrease angioedema and urticaria. Epinephrine, as a beta agonist, may cause bronchodilation and facilitate both positive inotropic and chronotropic cardiac activity. Moreover, the beta-receptor effect of epinephrine can increase the production of cAMP, which, as mentioned earlier, can decrease mediator release.

The usual recommendation is that epinephrine be given subcutaneously, since the intravenous administration of epinephrine at standard doses has caused the induction of arrhythmias, pulmonary edema, myocardial ischemia, and even infarction.[29,30] The generally accepted dose of subcutaneous epinephrine in adults is 0.3 to 0.5 mg of a 1:1000 concentration (0.3 to 0.5 ml) that can be repeated every 15 to 20 min.[30] In children, the recommended dose is 0.01 mg/kg of body weight of a 1:1000 dilution given subcutaneously every 15 to 20 min.[30] The use of intravenous epinephrine for the treatment of systemic anaphylaxis should be reserved for the patient in extremis. Intravenous administration should be done extremely cautiously, even in patients without a history of cardiovascular disease. A recommended dose to initiate treatment of intravenous

TABLE 14–6. Primary Medications Used in the Treatment of Anaphylaxis

Agent	Indications	Comment
Epinephrine	Bronchospasm, laryngeal edema, urticaria, angioedema, hypotension	First-line drug
Oxygen	Hypoxemia secondary to bronchoconstriction or hypoperfusion	Used to improve cellular oxygenation
Antihistamines	Urticaria, angioedema, hypotension	Not drugs of first choice; may block continuing mediator release
Corticosteroids	Bronchospasm, continuing urticaria and angioedema	Second-line drugs used to inhibit or reduce prolonged or late-phase reactions

epinephrine is 0.1 mg of a 1:1000 dilution of aqueous epinephrine mixed in 10 ml normal saline to result in a final dilution of 1:100,000.[30] This solution can then be infused over 5 to 10 min. An intramuscular injection of 0.3 ml of a 1:1000 concentration for a hypotensive patient may be considered when the patient has severe anaphylaxis but is not in extremis.

The probability of a fatal reaction from anaphylaxis is increased when epinephrine is not instituted early in the management of a reaction.[27] The risk of giving epinephrine for anaphylaxis is far less than the risk of untreated anaphylaxis.

OXYGEN

Oxygen should be administered to all patients with moderate to severe anaphylactic shock. This is essential to improve cellular oxygenation.[25] If the patient has bronchospasm, the oxygen should be administered at high enough flows to sustain a P_{O_2} over 60 mmHg (preferably 80 to 100 mmHg).[31] If a patient is hypotensive, oxygen should be administered to ensure adequate oxygenation of the hypoperfused tissues.

ANTIHISTAMINES

As mentioned earlier, histamine is a major mediator of anaphylactic reactions. Its effects are mediated through both H_1 and H_2 receptors. Antihistamines block the actions of histamine at these receptors. By the time anaphylaxis is diagnosed, it is usually too late for an antihistamine's blocking effect to be useful, and for this reason, antihistamines are not the drugs of first choice in treating anaphylaxis. Antihistamines, however, do seem to be useful when continuing mediator release is occurring.

H_1 antihistamines have been a widely used treatment for patients with allergic reactions. The most common H_1 antagonist used is diphenhydramine, 25 to 50 mg given intramuscularly. There has been some debate over whether H_2 receptor antagonists (e.g., cimetidine, 300 mg slowly, intravenously) are also useful. Some investigators have found that H_2 receptor antagonists help suppress allergic reactions.[32] Other investigators have found that a combined H_1 and H_2 blockade is more effective in the prevention of anaphylaxis but have been unable to verify that this combination is effective in the treatment of anaphylaxis.[33] Finally, still other investigators have found that adding H_2 antagonists to pretreatment regimens causes an increase of anaphylactic reactions.[34] Further research is necessary to determine the exact role of H_2 antagonists in the treatment of anaphylaxis.

CORTICOSTEROIDS

Systemic glucocorticoids are another class of second-line drug in an acute anaphylactic emergency. They are useful in biphasic and prolonged anaphylaxis. Systemic glucocorticoid therapy can suppress experimentally induced second-phase reactions in the lung, nose, and skin. Glucocorticoids have no influence on the initial anaphylactic reaction.[24] Steroids are helpful in treating prolonged bronchospasm and controlling continuing urticaria and angioedema. The initial dose of cortisone is equivalent to 60 mg prednisone.[31] The onset of action is usually 4 to 6 h after administration of the drug.

SPECIFIC INTERVENTIONS

Each patient's anaphylactic manifestations are unique. The specific interventions used to resuscitate the patient depend on which anaphylactic symptoms predominate and the severity of the symptoms.

If anaphylaxis is secondary to the injection of venom or a drug, a tourniquet should be placed on the extremity. The insect's stinger should be removed, if possible. A small dose of epinephrine (0.1 to 0.2 ml of 1:1000 dilution) should be administered subcutaneously at the site of the inoculation to reduce the local absorption of the antigen.[7]

In mild cases of anaphylaxis, subcutaneous epinephrine alone should control the symptoms. If the patient has urticaria and/or angioedema, diphenhydramine can be added for symptomatic relief. With more severe reactions, more directed measures must be undertaken.

UPPER AIRWAY OBSTRUCTION

When upper airway obstruction due to laryngeal or oropharyngeal edema occurs (the patient feels a lump in his or her throat, has hoarseness, or develops stridor), aerosolized epinephrine may be used in addition to subcutaneous epinephrine in an effort to reduce local edema. Neck extension and placement of an oropharyngeal airway can help relieve the symptoms. If the obstruction continues to progress, immediate endotracheal intubation is indicated. A smaller than normal endotracheal tube may be needed because of the edema. If intubation is not possible, a cricothyroidotomy should be performed to establish an adequate airway so that the patient can be ventilated. A 14-gauge needle can be inserted into the cricothyroid membrane for temporary use by someone not experienced in intubation or cricothyroidotomy.

LOWER AIRWAY OBSTRUCTION

The treatment of lower airway obstruction during anaphylaxis is very similar to the treatment of severe acute asthma. The initial management consists of subcutaneous epinephrine and oxygen administration. Inhaled bronchodilators may be used. Aminophylline may be given intravenously (using a loading dose of 6 mg/kg over 30 min, followed by a maintenance infusion of 0.3 to 0.9 mg/kg/h).[1] Lower infusion rates are suggested for older patients, for patients on other medications that would reduce theophylline metabolism, for patients with hepatic dysfunction, and for patients with congestive heart failure. Higher infusion rates are reserved for younger patients or patients who smoke. Serial theophylline level determinations should guide dosage when the patient is stabilized. Nausea, vomiting, and cardiac dysrhythmias are some of the early signs of theophylline toxicity that warrant halting theophylline infusion.

When the initial management of bronchospasm does not control the symptoms, intubation and positive-pressure ventilation may be necessary. Peak pressures on the ventilator are often quite high as a result of severe bronchoconstriction. In some refractory cases of severe bronchospasm, halothane (cautious use with epinephrine), ketamine, and endobronchial procaine have been used successfully to decrease the bronchospasm.[28,39] Perihilar infiltration with local anesthetic and open lung massage also have been used to treat refractory bronchospasm.[35] Ultimately, cardiopulmonary bypass can be used until the bronchospasm resolves.[25,35]

HYPOTENSION

The optimal treatment of hypotension in anaphylaxis is also centered on subcutaneous epinephrine. Epinephrine is usually sufficient to restore vascular tone and normal vascular permeability. It also effectively restores normal cardiac function. In addition to epinephrine, it is often necessary to administer intravenous fluids rapidly to help support the blood pressure. Normal saline can be administered at a rate of up to 100 ml/min up to 3 liters in adults. Crystalloid solutions are effective; however, colloid solutions may be effective in patients who have lost plasma through increased vascular permeability. Trendelenburg position is indicated. Antihistamines also may be effective, though, as noted in the section on their use, the timing of their administration is generally crucial to their effectiveness.

If epinephrine and fluids are not sufficient to raise the blood pressure, vasopressors may be needed. Norepinephrine is the most consistently effective vasopressor used in anaphylaxis.[31] Four milliliters of a 1-mg/ml solution of norepinephrine should be added to 1000 ml 5% dextrose to yield a 4-μg/ml solution. The infusion rate in adults should be started at 8 to 12 μg/min (or 2 to 3 ml/min). The infusion rate can be adjusted to allow the systolic blood pressure to be maintained at 80 to 100 mmHg.

In a patient exhibiting cardiac contractility disorders, epinephrine remains the drug of first choice. If alpha-adrenergic agonist effects are undesirable, isoproterenol may be given. In adults, isoproterenol is diluted to 2 μg/ml by dissolving 1 mg isoproterenol in 500 ml 5% dextrose solution. This solution is infused at a rate of 0.25 to 2.50 ml/min or 0.5 to 5 μg/min. The speed of the infusion is titrated to the patient's heart rate and clinical response.

CONCOMITANT USE OF BETA ANTAGONISTS

Occasionally, patients being treated with beta blockers develop anaphylaxis.[36–42] Some authors believe that these patients may have a more severe and protracted course.[36–41] Such patients may develop bradycardia associated with an undetectable blood pressure and be slow to respond to conventional therapy for anaphylaxis. Toogood,[36] for example, believes that beta blockade changes the pharmacotherapeutic actions of epinephrine and other adrenergic drugs used in treating anaphylaxis. He feels that a beta antagonist would block the expected beta$_1$ and beta$_2$ antianaphylactic actions of epinephrine, causing unopposed alpha-adrenergic and reflex vagotonic effects leading to augmented mediator release, bronchoconstriction, and bradycardia.[36] Jacobs et al.[37] believe that beta-blocking agents may potentiate anaphylaxis by inhibiting adenylate cyclase, which would therefore lower the level of intracellular cAMP and decrease the threshold of mediator release. They suggest that the beta antagonist can blunt the normal endogenous beta-adrenergic response to hypotension and cause unopposed cholinergic action, leading to bradycardia.[37] Other authors feel that calcium channel blockers may worsen anaphylaxis complicated by beta blockade.[38] However, a prospective study of 952 patients by Greenberger et al.[42] found no increased incidence of anaphylactoid reactions to radiocontrast media in patients receiving beta blockers or calcium channel blockers. This group also found that the reactions in patients on beta-adrenergic blocking agents were usually mild.[42]

In patients receiving beta-blocking medication and suffering anaphylaxis, it is important to initiate treatment aggressively. In some case reports of patients suffering prolonged anaphylaxis while being treated with beta blockers, initially inadequate treatment may have accounted for the protracted course.[37,40] Epinephrine should be used initially, but higher doses of epinephrine may be required. Glucagon may be injected intravenously (1-mg bolus) to counteract hypotension.[39] Glucagon is a polypeptide hormone with strong inotropic and chronotropic actions whose adrenergic activity is only minimally antagonized by beta blockade. These cardiac effects may be critical, since many people requiring beta antagonists have underlying heart disease and a limited cardiac reserve. Moreover, hypotension refractory to intravenous fluids, epinephrine, and vasopressors may respond to application of a military antishock trouser.[40]

SUBSEQUENT CARE

Once stabilized from an episode of acute anaphylaxis, patients may need to be monitored for 24 h, depending on the severity of the episode and the clinical situation, because relapses are possible. Patients should continue to receive corticosteroids and antihistamines during hospitalization. These medications can be slowly tapered upon discharge. It then becomes essential to search for the cause of anaphylaxis, because prevention of another episode is the best treatment. An allergy consultation may help to determine the incriminating agent.

PROPHYLAXIS OF CERTAIN CAUSES OF ANAPHYLAXIS

DRUG-INDUCED ANAPHYLAXIS

Anaphylaxis secondary to therapeutic medications is common. Once the cause has been determined, it is important for the patient to avoid the drug allergen and cross-reacting agents. If an offending drug is essential, skin testing, when available, can be instituted to assess whether the patient continues to have IgE antibody against the drug. Skin testing is applicable for high-molecular-weight proteins, such as insulin and chymopapain, and for low-molecular-weight substances that can form haptens with human proteins, such as the major and minor determinants of penicillin.[43] Many drugs that are simple chemicals cause irritant reactions when used for skin testing, so skin testing is not applicable with these medications.

If skin testing is not practical for a drug because of its structure or because the reaction elicited is not mediated by IgE, test dosing of the drug can be performed. Test dosing is the cautious administration of a drug to determine the patient's allergic status. Low doses of a drug are given at first to assess for a minor reaction which can be treated rapidly. If no reaction occurs, the dose may be gradually increased until the full dose is given.

If a drug allergy clearly exists but the drug is essential, desensitization can be performed. The goal of desensitization is to neutralize, gradually and in a controlled environment, the IgE antibodies specific for the agent while avoiding a massive outpouring of mediators. Desensitization is achieved by carefully administering incremental doses over a relatively short period of time. The patient must be monitored closely, with emergency therapy constantly available. This procedure should be done only by persons with training and with appropriate notification of the patient and his or her family. This is a highly dangerous process.

RADIOCONTRAST MEDIA

The infusion of radiocontrast media also may lead to anaphylactoid reactions. These are non-IgE-mediated reactions that do not occur with every infusion of radiocontrast media following a procedure with a reaction. A pretreatment regimen that is known to decrease the risk of a repeat reaction has been devised for patients with a history of reaction to radiocontrast media. This regimen consists of premedicating the patient with prednisone, 50 mg, at 13, 7, and 1 h prior to the procedure and diphenhydramine, 50 mg, and ephedrine, 25 mg (if not contraindicated), 1 h prior to the procedure.[44] Often a similar pretreatment regimen has been useful in allowing administration of plasma in patients who have experienced an immediate generalized reaction following a transfusion.[10]

FOOD-RELATED ANAPHYLAXIS

The primary prevention of food anaphylaxis is avoidance of the incriminating food. Patients should carefully read the ingredient list on food preparations. They also should ask about all ingredients used in restaurants. Food-allergic patients should carry epinephrine-containing syringes and should be shown how to self-administer the epinephrine at the first sign of an allergic reaction.

INSECT STINGS

After a patient has an anaphylactic reaction to the venom of a member of the Hymenoptera order, skin testing can be performed to determine against which specific insect the patient has IgE. Patients who had a severe systemic anaphylactic reaction after an insect sting and who demonstrate IgE against the venom receive benefit from venom immunotherapy.[8] These patients should carry epinephrine-containing syringes for self-administration in the event they are stung again. These patients should be instructed to avoid being stung by wearing closed shoes and long pants. Moreover, they should not wear perfumes or brightly colored clothing when at risk.

EXERCISE-INDUCED ANAPHYLAXIS

Exercise-induced anaphylaxis usually does not occur with every exertion. Prevention is aimed at modifying the exercise program of susceptible patients.[13] This can be accomplished by decreasing the intensity of exertion, avoiding exercise on warm and humid days, and halting exercise at the slightest sign of itching. These patients also should avoid exercising immediately after eating. They should carry epinephrine that can be self-administered while exercising and should always exercise with a companion who can help treat the anaphylaxis should it occur.

IDIOPATHIC ANAPHYLAXIS

An acute episode of idiopathic anaphylaxis should be treated in the same manner as anaphylaxis of a known etiology (Table 14–7). When patients feel an attack beginning, they should immediately take prednisone, 60 mg orally, an antihistamine (usually hydroxyzine hydrochloride, 25 mg, or diphenhydramine hydrochloride, 50 mg), self-inject epinephrine, 0.3 ml of 1:1000 solution subcutaneously, and proceed to the nearest emergency room for further treatment.[15]

If a patient has frequent life-threatening episodes (occurring at least six times a year) or very severe episodes, it is suggested that he or she be placed on main-

TABLE 14–7. Suggested Treatment for Idiopathic Anaphylaxis

Type of Idiopathic Anaphylaxis Episode	Treatment
Acute episode (with both frequent and infrequent episodes)	Patient to self-medicate with: 1. Epinephrine, 0.3 cc of 1 : 1000 solution, subcutaneously 2. Antihistamine (hydroxyzine hydrochloride, 25 mg, orally, or diphenhydramine hydrochloride, 50 mg, orally) 3. Prednisone, 60 mg, orally Patient to then proceed to nearest emergency room
Frequent episodes (greater than or equal to six times a year) or very severe episodes	Prednisone, 60–100 mg, orally, for at least 1 week or until signs and symptoms are controlled and then convert to every other day prednisone, 60–100 mg, and cautiously taper (5–10 mg per month) Continuous antihistamines (e.g., hydroxyzine hydrochloride, 25–50 mg, three times a day) Continuous sympathomimetic agents (ephedrine hydrochloride, 25 mg, or albuterol sulfate, 2 mg, orally, three times a day)

tenance therapy with a slowly tapering course of prednisone.[15,45] The patient should be treated with prednisone, 60 to 100 mg, every morning for 1 week or until the signs and symptoms of anaphylaxis are controlled. The daily dose of prednisone is then converted to an alternate-day regimen and then tapered by no greater than 5 to 10 mg a dose per month. These patients also should be maintained on antihistamines (e.g., hydroxyzine hydrochloride, 25 mg) three times a day and oral sympathomimetics (e.g., albuterol sulfate, 2 mg) three times a day. This prophylactic treatment has been shown to improve the outcome in patients with idiopathic anaphylaxis.[45]

SUMMARY

Anaphylaxis is the most severe form of allergic disease. It involves the respiratory and cardiovascular systems, skin, and gastrointestinal tract. There are numerous causes of anaphylactic reactions, both IgE-mediated and non-IgE-mediated. The release from mast cells and basophils of histamine, prostaglandins, leukotrienes, and other mediators brings about the systemic symptoms. The primary treatment for anaphylaxis is subcutaneous epinephrine. Avoidance of inciting agents or defining and managing idiopathic anaphylaxis are the key to preventing further episodes of this potentially fatal syndrome.

REFERENCES

1. Bochner BS, Lichtenstein LM: Current concepts: Anaphylaxis. *N Engl J Med* 324:1785, 1991.
2. Portier MM, Richet C: De L'action anaphylactique de certains venins. *CR Soc Biol (Paris)* 54:170, 1902.
3. Sheffer AL: Anaphylaxis. *J Allergy Clin Immunol* 75:228, 1985.
4. Wasserman SI, Marquardt DL: Anaphylaxis. In E Middleton, CE Reed, EF Ellis, et al (eds): *Allergy: Principles and Practice,* 3d ed. St. Louis, Mosby, 1988, chap 55, pp 1365–1376.
5. Boston Collaborative Drug Surveillance Program: Drug-induced anaphylaxis. *JAMA* 224:613, 1973.
6. Valentine MD, Schuberth KC, Kagey-Sobotka A, et al: The value of immunotherapy with venom in children with allergy to insect stings. *N Engl J Med* 323:1601, 1990.
7. Kaliner MA: Anaphylaxis. *NER Allergy Proc* 5:324, 1984.
8. Valentine MD, Lichtenstein LM: Anaphylaxis and stinging insect hypersensitivity. *JAMA* 258:2881, 1987.
9. Yuninger JW, Sweeney KG, Sturner WQ, et al: Fatal food-induced anaphylaxis. *JAMA* 260:1450, 1988.
10. Greenberger PA: Plasma anaphylaxis and immediate type reactions. In EC Rossi, TL Simon, GS Moss (eds): *Principles of Transfusion Medicine.* Baltimore, Williams & Wilkins, 1991, chap 70, pp 635–639.
11. Szczeklik A: Adverse reactions to aspirin and nonsteroidal anti-inflammatory drugs. *Ann Allergy* 59:113, 1987.
12. Szczeklik A, Gryglewski RJ, Czerniawska-Mysik G: Relationship of inhibition of prostaglan-

din biosynthesis by analgesics to asthma attacks in aspirin-sensitive patients. *Br Med J* 1:67, 1975.

13. Sheffer AL, Austen KF: Exercise-induced anaphylaxis. *J Allergy Clin Immunol* 73:699, 1984.

14. Casale TB, Keahey TM, Kaliner M: Exercise-induced anaphylactic syndromes: Insights into diagnostic and pathophysiologic features. *JAMA* 255:2049, 1986.

15. Wong S, Dykewicz MS, Patterson R: Idiopathic anaphylaxis: A clinical summary of 175 patients. *Arch Intern Med* 150:1323, 1990.

16. Orfan N, Stoloff R, Harris K, Patterson R: Idiopathic anaphylaxis: Total experience with 225 patients. *Allergy Proc* 13:35, 1992.

17. Wiggins CA, Dykewicz MS, Patterson R: Idiopathic anaphylaxis: A review. *Ann Allergy* 62:1, 1989.

18. Carolson RW, Bowles AL, Haupt MT: Anaphylactic, anaphylactoid and related forms of shock. *Crit Care Clin* 2:347, 1986.

19. White MV: The role of histamine in allergic diseases. *J Allergy Clin Immunol* 86:599, 1990.

20. Wasserman SI: Mediators of immediate hypersensitivity. *J Allergy Clin Immunol* 72:101, 1983.

21. Irani AA, Schechter NM, Craig SS, et al: Two types of human mast cells that have distinct neutral protease compositions. *Proc Nat Acad Sci USA* 83:4464, 1986.

22. Serafin WE, Austen KF: Mediators of immediate hypersensitivity reactions. *N Engl J Med* 317:31, 1987.

23. Schwartz LB, Metcalfe DD, Miller JS, et al: Tryptase levels as an indicator of mast-cell activation in systemic anaphylaxis and mastocytosis. *N Engl J Med* 316:1622, 1987.

24. Stark BJ, Sullivan TJ: Biphasic and protracted anaphylaxis. *J Allergy Clin Immunol* 78:76, 1986.

25. Fisher M: Anaphylaxis. *Disease-A-Month* August:458, 1987.

26. Smith PL, Kagey-Sobotka A, Bleecker ER, et al: Physiologic manifestations of human anaphylaxis. *J Clin Invest* 66:1072, 1980.

27. Netzel MC: Anaphylaxis: Clinical presentation, immunologic mechanisms and treatment. *J Emerg Med* 4:227, 1986.

28. Fisher MM: Clinical observations on the pathophysiology and treatment of anaphylactic cardiovascular collapse. *Anesth Intensive Care* 14:17, 1986.

29. Patterson R, Dykewicz MS, Perry JM: Iatrogenic pseudoanaphylaxis. *J Allergy Clin Immunol* 79:24, 1987.

30. Barach EM, Nowak RM, Lee TG, Tomlanovich MC: Epinephrine for treatment of anaphylactic shock. *JAMA* 251:2118, 1984.

31. Sullivan TJ: Systemic anaphylaxis. In LM Lichtenstein, AS Fauci (eds): *Current Therapy in Allergy, Immunology and Rheumatology*, 3d ed. Toronto, Decker, 1988, pp 91–98.

32. Mayumi H, Kimura S, Asano M, et al: Intravenous cimetidine as an effective treatment for systemic anaphylaxis and acute allergic skin reactions. *Ann Allergy* 58:447, 1987.

33. Lieberman P: The use of antihistamines in the prevention and treatment of anaphylaxis and anaphylactoid reactions. *J Allergy Clin Immunol* 86:684, 1990.

34. Greenberger PA, Patterson R, Tapio CM: Prophylaxis against repeated radiocontrast media reactions in 857 cases: Adverse experience with cimetidine and safety of β-adrenergic antagonists. *Arch Intern Med* 145:2197, 1985.

35. Fisher MM, Baldo BA: Acute anaphylactic reactions. *Med J Aust* 149:37, 1988.

36. Toogood JH: Risk of anaphylaxis in patients receiving beta-blocker drugs. *J Allergy Clin Immunol* 81:1, 1988.

37. Jacobs RL, Rake GW, Fournier DC, et al: Potentiated anaphylaxis in patients with drug-induced beta adrenergic blockade. *J Allergy Clin Immunol* 68:125, 1981.

38. Kivity S, Yarchovsky J: Relapsing anaphylaxis to bee sting in a patient treated with β-blocker and Ca blocker (letter). *J Allergy Clin Immunol* 85:669, 1990.
39. Zaloga GP, Delacey W, Holmboe E, Chernow B: Glucagon reversal of hypotension in a case of anaphylactoid shock. *Ann Intern Med* 105:65, 1986.
40. Bickell WH, Dice WH: Military antishock trousers in a patient with adrenergic resistant anaphylaxis. *Ann Emerg Med* 13:189, 1984.
41. Lang DM, Alpern MB, Visintainer PF, Smith ST: Increased risk for anaphylactoid reaction from contrast media in patients on β-adrenergic blockers with asthma. *Ann Intern Med* 115:270, 1991.
42. Greenberger PA, Meyers SN, Kramer BL, Kramer BL: Effects of beta-adrenergic and calcium antagonists on the development of anaphylactoid reactions from radiographic contrast media during cardiac angiography. *J Allergy Clin Immunol* 80:698, 1987.
43. Patterson R: Diagnosis and treatment of drug allergy. *J Allergy Clin Immunol* 81:380, 1988.
44. Greenberger PA, Patterson R: Adverse reactions to radiocontrast media. *Prog Cardiovasc Dis* 31:239, 1988.
45. Wong S, Yarnold PR, Yango C, et al: Outcome of prophylactic therapy for idiopathic anaphylaxis. *Ann Intern Med* 114:133, 1991.

15

POISONING AND OVERDOSE

Glendon C. Henry
Robert S. Hoffman
Lewis R. Goldfrank

Patients present to health care facilities with poisonings from multiple etiologies.[1] Although a child who ingests his or her parent's cardiac medicine may have consequential toxicity, children are more apt to be minimally poisoned from chewing on a readily available household plant or by tasting a bottle of cleaning fluid.[1] Adults, however, are more likely to suffer serious toxicity as a result of intentional drug overdoses and adverse reactions to illicit drugs.[1] Fortunately, most poisonings or overdoses result in neither significant morbidity nor mortality, and most reports to poison centers are neither poisonings nor overdoses but are merely classified as exposures.[1] The 1991 American Association of Poison Control Centers (AAPCC) reported 612 deaths out of 1.7 million exposures, the majority of which were accidental.[1] A brief analysis of some of these data demonstrates that the substances responsible for the most exposures, such as household cleaning products, are not the products that cause the greatest toxicity, resulting in only 25 deaths.[1] Another example of this dissociation in frequency of exposure is found in that of house plants, where 10,689 philodendron and dieffenbacia exposures resulted in no deaths. In comparison, of the 6527 reports of aminophylline/theophylline ingestions, 36 patients died. Poisoning can occur at anytime in one's life, but the route of the poisoning, the etiology, and the agent usually vary as the age of the patient changes.[2,3] Young children may be poisoned after licking the cap of a household product. Adults, however, frequently present after ingesting substantial quantities of their own medications in a suicide attempt or after smoking or injecting a drug in an attempt to alter their state of consciousness.

Children under age 6 are more often exposed accidentally than either teenage or adult patients and usually have a more benign clinical course.[2,3] The explanations for the benignity of pediatric exposures are multifactorial: (1) The exposures are usually accidental and commonly associated with small amounts of drugs/toxins, (2) children are usually without underlying medical disorders, and (3) children usually present to the hospital promptly, often within 1 to 2 h after an exposure.[4]

Teenagers and adults, on the other hand, when presenting with an acute overdose, are more likely to have intentionally ingested the agent as a form of substance abuse or suicide.[1] This intent often results in an exposure to large amounts of a toxin or multiple toxins.[1] These patients typically present to the hospital at a later stage, often more than 3 h following the ingestion.[5] This delay and the associated progression of intoxication limit the efficacy of gastric decontamination and other early interventions that may be possible in children.

While the patient's history is very important to guide management of the poisoned or overdosed patient, it is often inaccurate.[6] While a misleading data base is expected in a substance abuser or a suicidal patient, it also may be present in pediatric intoxications. The parent in distress may not review all the potential toxins in the child's environment prior to the arrival in the emergency department. Although overdoses in children usually involve one drug,[1] the parent may not accurately recall how many pills or how much liquid was in the bottle at the time of ingestion. This qualitative assay is usually further complicated by the inability to estimate how much liquid or how many pills spilled onto the floor or the child. In addition, the history may not be accurate because of child abuse, neglect, or a Munchausen's syndrome by proxy.[7–10] In the adult overdose, the history should be considered suspect, unless the overdose results from an iatrogenic error or overmedication secondary to a misunderstanding of the physician's or pharmacist's instructions. These major obstacles can make management of the poisoned or overdosed patient a challenging endeavor.

The problems of a delayed presentation and an inaccurate history may be alleviated by the clinician by utilizing the vital signs and physical examination to define a precise toxicologic syndrome, or toxidrome. Some of the valuable and distinct toxidromes that can be utilized are shown in Table 15–1. The presence of a mixed toxic exposure, a concomitant or confounding medical problem, or a delayed presentation may make it difficult or impossible for an absolute diagnosis to be made. For example, a patient with an opioid intoxication may manifest an altered mental status, decreased respirations, and miotic pupils, but when the same patient becomes hypoxic, the pupils may dilate, suggesting either a mixed overdose, another toxin, or a complication of hypoxia. A patient with a phenobarbital overdose may have a similar clinical presentation to that of an individual with an opioid overdose. Both overdoses can lead to decreased blood pressure, heart and respiratory rates, and temperature, whereas in the patient with a phenobarbital overdose the pupils are usually not miotic. The availability of the pure opioid antagonist naloxone, with both diagnostic and therapeutic effects, allows the clinician to differentiate between the two types of overdoses without placing the patient at additional risk.[11–13]

The physician is frequently unable to make a precise diagnosis while the patient is in the emergency department. This may not be necessary, since broad groupings of intoxication, such as opioids, CNS stimulants, or sedatives, are often adequate. In the adult patient, a further confounding problem is that overdoses frequently result from multiple drug exposures, thereby making exact diagnoses more difficult.[1] In addition, commonly available medications (e.g., acetaminophen) may have no distinct early clinical findings. Therefore, the

TABLE 15–1. Classic Presentations of Pure Toxicologic Syndromes (Toxicdromes). (Cocaine is used as a representative sympathomimetic agent)

Toxin	Vital Signs	Mental Status	Symptoms	Clinical Findings	Lab Findings
Anticholinergics	Tachycardia, hypotension, hypertension, hyperthermia	Altered (agitation, lethargy to coma)	Blurred vision, confusion	Dry mucous membranes, mydriasis, diminished bowel sounds, urinary retention	ECG abnormalities, widened QRS complex
Opioids	Hypotension, bradycardia, hypoventilation, hypothermia	Altered (lethargy to coma)	Intoxication	Miosis, absent bowel sounds	Abnormal ABGs
Organophosphates/carbamates	Bradycardia/tachycardia, hypotension, hyperventilation/hypoventilation	Altered (lethargy to coma)	Diarrhea, abdominal pain, blurred vision, vomiting	Salivation, diaphoresis, lacrimation, urination, defecation, miosis, seizures	Abnormal RBC & plasma cholinesterase activity
Sedative-hypnotics	Hypotension, hypoventilation, hypothermia	Altered (lethargy to coma)	Intoxication	Hyporeflexia, bullae	Abnormal ABGs
Cocaine	Hypertension, tachycardia, hyperthermia	Altered (anxiety, agitation, delirium)	Hallucinations	Mydriasis, tremor, perforated nasal septum, diaphoresis, seizures	ECG abnormalities, increased CPK

Source: Adapted from *Goldfrank's Toxicologic Emergencies*, 4th ed. Norwalk, CT, Appleton & Lange, 1990. Used with permission.

TABLE 15–2. Differential Diagnosis of Toxicologic Causes of Altered Vital Signs

Blood Pressure	Temperature
Hypotension	Hyperthermia
Anticholinergics	Amphetamines
Arsenic (acute)	Anticholinergics
Beta blockers	Arsenic (acute)
Calcium channel blockers	Cocaine
Clonidine	Cyclic antidepressants
Cyclic antidepressants	LSD
Digitalis	Phencyclidine
Disulfiram/ethanol	Phenothiazines
Iron	Salicylates
Isopropyl alcohol	Theophylline
Lithium	Hypothermia
Mercury	Carbon monoxide
Methanol	Hypoglycemic agents
Opioids	Opioids
Organophosphates/carbamates	Phenothiazines
Phenothiazines	Sedative-hypnotics
Sedative-hypnotics	**Respiration**
Theophylline	Hypoventilation
Hypertension	Barbiturates
Amphetamines	Botulism
Anticholinergics	Clonidine
Cocaine	Ethanol
Lead	Isopropyl alcohol
Phencyclidine	Opioids
Pulse	Organophosphates/carbamates
Bradycardia	Sedative-hypnotics
Beta blockers	Hyperventilation
Calcium channel blockers	Ethylene glycol
Clonidine	Methanol
Digitalis	Organophosphates/carbamates
Opioids	Salicylates
Organophosphates/carbamates	Theophylline
Tachycardia	
Amphetamines	
Anticholinergics	
Arsenic (acute)	
Cocaine	
Cyclic antidepressants	
Disulfiram/ethanol	
Ethylene glycol	
Iron	
Organophosphates/carbamates	
Phencyclidine	
Phenothiazines	
Theophylline	

Source: Adapted from *Goldfrank's Toxicologic Emergencies,* 4th ed. Norwalk, CT, Appleton & Lange, 1990. Used with permission.

physician must always consider this agent as a prototype of a potential intoxication that must remain in the toxicologic differential diagnosis until excluded by laboratory assay. For these reasons, it is imperative that the history be obtained from friends, family, or anyone that may be able to assist. The family member or friend may be able to give a history of previous drug abuse, depression, or suicide. It may be important for the family or friend to return to the home to look for drug paraphernalia or to check for such things as insecticides, rat poisons, empty pill bottles, other agents, or containers that might alter the management strategy. The physician should question the ambulance team or the individuals who brought the patient to the hospital. These individuals may be able to give a history of agents that they have reason to believe were involved in the accident or overdose. They may describe the initial condition and early clinical course of the patient which may help guide clinical management.

As the initial information is being collected, the airway and ventilatory capacity of the patient should be assessed. In the compromised patient, this evaluation and the establishment of an intravenous line must be performed before the complete physical examination. The physical examination must always begin with an assessment of the patient's vital signs. In the overdosed patient who may be defiant, belligerent, or seizing, determination of the temperature may be difficult and, unfortunately, is often deferred. A rectal temperature should be taken in all patients. Hypothermia or hyperthermia should be noted. A rectal probe capable of measuring temperature extremes from 66 to 120°F (18.9 to 48.9°C) should be inserted for continuous monitoring. An elevated temperature may offer a clue to ingestions such as salicylates or central nervous system stimulants, while mild hypothermia is associated with opioid or sedative-hypnotic intoxication. Similarly, while cocaine or amphetamine abuse leads to increased blood pressure, calcium channel blockers or beta blockers may lower blood pressure precipitously. The heart rate also can be used to help formulate a differential diagnosis, since cocaine and amphetamines cause tachycardia, while clonidine and beta blockers lead to bradycardia. The respiratory pattern also may help in diagnosis. Opioids cause a decreased respiratory rate, while salicylates increase the rate and depth of respiration[14–15] (Table 15–2). The physician must look for "track" marks or other telltale findings of parenteral drug abuse. Battle's sign, raccoon's eyes, or a perforated tympanic membrane may be the only indications of severe head trauma, which is common among drug abusing patients.

INITIAL MANAGEMENT

ADMINISTRATION OF OXYGEN, THIAMINE, GLUCOSE, AND NALOXONE

OXYGEN

Many patients are poisoned from drugs that cause respiratory compromise. Hypoxic patients may present with an altered mental status, seizures, agitation, or coma. Hypoxia can rapidly result in central nervous system or myocardial ischemia. Increasing the oxygen tension can reverse these complications before permanent damage has occurred. The use of high-flow supplemental oxygen is rarely contraindicated in the overdosed or poisoned patient. The only concern is the patient with chronic obstructive pulmonary disease (COPD). The respiratory drive of such a patient may be blunted by high-flow oxygen. All other patients should receive supplemental oxygen. In patients who are awake and alert, oxygen at 4 liters/min via a nasal cannula is usually adequate. Patients who have decreased respiratory rate and poor tissue perfusion should initially be placed on a 100% nonrebreathing face mask and then be evaluated for possible endotracheal intubation.

THIAMINE

Most health care providers are familiar with the use of thiamine in the alcoholic patient presenting with an altered mental status. While this alteration of consciousness may result directly from ethanol, these patients are also at high risk to develop Wernicke's encephalopathy (altered mental status, ophthalmoplegia, and ataxia) secondary to thiamine deficiency.[16] These neurologic manifestations are often reversible,[16] but if left untreated, they may progress to Korsakoff's psychosis, a condition which is usually irreversible.[16] Pregnant patients with hyperemesis gravidarum, chronically malnourished patients, patients with acquired immune deficiency syndrome (AIDS), patients receiving hyperalimentation, and acutely malnourished or fad-dieting patients also may be thiamine deficient. The initial thiamine dosage is 100 mg, which can be given either intravenously (preferably) or intramuscularly. For patients who are suspected of thiamine depletion, supplemental thiamine treatment at the same dosage of 100 mg should continue on a daily basis. Thiamine should always be given to prevent the precipitation of an acute Wernicke's encephalopathy when dextrose is administered to any patient who may have impaired metabolism.[17] This is done because of thiamine's essential nature as a cofactor in the intermediate metabolism of glucose.

GLUCOSE

The administration of glucose is required for any patient with a mental status change or neurologic deficit. Although a more restricted use of glucose may be beneficial in certain cerebrovascular catastrophes, the use of various brands of dextrose finger-stick assays may not be entirely reliable in the determination of hypoglycemia under conditions such as extreme cold,[18] package impairment or neglect,[18] or the use of venous as opposed to capillary blood.[19–21] Because any global or focal neurologic deficit may be secondary to hypoglycemia,[22] patients presenting with neurologic symptoms should be given an adequate trial of dextrose. In the adult patient, this is given as 1 g/kg of $D_{50}W$ (50% dextrose in water). Children also should receive 1 g/kg, but it should be given in a more dilute form, such as $D_{20}W$ or $D_{25}W$ (20 to 25% dextrose in water). Larger doses may be necessary for partial responders. If the patient has not been hypoglycemic for an extended period of time, the response will usually be very rapid.[23] With prolonged hypoglycemia, however, the response may be either delayed, partial, or both. If the patient responds with resolution of neurologic deficits, the use of a $D_{10}W$ (10% dextrose) intravenous solution with frequent glucose monitoring should be instituted, as well as the addition of oral caloric intake as soon as possible.

NALOXONE

Naloxone should be utilized for patients with respiratory or central nervous system depression related to opioid intoxication or of an unknown etiology. When naloxone is given to a patient with a multiple drug ingestion including an opioid (or to one who has been maintained on methadone or addicted to another opioid), withdrawal may occur. Ensuing nausea and vomiting increases the potential for aspiration pneumonitis. The patient should be given an initial naloxone dose of 2 mg by the intravenous route[24] and then monitored for increased respiratory rate, improvement of mental status, and pupillary dilation. If there is no response to the initial dose, additional naloxone should be administered. If there is no response by the time 10 mg naloxone has been given over a short period of time, the diagnosis of opioid-induced mental status change or respiratory depression should be questioned. Patients who respond should be started on a continuous naloxone infusion. Continuous infusions are necessary because the duration of effect of naloxone is usually 30 to 60 min, which is much shorter in duration than the agents under treatment. This infusion can be prepared by giving the patient approximately two-thirds of the amount of naloxone initially needed to improve the patient's mental or respiratory status over 1 h.[25] Thus a patient who required 3 mg naloxone to restore consciousness can be placed on a 2-mg/h continuous infusion. This dose should be adjusted as needed, based on the patient's clinical status.

GASTROINTESTINAL DECONTAMINATION

There are many questions as to how best to manage the gastrointestinal decontamination of poisoned or overdosed patients. Some practitioners currently believe that gastric emptying is of little or no value.[5,26] Others utilize lavage,[27] syrup of ipecac, activated charcoal, or a polyethylene glycol electrolyte lavage solution alone or in combination to decontaminate patients.[28] The critical questions relate to the need for gastrointestinal decontamination and which procedures are best. Any patient with a potentially toxic ingestion should be decontaminated, unless there is a clear contraindication, such as a caustic ingestion. The procedure that is then implemented depends on several factors: (1) Does the drug/toxin cause a change in mental status? (2) Will the pill pass up the orogastric tube? (3) Does the drug/toxin bind to activated charcoal? (4) Is the drug/toxin available for enterohepatic recirculation in the bile, or does it lend itself to enteroenteric recirculation and adsorption with multiple-dose activated charcoal? It must be determined whether or not this ingestion is a toxic ingestion. If it is not, then there is no need to perform decontamination, since all these methods have potential complications. A child who ingests his or her parent's unused bottle of penicillin should be observed. In contrast, the patient who ingests even a very small amount of mercuric chloride should be managed as though a life-threatening ingestion has occurred, because this toxin can cause death even after very small ingestions. When the history is unreliable, the patient should be decontaminated, assuming that there has been a serious ingestion. In making the decision with regard to decontamination, it must be considered whether or not the agent is still accessible for decontamination. If the toxic substance was ingested many hours before clinical evaluation, it may already have been absorbed into the systemic circulation. Therefore, lavage or ipecac-induced emesis may be of little benefit, unless the toxin has an intrinsic mechanism that delays gastric emptying (e.g., an anticholinergic agent). If there is a possibility that the toxin is still present in the gut, then lavage or ipecac-induced emesis may be beneficial. The use of activated charcoal also may be warranted if the toxin can be adsorbed to the charcoal. Some agents, such as the toxic alcohols[29] and small charged substances such as lithium,[30] are not easily adsorbed to activated charcoal. The use of repetitive-dose activated charcoal may be beneficial because some toxins exhibit enterohepatic recirculation. These toxins are secreted into bile and ultimately the gastrointestinal tract, where they can be adsorbed to activated charcoal. Other toxins, such as phenobarbital, diffuse back into the gut by enteroenteric recirculation and can be adsorbed to activated charcoal.[31]

SYRUP OF IPECAC

Syrup of ipecac is a useful emetic. It acts through both a local and a central mechanism. Gastric irritation and stimulation of the chemoreceptor trigger zone[32,33] combine to produce emesis, typically within 30 min.[4,34] Vomiting secondary to ipecac usually terminates within 1 h.[35] One of the disadvantages of ipecac is that even after the vomiting has stopped, the patient may remain nauseated and thereby prevent the physician from using an oral antidote such as N-acetylcysteine or activated charcoal. In one study, an average of 2.2 h was required before activated charcoal could be administered to patients who had received ipecac.[5] A substantial controversy remains as to the efficacy of syrup of ipecac, since varied studies show that toxin removal ranges from 10 to 60 percent.[36-38] The main determinant of toxin removal is the amount of time after ingestion that precedes ipecac use. As the time delay increases, the percentage of removal decreases.[37,39] Therefore, ipecac may be best suited for home administration. In the home setting, patients who ingest a toxin can be given ipecac immediately after consultation with the poison center. This telephone communication is necessary to ensure that no contraindication to ipecac use exists (Table 15-3). Adult patients should be given 30 ml ipecac. Children 6 months to 1 year of age should be given 10 ml, and those 1 to 5 years of age should be given 15 ml. Above age 5, children can receive the adult dose. Ipecac should not be utilized in children under 6 months of age. The administration of ipecac can be followed with 100 to 250 ml water, depending on the size of the patient. If there is no emesis within 20 to 30 min, the ipecac dose may be repeated. If this fails, then the patient should be lavaged with an orogastric tube for toxin removal if this is clinically appropriate.

Although ipecac remains the treatment of choice for gastric emptying in the home, its use in the hospital has decreased. The use of lavage also has decreased,

TABLE 15–3. Guide to the Administration of Syrup of Ipecac

Dose
  Adult
    30 ml (2 tbsp)
  Children
    6–12 months, 10 ml (2 tsp)
    1–5 years, 15 ml (1 tbsp)
    Over 5 years, 30 ml (2 tbsp)
    One additional dose (a second dose) may be given if the patient has not vomited
      within 30 min
Contraindications
  Child less than 6 months of age
  Nontoxic ingestion
  Comatose patient
  Patient experiencing seizures
  Any patient expected to rapidly deteriorate
  Ingestion of a strong acid or alkali
  When vomiting will delay administration of an oral antidote
  Compromised gag reflex
  Patient with a hemorrhagic diathesis (cirrhosis, varices, thrombocytopenia)
  Concomitant ingestion of sharp, solid materials (thermometer, glass, nails, razor blades)
  Evidence of significant vomiting prior to ipecac utilization
  Any patient with an accidental "pure" petroleum distillate or turpentine ingestion, or
    any patient who is symptomatic (pulmonary, neurologic, cardiac) following a hydro-
    carbon ingestion.

Source: Adapted from *Goldfrank's Toxicologic Emergencies,* 4th ed. Norwalk, CT, Appleton & Lange, 1990. Used with permission.

whereas the frequency and variety of indications for the use of activated charcoal have increased dramatically. Because orogastric lavage has specific limitations, however, ipecac remains valuable in the emergency department in specific instances, such as the patient who has ingested iron tablets that are too large to pass through the lavage tube and yet not effectively bound to activated charcoal.

LAVAGE

Lavage with a no. 36 to 42 French orogastric tube can be used to rapidly empty the stomach following an overdose. Although the orogastric tube is valuable for liquid ingestions, many pills will not pass through its orifice. When performing lavage, two people are usually required at the bedside, one to perform the lavage and the other to maintain control of the airway. The patient should be placed in the left lateral decubitus position and then lavaged with small aliquots of saline; 50- to 200-ml increments are administered until the return is clear (Table 15–4). All forms of gastric decontamination are most efficacious when performed shortly after the ingestion. Following gastric lavage, the physician is immediately able to instill activated charcoal, *N*-acetylcysteine, or any other oral antidote without concern about a substantial delay resulting from ipecac-induced nausea or emesis.

TABLE 15–4. Guide for Performing Orogastric Lavage

Tube
  Adult/adolescent
    Large-bore orogastric Lavacuator hose, 36 to 40 French
  Children
    16 to 28 French orogastric-type tube
Procedure
  1. Endotracheal or nasotracheal intubation should precede gastric lavage in the unconscious or seizing patient, with or without an absent gag reflex.
  2. If the patient can tolerate intubation without trauma, the patient merits intubation. In any case, the airway must be meticulously protected. (Vomiting commonly follows lavage.)
  3. The proper length of the tube that will be passed is measured and marked before insertion. Once the tube is introduced, confirmation of position of the tube in the stomach is essential.
  4. The patient should be kept in the left lateral decubitus position.
  5. A saline lavage solution initiated with 200 ml aliquots should be instilled in an adult (or 50–100 ml aliquots in a child).
  6. This should be continued for at least several liters of lavage in an adult or until no particulate matter is seen and the efferent lavage solution is clear.
  7. The tube should be used for instillation of activated charcoal and a cathartic.
Contraindications
  Strong acid or alkali ingestion
  Significant hemorrhagic diathesis (relative contraindication)
  Nontoxic ingestion

Source: Adapted from *Goldfrank's Toxicologic Emergencies*, 4th ed. Norwalk, CT, Appleton & Lange, 1990. Used with permission.

ACTIVATED CHARCOAL

Activated charcoal has become the most useful agent available in the treatment of the overdosed patient. The charcoal is activated by steaming burnt organic material to remove other adsorbed materials. The use of activated charcoal is based on two approaches to decontamination. The first approach achieves a*d*sorption of material from the gastrointestinal tract before a*b*sorption occurs. This is accomplished by administering the charcoal as soon as possible after the toxin has been ingested.[40,41] The second approach blocks the enteroenteric[31] or enterohepatic[42] recirculation, enhancing the elimination of a drug or toxin and thus achieving adsorption before reabsorption. Although during enteroenteric and enterohepatic recirculation activated charcoal does not come in contact with large quantities of the drug or toxin, the presence of a high concentration gradient between the blood and the gastrointestinal tract can be utilized effectively for drugs such as phenobarbital,[31] digoxin, and theophylline.[43,44] Drugs that undergo enterohepatic circulation, such as imipramine and amitriptyline, are metabolized in the liver, with the resultant active metabolites excreted in the bile. There they are readily accessible to charcoal adsorption as they pass through the intestine. The gastrointestinal tract serves as a semipermeable membrane, and the activated charcoal binds the toxin as it crosses the membrane, thereby maintaining a low concentration in the gut and a high concentration gradient. Following enterohepatic or enteroenteric recirculation, the concentration is much less on the luminal side of the gut; therefore, the drug will continue to passively diffuse back into the gut from the blood and can be bound by activated charcoal and eliminated from the body.

Charcoal has a variable capacity to bind different toxins. It is relatively ineffective at binding small molecules, such as alcohols,[29,45] lithium,[30] cyanide, and most of the heavy metals.[45] Activated charcoal is, in general, less effective in binding ionized molecules.[46] Commonly used drugs, such as acetaminophen and theophylline, have excellent adsorption. It is recommended that the initial loading dose by 1 g/kg of activated charcoal. This dose can then be followed by an additional dose at 0.5 g/kg at variable intervals, depending on how much total activated charcoal is needed. This total will vary, but the goal is to achieve at least a 10:1 ratio of activated charcoal to toxin.[47] A massive drug overdose of a product such as theophylline may require hourly activated charcoal. If the patient ingested 100 (300-mg) tablets of theophylline, the total amount of activated charcoal needed to achieve a 10:1 ratio would be 300 g. Even if 100 (0.25-mg) digoxin pills were ingested, the amount of activated charcoal needed might be as little as 250 mg, but a dose of 1 g/kg should still be given as a minimal dose. The administration of activated charcoal for a toxin that may not be well adsorbed to charcoal is still warranted. For example, mercuric chloride is poorly bound to charcoal and may require an activated charcoal to mercuric chloride ratio of 25:1 to have any significant adsorption. The toxicity of mercuric chloride is of such concern, however, that even if a small amount can be adsorbed, this potential adsorption should be considered consequential. A loading dose of 1 g/kg of body weight of activated charcoal in a 70-kg man could potentially adsorb approximately 3 g mercuric chloride. This is the equivalent of three to five lethal doses.

Certain relative contraindications apply to the use of activated charcoal. Activated charcoal should not be used in the patient with gastric obstruction of any etiology. Activated charcoal also may not be warranted in caustic ingestions if gastrointestinal perforation has occurred or if endoscopy is imminent, since activated charcoal hampers the use of this diagnostic modality by obscuring visualization. Patients who require activated charcoal and who continue to be nauseated or vomit may benefit from an antiemetic such as metoclopramide before activated charcoal use. Unlike the phenothiazines, which may lower the seizure threshold and decrease gut motility, metoclopramide does not lower the seizure threshold and enhances gut motility. The dosage is 0.1 mg/kg intravenously initially, and this can be repeated, if necessary, up to a total dose of 1 mg/kg of body weight. Alternatively, the patient may have a nasogastric tube placed and the activated charcoal dripped in slowly by continuous infusion.

CATHARTICS

The benefits of cathartics are not as well quantified as those of lavage, emesis, or activated charcoal. Cathartics increase gut motility and decrease drug transit time through the gut, thereby allowing a drug less opportunity for absorption.[48] Despite the fact that only a few studies have shown the benefit of cathartics, they are routinely administered to poisoned patients after the initial dose of activated charcoal.[49–52] Currently, the three cathartics used are sorbitol, magnesium citrate, and magnesium sulfate. Sorbitol is considered the cathartic of choice. Its use avoids the possibility of hypermagnesemia associated with the magnesium cathartics. The sweet taste of sorbitol may make activated charcoal more palatable. The dosage is 0.5 to 1 g/kg of a 70% sorbitol solution. The lower dosage may be as effective and result in fewer complications. In young children, however, magnesium-containing cathartics may cause less volume depletion and therefore be easier to tolerate. For magnesium citrate, the dosage is 4 ml/kg up to a maximum 300 ml, while magnesium sulfate dosing is 250 mg/kg up to 30 g. The magnesium salts are contraindicated in patients with renal failure. In addition, no cathartic should be utilized in any patient with severe diarrhea, intestinal obstruction, or adynamic ileus. Severe electrolyte disturbances and dehydration may result if more than one dose of a cathartic is used[53-55] (Table 15–5).

WHOLE BOWEL IRRIGATION

Whole bowel irrigation (WBI) is based on a simple principle. If a drug is moved rapidly out of the body, it cannot be absorbed. WBI is performed with a high-molecular-weight polyethylene glycol–balanced electrolyte solution (PEG-ELS). It is an isotonic and iso-osmolar solution that is neither absorbed, nor leads to fluid or electrolyte shifts.[56] PEG-ELS has been used successfully in the treatment of overdoses of iron[57] and sustained lithium pills,[58] as well as in "body packers" (individuals who purposefully ingest bags of cocaine or heroin in an effort to smuggle them into a country).[59] The WBI procedure requires that the patient

TABLE 15–5. Guide for the Use of Cathartics

	Dose
Adults and children	
Magnesium citrate	4 ml/kg to 300 ml per dose
Magnesium sulfate	250 mg/kg up to 30 g
Sorbitol	½–1 g/kg (0.5 g/kg in children, with a maximum 50 g of 35% concentrate in children over 1 year)

Precautions

Not warranted in routine management of trivial ingestions in children.
Do not use phospho-soda preparations in children.
Do not use repetitive doses of magnesium containing cathartics.
Sorbitol administration in children should be used cautiously, with attention paid to fluid and electrolyte status.
Do not use repetitive doses of cathartics in children.
Oil-based cathartics should not be used because of the risks of aspiration and enhanced toxin absorption.

Contraindications

Adynamic ileus
Diarrhea
Abdominal trauma
Intestinal obstruction
Renal failure (magnesium sulfate or citrate)

Source: Adapted from *Goldfrank's Toxicologic Emergencies*, 4th ed. Norwalk, CT, Appleton & Lange, 1990. Used with permission.

ingest a large amount of fluid for an extended period of time. For the adult, this consists of 2 liters/h and for the child about 500 ml/h. PEG-ELS may be particularly useful in the management of overdoses of drugs/toxins that are not well adsorbed to activated charcoal. The use of PEG-ELS in the "body packer" may remove packets of drugs before they rupture. Following clearance of the gut with PEG-ELS, it may be easier to perform an upper gastrointestinal series with a small bowel study. This approach may be indicated to determine if packets persist in the gut. Minor complications such as bloating, rectal irritation, and abdominal distension have been reported. Another concern with the use of WBI is the possibility that activated charcoal may not be as efficacious when used concomitantly with WBI, since the PEG-ELS also seems to bind to activated charcoal, thus decreasing its efficacy.[60] These issues have only been studied in vitro, but their implications are of concern and merit further evaluation.

The contraindications to the use of PEG-ELS for WBI include patients with caustic ingestions, possible gastrointestinal perforation, and the presence of bowel obstruction. Continuous observation and sequential radiographs are therefore required in the patient receiving WBI.

In summary, the procedure used for decontamination must be individualized for each patient, the toxin, and the history of ingestion. Mastery of the basic principles necessary to utilize each modality of decontamination is essential to treat poisoned or overdosed patients. By answering a few general questions, the physician will be able to determine if gastric emptying is warranted and which modality will serve the particular patient best. Initiating the evaluation with the

TABLE 15–6. Decision Analysis for the Use of Gastric Emptying in the Poisoned Patient

No Gastric Emptying

Ingestion of nontoxic agents—
Trivial ingestions of toxic agents—based on history, course
Agent unlikely to remain in stomach—alcohols, acetaminophen
Agents of low lethality, well adsorbed to charcoal for which charcoal:drug excess easily achieved (unless massive amount, early presentation)—benzodiazepines, clonidine
Prior post-repeated spontaneous vomiting
Gastric emptying more dangerous than risk of absorption—most caustics, combative patient with low-risk ingestion

Ipecac More Likely To Be of Value

Home use
Agents too large to pass through lavage tube
Infants and young children

Lavage More Likely To Be of Value

Absence of airway protective reflexes due to seizures, cardiovascular collapse, or altered mental status—many causes
Imminent potential loss of airway protective reflexes—cyclic antidepressants, isoniazid, propoxyphene, camphor, propranolol, cyanide, strychnine, and others
Agents for which early activated charcoal is important—nearly all cases, particularly theophylline and sedative-hypnotics
Liquids

Source: Adapted from *Goldfrank's Toxicologic Emergencies,* 4th ed. Norwalk, CT, Appleton & Lange, 1990. Used with permission.

basic question of whether or not the ingestion is a potentially dangerous one is essential. The clinician must then determine whether or not the toxin can be removed by gastric emptying. The next decision may be whether syrup of ipecac or gastric lavage is better or actually indicated. This question may best be answered by the size of the pills, tablets, or capsules and the potential for the toxin to cause a change in mental status and ultimately alter airway control. Additional pertinent questions that must be answered to most effectively achieve gastrointestinal decontamination include: How well is the substance bound to activated charcoal? Is there an oral antidote for the toxin or drug? Should the dosage of activated charcoal be repeated? Is the use of a cathartic necessary? Would WBI be useful? After answering all or some of these questions, the physician will be able to determine an appropriate strategy for gastric emptying in almost every patient (Table 15–6).

LABORATORY EVALUATION

Although in certain specific instances a toxicologic diagnosis can and should be made by utilizing the toxicology laboratory, this is rarely done during the initial emergency department management.[61] In the emergency department, one can usually rely on assessment of the clinical presentation. Many physicians misunderstand the limitations of their laboratory and possess unreasonable expectations. When sending a "tox screen," it must be known what the laboratory is capable of doing and how rapidly the results will be available.[62,63] Quantitative levels are of importance in the acute management of the following specific ingestions: acetaminophen, carbon monoxide, digoxin, ethylene glycol, lithium, methanol, methemoglobin-forming agents, theophylline, and salicylates. These agents may or may not result in characteristic clinical manifestations and necessitate treatment with special methods, depending on the level.

Alternatively, the patient who has overdosed on a benzodiazepine and has a blood level that is four to five times the "therapeutic level" will be managed in the same manner as the patient who has a "therapeutic level" even if they are both comatose. The reason for the lack of utility of this level is that the LD_{50} for oral benzodiazepines is very high and little or no correlation exists between the measured level and the toxicity of the benzodiazepines. This is not the case for such toxins as salicylates or theophylline. In an acetaminophen overdose, for example, clinical manifestations are limited, and it is useless for the physician to send a urine toxicology screen for acetaminophen. If the result is positive, a blood acetaminophen level will certainly be required to determine the risk of toxicity. The potential benefits of sending a specimen of blood, urine, or, rarely, gastric contents should be thoroughly understood and discussed with your toxicology laboratory. There are thousands of toxins and only a very small number of laboratory analyses that can be performed in any particular laboratory and fewer yet in the typical hospital setting. When a specimen is sent to the laboratory, the clinician must know what questions he or she is asking and whether the laboratory can perform an analysis that answers the questions. If a patient has used cocaine within the last several hours, a screen that looks for cocaine itself may be negative, while an assay of cocaine metabolites would probably be positive. The sensitivity of each specific test must be understood. For example, if a test is too sensitive, it may result in a large number of false-positive results. If a test is too specific for a particular toxin, it may not recognize as present other similar toxins representative of the same class or family. At this level of specificity, a different test would be required for every toxin, thereby substantially increasing the cost of detecting each toxin.

One of the best clinical examples is the presence of a negative toxicology screen for opioids in a patient who has been awakened and is fully alert following a dose of the pure opioid antagonist naloxone. The clinician can be certain that an opioid was used because of the clinical response, despite the fact that laboratory results for the test requested are negative. The interpretation is critical: Either the drug was used in such small amounts that the test was quantitatively insensitive, or the test was too specific to recognize the opioid in question. Another problem results from the inability of a positive test to determine when the toxin was most recently used. For instance, certain cocaine metabolites can be recognized in the urine of a chronic abuser for up to 3 weeks following utilization.[64] Thus a positive test never confirms intoxication; it only confirms use or exposure. The diagnosis of intoxication is made on clinical grounds.

Although the generic urine toxicology screen is neither useful nor recommended in the emergency department, medicolegally, it may be helpful. Besides requesting specific drug levels, there are additional laboratory data that can be very useful to the physician on an emergent basis. As the physician is placing the intravenous line, blood can be drawn for determination of electrolytes, glucose, blood urea nitrogen (BUN), creatinine, and osmolality. The ECG may be very important and should be done soon after the intravenous line is placed. The patient's acid-base status can be evaluated by calculation of the anion gap: Na^+ (mEq/liter) $-$ [Cl^- (mEq/liter) $+$ $HCO3^-$ (mEq/liter)], with normal being 8 to 12 mEq/liter. A determination of the osmolal gap should be made, being equal to the measured freezing point osmolality minus the calculated osmolarity. The calculated osmolarity (mosmol/liter) is equal to [$2Na^+$ (mEq/liter) $+$ BUN (mg%)/2.8 $+$ glucose (mg%)/18]. The normal calculated osmolarity is 280 to 295 mosmol/liter. A difference of more than 10 mosmol/liter between the measured and calculated values is considered abnormal. The determination of the osmolality may be important if a toxic alcohol ingestion is suspected. The arterial blood gas can be used to quickly determine the patient's minute-to-minute metabolic status and may be the first clue to an acid-base abnormality.

BEDSIDE CLUES AND RAPID TESTS

Bedside clues and testing can help the physician establish a diagnosis. The first effort is to group the vital signs into possible toxidromes (toxic syndromes), although this is more difficult in a mixed overdose. The physician should become familiar with characteristic odors. The minty odor of oil of wintergreen, when noted in the patient presenting with tinnitus, decreased hearing, and a respiratory alkalosis, should alert the physician to a significant methylsalicylate overdose.[65] In the patient with an altered mental status, the odor of a new car or a shower curtain on his or her breath should suggest an etchlorvynol (Placydil) overdose.[65] In the patient with rales, frothy sputum, respiratory distress, diarrhea, profuse sweating, the odor of garlic on his or her breath should suggest the diagnosis of an organophosphate exposure.[65] Other typical odors of importance include that of russet apples or ketones, suggesting diabetic ketoacidosis.[65] The odor of bitter almonds may be associated with cyanide poisoning,[65] although it must be remembered that a significant portion of the population will not have the ability to detect this odor.[66]

Physical examination of the blood of the patient who presents with respiratory or cardiac symptoms and cyanosis is another useful bedside aid. If the blood appears chocolate brown, the diagnosis of methemoglobinemia should be considered.[67] Although this diagnosis probably can be confirmed clinically if the patient's cyanosis does not respond to high-flow oxygen, the cooximeter-determined methemoglobin level is the definitive assay. The appropriate treatment is methylene blue in a dose of 1 to 2 ml of a 1% solution when clinically indicated.[68]

A Woods (ultraviolet) lamp, typically used for the detection of corneal abrasions or fungal infections, also may be useful if ethlyene glycol has been ingested. Some antifreezes have fluorescein added so that radiator leaks can be easily identified. When viewed under a Woods lamp, these fluorescein-marked ethylene glycol antifreezes will glow, as will the patient's urine if the product has been ingested. Since not all radiator antifreezes have fluorescein in them, a negative test does not mean the patient did not ingest ethylene glycol.

Use of a urine dipstick to look for urine or serum ketones is also of toxicologic importance. A positive test for ketones may result from diabetic ketoacidosis, salicylates,[69] isopropyl alcohol,[70] acetone, or alcoholic ketoacidosis. At the same time, the presence of ketones may be used to help eliminate the other two major toxic alcohol ingestions (ethylene glycol and methanol), which do not produce ketones upon metabolism. Similarly, the ferric chloride test is a very sensitive and specific assay for the presence of salicylates, although it will not determine if a patient has salicylism. The test is performed by adding 2 to 3 drops of a 10% ferric chloride to 1 ml of urine. The urine will turn purple if acetylsalicyclic acid or phenylpyruvic acid is present in the urine sample.[71] There are occasional false-positive reactions (if methyldopa or a phenothiazine is ingested) but very few false-negative reactions. If a ferric chloride test on the urine is positive, a salicylate determination should be done by the laboratory.

The urine dipstick also can help make the diagnosis of myoglobinuria or hemoglobinuria if positive for blood in the absence of red blood cells on microscopic analysis. The differentiation of myoglobinuria and hemoglobinuria can be then made by centrifuging the serum and noting if the supernatant is red. Myoglobin, which is one-fourth the size of hemoglobin at approximately 16,000 Da, is easily filtered in the renal tubules and yields a clear supernatant, whereas hemoglobin will not be easily filtered and imparts its red color to the supernatant. The early detection of the presence of rhabdomyolysis is critical to the appropriate management of muscle injury and the prevention of acute tubular necrosis.

Further microscopic evaluation of the urine may reveal rhomboid or needle-shaped calcium oxalate crystals, which may be present in patients who have ingested ethylene glycol,[72,73] although they have been reported to be absent even in the presence of large ingestions of glycol.[74] Therefore, even if both bedside tests (Woods lamp and microscopic urine evaluation) are negative, ethylene glycol levels should still be determined if there is suspicion of a glycol ingestion.

Another very important bedside test is the use of the electrocardiogram (ECG) for assessing the consequences of a possible tricyclic antidepressant (TCA) overdose. Besides the presence of a tachycardia,[75,76] these patients also frequently develop subtle ECG abnormalities. Some of these changes include a right axis deviation, which consists of an S wave in leads I and aVL, and an R wave in aVR.[76] These changes occur because the smaller right fascicle may be poisoned more easily than the left.[76] As toxicity increases, a widened QRS complex may develop.[79] In TCA poisoning, the width of the QRS complex is directly correlated with the risk of ventricular arrhythmias and seizures.[77] The recognition of this abnormality is essential, since therapy with sodium bicarbonate is indicated and may be highly effective.[78,79] It has been shown that this condition can be treated with sodium bicarbonate[79] or sodium chloride[80] or by hyperventilation.[81] Neither of these latter two therapies are as effective as sodium bicarbonate in the reversal of the conduction abnormalities associated with TCA toxicity.[80,82]

When a blood sample is sent to the laboratory, the patient's condition must be considered if the toxicologic results are to be of value. The time of ingestion, prior exposure to a drug or toxin, or dependency on a particular drug or drug group will each result in a different clinical pattern and complicate the interpretation of a laboratory value. The units of the drug being monitored must be known in the particular laboratory employed, since the units utilized may not be the same as those used in a standard textbook. It would be a grave mistake to have a laboratory report a 4-h acetaminophen level in a particular patient as 35 mg/dl and have this level be considered nontoxic. This might occur because most clinicians expect acetaminophen levels to be reported in micrograms per milliliter. In reality, this particular level is equivalent to 350 μg/ml and would be toxic at 4 h, having a substantial risk of hepatotoxicity and necessitating antidotal therapy.[83,84] The normal range for each agent of the particular laboratory should be ascertained, and the units of unfamiliar drug results must be checked.

Antidotal treatment may be warranted under certain circumstances before a definitive diagnosis has been made. A patient with a significant acetaminophen ingestion presenting 8 h after ingestion should receive N-acetylcysteine at the time of presentation, while the level determination is pending in the laboratory, because any delay in treatment may lead to an increased risk for hepatotoxicity.[85] Similarly, the patient with a consequential theophylline overdose should immediately receive repetitive doses of activated charcoal, and the nephrology service notified that charcoal hemoperfusion may be needed.[44,86,87] Treatment is often required before definitive diagnosis when the ingestion of a toxic alcohol is considered, since both ethylene glycol and methanol ingestions may have delayed clinical manifestations and toxicity.[88] If a history exists that these toxins were ingested, it is prudent to send a sample to the laboratory immediately and to start the patient on an intravenous ethanol infusion in order to block the conversion of either agent to its toxic metabolites.[89–92] One should simultaneously inform the nephrology service of the patient's potential need for hemodialysis. The patient should be started on folinic acid, 50 mg every 4 h, in the case of a methanol ingestion[93] or pyridoxine, 50 mg, and thiamine, 100 mg, every day for an ethylene glycol ingestion.[94] In this same regard, the patient with possible carbon monoxide intoxication should be given 100% oxygen while awaiting the result of carboxyhemoglobin level determination.[95,96]

THERAPY

URINARY pH CONTROL

Urinary pH manipulation is an important method of enhancing drug elimination for a select group of toxins. The concept of enhancement of toxin removal with forced diuresis is dependent on a toxin having significant renal elimination. Forced diuresis, however, has not proven beneficial, except when combined with urine pH manipulation. Therefore, forced diuresis is neither efficacious nor appropriate as a technique of management because it does not increase the rate of excretion and may lead to the potential complications of fluid overload, including congestive heart failure, cerebral edema, and electrolyte disturbances.

The alteration of the urine pH, either making the urine more alkaline or acidic, offers the opportunity to change the ratio of the ionized/non-ionized fraction of a toxin. Toxins that are in their ionized state in the urine do not cross the renal tubular membrane and are therefore trapped in the urine. Weak bases and weak acids are theoretically most amenable to pH manipulation. In order for pH manipulation to be efficacious, the toxin must have a pK_a that is in the range of urine pH. The pK_a is the pH at which half the toxin is in the ionized (polar) state and half is in the non-ionized state. If the pH of the urine can be manipulated so that more toxin can be in the ionized form, then reabsorption will decrease and more of toxin will be trapped in the urine and eliminated. Substances that are weak acids are more readily ionized in alkaline solutions, and the converse is true for substances that are weak bases.

Although urinary acidification had been recommended previously to enhance elimination of toxins such as phencyclidine[97] and amphetamines,[98] it is now generally believed that the risks of urinary acidification outweigh any potential benefit. One reason is that the agents in question may result in rhabdomyolysis and myoglobinuria. Acute tubular necrosis, a potential complication of rhabdomyolysis, may be exacerbated by urinary acidification by enhancing tubular deposition of myoglobin. Urinary alkalinization can be used to enhance the elimination of salicylates,[99,100] phenobarbital,[101] chlorpropamide,[102] and chlorphenoxy herbicides.[103] Alkalinization is achieved by raising the urinary pH to 7.5 to 8.0.[104,105] An initial bolus of about 1 to 2 mEq/kg of sodium bicarbonate is usually sufficient to achieve this goal.[104] Urinary alkalinization cannot be achieved effectively in the presence of hypokalemia.[106,107] In the presence of hypokalemia, the kidney conserves potassium and excretes a hydronium ion. Urinary alkalinization is particularly useful in the presence of salicylate overdoses. Salicylate is a weak acid with a pK_a of about 3.5, and it becomes more readily trapped in the ionized state as the urine pH reaches the 7.5 range, thereby enhancing its excretion. Although acetazolamide is another agent that can be used to alkalinize the urine, it is not generally utilized because urinary alkalinization is accomplished at the cost of a systemic acidification and potential acidemia.[108,109] While this may have a salutary effect on the urinary ion trapping of drugs such as salicylates, it may concomitantly result in more of the drug entering tissue spaces, such as the brain,[110] as the developing pH gradient allows for enhanced tissue ion trapping. Potential complications of alkalinization include the loss of enzymatic efficacy if alkalemia ensues,[106] the risk of congestive heart failure if a large sodium load is administered to achieve alkalinization,[111] and the risk of shifting the oxyhemoglobin dissociation curve to the left, decreasing the unloading of oxygen at the tissue level. Careful monitoring of the serum pH, the patient's fluid status, and oxygenation are therefore warranted. The goal of alkalinization is to maintain the serum pH at 7.5 to 7.55.[105] After the initial bolus of sodium bicarbonate, approximately 150 mEq can be placed in 1 liter of D_5W and infused at twice the maintenance rate.

Sodium bicarbonate plays a special role in the management of overdoses of tricyclic antidepressants (TCA) and other drugs with sodium channel blocking properties.[112-114] These agents include the type IA antiarrhythmic agents (quinidine and procainamide),[115] flecainide,[116] cocaine,[117] and, in theory, carbamazepine and the antiviral agent amantadine. In these overdoses, sodium bicarbonate is used to achieve serum alkalinization. Simultaneously, the infusion of a large sodium load may achieve partial reversal of the sodium channel blockade.[118] An additional beneficial mechanism may be due to an increased binding of the TCA to protein at a higher pH. This may permit less TCA to be bound to tissue receptors and decrease myocardial binding, thereby limiting toxicity.[113]

EXTRACORPOREAL TECHNIQUES

Hemodialysis and charcoal hemoperfusion are effective methods of extracorporeal toxin removal, whereas peritoneal dialysis has minimal utility for the patient with an overdose. The potential role of continuous arterial-venous hemofiltration, a new form of extracorporeal drug removal, is currently under investigation in medical toxicology. When using any of these techniques, it is important to maintain the patient's endogenous elimination processes. Therefore, the urine output should be maintained at an optimal level to ensure the maximum clearance of the drug. At the same time, activated charcoal should be given as indicated.

Hemodialysis, charcoal hemoperfusion, and hemofiltration utilize the principle of passing blood through an extraction system consisting of a dialyzer, an activated charcoal cartridge, and a hemofilter, respectively. Catheters are inserted on both the arterial and venous sides of the circulatory system, and as the blood leaves the arterial side, it passes through the specific extraction system before arriving on the venous side. Prior to deciding that a patient should receive hemodialysis or charcoal hemoperfusion, several questions must be answered: Will the toxin cause any systemic toxicity? Can the toxin be removed by an extracorporeal technique? Is this procedure the best and safest way to manage the patient? Can the patient tolerate the appropriate procedure? In critically ill patients or those who have ingested consequential toxins, it is very important to consider these extracorporeal removal methods as early as possible, while the patient remains stable or prior to such deterioration that the patient can no longer tolerate the procedure.

Important considerations relating to toxin dialyzability are the size of the toxin, its protein binding, the ionic state of the toxin, and the volume of distribution of the toxin.[119] Under ideal conditions, these characteristics will determine the amount of toxin that is removed. In patients who are hypotensive, the efficacy of toxin removal will be diminished because blood flow will be decreased, thereby reducing the amount of toxin exposed to activated charcoal or the dialysate fluid. Less consequential factors in the removal process that should be considered include the pK_a of the molecule and the properties of the dialyzer or activated charcoal to be utilized. As the toxin's molecular weight approaches 500 Da, clearance decreases.[119] Small, uncharged, non-protein-bound molecules are better cleared by hemodialysis than by hemoperfusion. Since most toxins weigh less than 500 Da, this is not a common limiting factor. A small, highly protein-bound drug, such as phenytoin (mol. wt. 252) is not removed particularly well by either hemodialysis or hemoperfusion. The ionic state of the toxin is important, since uncharged particles cross cell membranes, while charged substances remain in the plasma and are therefore best removed by extracorporeal techniques. A fourth characteristic of importance, the volume of distribution, is a theoretical value defining the apparent space that would be required to contain the total body drug load. The *volume of distribution* (V_d) is defined as the total amount of drug in the body divided by the serum drug concentration. A small volume of distribution indicates that the drug is located in the vascular compartment, whereas drugs that have large volumes of distribution exist to a greater extent outside the vascular compartment, in the tissues. Drugs that have large volumes of distribution (greater than or equal to 1 liter/kg) are not readily available to extracorporeal removal processes. The dialysis of drugs such as the tricyclic antidepressants is neither indicated clinically, for the response could not be rapid enough, nor efficacious, due to the agent's large volumes of distribution and inaccessibility to the procedure.

While hemodialysis plays a significant role in removing some toxins, hemoperfusion results in better clearance of those substances which bind to activated charcoal.[120] An exception to this approach is in salicylate intoxication, where hemodialysis is employed even though charcoal hemoperfusion may remove the toxin more efficaciously. In this case, the amount of salicylate in the body is only part of the problem. The intoxication results in severe fluid and electrolyte abnormalities, as well as other metabolic disturbances.[121-123] Although hemoperfusion would presumably decrease the drug concentration more rapidly than hemodialysis, immediately life-threatening fluid and electrolyte problems would not be ameliorated. Hemodialysis is therefore the procedure of choice in salicylate overdoses.

Hemodialysis is most effective for small, water-soluble molecules. Hemodialysis depends on passing the patient's blood over a semipermeable membrane against a concentration gradient in the dialysate. Since the concentration of the toxin is higher in the blood than in the dialysate, the toxin will passively flow into the dialysate and be cleared from the body. Effective tissue perfusion is also required. Effective tissue perfusion is dependent on the ability to pump blood with a reasonable blood pressure to the dialysis machine, as well as on the quality of the dialyzer. Hemodialysis is commonly used for salicylates and toxins not well adsorbed to charcoal, such as lithium[30] and the toxic alcohols (methanol and ethylene glycol).[124-126] Although many other agents (e.g., phenobarbital or acetaminophen) can be removed by hemodialysis, the benefit is limited, recovery may not be enhanced, and the risks of the procedure are significant.

Problems associated with the loss of electrolytes can be prevented by making the dialysate fluid close to the physiologic characteristics of electrolytes and pH, thereby eliminating a concentration gradient for electrolytes. This approach necessitates careful analysis of the patient's serum electrolytes during dialysis. Other problems may result from the fact that hemodialysis necessitates a large intravenous line that may result in bleeding, thrombosis, hematoma formation, and infection.[127] These problems can be exacerbated by the requirement for anticoagulation during dialysis. Dialysis also may result in platelet destruction with subsequent thrombocytopenia.[128] Another major complication can be the development of hypotension as dialysis is initiated.[127]

Successful hemoperfusion does not require that a toxin be highly soluble in water. Larger, protein-bound molecules are also effectively removed.[120] The primary requirement for toxin removal by hemoperfusion is that the agent bind to activated charcoal. Although many toxins can be removed by hemodialysis, few agents are routinely treated with this technique because of the risk/benefit analysis and a limited understanding of efficacy. Hemoperfusion is used most commonly in the treatment of severe theophylline overdoses.[127,130] Theophylline binds well to activated charcoal, and there are not usually severe electrolyte abnormalities that would require correction by hemodialysis. Other agents that are theoretically perfusable but rarely treated in this fashion include phenobarbital, methotrexate, and phenytoin.[127,136] The complications of hemoperfusion, like those seen with hemodialysis, may include hypotension and depletion of electrolytes, particularly calcium.[132] Infection, bleeding from the puncture site, hematoma formation, and the risk of heparinization remain of concern.[127]

Although peritoneal dialysis has been used for toxicologic problems in the past, its rate of clearance is rather small, and it is rarely, if ever, clinically indicated or efficacious.[119,128] This procedure is not recommended. It lacks efficacy, and the aforementioned modalities are much more reliable and effective. The one instance where peritoneal dialysis might become beneficial is when a patient has a delayed or prolonged transfer to another institution to accomplish either hemodialysis or hemoperfusion. Under these conditions, it might be worthwhile to begin peritoneal dialysis while enroute as a temporizing measure.

ANTIDOTES

Numerous antidotes are available to the physician on an emergent basis (Table 15–7). Some of the more important agents, including oxygen, naloxone, glucagon, pyridoxine, digoxin-specific antibody (Fab) fragments, N-acetylcysteine, and physostigmine, will be discussed in depth.

Oxygen is used generically in the treatment of hypoxia. As an antidote, it is specifically indicated for carbon monoxide (CO) poisoning. In the CO-poisoned patient, oxygen has two important effects: It decreases the tissue hypoxia induced by CO, and it displaces CO from hemoglobin, thereby shorting the half-life of carboxyhemoglobin and decreasing the toxic effects.[133,136]

Naloxone, a pure opioid antagonist, is a competitive inhibitor at the opioid receptor site and can thereby reverse associated adverse effects such as respiratory depression, miosis, and central nervous system depression. All patients with respiratory depression of any etiology should be given a trial of these two agents.

TABLE 15–7. A Comprehensive List of Antidotes that Should Be Available for the Treatment of Poisoned Patients*

Therapeutic Agent	Uses
Activated charcoal	General (adsorbent, "gastrointestinal dialysis")
Antivenin (Crotalidae), Polyvalent (Wyeth)	Crotalid snake bites
Antivenin (*Latrodectus mactans*) (MSD)	Black widow spider bites
Atropine	Bradydysrhythmias, cholinesterase inhibitors (organophosphates, physostigmine)
	Mushrooms: clitocybe, inocybe
Botulinal antitoxin (ABE-trivalent)	Botulism (available from local health department or Centers for Disease Control)
Calcium chloride	Oxalates, fluoride, hydrofluoric acid, ethylene glycol, calcium channel blockers, black widow spider bites, magnesium
Calcium gluconate	Hydrofluoric acid burns, black widow spider bites
Cyanide kit (amyl nitrite, sodium nitrite, sodium thiosulfate)	Cyanide, hydrogen sulfide
Deferoxamine mesylate (Desferal)	Iron
Dextrose in water (50%), (20%)	Hypoglycemic agents, patients with altered mental status
Diazepam (Valium)	Seizures, severe agitation, stimulants
Digoxin specific antibodies (Digibind)	Digoxin, digitoxin, and other cardiac glycosides
Dimercaprol (BAL, British anti-lewisite)	Arsenic, mercury, gold, lead
Diphenhydramine (Benadryl)	Extrapyramidal reactions (antipsychotics), allergic reactions
Dopamine HCl	Hypotension
Edrophonium chloride (Tensilon)	Anticholinergic agents, diagnostic test (myasthenia gravis)
Ethanol injection 100% for dilution or 10%	Methyl alcohol, ethylene glycol
Ethylenediaminetetraacetic acid (Calcium EDTA)	Lead, zinc, and other heavy metals
Folinic acid/folic acid	Methyl alcohol, methotrexate
Glucagon	Beta blockers, calcium channel blockers, oral hypoglycemics
Haloperidol (Haldol)	General (as a major tranquilizer)
Ipecac, syrup of	Emetic
Magnesium sulfate (Epsom salts) or magnesium citrate	General cathartic

Agent	Indication
Magnesium sulfate injection	Digitalis, hydrofluoric acid
Methylene blue (1% solution)	Methemoglobinemia
N-acetylcysteine (Mucomyst)	Acetaminophen
Naloxone hydrochloride (Narcan)	Opioids (agonists, partial agonists/antagonists)
Niacinamide	Vacor rodenticide
Nitroprusside	Antihypertensive, ergotamines
Norepinephrine (Levarterenol)	Hypotension (preferred for tricyclic antidepressants), alpha blockers
Oxygen	Carbon monoxide, cyanide, hydrogen sulfide
{Oxygen, hyperbaric}	
d-Penicillamine	Copper, lead, mercury, arsenic
Phenobarbital	General (as anticonvulsant, sedative)
Phenytoin injection	General (an anticonvulsant, antiarrhythmic)
Physostigmine salicylate (Antilirium)	Anticholinergic agents
Polyethylene glycol (Golytely)	General (gastric decontamination)
Pralidoxime chloride (2-PAM-chloride) (Protopam)	Acetyl cholinesterase inhibitors (organophosphates and carbamates)
Protamine sulfate injection	Heparin
Pyridoxine hydrochloride	Ethylene glycol, isoniazid, monomethylhydrazine containing mushrooms
Sodium bicarbonate (5% solution)	Iron, ethylene glycol, methanol, salicylates, tricyclic antidepressants, phenobarbital, quinidine, chlorpropamide
Sorbitol	General (cathartic); sweetener for activated charcoal
Starch	Iodine
Thiamine hydrochloride	Thiamine deficiency, ethylene glycol
Vitamin K$_1$ (Aquamephyton)	Oral anticoagulants

*Each emergency department should have all the above agents readily available to its staff. Some of these antidotes may be stored in the pharmacy, others may be available from the Centers for Disease Control, but the precise mechanism for locating each one must be known by each staff member.

Source: Adapted from *Goldfrank's Toxicologic Emergencies,* 4th ed. Norwalk, CT, Appleton & Lange, 1990. Used with permission.

GLUCAGON

Glucagon is a natural polypeptide hormone that can be used in the treatment of patients with beta-blocker or calcium channel blocker overdoses, as well as for the management of certain hypoglycemic patients. Patients with either beta-blocker or calcium channel blocker overdoses can present with altered mental status, hypotension, bradycardia, decreased cardiac output, and arrhythmias.[135–139] The toxicity from these agents may be resistant to conventional therapy, such as atropine, and inotropic agents, such as dopamine, dobutamine, or epinephrine. Glucagon at high doses may increase myocardial cAMP,[140] leading to increased myocardial inotropic and chronotropic effects.[141–144] This increase in cAMP occurs through a non-beta-mediated pathway.[142] The initial glucagon bolus should be 50 µg/kg, given over a 1- to 2-min interval. If there is no clinical response, then the bolus can be increased up to 145 µg/kg (approximately 10 mg in a 70-kg person).[139] If a favorable clinical response is achieved, then an infusion can be started to maintain the desired effect. The hourly infusion dosage should be the same amount utilized to obtain initial improvement, usually in the range of 1 to 5 mg/h.[146,147] Complications of the use of glucagon include nausea, vomiting, allergic reactions, hyperglycemia, and hypokalemia.

DIGOXIN-SPECIFIC ANTIBODIES (Fab)

Digibind (digoxin-specific antibodies, Fab) has revolutionized the approach to the patient with digoxin intoxication or overdose. These Fab fragments are the smallest effective component of sheep antibodies created after chronic immunization with digoxin bound to bovine serum albumin. The Fab fragments are capable of reversing all the toxic effects of digoxin overdose. Acute overdose with digoxin can present with nausea and vomiting, altered mental status, and diverse cardiac arrhythmias.[147,148] Each vial (40 mg) of Digibind is capable of binding 0.6 mg digoxin. After the binding of digoxin to Digibind, digoxin is inactivated and can no longer exert myocardial or systemic toxicity.[149] The dosage of Digibind is dependent on the digoxin burden and the clinical status of the patient. Once Digibind has been employed, the serum digoxin level can no longer be considered reliable, since the level reported by the laboratory is that of both the bound and unbound digoxin.[150]

N-ACETYLCYSTEINE

Since its approval by the Food and Drug Administration in 1985, N-acetylcysteine (NAC) has dramatically altered the management of acetaminophen overdoses and decreased morbidity and mortality. It is believed that the hepatic and infrequent renal toxicity induced by acetaminophen may be secondary to the increased formation of a toxic metabolite, N-acetyl-p-benzoquinoneimine (NAPQI).[151] In overdose, acetaminophen depletes hepatic glutathione, which is required to detoxify NAPQI. NAC is felt to prevent toxicity by (1) replacing depleted glutathione,[152] (2) increasing the amount of acetaminophen that is sulfated, thereby decreasing the use of the toxic pathway,[153] (3) increasing glutathione synthesis,[154] and (4) acting as an antioxidant and decreasing the amount of inflammation.[155] An acetaminophen (APAP) level should be obtained no earlier than 4 h after ingestion, and treatment should be initiated if this APAP level exceeds the lower limit for the appropriate time period on the Rumack-Matthew nomogram. Individuals to be treated should be given a loading dose of NAC and then 17 subsequent doses every 4 h. The loading dose is 140 mg/kg, and the subsequent doses are 70 mg/kg. NAC is most efficacious if given within the first 8 h after the overdose.[85] Treating every patient before a level has been determined may lead to unnecessary therapy, but the initiation of therapy after ingestion should certainly not exceed 8 h, since toxicity may increase. Benefits from NAC have been demonstrated up to 24 h after ingestion,[85] and even those patients with hepatic encephalopathy may benefit from treatment no matter how substantial a delay has occurred.[156] This suggests that NAC may have mechanisms of action as an antidote in addition to those mentioned above.

PYRIDOXINE

Pyridoxine (vitamin B_6) is a water-soluble vitamin that is essential for many enzymatic reactions. Functional pyridoxine deficiency and subsequent seizures may result from isoniazid or monomethylhydrazine toxicity.[157,158] The effects of these agents include inhibition of pyridoxine kinase, the enzyme that transforms pyridoxine to its active form,[159] and binding to pyridoxine phosphate. This binding leads to a decrease in pyridoxine concentration by facilitating its excretion.[159] These two mechanisms lead to decreased transformation of glutamic acid to gamma-aminobutyric acid (GABA).[159] GABA is the major inhibitory neurotransmitter in the central nervous system. Decreased GABA levels may result in seizures. Chin et al.[160] showed that pyridoxine and the GABA agonist diazepam were effective and synergistic when given to dogs with seizures induced by isoniazid (INH). A patient who presents with seizures that are unresponsive to standard interventions should be given an empiric dose of 5 g pyridoxine (70 mg/kg) intravenously.[161] If INH is thought to be the cause of the seizures, then the patient should receive 1 g pyridoxine for every gram of INH taken.[162] If the amount ingested is unknown, then the patient should receive 5 g (70 mg/kg) pyridoxine as an initial intravenous dose. In either case, the patient also should receive diazepam with the pyridoxine.[156,157] No single dose of pyridoxine should exceed 375 mg/kg because pyridoxine toxicity may occur.

PHYSOSTIGMINE

Physostigmine is a acetylcholinesterase inhibitor that can cross the blood-brain barrier and has analeptic properties. It is currently recommended for severe anticholinergic poisoning, particularly in patients with peripheral signs of anticholinergic poisoning such as hyperthermia, flushed dry skin and dry mucous membranes, dilated pupils, decreased bowel sounds, and urinary retention. If these anticholinergic manifestations are present and the patient has severe signs of anticholinergic poisoning, such as agitation, hallucinations, or seizures with a normal QRS and no arrhythmias, physostigmine use may be warranted.[163] The adult patient should be treated with 2 mg; the child with 0.02 mg/kg given over a 2- to 3-min period.[164] The dose can be repeated if no cholinergic manifestations are noted and the anticholinergic signs persist. Because of the cholinergic side effects of bronchorrhea, seizures, asystole,[165] and respiratory arrest, extreme caution in patient selection should be employed.

PSYCHIATRIC ASSESSMENT

Not all patients who present for treatment secondary to a drug overdose are suicidal. The patient who abuses cocaine or some other illicit agent on a chronic basis may suffer a serious adverse effect and present for this reason. Substance abusers, as well as suicidal patients, are in need of psychiatric evaluation and eventual psychosocial support. While these patients may not be in need of medical admission, they may warrant psychiatric admission to meet their needs and break the cycle of dependency and depression. While awaiting psychiatric evaluation, these patients should be kept under clinical surveillance, since their behavior may be erratic and result in another suicide attempt. The first physician to see the patient should obtain as much of the history as possible. The physician or the nurse should assess the seriousness of the suicide attempt while comforting the patient and creating a nonthreatening environment. Once these patients have been treated by the medical staff, a psychiatric assessment must be accomplished before hospital discharge. If admitted to the hospital, the patient should be observed closely until the psychiatric evaluation has been completed.

ADMISSION TO THE INTENSIVE CARE UNIT

The majority of emergency department patients with either an overdose or toxic exposure will be seen and discharged.[166] Most of those admitted to the hospital will require neither special monitoring nor intensive care,[166] although almost all will need psychosocial assessment. The actual challenge in the management of these patients lies in deciding which individuals warrant intensive care unit (ICU) admission. Unlike patients with medical and surgical pathology, where admission to the ICU is determined by the patient's clinical data on presentation to the hospital,[166,167] an ICU admission for a poisoned patient may be based on the potential manifestations of the toxin in question. Many of the toxins and drugs that patients are exposed to may not manifest their most serious toxicity at the time of presentation. The physician must be cognizant not only of the acute complications of these toxins but also of possible delayed toxicity.

The poisoned patient who presents after an acute or chronic overdose with altered vital signs secondary to the ingestion should be evaluated for ICU admission in the same manner as a medical or surgical patient. Therefore, decision regarding a hypotensive and bradycardic patient who has ingested a beta blocker is easy. Any patient with abnormal electrolytes from a methanol or ethylene glycol ingestion or electrocardiographic changes produced by a digoxin ingestion should be admitted to the ICU on presentation. Patients with depressed respirations from opioids or severe hypertension from amphetamines should be admitted to the ICU. Unfortunately, most overdoses do not present with these clear-cut indications for admission, and therefore the decision-making process becomes more complex.

Several studies have utilized physiologic parameters to determine if a patient requires ICU monitoring.[168,169] These studies have been limited to medical conditions with well-defined clinical courses. Brett et al.[170] attempted to predict the need for ICU monitoring for poisoned patients, but these researchers eliminated patients who had ingested or been exposed to drugs with known delayed toxic manifestations. Those patients with monoamine oxidase inhibitor overdose[171] or ingestions of extended-release preparations such as theophylline[172] or verapamil[135] were excluded. The study looked at patients who had ingested agents such as ethanol, barbiturates, and diazepam, which actually allowed for early determination of the need for intensive care.

Although there are no prospective studies with regard to the need for ICU care, some guidelines may be helpful. The physician must have a knowledge of the toxin's acute, subacute, and chronic manifestations. This may require consultation with the local or regional poison center to define the delayed clinical manifestations. Patients are candidates for ICU monitoring if the delayed toxicity involves the respiratory, central nervous, or cardiovascular systems in any way that may lead to morbidity and mortality if the patient is not effectively monitored. Patients who require invasive monitoring, have extensive end-organ dysfunction, or require mechanical or chemical support of any of their major organ systems also should be monitored in an ICU setting. Patients with potential for airway compromise, such as caustic ingestions, should be monitored in the ICU until their airway and esophagus can be visualized directly for risk assessment and therapeutic staging. Patients with toxic exposures and unexplained abnormalities of vital signs also should be monitored. Examples include the patient with a TCA overdose, a mild tachycardia, and a widened QRS complex.[173,174] Another example is the patient with a hydrocarbon ingestion, a tachycardia, and tachypnea, who may have an aspiration pneumonia and warrant close observation in the ICU. This approach may appear ill-defined, but it must be remembered that many poisonings have unpredictable courses due to unknown ingestions and extreme patient variability. Many overdoses result from mixed ingestions, and one drug may initially mask the effects of another agent whose toxicity may be delayed. Lomotil (atropine and diphenoxylate) is a prime example of such a combination. The physician should approach the acutely poisoned patient as if he or she were a time bomb. Until one is sure that the "bomb" has been defused, it may be best to monitor the patient carefully in an area where close observation can be conducted at all times. Fortunately, most of the severe toxicity in overdosed or poisoned patients will occur within 24 h of presentation. For this reason, these patients can usually be discharged from the ICU after a limited period of observation.

CONCLUSION

The acutely poisoned or overdosed patient can present at any stage of life. Many patients present with mixed overdoses and may offer a partial or inaccurate history to the physician. Because of the multitude of toxins that are available, diagnosis can be challenging. The physician must perform a meticulous physical examination and combine these skills with a guided use of the laboratory in an attempt to determine the etiology of the poisoning. Unfortunately, it is not easy to determine the etiology of most poisonings. This is especially true when patients present for other reasons, such as associated trauma. Because some overdoses can present with minimal initial clinical findings that may progress to catastrophic events, the initial management should be similar to the trauma approach, where airway, breathing, and circulation are always established and monitored aggressively. An intravenous line should be placed, and appropriate laboratory studies should be initiated regardless of the presenting clinical picture. If any doubt exists, a call to a regional or local poison center is warranted so that not only the acute but also the delayed pharmacology and toxicology of the particular agent can be ascertained. Fortunately, most poisonings are benign, and with good supportive care and basic medical management, these patients will not suffer substantial morbidity or mortality.

REFERENCES

1. Litovitz TL, Schmitz BF, Bailey KM: Annual report of the American Association of Poison Control Centers national data collection system. *Am J Emerg Med* 8:394, 1990.
2. Clements FW, Southby R, Rowlands JB, et al: Analysis of deaths from accidental poisonings in children aged under 5 years. *Med J Aust* 2:649, 1963.
3. Buffoni L, Roboa E, Galletti A, et al: Epidemiological aspects of poisoning in children observed over a 10 year period. *Clin Toxicol* 18:1149, 1981.
4. Robertson WO: Syrup of ipecac: A slow or fast emetic? *Am J Dis Child* 103:136, 1962.
5. Kulig K, Bar-OR D, Cantrill SV, et al: Management of acutely poisoned patients without gastric emptying. *Ann Emerg Med* 14:562, 1985.
6. Wright N: An assessment of the unreliability of the history given by self-poisoned patients. *Clin Toxicol* 16:381, 1980.
7. Dine MS, McGovern ME: International poisoning of children: An overlooked category of child abuse. Report of seven cases and review of literature. *Pediatrics* 70:32, 1982.
8. Shnaps Y, Frand M, Rotem Y, et al: The chemically abused child. *Pediatrics* 68:119, 1981.
9. McClung HJ, Murray R, Braden NJ, et al: Intentional ipecac poisoning in children. *Am J Dis Child* 142:637, 1988.
10. Berkner P, Kastner T, Skolnick L: Chronic ipecac poisoning in infancy: A case report. *Pediatrics* 82:384, 1988.
11. Leach M: Naloxone: A new therapeutic and diagnostic agent for emergency use. *J Am Coll Emerg Physicians* 2:21, 1973.
12. Evans LE, Swainson CP, Roscoe P, et al: Treatment of drug overdosage with naloxone: A specific narcotic antagonist. *Lancet* 1:452, 1973.
13. Martin WR: Naloxone. *Ann Intern Med* 85:765, 1976.
14. Ring T, Andersen PT, Knudsen F, et al: Salicylate-induced hyperventilation. *Lancet* 1:1450, 1985.
15. Reed JR, Palmisano PA: Central nervous system salicylate. *Clin Toxicol* 8:623, 1975.
16. Reuler JB, Girard DE, Cooney TG: Wernicke's encephalopathy. *N Engl J Med* 312:1035, 1985.
17. Watson AJS, Walker JF, Tomkin GH, et al: Acute Wernicke's encephalopathy precipitated by glucose loading. *Ir J Med Sci* 150:301, 1981.
18. Rasaiah B: Self-monitoring of the glucose level: Potential sources of inaccuracy. *Can Med Assoc J* 132:1357, 1985.
19. Foster GL: Carbohydrate metabolism: Some comparison of blood sugar concentrations in venous blood and in finger blood. *J Biol Chem* 55:291, 1923.
20. Hecht A, Weisenfeld S, Goldner MG: Factors influencing oral glucose tolerance: An experience with chronically ill patients. *Metabolism* 10:712, 1961.
21. Somogyi M: Studies of arteriovenous difference in blood sugar: Effect on alimentary hypoglycemia on rate of extrahepatic glucose assimilation. *J Biol Chem* 174:189, 1948.

22. Andrade R, Mathew V, Morgenstern MJ, et al: Hypoglycemic hemiplegic syndrome. *Ann Emerg Med* 13:529, 1984.
23. Arky RA, Veverbrants E, Abramson TA: Irreversible hypoglycemia. *JAMA* 206:575, 1968.
24. Weisman RS: Antidotes in depth: Naloxone. In *Goldfrank's Toxicologic Emergencies,* 4th ed. Norwalk CT, Appleton & Lange, 1990, p 444.
25. Goldfrank L, Weisman RS, Errick JK, et al: A dosing nomogram for continuous infusion intravenous naloxone. *Ann Emerg Med* 15:566, 1986.
26. Tenenbein M, Cohen S, Sitar DS: Efficacy of ipecac-induced emesis, orogastric lavage, and activated charcoal for acute drug overdose. *Ann Emerg Med* 16:838, 1987.
27. Auerbach PJ, Osterloh J, Braun O, et al: Efficacy of gastric emptying: Gastric lavage versus emesis induced with ipecac. *Ann Emerg Med* 15:692, 1986.
28. Merigian KS, Woodword M, Hedges J, et al: Prospective evaluation of gastric emptying in the self poisoned patient. *Am J Emerg Med* 8:479, 1990.
29. Minocha A, Herold DA, Barth JT, et al: Activated charcoal in oral ethanol absorption: Lack of effect in humans. *J Toxicol Clin Toxicol* 24:225, 1986.
30. Elendeninn NJ, Pond SM, Kaysen G, et al: Potential pitfalls in the evaluation of the usefulness of hemodialysis for the removal of lithium. *J Toxicol Clin Toxicol* 19:341, 1982.
31. Berg MJ, Berlinger WG, Goldberg MJ, et al: Acceleration of the body clearance of phenobarbital by oral activated charcoal. *N Engl J Med* 307:642, 1982.
32. Habib MS, Harkiss KJ: Quantitative determination of emetine and cephaeline in ipecacaunha root. *J Pharm Pharmacol* 21:557, 1969.
33. Stewart J: Effects of emetic and cathartic agents on the gastrointestinal tract and the treatment of toxic ingestion. *J Toxicol Clin Toxicol* 20:199, 1983.
34. Meester WD: Emesis and lavage. *Vet Human Toxicol* 22:225, 1980.
35. Rauber AP, Marconcelli RD: Two studies on the duration of emesis induced by therapeutic doses of syrup of ipecac. *Vet Human Toxicol* 24:60, 1982.
36. Corby DG, Decker WJ, Moran MJ, et al: Clinical comparison of pharmacologic emetics in children. *Pediatrics* 42:361, 1968.
37. Abdallah AH, Tye A: A comparison of the efficacy of emetic drugs and stomach lavage. *Am J Dis Child* 113:571, 1967.
38. Arnold FJ, Hodges JB, Barta RA, et al: Evaluation of the efficacy of lavage and induced emesis in treatment of salicylate poisoning. *Pediatrics* 23:286, 1959.
39. Neuvonen P, Varitiainen M, Tokola O: Comparison of activated charcoal and ipecac syrup in prevention of drug absorption. *Eur J Clin Pharmacol* 24:557, 1983.
40. Levy G: Gastrointestinal clearance of drugs with activated charcoal. *N Engl J Med* 307:676, 1982.
41. Neuvonen P, Olkkola K: Oral activated charcoal in the treatment of intoxications. *Med Toxicol* 3:33, 1988.
42. Storstein L: Studies on digitalis: III. Biliary excretion and enterohepatic circulation of digitoxin and its cardioactive metabolite. *Clin Pharmacol Ther* 17:313, 1975.
43. Berlinger WG, Spector R, Goldberg MJ, et al: Enhancement of theophylline clearance by oral activated charcoal. *Clin Pharmacol Ther* 33:351, 1983.
44. True RJ, Berman JM, Mahutte CK: Treatment of theophylline toxicity with oral activated charcoal. *Crit Care Med* 12:113, 1984.
45. Jones J, McMullen MJ, Dougherty J, et al: Repetitive doses of activated charcoal in the treatment of poisoning. *Am J Emerg Med* 5:305, 1987.
46. Anderson HA: Experimental studies on the pharmacology of activated charcoal: II. The effect of pH on the adsorption of charcoal from aqueous solutions. *Acta Pharmacol Toxicol* 3:199, 1947.
47. Olkkola K: Effect of charcoal-drug ratio on antidotal efficacy of oral activated charcoal in man. *Br J Clin Pharmacol* 19:767, 1985.

48. Keller RE, Schwab RA, Krenzelok EP: Contribution of sorbitol combined with activated charcoal in prevention of salicylate absorption. *Ann Emerg Med* 19:654, 1990.

49. Riegel JM, Becker CE: Use of cathartics in toxic ingestions. *Ann Emerg Med* 10:254, 1981.

50. Chin L, Picchioni A, Gillespie T: Saline cathartics and saline cathartics plus activated charcoal as antidotal treatments. *Clin Toxicol* 18:865, 1981.

51. Stetris IS, Mowry JB, Czajka PA, et al: Saline catharsis: Effect on aspirin bioavailability in combination with activated charcoal. *J Clin Pharmacol* 22:59, 1982.

52. Goldberg MJ, Spector R, Park GD, et al: The effect of sorbitol and activated charcoal on serum theophylline concentration after slow release theophylline. *Clin Pharmacol Ther* 41:108, 1987.

53. Mordes JP, Wacker WEC: Excess magnesium. *Pharm Rev* 29:273, 1978.

54. Smilkstein MJ, Smolinske SC, Kulig KW, et al: Severe hypermagnesemia due to multiple dose cathartic therapy. *West J Med* 148:208, 1988.

55. Farley TA: Severe hypernatremic dehydration after use of an activated charcoal-sorbitol suspension. *J Pediatr* 109:719, 1986.

56. Davis G, Santa Ana C, Morawski S, et al: Development of a lavage solution with minimal water and electrolyte absorption or secretion. *Gastroenterology* 78:991, 1980.

57. Tenenbein M: Whole bowel irrigation in iron poisoning. *J Pediatr* 111:142, 1987.

58. Smith SW, Ling LJ, Halstenson CE: Whole bowel irrigation as a treatment for acute lithium overdose. *Ann Emerg Med* 20:536, 1991.

59. Hoffman RS, Smilkstein MJ, Goldfrank LR: Whole bowel irrigation and the cocaine body-packer: A new approach to a common problem. *Am J Emerg Med* 8:523, 1990.

60. Kirshenbaum LA, Sitar DS, Tenenbein M: Interaction between whole bowel irrigation solution and activated charcoal: Implications for the treatment of toxic ingestions. *Ann Emerg Med* 19:1129, 1990.

61. McCarron MM: The role of the laboratory in treatment of the poisoned patient: A clinical perspective. *J Anal Toxicol* 7:142, 1983.

62. Helper BR, Sutheimer CA: The role of the toxicology laboratory in emergency medicine, II. *J Toxicol Clin Toxicol* 22:503, 1984.

63. Helper BR, Sutheimer CA, Sunshine I: Role of toxicology laboratory in the treatment of acute poisoning. *Med Toxicol* 1:61, 1986.

64. Weiss RD, Gawin FH: Protracted elimination of cocaine metabolites in long-term, high-dose cocaine abusers. *Am J Med* 75:879, 1988.

65. Goldfrank LR, Flomenbaum NE, Lewin NA, et al: *Goldfrank's Toxicological Emergencies,* 4th ed. Norwalk, CT, Appleton & Lange, 1990, p 620.

66. Kirk RL, Stenhouse NS: Ability to smell solutions of potassium cyanide. *Nature* 171:698, 1953.

67. Henretig FM, Gribetz B, Kearney T, et al: Interpretation of color change in blood with varying degree of methemoglobinemia. *J Toxicol Clin Toxicol* 26:293, 1988.

68. Harvey JW, Keitt AS: Studies of the efficacy and potential hazards of methylene blue therapy in aniline-induced methemoglobinemia. *Br J Haematol* 54:29, 1983.

69. Done AK: Drug intoxication. *Pediatr Clin North Am* 7:235, 1960.

70. Lacouture PG, Wason S, Abrams A, et al: Acute isopropyl alcohol intoxication: Diagnosis and management. *Am J Med* 75:680, 1983.

71. Weisberg HF: Water and electrolytes. In I Davidson, BB Wells (eds): *Clinical Diagnosis by Laboratory Methods.* Philadelphia, Saunders, 1962, p 456.

72. Turk J, Morrell L, Avioli LV: Ethylene glycol intoxication. *Arch Intern Med* 146:1601, 1986.

73. Terlinsky AS, Grochowski J, Geoly KL, et al: Identification of atypical calcium oxalate crystalluria following ethylene glycol ingestion. *Am J Clin Pathol* 76:223, 1981.

74. Haupt MC, Zull DN, Adams SL: Massive ethylene glycol poisoning without evidence of crystalluria: A case for early intervention. *J Emerg Med* 6:295, 1988.

75. Frommer DA, Kulig K, Marx JA, et al: Tricyclic antidepressant overdose. *JAMA* 257:521, 1987.
76. Niemann JT, Bessen HA, Rothstein RJ, et al: Electrocardiographic criteria for tricyclic antidepressant cardiotoxicity. *Am J Cardiol* 57:1154, 1986.
77. Boehnert MT, Lovejoy FH: Value of the QRS duration versus the serum drug level in predicting seizures and ventricular arrhythmias after an acute overdose of tricyclic antidepressants. *N Engl J Med* 313:474, 1985.
78. Pentel P, Benowitz N: Efficacy and mechanism of action of sodium bicarbonate in the treatment of desipramine toxicity in rats. *J Pharmacol Exp Ther* 230:12, 1984.
79. Malloy DW, Penner SB, Rabson J, et al: Use of sodium bicarbonate to treat tricyclic antidepressant induced arrhythmias in a patient with alkalosis. *Can Med Assoc J* 130:1457, 1984.
80. Pentel P, Benowitz N: Tricyclic antidepressant poisoning: Management of arrhythmias. *Med Toxicol* 1:101, 1986.
81. Bessen HA, Neiman JT: Improvement of cardiac function after hyperventilation in tricyclic antidepressant overdose. *J Toxicol Clin Toxicol* 23:537, 1985.
82. Sasyniuk BI, Jhamandas V, Valois M: Experimental amitriptyline intoxication: Treatment of cardiac toxicity with sodium bicarbonate. *Ann Emerg Med* 15:1052, 1986.
83. Rumack BH, Peterson RC, Koch GG, et al: Acetaminophen overdose: 662 cases with evaluation of oral acetylcysteine treatment. *Arch Intern Med* 144:380, 1981.
84. Prescott LF, Roscoe P, Wright N, et al: Plasma paracetamol half-life and hepatic necrosis in patients with paracetamol overdosage. *Lancet* 1:519, 1971.
85. Smilkstein MJ, Knapp GL, Kulig KW, et al: Efficacy of oral *N*-acetylcysteine in the treatment of acetaminophen overdose: Analysis of the national multicenter study (1976–1985). *N Engl J Med* 319:1557, 1988.
86. Shannon M, Amitai Y, Lovejoy FH: Multiple dose activated charcoal for theophylline poisoning in young infants. *Pediatrics* 80:368, 1987.
87. Gal P, Miller A, McCue JD: Oral activated charcoal to enhance theophylline elimination in an acute overdose. *JAMA* 251:3130, 1984.
88. Brown CG, Trumbull D, Klein-Schwartz W, et al: Ethylene glycol poisoning. *Ann Emerg Med* 12:501, 1983.
89. Kulig K, Duffy JP, Linden CH, et al: Toxic effect of methanol, ethylene glycol and isopropyl alcohol. *Top Emerg Med* 6:14, 1984.
90. Linnenvuo-Laitinen M, Huttunen K: Ethylene glycol intoxication. *J Toxicol Clin Toxicol* 24:167, 1986.
91. Peterson CD: Oral ethanol doses in patients with methanol poisoning. *Am J Hosp Pharm* 38:1024, 1981.
92. McCoy HG, Cipolle RJ, Ehlers SM, et al: Severe methanol poisoning: Application of a pharmacokinetic model for ethanol therapy and hemodialysis. *Am J Med* 67:804, 1979.
93. Osterloh JD, Pond SM, Grady S, et al: Serum formate concentrations in methanol intoxication as a criterion for hemodialysis. *Ann Intern Med* 104:200, 1986.
94. Jacabsen D, Hewlett TP, Webb R, et al: Ethylene glycol intoxication: Evaluation of kinetics and crystalluria. *Am J Med* 84:145, 1988.
95. Burney RE, Wu S, Nemiroff MJ, et al: Mass carbon monoxide poisoning: Clinical effects and results of treatment in 184 victims. *Ann Emerg Med* 11:394, 1982.
96. Myers RAM, Snyder SK, Emhoff TA: Subacute sequelae of carbon monoxide poisoning. *Ann Emerg Med* 14:1163, 1985.
97. Aronow R, Done AK: Phencyclidine overdose: An emerging concept of management. *J Am Coll Emerg Physicians* 7:56, 1978.
98. Gary NE, Saidi P: Methamphetamine intoxication: A speedy new treatment. *Am J Med* 64:537, 1978.

99. Morgan AG, Polak A: The excretion of salicylate in salicylate poisoning. *Clin Sci* 41:475, 1971.

100. Prescott LF, Balali-Mood M, Critchley JAJH, et al: Diuresis or urinary alkalinization for salicylate poisoning? *Br Med J* 285:1383, 1982.

101. Linton AL, Luke RG, Briggs JD: Methods of forced diuresis and its application in barbiturate poisoning. *Lancet* 2:377, 1967.

102. Neuvonen PJ, Karkkainen S: Effects of charcoal, sodium bicarbonate and ammonium chloride on chlorpropamide kinetics. *Clin Pharmacol Ther* 33:386, 1983.

103. Prescott LF, Park J, Darrien I: Treatment of severe 2,4-D and mecoprop intoxication with alkaline dieresis. *Br J Clin Pharmacol* 7:111, 1979.

104. Temple AR: Acute and chronic effects of aspirin toxicity and their treatment. *Arch Intern Med* 141:364, 1981.

105. Snodgrass W, Rumack BH, Peterson RG, et al: Salicylate toxicity following therapeutic doses in children. *J Clin Toxicol* 18:247, 1981.

106. Lawson AA, Proudfoot AT, Brown SS, et al: Forced diuresis in the treatment of acute salicylate poisoning in adults. *Q J Med* 38:31, 1969.

107. Whitten CF, Kesaree NM, Goodwin JF: Managing salicylate poisoning in children. *Am J Dis Child* 101:178, 1961.

108. Feuerstein RC, Finberg L, Fleishman E: The use of acetazolamide in the therapy of salicylate poisoning. *Pediatrics* 25:215, 1960.

109. Cowan RA, Hartnell GG, Cowdell CP, et al: Metabolic acidosis induced by carbonic anhydrase inhibitors and salicylates in patients with normal renal function. *Br Med J* 289:347, 1984.

110. Buchanan N, Kandig H, Eyberg C: Experimental salicylate intoxication in young baboons. *J Pediatr* 86:225, 1975.

111. Segar WE: The critically ill child: Salicylate intoxication. *Pediatrics* 44:440, 1969.

112. Brown TCK: Sodium bicarbonate treatment for tricyclic antidepressant. *Med J Aust* 2:380, 1976.

113. Brown TCK, Barker GA, Dunlop ME, et al: The use of sodium bicarbonate in the treatment of tricyclic antidepressant induced arrhythmia. *Anesth Intensive Care* 1:203, 1973.

114. Sasyniuk BI, Jhamandas V: Experimental amitriptyline intoxication: Treatment of cardiac toxicity with sodium bicarbonate. *Ann Emerg Med* 15:1052, 1986.

115. Wasserman F, Rodensky PL, Dick MM, et al: Successful treatment of quinidine and procainamide intoxication. *N Engl J Med* 259:757, 1958.

116. Pentel PR, Goldsmith SR, Salerno DM, et al: Effect of hypertonic sodium bicarbonate on encainide overdose. *Am J Cardiol* 57:878, 1986.

117. Beckman KJ, Parker RB, Hariman RJ, et al: Hemodynamic and electrophysiological actions of cocaine: Effects of sodium bicarbonate as an antidote in dogs. *Circulation* 83:1799, 1991.

118. Gaultier M: Sodium bicarbonate and tricyclic-antidepressant poisoning. *Lancet* 2:1258, 1976.

119. Blye E, Lorch J, Cartell S: Extracorporeal therapy in the treatment of intoxication. *Am J Kidney Dis* 3:321, 1984.

120. Rosenbaum JL, Winsten S, Kramuer MS, et al: Resin hemoperfusion in the treatment of drug intoxication. *Trans Am Soc Artif Intern Organs* 16:134, 1970.

121. Proudfoot AT, Brown SS: Acidaemia and salicylate poisoning in adults. *Br Med J* 2:547, 1969.

122. Gabow PA, Anderson RJ, Potts DE, et al: Acid-base disturbances in the salicylate intoxicated adult. *Arch Intern Med* 138:1481, 1978.

123. Temple AR, George DJ, Thompson JA: Salicylate poisoning complicated by fluid retention. *Clin Toxicol* 9:61, 1976.

124. Jorgensen HE, Wieth JO: Dialyzable poisons: Haemodialysis in the treatment of acute poisoning. *Lancet* 1:81, 1963.

125. McCoy HG, Cipolle RJ, Ehlers SM, et al: Severe methanol poisoning. Application of a pharmacokinetic model for ethanol therapy and hemodialysis. *Am J Med* 67:804, 1979.

126. Parry MF, Wallach R: Ethylene glycol poisoning. *Am J Med* 57:143, 1974.

127. Pond SM: Diuresis, dialysis and hemoperfusion: Indications and benefits. *Emerg Med Clin North Amer* 2:29, 1984.

128. Winchester JF: Evaluation of artificial organs: Extracorporeal removal of drugs. *Artif Organs* 10:316, 1986.

129. Rosenbaum JL, Weinstein S, Kramer MS, et al: Resin hemoperfusion in the treatment of drug intoxication. *Trans Am Soc Artif Intern Organs* 16:134, 1970.

130. Park GD, Spector R, Roberts RJ, et al: Use of hemoperfusion for treatment in theophylline intoxication. *Am J Med* 74:961, 1983.

131. Gibson TP, Reich SD, Krumlovsky FA, et al: Hemoperfusion for methotrexate removal. *Clin Pharmacol Ther* 23:351, 1978.

132. Cutler RE, Farland SC, Hammond PG, et al: Extracorporeal removal of drugs and poisons by hemodialysis and hemoperfusion. *Annu Rev Pharmacol Toxicol* 27:169, 1987.

133. Ilano AL, Raffin TA: Management of carbon monoxide poisoning. *Chest* 97:165, 1990.

134. Kumar S: Hyperbaric oxygen in treatment of carbon monoxide poisoning. *Br Med J* 289:1315, 1984.

135. Da silva O, De Melo RA, Filho JP: Verapamil acute self-poisoning. *Clin Toxicol* 14:361, 1979.

136. Candell J, Valle V, Soler M, et al: Acute intoxication with verapamil. *Chest* 75:200, 1979.

137. Shover SW, Bocchino V: Massive diltiazem overdose. *Ann Emerg Med* 15:1221, 1986.

138. Salberg MR, Gallagher EJ: Propranolol overdose. *Ann Emerg Med* 4:26, 1980.

139. Frishman W, Jacob H, Eisenberg E, et al: Clinical pharmacology of the beta-adrenergic blocking drugs: 8. Self poisoning with beta-adrenoceptor blocking agents. Recognition and management. *Am Heart J* 98:798, 1979.

140. Levey GS, Epstein S: Activation of adenyl cyclase by glucagon in cat and human heart. *Circ Res* 24:151, 1969.

141. Robson RH: Glucagon for beta blocker poisoning. *Lancet* 1:1357, 1980.

142. Kosinski EJ, Malidzak GS, et al: Glucagon and isoproterenol in reversing propranolol toxicity. *Arch Intern Med* 132:840, 1973.

143. Zaloga G, Malcolm D, Holaday J, et al: Glucagon reverses the hypotension and bradycardia of verapamil overdose in rats. *Crit Care Med* 13:273, 1985.

144. Zaritsky AL, Horowitz M, Chernow B: Glucagon antagonism of calcium channel blocker induced myocardial dysfunction. *Crit Care Med* 16:246, 1988.

145. Weinstein TC: Recognition and management of poisoning with beta-adrenergic blocker agents. *Ann Emerg Med* 13:1123, 1984.

146. Peterson DC, Leeder S, Sterner S: Glucagon therapy for beta-blocker overdose. *Drug Intell Clin Pharmacol* 18:394, 1984.

147. Sharff J, Bayer M: Acute and chronic digitalis toxicity: Presentation and treatment. *Ann Emerg Med* 11:327, 1982.

148. Bigger J: Digitalis toxicity. *J Clin Pharmacol* 25:514, 1985.

149. Smith TW, Haber E, Yeatman L, et al: Reversal of advanced digoxin intoxication with Fab fragments of digoxin-specific antibodies. *N Engl J Med* 294:797, 1976.

150. Lemon M, Andrews DJ, Binks AM, et al: Concentration of free serum digoxin after treatment with antibody fragments. *Br Med J* 295:1520, 1987.

151. Corcoran GB, Mitchell JR, Vaishnav YN, et al: Evidence that acetaminophen and *N*-hydroxyacetaminophen form a common arylating intermediate, *N*-acetyl-*p*-benzoquinoneimine. *Mol Pharmacol* 18:536, 1980.

152. Buckpitt AR, Rollins DE, Mitchell JR: Varying effects of sulfhydryl nucleophiles on acetaminophen oxidation and sulfhydryl adduct formation. *Biochem Pharmacol* 28:2941, 1979.

153. Lin JH, Levy G: Sulfate depletion after acetaminophen administration and replenishment by infusion of sodium sulfate of *N*-acetylcysteine in rats. *Biochem Pharmacol* 30:2723, 1981.

154. Miners JO, Drew R, Brikett DJ: Mechanism of action of paracetamol protective agents in mice in vivo. *Biochem Pharmacol* 33:2995, 1984.

155. Mitchell JR: Acetaminophen toxicity. *N Engl J Med* 319:1601, 1988.

156. Harrison PM, Wendon JA, Gimson AE, et al: Improvement by acetylcysteine of hemodynamics and oxygen transport in fulminant hepatic failure. *N Engl J Med* 324:1852, 1991.

157. Chin L, Sievers ML, Laird HE, et al: Evaluation of diazepam and pyridoxine as antidotes to isoniazid intoxication in rats and dogs. *Toxicol Appl Pharmacol* 45:713, 1978.

158. George ME, Pinkerton MK, Back KC: Therapeutics of monomethylhydrazine intoxication. *Toxicol Appl Pharmacol* 63:201, 1982.

159. Holtz P, Palm D: Pharmacological aspects of vitamin B_6. *Pharmacol Rev* 16:113, 1964.

160. Chin L, Sievers ML, Herrier RN, et al: Potentiation of pyridoxine by depressant and anticonvulsants in the treatment of acute isoniazid intoxication in dogs. *Toxicol Appl Pharmacol* 58:504, 1981.

161. Blanchard P, Yao J, McAlpine D, et al: Isoniazid overdose in the Cambodian population of Olmsted County, Minnesota. *JAMA* 256:3131, 1986.

162. Wason S, Lacouture PG, Lovejoy FH: Single high dose pyridoxine treatment for isoniazid overdose. *JAMA* 246:1102, 1981.

163. Burks JS, Walker JE, Rumack BH, et al: Tricyclic antidepressant poisoning. *JAMA* 230:1405, 1974.

164. Physostigmine Package Insert. 1991. Forest Pharmaceuticals, Incorporation, Professional Service Department, 2510 Metro Blvd. St. Louis, MO, 63043.

165. Pentel P, Peterson CD: Asystole complicating physostigmine treatment of tricyclic antidepressant overdose. *Ann Emerg Med* 9:588, 1980.

166. Ron A, Aronne LJ, Kalb PE, et al: The therapeutic efficacy of critical care units: Identifying subgroups of patients who benefit. *Arch Intern Med* 149:338, 1989.

167. Charlson ME, Sax FL, MacKenzie CR, et al: Assessing illness severity: Does clinical judgment work. *J Chron Dis* 39:439, 1986.

168. Knaus WA, Draper EA, Wagner DP, et al: Apache II: A severity of disease classification system. *Crit Care Med* 13:818, 1985.

169. Kruse JA, Thill-Baharozian MC, Carlson RW: Comparison of clinical assessment with Apache II for predicting mortality: Risk in patients admitted to a medical intensive care unit. *JAMA* 260:1739, 1988.

170. Brett AS, Rothschild N, Gray R, et al: Predicting the clinical course in intentional drug overdose. *Arch Intern Med* 147:133, 1987.

171. Linden CH, Rumack BH: Monamine oxidase inhibitor overdose. *Ann Emerg Med* 13:1137, 1984.

172. Connell JMC, McGeachie JF, Knepil J, et al: Self poisoning with sustained release aminophylline: Secondary rise in serum theophylline concentration after charcoal hemoperfusion. *Br Med J* 248:943, 1982.

173. Tokarski GF, Young MJ: Criteria for admitting patients with tricyclic antidepressant overdose. *J Emerg Med* 6:121, 1988.

174. Callaham M, Kassel D: Epidemiology of fatal tricyclic antidepressant ingestion: Implications for management. *Ann Emerg Med* 14:1, 1985.

16

BURN RESUSCITATION

Robert L. Waguespack
Loring W. Rue, III
Basil A. Pruitt, Jr.

Although the precise incidence of thermal injury is unknown, it has been estimated that over 2 million Americans sustain burns annually. Approximately 300 burn patients per million population per year require in-hospital care as a result of their thermal injury, and 82 individuals per million population per year have injuries of such significance that care is best undertaken in a designated burn care facility.

Thermal trauma is characterized by the rapid development of massive burn wound edema. This fluid is primarily derived from the circulating plasma volume. Continued loss of intravascular volume mandates intravenous fluid administration to counter physiologic derangements and to prevent the onset of shock. Extensive clinical and laboratory investigation has yielded many resuscitation stratagems to preserve organ perfusion and function. In addition to improved wound care, respiratory support, and nutritional management, physiologic resuscitation of the burn victim has led to marked improvement in patient outcome during the past two decades.

PATHOPHYSIOLOGY

The burn patient has been termed the universal model of trauma in that "a reproducible, readily quantifiable, local injury evokes a global systemic response the magnitude and duration of which are proportional to the extent of injury."[1] Thermal contact of sufficient duration and intensity leads to the development of areas of protein coagulation and cellular death referred to as the *zone of coagulation* or *necrosis*. This necrotic zone involves the entirety of the dermis in full-thickness burns and a variable depth of dermis in partial-thickness injuries. Areas of lesser cellular damage have been designated the *zones of stasis* and *hy-*

561

peremia and are oriented as concentric rings of tissue surrounding the contact point. With adequate fluid resuscitation, the attenuated perfusion associated with the zone of stasis resolves and ischemic conversion is obviated[2] (Fig. 16–1).

Edema in the burn wound in the first 3 to 4 h after injury is primarily dependent on perfusion pressure and thereafter predominantly the result of increased capillary permeability. Although not completely understood, the mechanism by which burn wound edema develops is the result of a complex interaction of cellular compounds released by thermally injured tissue. These compounds include histamine, serotonin, and various inflammatory mediators, such as leukotrienes and prostaglandins. Activation of both the complement and coagulation cascades is involved as well. Additionally, these inflammatory mediators influence neutrophil activation and chemotaxis. Subsequent release of cytotoxic granulocyte lysosomal products and oxygen radicals at the site of tissue damage further contribute to alterations in function, both locally and systemically.

Edema formation is also noted in unburned tissue following extensive thermal injury. Montero et al.,[3] using an ovine model of thermal injury, demonstrated significant alteration in vascular permeability in uninjured tissue by demonstrating a twofold increase in the ratio of lymph to plasma protein emanating from uninjured extremities. Reid et al.,[4] using radiolabeled albumin as a marker of protein flux in rodents, also demonstrated a threefold increase in extravasation of albumin in uninjured tissue following a 40 percent total body surface area (TBSA) burn. However, Demling et al.[5] were unable to demonstrate a change in lymph/serum protein ratios in an uninjured sheep extremity, suggesting an absence of permeability changes. Nevertheless, despite conflicting reports, edema is noted in unburned tissue following burn injury. It is most likely a consequence

ZONES OF THERMAL INJURY

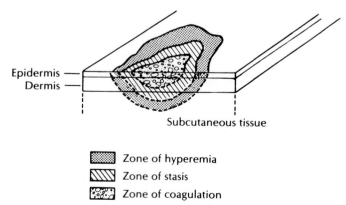

Epidermis —
Dermis —

Subcutaneous tissue

▨ Zone of hyperemia
▨ Zone of stasis
▨ Zone of coagulation

FIG. 16–1. Concentric rings of cellular damage or death result from thermal injury. With prompt and appropriate fluid resuscitation, perfusion is restored to the zone of stasis, thus limiting cellular death.

of combined osmotic and volume effects associated with the administration of large volumes of crystalloid fluid required for burn resuscitation.

The pathophysiologic response following burn injury is biphasic, much like Cuthbertson's original description of the biphasic response to long bone fractures, the model used in 1939 to study the metabolic response to trauma.[1] Cuthbertson's "ebb phase" is seen in the early postburn period and is marked by generalized organ hypofunction as a consequence of diminished cardiac output (Table 16–1). Intimately associated with this diminution in cardiac output is an increase in the systemic vascular resistance, which occurs as a result of activation of the neurohormonal stress response. In addition to the increased afterload, alterations in vascular permeability and subsequent intravascular hypovolemia decrease preload and further reduce cardiac output and organ perfusion. Most studies have attributed the depression in cardiac performance seen in this early period to an impairment of left ventricular end-diastolic volume, which is consistent with a hypovolemic state. An improvement in cardiac performance can be achieved with adequate fluid resuscitation. Although some investigators have attributed the postburn diminution in cardiac output to a circulating myocardial depressant factor, efforts to characterize this agent have been inconclusive.[6,7]

With adequate volume repletion, hemodynamic performance improves. As plasma volume increases during the second 24 h following injury, cardiac performance increases to supranormal levels. This hyperdynamic state, correlating with Cuthbertson's "flow phase" after injury, is felt to be fueled by elevated serum levels of the stress hormones cortisol, glucagon, and epinephrine. In fact, this hyperdynamic state can be replicated in normal individuals when these stress hormones are infused at concentrations similar to those seen following mild to moderate trauma.[8]

Paralleling the changes in cardiovascular function are decreases in renal blood flow and glomerular filtration rate in the early postburn period. The diminution in cardiac output, hypovolemia, and increased peripheral vascular resistance all contribute to impaired renal function and relative oliguria seen in the early post-injury period. Marked delay or inadequacy of fluid administration may lead to acute tubular necrosis. Following successful resuscitation and evolution into the hyperdynamic phase, a modest diuretic response is encountered. This is most

TABLE 16–1. A Characteristic Biphasic Response to Thermal Injury Is Seen, with Effects Manifested in All Organ Systems

Organ System	Early Change (Phase 1)	Later Response (Phase 2)
Cardiovascular	Hypovolemia	Hyperdynamic state
Pulmonary	Hypoventilation	Hyperventilation
Central nervous	Agitation	Obtundation*
Endocrine	Catabolic effects	Anabolic effects
Gastrointestinal	Ileus	Hypermotility
Urinary	Oliguria	Diuresis
Skin	Hypoperfusion	Hyperemia

*Usually associated with septic or metabolic complications.

prominent with resorption of burn-associated edema; however, the diuretic response is modified somewhat by large evaporative fluid losses occurring through the wound surface. Additionally, as a consequence of increased renal blood flow and glomerular filtration rate associated with the supranormal levels of cardiac output, an increased rate of renal drug clearance occurs, and appropriate dosing adjustments become necessary.[9]

Even in the absence of inhalation injury, thermal injury influences the pulmonary system. Most notable is an increase in the pulmonary vascular resistance to a greater extent and duration than that noted in the systemic vasculature, a phenomenon likely mediated by the release of vasoactive amines. Although causing an increase in right ventricular afterload and concomitant right ventricular strain, the net effect may be protective to the lungs by avoiding the early development of pulmonary edema during resuscitation.[10] Demling et al.,[11] using an ovine model to assess changes in lung edema and the influence of vasoactive mediators in the early postburn period, noted that although there was an increase in lung lymph flow, the pulmonary lymphatics were normally able to handle this increased flux. In addition, there was no evidence of increased pulmonary capillary permeability in animals not subjected to inhalation injury. Using the same model, the authors examined the levels of various inflammatory mediators and noted that thromboxane A_2 levels were significantly elevated, with peak levels occurring at 18 to 20 h after the burn.[11] It was concluded that this agent, having potent vasoconstrictive and bronchoconstrictive properties, may be an integral cause for the increased pulmonary vascular resistance and decreased pulmonary compliance seen following injury.

In addition to the compliance-induced increased work of breathing, an increase in minute ventilation is seen in the early postburn phase. Immediately following burn injury, there is little change in minute ventilation; however, with fluid resuscitation, minute ventilation progressively increases and, in fact, increases in proportion to burn size. This exaggerated minute ventilation is thought to be a further reflection of postburn hypermetabolism. The combination of these factors may lead to an inadequate ventilation by the patient with extensive burn injury and may necessitate intubation and mechanical ventilation for respiratory support.

Gastrointestinal motility is typically impaired following extensive thermal injury, particularly when the burn involves more than 20 percent of the total body surface area (TBSA). Typically, the gastrointestinal response includes ileus and requires the placement of a nasogastric tube to prevent emesis and possible aspiration. Because of the generalized organ hypoperfusion seen following thermal injury, splanchnic blood flow may be compromised prior to adequate resuscitation. McElwee et al.[12] demonstrated that this ischemic phenomenon resulted in focal gastric mucosal damage which may lead to the development of superficial erosions in the stomach and duodenum. McAlheny et al.[13] reported the presence of these lesions endoscopically in fully 86 percent of patients sustaining burns greater than 35 percent TBSA. Without adequate protective measures, such as the administration of H_2 receptor blockers and antacid titration of gastric pH to levels above 4, frank ulcerations and gastrointestinal hemorrhage, as described by Curling in 1842, may occur.

The thermally injured patient manifests the characteristic metabolic response to injury. Immediately after the burn there is a transient decrease in the metabolic rate. However, as resuscitation proceeds and the hormonal milieu is altered in such a way that catabolic hormones predominate, energy requirements increase significantly. Serum levels of catecholamines, glucagon, and cortisol increase, whereas the anabolic hormones insulin and triiodothyronine decrease. The increased energy requirement is proportional to burn size and is associated with negative nitrogen balance and increased glucose flux.[8] At this institute, a recent analysis by indirect calorimetry has determined a linear relationship between caloric needs and extent of burn. This study noted a lesser overall metabolic elevation than the previously described curvilinear association peaking at 2 to 2½ times the basal metabolic requirement for patients suffering burns exceeding 50 percent TBSA. This difference may reflect changes in wound management and a decrease in septic complications when compared with earlier studies. These observations underscore the need to measure metabolic rate in order to provide adequate quantities of nutritional supplementation to the thermally injured patient. As the burn wounds are closed, hormonal levels return toward normal. Periodic reassessment of nutritional requirements is therefore important in order to avoid overfeeding of the patient and associated complications.

Thermal injury also induces a generalized impairment of the immune system, subjecting the patient to increased susceptibility to infection. Not only is there an obvious destruction of the cutaneous barrier to infection but also a systemic impairment of the immune system. This is manifested by decreased immunoglobulin levels and impaired neutrophil chemotaxis, phagocytosis, and cytotoxicity.[14] Alterations in lymphocyte subpopulations also have been described, as has decreased lymphocyte production of interleukin 2 (IL-2). The magnitude of these effects is related to the extent of burn and may further increase the patient's susceptibility to infection.[15,16] Reticuloendothelial system suppression following burn injury results in diminished fibronectin levels, which are associated with impaired opsonic capability and decreased bacterial clearance.[17]

Elements of the hematopoietic system are often destroyed as a consequence of thermal injury, and the magnitude of this destruction appears directly proportional to burn size. Patients sustaining full-thickness burn injury often have immediate red blood cell destruction in the areas of the involved microvasculature. Clearance of damaged red cells and frequent phlebotomy necessary for patient monitoring may account for as much as 8 to 12 percent loss of the circulating red cell mass per day during the first postburn week. Successful resuscitation results in increases in fibrin split products and decreases in platelet count and fibrinogen levels. However, with time, fibrinogen, factors V and VIII, and platelet counts increase to supranormal levels, as reported by Curreri et al.[18]

Resuscitation measures are employed to minimize and correct these pathophysiologic responses to burn injury. Only by maintenance of vital organ perfusion and function can the adverse physiologic consequences of burn injury be obviated.

HISTORICAL PERSPECTIVE

The earliest written records of burn care are found in the Smith and Ebers papyri from 1600 B.C. Egypt. They described the various agents that the ancient Egyptians used for the topical treatment of burn injury, but no mention was made of the treatment of burn shock. Although many earlier writings described the great thirst seen in acutely burned patients, it was not until 1828 that Baron Dupuytren reported the first statistical study of burn injury and made reference to the importance of fluid therapy in the management of burn patients. Not until the end of the nineteenth century was intravenous fluid replacement advocated, first by Tommasoli in Sicily and subsequently by Parascondolo from Italy, both of whom described the use of saline infusions for patients sustaining severe burn injury.

Underhill and colleagues[18a] at Yale University reported their experience in treating 20 severely burned patients from the Rialto Theatre fire of 1921. This study was a thorough examination of several of the patients' physiologic indices, including hemoglobin, hematocrit, blister fluid chloride levels, and serum chloride levels. On the basis of their studies, the authors concluded that hypovolemia, as a consequence of fluid and electrolyte shifts, was the cause of burn shock, not the release of toxins, as had been believed previously. These findings were further reinforced by Cope and Moore's experience[19] with patients burned in the Cocoanut Grove fire of 1942. These authors studied a large number of burn patients and advanced our understanding of the fluid, electrolyte, and protein derangements that are produced by thermal injury. Like Underhill and associates, they demonstrated that hypovolemia occurred not only through the loss of fluid via the burn wound itself but also from internal fluid shifts. Their observations led to the development of the first widely utilized resuscitation formula for burn patients, the "burn budget formula." This resuscitation stratagem employed various quantities of crystalloid solutions (lactated Ringer's, 5% dextrose in water, and 0.45% normal saline) and colloid-containing fluids that were administered during the initial 48 h following the burn.[19]

In 1952, as a result of a 5-year collaborative effort of laboratory research and clinical trials between the U.S. Army Medical Research and Development Command and the Medical College of Virginia, the Evans formula of resuscitation was introduced.[20] This formula established a more uniform approach to burn resuscitation and was the first formula to consider body size and extent of burn in the calculation of fluid needs. Again, both colloid and crystalloid solutions were employed during the initial 48 h after injury.

Reiss et al.[21] introduced the Brooke formula for resuscitation in 1953, which was a modification of the Evans formula and was based on data from the records of surviving patients treated at the U.S. Army Surgical Research Unit. Like the Evans formula, body size and burn extent were considered; however, an upper limit of burn size for calculation purposes was set at 50 percent TBSA. It was noted that surviving patients had been given a preponderance of salt-containing fluids, specifically in a 3:1 ratio of crystalloid to colloid solutions, and consequently, the Evans formula was modified to meet this crystalloid/colloid ratio.

The original Brooke formula consisted of colloid-containing fluids, electrolyte solutions, and daily maintenance fluids. Specifically, colloid in the form of blood, plasma, or other plasma expanders was administered in volumes of 0.5 ml/kg of body weight per percentage of TBSA burned. Electrolyte solution in the form of lactated Ringer's solution was provided in volumes of 1.5 ml/kg of body weight per percentage of TBSA burned. Additionally, maintenance fluids were administered in the form of 5% dextrose in water or lactated Ringer's solution depending on the severity of injury, with the recommendation that complete restriction of electrolyte-free solutions be adhered to for patients with extensive deep burns. One-half the calculated fluid volume was administered to patients during the first 8 h following burn injury, and the remainder was infused over the ensuing 16 h. Subsequently, in the second 24-h period, one-half the colloid and electrolyte solutions administered during the initial 24 h was provided to the patient, as well as daily maintenance fluids in the form of 5% dextrose in water.

Reckler et al.,[22] in a retrospective review of patients treated with this resuscitation regimen, noted that the original Brooke formula satisfactorily predicted the required fluid volume for patients with burn sizes less than 50 percent TBSA. Patients with larger burns, however, required more fluid than the formula predicted. The effectiveness of the Brooke resuscitation formula was supported by clinical experience and detailed hemodynamic studies of patients. It was noted in clinical studies that an average 20 percent decrease in blood and plasma volume occurred following burn injury, and the implementation of the Brooke resuscitation strategy defended against further intravascular volume loss during the first 24 h after the burn. During the second 24 h, this formula progressively restored plasma volume and essentially completed volume restoration by the fifty-fourth postburn hour.

Moylan et al.,[23] using a canine model of scald injury, evaluated the contribution of volume, sodium, and colloid to the restoration of cardiac output during the initial 12 h following injury. In this study, various combinations of fluid volumes and the sodium and colloid content of these fluids were administered to injured dogs beginning 1 h after burn and continued at a constant rate for the ensuing 11 h. It was noted that in untreated control animals, cardiac output decreased by as much as 30 percent within 6 h following injury. When various combinations of resuscitation fluids were administered, it was noted that statistically significant improvement in cardiac output could be attributed to volume and sodium administration. Colloid, however, had no influence on cardiac output during the initial 12 h following injury. This laboratory result complemented Pruitt's earlier clinical observation that colloid had minimal effect on the intravascular fluid balance during early resuscitation of burn patients.

In the latter half of the first 24 h, capillary permeability returns toward normal. Consequently, it was observed that during the initial 24 h following burn injury, colloid-containing fluids were retained in the circulation to no greater extent than equal volumes of colloid-free electrolyte solutions. During the second 24 h, when the capillary leak had decreased, colloid-containing fluids were more optimally retained intravascularly than colloid-free solutions. Furthermore, Baxter[24] demonstrated that during the second 24 h following burn, colloid-containing solutions facilitated intravascular volume repletion more efficiently and with smaller volumes than crystalloid solutions. These observations led to modifications of the Brooke formula. Crystalloid solutions are used exclusively during the initial 24 h following burn injury if resuscitation proceeds uneventfully, and a combination of crystalloid and colloid is employed during the second 24 h. Again, the modified Brooke resuscitation formula emphasized fluid delivery rates based on the extent of cutaneous burn and the patient's weight.

Additional resuscitation stratagems have been proposed which confine fluid administration in the first 24 h to colloid-free fluids (Table 16–2). In 1974, Bax-

TABLE 16–2. Commonly Used Burn Resuscitation Formulas for Adult Patients

Formula	Electrolyte-Containing Solution	Colloid-Containing Fluid Equivalent to Plasma	Glucose in Water
First 24 Hours			
Evans	Normal saline 1.0 ml/kg/% TBSA	1.0 ml/kg/% TBSA	2000 ml
Brooke	Lactated Ringer's 1.5 ml/kg/% TBSA	0.5 ml/kg/% TBSA	2000 ml
Parkland	Lactated Ringer's 4.0 ml/kg/% TBSA	—	—
Hypertonic saline solution	Volume of fluid required to maintain hourly urinary output of 30 ml	—	—
Modified Brooke	Lactated Ringer's 2.0 ml/kg/% TBSA	—	—
Second 24 Hours			
Evans	One-half of first 24-h requirement	One-half of first 24-h requirement	2000 ml
Brooke	One-half to three-quarters of first 24-h requirement	One-half to three-quarters of first 24-h requirement	2000 ml
Parkland	—	20 to 60% of calculated plasma volume	As needed to maintain urinary output
Hypertonic saline solution	One-third isotonic salt solution orally up to 3500 ml limit	—	—
Modified Brooke	—	0.3 to 0.5 ml/kg/% TBSA	As needed to maintain urinary output

ter et al.[25] proposed the Parkland formula of resuscitation, which called for administration of lactated Ringer's solution in a volume of 4 ml/kg per percent of TBSA burned in the initial 24 h. In the second 24 h, this resuscitation stratagem called for the administration of colloid in volumes of between 20 and 60 percent of the calculated plasma volume. In addition, 5% dextrose in water was administered as necessary to maintain an adequate urinary output.

In an attempt to reduce the volume of fluid administration during the resuscitation phase and to minimize consequent edema formation, Monafo[26] and others[27] reported the use of hypertonic crystalloid solutions for the resuscitation of burn patients. These fluids were felt to be particularly beneficial in patients who were volume sensitive, such as those at the extremes of age and patients with preexisting cardiopulmonary disease. Reports of these early clinical trials claimed that significantly smaller volumes of resuscitation fluid were required with a similar sodium load and a satisfactory outcome when compared with standard crystalloid resuscitation. Additionally, proponents have claimed that hypertonic lactated saline solutions induce a higher urinary output, minimize the fractional retention of sodium, diminish the need for escharotomy, and decrease the incidence of ileus.

Hypertonic fluid resuscitation appears to produce its effect by the delivery of a high-osmolar solution, giving rise to a rapid shift of fluid from the intracellular compartment into the vasculature and thereby expanding plasma volume. Consequently, intracellular dehydration and hypernatremia appear to be major limitations to the use of these resuscitation fluids. Intracellular dehydration in excess of 15 percent appears to be associated with impaired cellular function. Additionally, serum sodium concentrations in excess of 160 mEq/liter may exceed physiologic tolerance and necessitate the administration of hypotonic fluids. The provision of additional intravenous fluid would appear to defeat the claimed advantages of using these hypertonic saline solutions. In fact, when conventional resuscitation stratagems are compared with hypertonic saline resuscitation regimens, no difference in the total amounts of sodium or volume administered can be appreciated. Gunn et al.[28] randomized 51 adult burn patients to resuscitation with either lactated Ringer's solution or 514-mosmol hypertonic saline. At the termination of the resuscitation period, there was no difference in the volume of fluid administered, although the hypertonic saline patients received twice the amount of sodium of patients receiving standard resuscitation.

Furthermore, many investigators have shown that these hypertonic solutions are only transiently beneficial to cardiovascular performance. Onarheim et al.[29] studied an ovine model of thermal injury in which they compared bolus therapy of 4 ml/kg of 7.5% sodium chloride and 6% dextran 70 with an equivalent volume of physiologic saline. Following the initial boluses, resuscitation continued with lactated Ringer's solution in sufficient volumes to maintain cardiac output, mean arterial pressure, and urinary output. While they demonstrated an initial rapid increase in cardiac output and mean arterial pressure in the hypertonic resuscitation fluid group, the effect was short-lived. Total fluid volumes administered subsequently were found to be similar, and no change in edema formation was appreciated. As a consequence of a review of the previously cited studies, it would appear that the hypertonic fluid resuscitation regimens are best reserved for patients with markedly impaired cardiovascular performance and may otherwise unnecessarily complicate fluid management in other critically burned patients. Bowser-Wallace et al.[30] support this view in their report of hypertonic saline resuscitation of a group of severely burned elderly patients. In this study, a significant decrease in volume load was seen without an increase in net sodium administration.

RESUSCITATION: INITIAL 24 H

As previously emphasized, modern burn resuscitation formulas are based on the patient's body size as expressed by weight in kilograms and the total extent of burn expressed as a percentage of the TBSA involved. Consequently, an accurate assessment of burn extent is essential for calculation of estimated resuscitative fluid requirements. Perhaps the most widely known method for estimating burn area is the "rule of nines." This method is quick and reasonably accurate, attributing 9 percent of the TBSA to various body parts (Fig. 16–2). This approach is modified in infants and children, in whom the head and neck account for a larger percentage of TBSA and the lower extremities comprise a smaller percentage. A more precise method of estimating burn size employs a standardized body surface area chart such as the Lund-Browder diagram, which assigns body surface area measurements to specific body parts depending on the patient's age (Fig. 16–3). Scattered irregular burn areas may be quantified by comparing such areas with the patient's palmar surface, which is equivalent to approximately 1 percent of the TBSA.

We advocate the use of the modified Brooke formula. For the adult patient, the initial 24-h fluid volume is calculated as 2 ml lactated Ringer's solution per kilogram of body weight per percentage of TBSA burned. As a consequence of the early massive fluid shifts occurring after injury, one-half of this calculated 24-h fluid need is scheduled to be administered during the first 8 h after the burn. The balance of fluid is provided over the ensuing 16 h. If the patient arrives at a treatment facility hours after injury, adjustments in the rate of fluid administration are made to ensure that half the calculated fluid needs are received in the first 8 h after the burn injury occurred. As with all resuscitation approaches, the calculated volumes are only estimates of resuscitation needs, and the actual fluid infusion rates are dependent on the patient's physiologic response.

Children have a greater body surface area per unit of body mass and consequently require relatively more resuscitation fluid than the adult patient.[31] For these patients, resuscitation is calculated as 3 ml lactated Ringer's solution per kilogram of body weight per percentage of TBSA burned. Again, as in the adult patient, half the fluid is infused over the initial 8 h after the injury, and the

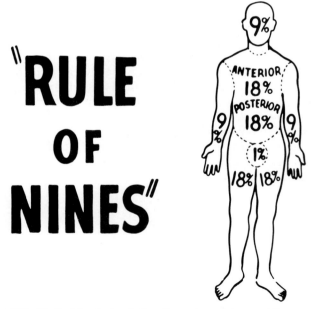

FIG. 16–2. The "rule of nines" may be used to rapidly assess the extent of thermal injury in adults.

BURN ESTIMATE AND DIAGRAM
AGE vs AREA

Area	Birth 1 yr	1 – 4 yr	5 – 9 yr	10 – 14 yr	15 yr	Adult	2°	3°	Total	Donor Areas
Head	19	17	13	11	9	7				—
Neck	2	2	2	2	2	2				—
Ant Trunk	13	13	13	13	13	13				
Post Trunk	13	13	13	13	13	13				
R Buttock	2½	2½	2½	2½	2½	2½				
L. Buttock	2½	2½	2½	2½	2½	2½				
Genitalia	1	1	1	1	1	1				
R U Arm	4	4	4	4	4	4				
L.U. Arm	4	4	4	4	4	4				
R L Arm	3	3	3	3	3	3				
L L Arm	3	3	3	3	3	3				
R Hand	2½	2½	2½	2½	2½	2½				
L Hand	2½	2½	2½	2½	2½	2½				
R Thigh	5½	6½	8	8½	9	9½				
L. Thigh	5½	6½	8	8½	9	9½				
R. Leg	5	5	5½	6	6½	7				
L. Leg	5	5	5½	6	6½	7				
R Foot	3½	3½	3½	3½	3½	3½				
L. Foot	3½	3½	3½	3½	3½	3½				
						TOTAL				

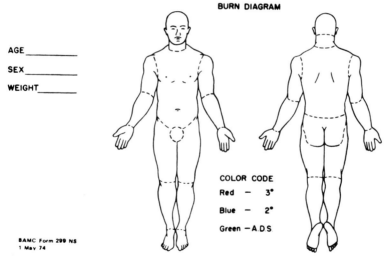

BURN DIAGRAM

AGE _____

SEX _____

WEIGHT _____

COLOR CODE

Red   —   3°

Blue   —   2°

Green — A.D.S

BAMC Form 299 NS
1 May 74

FIG. 16–3. The use of a burn diagram permits a more exact estimation of the extent of thermal injury. The surface areas of the head and lower extremities change significantly with age.

remainder is administered over the subsequent 16 h. In addition, provision of required maintenance fluid is important in the pediatric age group, particularly in small children, since frequently the calculated resuscitation needs may be insufficient to meet daily maintenance requirements. Maintenance fluids are provided in the form of 5% dextrose in 0.45% saline in quantities of 1500 ml/

TABLE 16–3. Pediatric Burn Resuscitation Formula

	First 24 Hours
Lactated Ringer's	3 ml/kg/% TBSA
5% dextrose in 0.5 normal saline	Maintenance rate
	Second 24 Hours
5% albumin in lactated Ringer's	0.3–0.5 ml/kg/% TBSA
5% dextrose in 0.5 normal saline	As necessary to maintain urinary output

m² of body surface (Table 16–3). Because of the smaller blood volume in children, administration of large quantities of hypotonic solutions is avoided so as to prevent the development of hyponatremia. Hyponatremia, if of severe enough magnitude and occurring with sufficient rapidity, may promote cerebral edema and even induce tonic-clonic seizure activity. Furthermore, dextrose-containing fluids are employed in burned infants in order to prevent or correct stress-induced hypoglycemia as a consequence of postinjury glycogen exhaustion.

MONITORING RESUSCITATION ADEQUACY

The modified Brooke formula, like all resuscitation formulas, serves only as a guide to fluid administration. The actual rate of intravenous fluid infusion is dependent on the patient's physiologic response to resuscitation. Consequently, achieving the goal of resuscitation, namely, the maintenance of adequate organ perfusion and function, necessitates repeated, scheduled assessment of the patient's general status and hemodynamic response. The hourly urinary output, which reflects glomerular filtration, renal perfusion, and cardiac output, is monitored as an indirect index of blood volume.

In the adult patient, urinary outputs of between 30 to 50 ml/h are considered to reflect adequate renal perfusion and satisfactory progress of the resuscitative effort. For the pediatric patient weighing less than 30 kg, urinary outputs of 1 ml/kg of body weight per hour are felt to reflect adequate renal perfusion. Urinary outputs exceeding these recommended guidelines are indicative of excessive fluid administration and mandate appropriate adjustment of intravenous fluid infusion rates. Care should be taken to exclude the possibility of an osmotically driven diuresis, which may be promoted by excessive glucose or protein in the urine. Alternatively, oliguria most commonly reflects inadequate fluid administration and should prompt an increase in the rate of fluid infusion until the recommended urinary output is achieved. As in the case of excessive urinary output, patients with oliguria should undergo fluid adjustments by 10 to 20 percent increments per hour until adequate physiologic indices are met. Patients not responding in the expected fashion to resuscitative efforts, particularly when the infusion rates approach that which would yield a total resuscitative volume of between 6 and 8 ml/kg per percentage of TBSA burned, may benefit from invasive hemodynamic monitoring, specifically with a flow-directed pulmonary artery catheter. In patients who demonstrate evidence of impaired myocardial performance, the addition of inotropic agents may augment the resuscitative effort (Fig. 16–4).

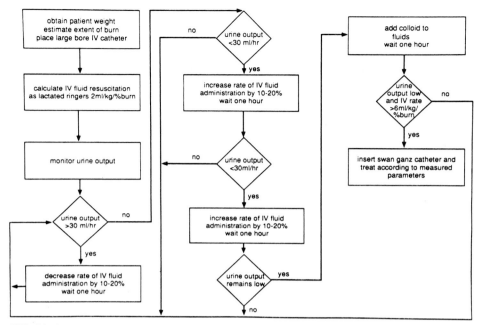

FIG. 16–4. Algorithm for fluid therapy for the first 24 h following thermal injury.

As well as ensuring vital organ perfusion, maintaining adequate peripheral perfusion is a mandatory aspect of resuscitation therapy. Circumferentially burned extremities are at risk for blood flow restriction as subeschar burn wound edema accumulates. Once the tissue pressure exceeds the venous and capillary pressures, nutrient blood flow to the distal extremity and subjacent areas is impaired, and if it is reduced significantly, cell death may occur. Elevation of the burned extremity and active exercise of the involved body part for 5 min/h are prophylactic measures which may be employed to avoid hazardous levels of edema formation.

Distal cyanosis, impaired capillary refill, neurologic deficits, and constant deep tissue pain are all indications of impaired extremity perfusion. However, these findings are relatively unreliable when compared with the use of a Doppler flow-meter, which gives a more precise assessment of peripheral perfusion.[32] Superficial palmar arch and posterior tibial artery pulses are routinely monitored for alterations in blood flow in the upper extremity and lower extremity, respectively. Progressive diminution in Doppler signal intensity in a patient with an adequate circulating blood volume is indicative of impaired tissue perfusion, and ischemic necrosis will result unless escharotomy is promptly performed.

Escharotomy can be performed as a bedside procedure, since the incisions are made through insensate full-thickness burns and anesthetic is unnecessary. Either the midlateral or midmedial line of the involved extremity is chosen as the site of the escharotomy incision. The incision extends from the distal to most proximal extent of full-thickness burn. Only the eschar need be incised to permit the wound edges to separate and relieve the tension in subjacent tissue. Minimal bleeding is encountered if the procedure is appropriately performed (Fig. 16–5).

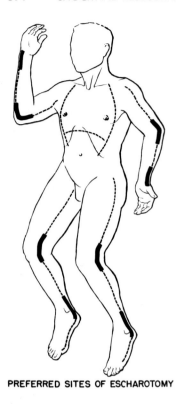

PREFERRED SITES OF ESCHAROTOMY

FIG. 16–5. Correct anatomic positioning of the patient is imperative prior to performing escharotomy. An escharotomy incision should be carried across any joint that is involved in a circumferential full-thickness burn, as indicated by the thickened lines.

Fasciotomies are only rarely required to restore peripheral perfusion and are most commonly needed in the setting of high-voltage electrical injury or concomitant crush injury. Unlike escharotomy, fasciotomies are best performed in the operating room with general anesthetic management.

SPECIAL RESUSCITATION CONCERNS

Evaluation of the extent of injury in patients with high-voltage electric injury is more difficult than in patients with flame or scald burns. In patients with electric injuries, a small cutaneous injury may be associated with extensive inapparent injury of underlying tissues. Contact with high-voltage electricity, typically defined as greater than 1000 V, causes tissue damage by the conversion of electrical energy to thermal energy. Joules law states that the power, or heat, is proportional to the amperage squared times the tissue resistance ($P = I^2R$). Although initially offering significant resistance to current flow, the skin, once damaged, permits easy flow of current to the underlying tissues. Upon electrical contact, the body behaves as a volume conductor, and consequently, the heat generated is proportional to the current flow per unit of cross-sectional area.[33] Extremities, therefore, tend to sustain severe injury, whereas truncal contacts rarely produce significant damage. The body functions as a volume radiator following cessation of current contact. Superficial tissues, therefore, cool rapidly and sustain less injury than the deeper structures, which tend to retain the heat.

Because the muscle and deeper tissues may sustain extensive injury while the overlying skin appears relatively unaffected, resuscitation formulas based on the extent of cutaneous injury alone may significantly underestimate the fluid needs of electric injury patients. In addition, myoglobin and/or hemoglobin may be liberated into the circulation as a consequence of tissue destruction in such patients. These hemochromogens may cause acute tubular necrosis if they are not eliminated promptly. Because these pigments precipitate more readily in an acidic solution and/or in the setting of a low glomerular filtration state, the initial fluid management is directed toward increasing the flow of urine and the urinary pH. Accordingly, intravenous fluid administration rates are increased so as to achieve hourly urine outputs of 75 to 100 ml. Additionally, intravenous sodium bicarbonate, given either as an infusion or in a bolus form, is administered to alkalinize the urine. If oliguria and pigmenturia persist despite these measures, an osmotic diuretic agent such as mannitol should be administered in a dose of 12.5 g/liter of intravenous fluid infused. Unfortunately, the use of these agents invalidates urinary output as an index of blood volume adequacy, and alternative indices of resuscitation adequacy must be monitored.

Inhalation injury is a common and potentially lethal concomitant insult associated with thermal injury. In a recent unpublished review at this institute, approximately 26 percent of all patients admitted during a 6-year period had sustained inhalation injury. Inhalation injury typically occurred in patients sustaining more extensive burn injury (average of 42 percent TBSA versus 18 percent TBSA). Inhalation injury is a chemical tracheobronchitis that occurs as a consequence of inhaling the products of incomplete combustion. It has been shown to be an independent, additive risk factor to the age- and burn size–related mortality, in some cases increasing the risk of death by as much as 20 percent. A recent review of patients with documented inhalation injury at this institute has revealed a 38 percent incidence of pneumonia in such patients.[34]

Various clinical reviews have indicated that inhalation injury is associated with increased fluid requirements beyond those expected during the initial 48 h following burn. Scheuler and Munster,[35] in a retrospective review of adult patients with burn sizes between 20 and 60 percent TBSA, found that patients with concomitant inhalation injury had an approximate 37 percent increase in resuscitation fluid requirements. However, excessive administration of intravenous fluids can lead to increased pulmonary microvascular hydrostatic pressure, potentially resulting in pulmonary edema. It is possible to administer the required resuscitation fluids in such a way that the risks of pulmonary insult are minimized while maintaining resuscitation adequacy. It is particularly important not to administer resuscitation fluids in bolus form but to provide them at a uniform rate of administration. Transient increases in pulmonary microvascular hydrostatic pressure may overwhelm the lung protective mechanisms and lead to pulmonary edema formation.

In addition to the previously cited physiologic reasons to avoid colloid in the initial 24 h, it is important to avoid premature administration of colloid to patients suffering concomitant inhalation injury. Goodwin et al.[36] demonstrated that delayed pulmonary edema was more common in patients receiving colloid-containing solutions in the first 24 h than those receiving only crystalloid solutions. Twenty percent of those patients receiving colloid in the initial 24 h developed pulmonary edema during the first postburn week as compared with only 5 percent of patients receiving only crystalloid solutions. Studies suggesting a lower incidence of pulmonary complications in patients resuscitated with colloids initially have, in general, been poorly controlled. Those studies are, at best, anecdotal and do not allow firm conclusions to be drawn as to the efficacy of colloids in preventing pulmonary complications during the early resuscitation phase.

RESUSCITATION: SECOND 24 H

During the second 24 h after a burn, the fluid requirements of the patient change. As the capillary leak resolves, protein and fluid losses into the wound significantly decrease. The goal of fluid therapy is the continued maintenance of organ perfusion and repletion of the plasma volume deficit with fluids that minimize both volume and sodium loading. Thus 5% dextrose in water is utilized to maintain an adequate urinary output. In addition, the plasma volume deficit is replaced with colloid in the form of albumin diluted to physiologic concentrations with either lactated Ringer's solution or normal saline administered in amounts proportional to the extent of burn. These colloid solutions minimize the volume requirements during the second 24 h after the burn. The modified Brooke formula recommends colloid replacement as follows:

Total Body Surface Area (TBSA) Burned (%)	Milliliters per Kilogram per Percent TBSA Burned
30–50	0.3
50–70	0.4
>70	0.5

The second 24-h fluid requirements for children are similar to those of the adult patient. Colloid repletion is as in the adult patient, however, crystalloid is infused in the form of 5% dextrose in 0.45% saline rather than sodium-free crystalloid solutions. As mentioned previously, because of the smaller blood volume in children, avoidance of large quantities of hypotonic solutions is imperative.

The fluid loss into the wound is markedly decreased in this phase, and overall volume requirements are in turn reduced. Fluid infusion rates are adjusted according to the patient's urinary output, with 30 to 50 ml/h being considered adequate. If the patient's urinary output is appropriate, the rate of electrolyte-free water is decreased by 25 to 50 percent. The hourly urinary output is monitored for the subsequent 3 h, and if output is maintained, the infusion rate is further reduced in stepwise fashion. These reductions should continue until the point at which the infusion rate is equal to the patient's estimated maintenance fluid rate (Fig. 16–6).

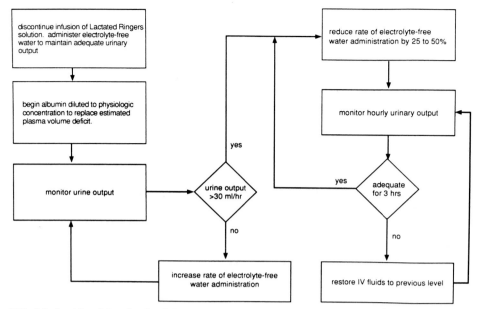

FIG. 16–6. Algorithm for fluid therapy for the second 24 h following thermal injury.

These maneuvers limit excessive salt and volume loading in this phase of resuscitation and thereby minimize the associated delayed complications.

POSTRESUSCITATION FLUID AND ELECTROLYTES

Following the initial 48 h after a burn, fluid management is adjusted in such a way as to assist the patient in excreting the large sodium and water load administered during the resuscitation phase. Ideally, the patient should return to his or her preburn weight by the eighth to tenth postburn day and should consequently lose approximately 10 to 12 percent of his or her resuscitative weight gain per day. Elimination of the water load is facilitated by the burn wound evaporative loss. An estimation of the total insensible water loss through the burn wound has been formulated by Warden et al.[37] to be

$$\text{Insensible water loss (ml/h)} = (25 + \% \text{ TBSA burned}) \times \text{TBSA (m}^2)$$

Excessive loss of free water can lead to the development of hypernatremia, the most common electrolyte abnormality seen in burn patients. Compounding the evaporative water loss, elevated levels of renin, angiotensin, and aldosterone promote overall sodium retention. The osmotic diuretic effects of excessive glucose or urea also can lead to dehydration and hypernatremia. Treatment of this electrolyte abnormality is based on the serum sodium level, the serum osmolarity, and the patient's body weight trends. The volume and composition of the infused fluids are adjusted as necessary to replete the free water deficit and compensate for the ongoing evaporative losses via the burn wound.

Hyponatremia is commonly seen immediately following fluid resuscitation as a result of the large volumes of lactated Ringer's solution and electrolyte-free water infused. This form of hyponatremia is typically asymptomatic and self-limited and, with an appropriate decrease in the rate of fluid administration, rapidly corrects. Transeschar sodium losses in patients treated with occlusive 0.5% silver nitrate soaks for antimicrobial control may produce hyponatremia. In patients in whom the serum sodium level is less than 120 mEq/liter and symptoms or signs of hyponatremia occur, the use of hypertonic saline infusions and/ or loop diuretics may be necessary in addition to the obligatory reduction of intravenous fluid infusion rates. Signs of cerebral edema or seizure activity may necessitate mechanical ventilatory support in an effort to reduce the arterial P_{CO_2} to 25 to 30 mmHg. The use of anticonvulsant medications may be required.

Cellular destruction and hemolysis immediately following the burn injury typically result in an elevation in the serum potassium concentration. In addition, metabolic acidosis associated with inadequate fluid resuscitation may promote hyperkalemia. Consequently, serum potassium supplementation is not indicated in the early management of the burn patient. Patients in whom the serum potassium level exceeds 5.5 mEq/liter may require the use of an ion-exchange resin such as Kayexalate (sodium polystyrene sulfonate) as well as the intravenous administration of sodium bicarbonate, glucose, and insulin to promote movement of potassium into cells. Patients demonstrating electrocardiographic changes may require the addition of intravenous calcium gluconate to counteract the adverse myocardial effects of hyperkalemia.

With mobilization of resuscitative fluids and entry into the postburn diuresis phase, hypokalemia may become a problem. The use of the topical antimicrobial mafenide acetate may further exacerbate hypokalemia by promoting kaliuresis. Careful monitoring of serum electrolytes and urinary potassium losses will help quantify the potassium replacement needs.

Serum calcium levels are also typically decreased following burn injury, particularly in patients with burn sizes greater than 30 percent TBSA. This finding is typically related to hypoalbuminemia and decreased calcium binding proteins rather than to an actual diminished ionized calcium level. Excessive use of antacids as prophylaxis against stress ulcerations also may cause symptomatic hypophosphatemia. Reduction in antacid doses, discontinuation of phosphate-binding antacids, and phosphate repletion all contribute to the resolution of this electrolyte abnormality. Finally, with adequate nutritional support, magnesium depletion and zinc deficiencies can be prevented, and the neuromuscular abnormalities and adverse wound healing effects associated with such electrolyte abnormalities can be avoided.

Continued investigation and further understanding of the pathophysiologic responses to burn injury may provide new insights into fluid resuscitation. The ultimate objective in the early management of the burn patient is vital organ preservation at the least immediate or delayed physiologic cost. The modified Brooke formula has been associated with the uncomplicated resuscitation of thousands of burned patients treated at the U.S. Army Institute of Surgical Research. A thorough understanding of the multiple organ system response to burn injury permits one to monitor resuscitation effectively and modify fluid management to meet the specific needs of the individual patient in a timely manner. Such an approach will minimize the incidence of complications related to fluid and electrolyte balance.

REFERENCES

1. Pruitt BA Jr: The Scudder oration on trauma, the universal trauma model. *Bull Am Coll Surg* 70(10):2, 1985.
2. Jackson DM: Second thoughts of the burn wound. *J Trauma* 9:839, 1969.
3. Montero KE, Lubbesmeyer HJ, Traber DL: Inhalation injury increases systemic microvascular permeability. *Surg Forum* 38:303, 1987.
4. Lund T, Reed RK: Microvascular fluid exchange following thermal skin injury in the rat: Changes in extravascular colloid osmotic pressure, albumin mass, and water content. *Circ Shock* 20(2):91, 1986.
5. Demling RH, Kramer G, Harms B: Role of thermal-induced hypoproteinemia on fluid flux and protein permeability in burned and nonburned tissue. *Surgery* 95(2):136, 1984.
6. Baxter CR, Cook WA, Shires GT: Serum myocardial depressant factor of burn shock. *Surg Forum* 17:1, 1966.
7. Cioffi WG, DeMeules JE, Gamelli RL: The effects of burn injury and fluid resuscitation on cardiac function in vitro. *J Trauma* 26(7):638, 1986.
8. Wilmore DW: Pathophysiology of the hypermetabolic response to burn injury. *J Trauma* 30 (suppl 12):S4, 1990.
9. Aulick LH, Goodwin CW, Becker RA: Visceral blood flow following thermal injury. *Ann Surg* 193(1):112, 1981.
10. Asch MJ, Feldman RJ, Waker HL: Systemic and pulmonary hemodynamic changes accompanying thermal injury. *Ann Surg* 178(2):218, 1971.
11. Demling RH, Wong C, Jin L: Early lung dysfunction after major burns: Role of edema and vasoactive mediators. *J Trauma* 25(10):959, 1985.
12. McElwee HP, Sirinek KR, Levine BA: Cimetidine affords protection equal to antacids in prevention of stress ulceration following thermal injury. *Surgery* 86(4):602, 1979.
13. McAlheny JC, Czaja AJ, Pruitt BA Jr: Antacid control of complications from acute gastrointestinal disease after burns. *J Trauma* 16(8):645, 1976.
14. Alexander JW, Wixson D: Neutrophil dysfunction and sepsis in burn injury. *Surg Gynecol Obstet* 130:431, 1970.
15. Teodorczyk-Injeyan JA, Sparkes BG, Peters WJ: Serum interleukin-2 receptor as a possible mediator of immunosuppression after burn injury. *J Burn Care Rehabil* 10(2):112, 1989.
16. Klimpel GR, Herndon DH, Stein MD: Peripheral blood lymphocytes from thermal injury patients are defective in their ability to generate lymphokine-activated killer cell activity. *J Clin Immunol* 8(1):14, 1988.
17. Solomkin JS: Neutrophil disorders in burn injury: Complement, cytokines, and organ injury. *J Trauma* 30(suppl 12):S80, 1990.
18. Curreri PW, Katz AJ, Dotin LN: Coagulation abnormalities in the injured patient. *Curr Top Surg Res* 2:401, 1970.
18a. Underhill FP: The significance of anhydremia in extensive superficial burns. *JAMA* 95:852, 1930.
19. Cope O, Moore FD: The redistribution of body water and the fluid therapy of the burned patient. *Ann Surg* 126(6):1010, 1947.

20. Evans EI, Purnell OJ, Robinette PW: Fluid and electrolyte requirements in severe burns. *Ann Surg* 135(6):804, 1952.

21. Reiss E, Stirman JA, Artz CP: Fluid and electrolyte balance in burns. *JAMA* 152:1309, 1953.

22. Reckler JM, Mason AD Jr: A critical evaluation of fluid resuscitation in the burned patient. *Ann Surg* 174:115, 1971.

23. Moylan JA, Mason AD Jr, Rogers PW: Postburn shock: A critical evaluation of resuscitation. *J Trauma* 13(4):354, 1973.

24. Baxter CR: Problems and complications of burn shock resuscitation. *Surg Clin North Am* 58(6):1313, 1978.

25. Baxter CR, Marvin J, Curreri PW: Fluid and electrolyte therapy of burn shock. *Heart Lung* 2(5):707, 1973.

26. Monafo WM: The treatment of burn shock by the oral and intravenous administration of hypertonic lactated saline solution. *J Trauma* 10(7):575, 1970.

27. Shimazaki S, Yoshioka T, Tanaka N: Body fluid changes during hypertonic lactated saline solution therapy for burn shock. *J Trauma* 17(1):38, 1977.

28. Gunn ML, Hansbrough JF, Davis JW: Prospective randomized trial of hypertonic sodium lactate versus lactated Ringer's solution for burn shock resuscitation. *J Trauma* 29(9):1261, 1989.

29. Onarheim H, Missavage AE, Kramer GC: Effectiveness of hypertonic saline–dextran 70 for initial fluid resuscitation of major burns. *J Trauma* 30(5):597, 1990.

30. Bowser-Wallace BH, Cone JB, Caldwell FT Jr: Hypertonic lactated saline resuscitation of severely burned patients over 60 years of age. *J Trauma* 25(1):22, 1985.

31. Graves TA, Cioffi WG, McManus WF: Fluid resuscitation of infants and children with thermal injury. *J Trauma* 28(12):1656, 1988.

32. Moylan JA, Inge WW Jr, Pruitt BA Jr: Circulatory changes following circumferential extremity burns evaluated by the ultrasonic doppler flowmeter: An analysis of 60 thermally injured limbs. *J Trauma* 11(9):763, 1971.

33. Hunt JL, Mason AD Jr, Masterson TS: The pathophysiology of acute electrical injuries. *J Trauma* 16(5):335, 1976.

34. Shirani KZ, Pruitt BA Jr, Mason AD Jr: The influence of inhalation injury and pneumonia on burn mortality. *Ann Surg* 205:82, 1987.

35. Scheulen JJ, Munster AM: The Parkland formula in patients with burns and inhalation injury. *J Trauma* 22(10):869, 1982.

36. Goodwin CW, Dorethy J, Lam V: Randomized trial of efficacy of crystalloid and colloid resuscitation on hemodynamic response and lung water following thermal injury. *Ann Surg* 197(5):520, 1983.

37. Warden GD, Wilmore DW, Rogers PW: Hypernatremic state in hypermetabolic burn patients. *Arch Surg* 106:420, 1973.

INDEX

INDEX

Page numbers in *italic* indicate figures; page numbers followed by "t" indicate tabular material.